Cross-Cultural Advancements in Positive Psychology

Volume 16

Series Editor

Antonella Delle Fave, University of Milano, Milano, Italy

The aim of the Cross Cultural Advancements in Positive Psychology book series is to spread a universal and culture-fair perspective on good life promotion. The series will advance a deeper understanding of the cross-cultural differences in well-being conceptualization. A deeper understanding can affect psychological theories, interventions and social policies in various domains, from health to education, from work to leisure. Books in the series will investigate such issues as enhanced mobility of people across nations, ethnic conflicts and the challenges faced by traditional communities due to the pervasive spreading of modernization trends. New instruments and models will be proposed to identify the crucial components of well-being in the process of acculturation. This series will also explore dimensions and components of happiness that are currently overlooked because happiness research is grounded in the Western tradition, and these dimensions do not belong to the Western cultural frame of mind and values.

More information about this series at https://link.springer.com/bookseries/8420

Lusilda Schutte • Tharina Guse • Marié P. Wissing
Editors

Embracing Well-Being in Diverse African Contexts: Research Perspectives

Springer

Editors
Lusilda Schutte
Africa Unit for Transdisciplinary Health Research, Faculty of Health Sciences
North-West University
Potchefstroom, South Africa

Tharina Guse
Department of Psychology
University of Pretoria
Pretoria, South Africa

Marié P. Wissing
Africa Unit for Transdisciplinary Health Research
North-West University
Potchefstroom, South Africa

ISSN 2210-5417 ISSN 2210-5425 (electronic)
Cross-Cultural Advancements in Positive Psychology
ISBN 978-3-030-85923-7 ISBN 978-3-030-85924-4 (eBook)
https://doi.org/10.1007/978-3-030-85924-4

This Springer imprint is published by the registered company Springer Nature Switzerland AG.
The registered company address is: Gewerbestrasse 11, 6330 Cham, Switzerland

Preface

When starting with this book project, we asked ourselves what the significance, contribution, and legacy of the volume should be. A possible response could link to the volume's theme: "*Embracing Well-being in Diverse Contexts*". The Cambridge English Dictionary (2021) defines *embracing* as "accepting something with great interest or enthusiasm"; *diverse* as "including many different types of people or things"; and *context* as "the situation within which something exists or happens, and that can help explain it". Well-being can be considered to relate to the feeling good and functioning well of individuals, groups, communities, and societies (e.g. Keyes, 2007; Keyes & Annas, 2009; Marujo & Neto, 2014). Adding this together, *embracing well-being in diverse contexts* may thus refer to understanding and promoting, with enthusiasm and great interest, the well-functioning of individuals, groups, communities, and societies, where the differences and variety of cultures and circumstances in which peoples' functioning is embedded are acknowledged and respected. In this case, the focus is specifically on work done in Africa.

Internationally, much of the work on well-being in the field of positive psychology has been done using samples from Western, Educated, Industrialised, Rich, and Democratic (WEIRD) countries (Henrich, Heine, & Norenzayan, 2010), especially in the early years of the field's development (Rao & Donaldson, 2015; Hendriks et al., 2019). Echoing this, Møller and Roberts (2017) observed that first studies on well-being in sub-Saharan Africa were done by non-Africans who uncritically applied their viewpoints and assessment instruments, developed elsewhere, to African samples. This is not unique to well-being research and practice, as much of psychology is built on research conducted in WEIRD countries (Henrich et al., 2010). In reaction, current debates on and discussions about the development of an African-centred psychology in terms of research, training, and practice are very prominent (e.g. Nobles, 2013, 2015; Nwoye, 2006, 2013, 2015; Mkhize, 2020). Against this backdrop, the significance, contribution, and legacy of the volume rest on two levels: (1) to present and promote context-sensitive and context-relevant discussions and empirical research on well-being in Africa which should ultimately impact well-being promotion locally and (2) to contribute diversity to global discourses on well-being.

In an attempt to achieve this, this volume presents 17 chapters that are divided into four sections. These will now be briefly introduced.

Part I foregrounds theoretical perspectives on well-being in Africa. In Chap. 1, Marié Wissing, Lusilda Schutte, and Christelle Liversage provide an overview of the development of positive psychology as a science over time and argue that a third wave of positive psychology is emerging, which is based on the assumption of a strong relational ontology, and that emphasises contextual embeddedness, interconnectedness, and post-disciplinarity. They illustrate how these tenets echo traditional African wisdom that accepts interconnectedness as a way of being and suggest that one way to deepen our understanding of well-being is to harmonise Western and African perspectives, with harmony and related facets being core to the conceptualisation of well-being. They propose that, while positive psychology is by name bound to the discipline of psychology, the third wave of positive psychology signifies the emergence of a new transdisciplinary scientific field of well-being studies, which is compared to “a butterfly leaving its cocoon”.

Angelina Wilson Fadiji, Itumeleng P. Khumalo, and Ncamisile Thumile Zulu propose in Chap. 2 an Africa(n)-centred positive psychology. After arguing that cross-cultural psychology is inadequate to explore well-being in context, they build on the assumptions of critical, cultural, and African psychology to describe an African-centred positive psychology that is critical, driven by theory, and supported by empirical evidence and that takes social and political context into consideration.

Concluding Part I, Elias Mpofu and Elias Machina propose in Chap. 3 that African culture followers’ social affiliation and cultural orientation (ranging from traditionalist to transitional to modern) may effect their health norms and health practices. They point to the need for research that investigates health norms and practices across the different cultural orientations, and pathways to the implementation of health activities and actions within and between the orientations. In this regard, they propose a research framework which could inform best practices and public health policy.

Part II comprises three chapters on the measurement of well-being in African samples. In Chap. 4, Richard Appiah, Marié P. Wissing, Angelina Wilson Fadiji, and Lusilda Schutte investigate the factorial validity of the Twi translation of the Mental Health Continuum – Short Form in a sample of rural Ghanaian adults, as well as the prevalence of positive mental health in this sample. A bifactor exploratory structural equation modelling model displayed best fit, and support was provided for use of the total scale score but not the subscale scores. A concerning high percentage of participants were languishing or reported moderate levels of positive mental health, indicating the need for context-relevant and appropriate interventions.

Sahaya G. Selvam, Joyce Wanjiru Kiige, and Jeketule Soko argue in Chap. 5 that hospitality is a neglected character strength, which is particularly salient in Africa. In three studies, they investigate Kenyan participants’ experiences and perceptions of hospitality, they present findings on the development and psychometric properties of the Tangaza Hospitality Scale, and they examine the correlations between hospitality and extraversion and well-being-related variables. They conclude that hospitality is an important topic for future well-being research, also in Africa.

Recognising the importance of relationships and relatedness in the African context, Amanda Cromhout, Lusilda Schutte, and Marié P. Wissing report on the factor structure of the Peer and Community Relational Health Indices in English- and Setswana-speaking South African adult samples in Chap. 6. Applying bifactor exploratory structural equation modelling, they found (after removal of some problematic items) preliminary support for the use of total scale scores, but not all subscale scores. They stress the necessity of taking cognisance of context and culture when measuring relational well-being and suggest that an emic approach should be applied in future research to develop culturally appropriate measures of relational well-being.

In nine chapters, Part III presents findings on the manifestations and dynamics of well-being among adolescents and emerging adults, students, and adults in Africa. First, in Chap. 7, Linda Theron and Michael Ungar present a single case study from South Africa to gain insights into how emerging adults who are unemployed and have no education or training account for their resilience despite the socio-ecological stressors they face. They find that the resilience process is informed by both personal and ecological resources. In the case under study, personal resources and self-reliance were foregrounded, probably in response to the ecological constrictions in the emerging adult's context. This highlights a pressing need for more attention to the socio-ecological environments of emerging adults.

Charles Magoba Muwonge, Annet Kembabazi, Gladys Nakalema, Margaret Ekatushabe, Diana Kwarikunda, Henry Kibedi, and Joseph Ssenyonga focus on the psychological well-being of young people in Uganda living with HIV in Chap. 8. They firstly examine the associations between psychological well-being and demographic variables in their sample, and secondly to what extent the association between social support and psychological well-being is mediated by self-esteem. Their findings show that strengthening the social support networks of young people living with HIV in Uganda (and wider) can improve their self-esteem and psychological well-being.

Hajara Baba, Joana Salifu Yendork, and Samuel Atindanbila explore in Chap. 9 protective resources that married girls in the Northern region of Ghana use to buffer against the negative impact of child marriage and that can facilitate positive outcomes. From qualitative interview data, they find that intrinsic resources, such as resilience attitudes, help-seeking and active coping strategies, and avoidance coping, as well as extrinsic resources such as interpersonal support networks, were used by participants. However, participants reported lack of access to community support systems and non-governmental organisations. A social justice approach when working with these girls and increasing access to external support systems are provided as recommendations.

Introducing a series of chapters focusing on student well-being, Irma Eloff, Sumari O'Neil, and Herbert Kanengoni explore the factors that students from a large South African residential university identify as contributing to their well-being in Chap. 10. The learning environment (physical environment and facilities on and around campus) and support structures (e.g. peers, family, lecturers and tutors, and medical facilities on campus) emerged as main themes. Security and safety emerged as a particularly important contextual factor from students' responses. Findings emphasise the responsibility that lies with higher education institutions to support the well-being of their students.

Next, in Chap. 11, Itumeleng P. Khumalo, Werner de Klerk, and Angelina Wilson explore the nature and role of meaning and hope in the goal setting of participants from a university of technology in South Africa. Two latent hope-meaning classes were identified: the majority of participants were assigned to the high hope, high meaning class and a small proportion to the low hope, search for meaning class. Goal themes included tertiary education, employment and career, mobility, secure accommodation, and support for family. The first two goal themes were driven by students' need for a better financial future and to support their families. Perceived obstacles to reach the goals included lack of resources, poor self-regulation, employment problems, fear of failure, and health problems. No distinction was detected between the content of goals and meaning for the two hope-meaning latent classes. The authors suggest that universities should not focus only on developing academic skills but also on providing social and material support as far as possible.

In another study among university students, this time from Angola, Rutnilson da Silva, Ana Maria Rocha, and Dilson Francisco investigate the relationships between virtues and character strengths, subjective well-being, and academic achievement (Chap. 12). Psychological well-being displayed higher levels of correlation with character strengths than emotional and social well-being. Love of learning was the only character strength that exhibited a significant positive correlation with academic achievement.

The final study among university students focuses on medical students from a Nigerian university, where Ephraim Chima Maduakor, JohnBosco Chika Chukwuorji, Peace N. Amanambu, and Chuka Mike Ifeagwazi examine the associations between attachment and psychological well-being, and whether self-efficacy mediated such relationships (Chap. 13). Their findings show that attachment style was associated with psychological well-being and that self-efficacy, which was negatively correlated with attachment avoidance, mediated the negative association between attachment avoidance and psychological well-being. The authors conclude that interventions are needed to promote students' self-efficacy.

In Chap. 14, Lusilda Schutte, Marié P. Wissing, Angelina Wilson Fadiji, Sonia Mbowa, Placidia Shoko, and Willem D. Schutte explore harmony as a quality of happiness in adult samples from South Africa and Ghana. Echoing African and other philosophical traditions, results revealed that harmony as a quality of happiness was experienced within and across levels of functioning (intrapersonal, interpersonal, transcendental, universal) and expressed as an intricate sense of wholeness, interconnectedness, and synergy. The authors conclude that harmony as a quality of happiness should be understood and promoted using context-sensitive, holistic, interdisciplinary approaches.

In the final chapter of Part III, Chap. 15, Christelle Liversage, Marié Wissing, and Lusilda Schutte evaluate the self-concordance model with reference to the wider interpersonal relationship life domain in a multicultural South African adult sample. Specifically, they investigate whether alignment between people's goals and meaning with reference to wider interpersonal relationships is associated with higher well-being levels. The self-concordance model was not supported in this study, pointing to the need for further exploration of the self-concordance model with reference to wider interpersonal relationships.

The last section of this volume, Part IV, considers well-being promotion interventions in Africa in two chapters. In Chap. 16, Tharina Guse presents a scoping review of positive psychological interventions in African contexts. While she finds that the most studies were done on a group level among South African adults, intervention evaluation studies also started emerging in other African countries. Most previous studies employed quantitative research designs. She highlights a gap in intervention research on children, adolescents, older adults, and clinical populations and recommends that future research should focus on adapting positive psychological interventions to fit the cultural context where it will be applied.

Finally, Izanette van Schalkwyk provides an overview of experiences and outcomes of a multidisciplinary well-being promotion programme in Chap. 17, based on positive psychology, which has been implemented in a high-risk South African community over the course of ten years. While the adverse effects of poverty and other structural problems remain apparent, the need for context-relevant well-being promotion activities is stressed.

In sum, important themes emerge in this volume. First, the contextual and cultural embeddedness of well-being is clear, and the need for building context-relevant, African-centred well-being science and evidence-based practices is highlighted. Linking to this, and as a second theme here, several contributions highlight the importance of social and ecological structures to the well-being of particularly vulnerable population groups. This implies that well-being promotion should not only be a psychological endeavour focused on the individual, but also a social and political one, impelling social systems, institutions, and governments to recognise their role and responsibility in well-being promotion. Third, the centrality of relatedness and interconnectedness in African conceptions, expressions, and experiences of well-being is evident, suggesting that well-being research and practice in Africa (and beyond) should take a holistic approach and involve multi-, inter-, and transdisciplinary team efforts. Overall, this volume not only contributes to a discussion and growing body of evidence on well-being science and practice in Africa, but also contributes to global discourses and debates, where it calls for recognition and appreciation of and sensitivity to diversity and nuance.

Potchefstroom, South Africa — L. Schutte
Pretoria, South Africa — T. Guse
Potchefstroom, South Africa — M. P. Wissing

References

Cambridge English Dictionary. (2021). Cambridge University Press. Retrieved from https://dictionary.cambridge.org/dictionary/english

Hendriks, T., Warren, M. A., Schotanus-Dijkstra, M., Hassankhan, A., Graafsma, T., Bohlmeijer, E., & de Jong, J. (2019). How WEIRD are positive psychology interventions? A bibliometric analysis of randomized controlled trials on the science of well-being. *The Journal of Positive Psychology, 14*(4), 489-501. https://10.1080/17439760.2018.1484941

Henrich, J., Heine,S. J., & Norenzayan, A. (2010). The weirdest people in the world? *Behavioral and Brain Sciences, 33,* 6–83.

Keyes, C .L. M. (2007). Promoting and protecting mental health as flourishing: A complementary strategy for improving national mental health. *American Psychologist, 62*(2), 95–108.

Keyes, C. L. M., & Annas, J. (2009). Feeling good and functioning well: distinctive concepts in ancient philosophy and contemporary science. *Journal of Positive Psychology, 4*(3), 197–201.

Marujo, H. A. & Neto, L. M. (Eds.) (2014). *Positive nations and communities.* Dordrecht, The Netherlands: Springer

Mkhize, N. (2020). African/Afrikan-centered Psychology. *South African Journal of Psychology*, 1–8. https://10.1177/0081246320972002

Møller, V., & Roberts, B. (2017). New beginnings in an ancient region: Well-being in Sub-Saharan Africa. In R. J. Estes, & M. J. Sirgy (Eds.). *The pursuit of human well-being: The untold global history* (pp. 161–215), Cham, Switzerland: Springer.

Nobles, W. W. (2013). Fundamental task and challenge of Black psychology. *Journal of Black Psychology, 39*(3), 292–299. http://10.1177/0095798413478072

Nobles, W. W. (2015). From black psychology to Sakhu Djaer: Implications for the further development of a Pan African Black psychology. *Journal of Black Psychology, 41*(5), 399–414. https://10.1177/0095798415598038

Nwoye, A. (2006). Remapping the fabric of the African self: A synoptic theory. *Dialectical Anthropology, 30*(1–2), 119–146. https://10.1007/s10624-005-5058-x

Nwoye, A. (2013). Àfrican psychotherapy. In A. Runehov & L. Oviedo (Eds.), *Encyclopedia of Sciences and Religions* (pp. 32–41). Berlin, Germany: Springer.

Nwoye, A. (2015). What is African psychology the psychology of? *Theory & Psychology, 25*(1), 96–116. https://10.1177/0959354314565116

Rao, M. A. & Donaldson, S. I. (2015). Expanding opportunities for diversity in positive psychology: An examination of gender, race, and ethnicity. *Canadian Psychology, 56*(3), 271–282. https://10.1037/cap0000036

Acknowledgements

As editors, we are extremely grateful to Amanda Cromhout who provided invaluable and impeccable editorial support during the final phases of the compilation of the volume, including handling correspondence with authors and reviewers, conducting technical editing and reference checking of all manuscripts, and compiling the full draft manuscript of the volume; to Sonia Mbowa who acted as editorial assistant for the first part of the project with incredible dedication, administrating the review process and conducting technical editing of earlier drafts of chapter manuscripts; and Placidia Shoko who assisted with technical editing of earlier drafts of selected chapter manuscripts.

The chapters in this book were double-blind peer-reviewed. In this regard, we gratefully acknowledge the support of the following scholars:

Richard Appiah
Kwaku Oppong Asante
Justin August
Bukola Victoria Bada
Anselm Berde
Petra Bester
Willem Boshoff
Shingairai Chigeza
JohnBosco Chika Chukwuorji
Nicoleen Coetzee
Amanda Cromhout
Werner de Klerk
Irma Eloff
Awie Greeff
Arnel Huisamen
Leon Jackson
Itumeleng P. Khumalo
Andreas Krafft

Vicki Koen
Peter Little
Christelle Liversage
Setagwa Mahlo
David Maree
Henri Mason
Sonia Mbowa
Inmaculada Montoya-Castilla
Brandon Morgan
Elias Mpofu
Lindi Nel
Werner Nell
Kamilla Rawatlal
Kleinjan Redelinghuys
Ana Rocha
Sahaya G Selvam
Placidia Shoko
Alena Slezáčková
Michael Temane
Chrizanne van Eeden
Leon van Niekerk
CJ van Zyl
Maretha Visser
Meghano Warren
Laura Weiss
Sarah White
Angelina Wilson Fadiji
Haorui Wu

Contents

Editors and Contributors

About the Editors

Lusilda Schutte Africa Unit for Transdisciplinary Health Research, Faculty of Health Sciences, North-West University, Potchefstroom, South Africa

Tharina Guse Department of Psychology, University of Pretoria, Pretoria, South Africa

Marié P. Wissing Africa Unit for Transdisciplinary Health Research, Faculty of Health Sciences, North-West University, Potchefstroom, South Africa

Contributors

Peace N. Amanambu Department of Psychology, University of Nigeria, Nsukka, Enugu State, Nigeria

Richard Appiah Africa Unit for Transdisciplinary Health Research, Faculty of Health Sciences, North-West University, Potchefstroom, South Africa
College of Health Sciences, University of Ghana, Accra, Ghana

Samuel Atindanbila Department of Psychology, University of Ghana, Accra, Ghana

Hajara Baba Department of Psychology, University of Ghana, Accra, Ghana

JohnBosco Chika Chukwuorji Department of Psychology, University of Nigeria, Nsukka, Enugu State, Nigeria
Department of Psychology, College of Sciences and the Health Professions, Cleveland State University, Cleveland, OH, USA
Promotion of Health and Innovation Lab (PHI), Network for Wellbeing, Nsukka, Enugu State, Nigeria

Amanda Cromhout Africa Unit for Transdisciplinary Health Research (AUTHeR), Faculty of Health Sciences, North-West University, Potchefstroom, South Africa

Rutnilson da Silva Universidade Católica de Angola, Luanda, Angola

Werner de Klerk Department of Psychology, North-West University, Potchefstroom, South Africa
COMPRES, North-West University, Potchefstroom, South Africa

Margaret Ekatushabe Department of Educational Foundations and Psychology, Mbarara University of Science and Technology, Mbarara, Uganda

Irma Eloff Department of Educational Psychology, University of Pretoria, Pretoria, South Africa

Dilson Francisco Universidade Católica de Angola, Luanda, Angola

Tharina Guse Department of Psychology, University of Pretoria, Pretoria, South Africa

Chuka Mike Ifeagwazi Department of Psychology, University of Nigeria, Nsukka, Enugu State, Nigeria

Herbert Kanengoni Department of Human Resource Management, University of Pretoria, Pretoria, South Africa

Annet Kembabazi Department of Educational Foundations and Psychology, Mbarara University of Science and Technology, Mbarara, Uganda

Itumeleng P. Khumalo Department of Psychology, University of the Free State, Bloemfontein, South Africa

Henry Kibedi Department of Work and Organizational Psychology, Kyambogo University, Kampala, Uganda

Joyce Wanjiru Kiige Tangaza University College, Nairobi, Kenya

Diana Kwarikunda Department of Educational Foundations and Psychology, Mbarara University of Science and Technology, Mbarara, Uganda
Department of Educational Sciences, University of Potsdam, Potsdam, Germany

Christelle Liversage Africa Unit for Transdisciplinary Health Research, Faculty of Health Sciences, North-West University, Potchefstroom, South Africa

Elias Machina Western Sydney University, Sydney, NSW, Australia

Ephraim Chima Maduakor Department of Psychology, University of Nigeria, Nsukka, Enugu State, Nigeria

Sonia Mbowa Africa Unit for Transdisciplinary Health Research, Faculty of Health Sciences, North-West University, Potchefstroom, South Africa

Elias Mpofu University of North Texas, Denton, TX, USA
University of the Witwatersrand, South Africa
University of Sydney, Sydney, NSW, Australia

Charles Magoba Muwonge Department of Educational Foundations and Psychology, Mbarara University of Science and Technology, Mbarara, Uganda

Gladys Nakalema Department of Educational Foundations and Psychology, Mbarara University of Science and Technology, Mbarara, Uganda

Sumari O'Neil Department of Human Resource Management, University of Pretoria, Pretoria, South Africa

Ana Maria Rocha Universidade Católica de Angola, Luanda, Angola

Lusilda Schutte Africa Unit for Transdisciplinary Health Research, Faculty of Health Sciences, North-West University, Potchefstroom, South Africa

Willem D. Schutte Centre for Business Mathematics and Informatics (BMI), Faculty of Natural Sciences, North-West University, Potchefstroom, South Africa

Sahaya G. Selvam Tangaza University College, Nairobi, Kenya

Placidia M. Shoko Africa Unit for Transdisciplinary Health Research, Faculty of Health Sciences, North-West University, Potchefstroom, South Africa

Jeketule Soko Tangaza University College, Nairobi, Kenya

Joseph Ssenyonga Department of Educational Foundations and Psychology, Mbarara University of Science and Technology, Mbarara, Uganda

Linda Theron Department of Educational Psychology, University of Pretoria, Pretoria, South Africa

Michael Ungar Resilience Research Centre, Dalhousie University, Halifax, NS, Canada

Izanette van Schalkwyk Africa Unit for Transdisciplinary Health Research (AUTHeR), Faculty of Health Sciences, North-West University, South Africa

Angelina Wilson Fadiji Department of Educational Psychology, Faculty of Education, University of Pretoria, Pretoria, South Africa
Africa Unit for Transdisciplinary Health Research, Faculty of Health Sciences, North-West University, Potchefstroom, South Africa

Marié P. Wissing Africa Unit for Transdisciplinary Health Research, Faculty of Health Sciences, North-West University, Potchefstroom, South Africa

Joana Salifu Yendork Department of Psychology, University of Ghana, Accra, Ghana

Ncamisile Thumile Zulu University of KwaZulu-Natal, Durban, South Africa

Part I
Theoretical Perspectives on Well-Being in Africa

Chapter 1
Embracing Well-Being in Diverse Contexts: The Third Wave of Positive Psychology and African Imprint

Marié P. Wissing, Lusilda Schutte, and Christelle Liversage

Abstract For a long time, well-being research had been driven from a Western perspective with a neglect of cultural and contextual variables. In this chapter we argue with reference to well-being research as manifested in positive psychology (PP) as a discipline, that contextual, metatheoretical and metadisciplinary perspectives need to be taken into account. Developments in PP over time are described, illustrating the importance of contexts and assumptions in understanding well-being, and how new assumptions in the third wave of PP resonate with old African wisdoms about interconnectedness as a core value in human lives. The first wave of PP focused on advocating for the positive in human functioning, many facets of well-being were differentiated in theory and empirical studies, while assuming a naturalist worldview and that findings from the West are globally applicable. The second wave showed that PP needs to take context, culture and negative facets of human life into account for understanding the nature and dynamics of well-being. The emerging third wave of PP is characterized by the acceptance of a strong relational ontology and trends towards contextualization, interconnectedness and post-disciplinarity. Harmonizing Western and African perspectives are indicated, and specifically also the understanding of well-being as harmony and harmonization. The third wave suggests a move to "well-being studies", instead of the disciplinary bound "positive psychology studies"—a butterfly leaving its cocoon.

Keywords African values · Development of disciplines · Diverse contexts · Worldviews · Third wave of positive psychology · Interconnectedness · Complexity · Post-disciplinarity

---

Some of the ideas on the third wave of positive psychology in this chapter had been presented at the *First Africa Positive Psychology Conference*, 4–7 April, 2018, Potchefstroom South Africa, and the *9th European Conference on Positive Psychology*, 27–30 June 2018, Budapest, Hungary.

M. P. Wissing (✉) · L. Schutte · C. Liversage
Africa Unit for Transdisciplinary Health Research, Faculty of Health Sciences, North-West University, Potchefstroom, South Africa
e-mail: Marie.Wissing@nwu.ac.za

L. Schutte et al. (eds.), *Embracing Well-Being in Diverse African Contexts: Research Perspectives*, Cross-Cultural Advancements in Positive Psychology 16,
https://doi.org/10.1007/978-3-030-85924-4_1

1.1 Introduction

In the past, psychology and positive psychology (PP) in particular, had neglected the role of worldviews, culture and context largely in efforts to understand human behavior, and tended to assume that perspectives and findings from the West apply globally. However, science develops continuously and in more recent times the skewedness of these assumptions became clear. More voices iterate that culture fair models and indigenous studies are needed. These insights mainly came from observed differences between the West and East Asian perspectives, and functioning in an African context was for a long time neglected. Lately this picture started to change, enriching both psychology and positive psychology, but insights are still scattered. In this chapter, developments in PP will be indicated, and it will be argued that the understanding of well-being needs to be informed by insights gained from diverse contexts. We will highlight how new developments in PP resonate with imprints from long existing African values. Positive psychology is only starting to make footprints in Africa, but the richness of African values already revealed imprints that make this context a fertile soil for well-being studies and flourishing of PP as a science—despite the prevailing existence of political strife, poverty and corruption. Africa has an abundance of cultures rich in art, spirituality, caring and sharing. Countries in Africa also have a shared collectivist orientation in which the individual is less important than the (in)group (Nwoye, 2017). However, nowadays collectivist and individualist orientations across many world regions tend to exist side by side in urban areas with a collectivist orientation more prevalent in rural and poorer areas (Philips & Wong, 2017).

Our methodological approach in this chapter is that of a purposive narrative and interpretative literature review with abstraction of broad trends (Onwuegbuzie & Frels, 2016). Slife et al. (2017) recently criticized psychology for the lack of attention to worldviews and recognition that these may differ in diverse contexts. The question is whether the same pertains to positive psychology, and if, or to what extent, changes can be noted in the development of thoughts in PP as shown in content focused on, methods used, and metatheoretical assumptions influencing focus and preferred methods, and in turn being influenced by context—also looking out for the African footprint. We noted signs of changes over time and propose that three phases can be distinguished. Our line of argumentation will be reflected in the structure of this chapter (cf. Jaakkola, 2020). Assumptions about the world, people, and proper methods to generate new knowledge, are typically implicit and need to be highlighted or detected and made explicit. Therefore, our aim was to detect, abstract and describe noted changes in focus, methods and worldview assumptions of PP over time, making the implicit explicit (cf. Kosterec, 2016) with the use of exemplars as found in PP literature, as well as juxtaposing it with developments and assumptions from African perspectives. Our approach to document tracking was purposive, and articles were selected to illustrate our argument about changes in PP thoughts and assumptions over time, and manifesting in what we named the third wave of PP. Of course the ideas presented here may also be influenced by our own worldviews and process of development in conceptualizations and foci. We thus do not claim that it is an "objective" reflection of the state of the art. However, we will illustrate, with use of the selected relevant literature (exemplars), changes in content, methods and assumptions, and especially highlight "markers" of what we note as an emerging "third wave" of positive psychology moving towards inter- and transdisciplinary well-being studies. These ideas will be linked to old African notions of interconnectedness among people, people and nature, the natural and the supranatural.

In the following text, we argue in Sect. 1.2 the problem of a neglect of attention to diverse contexts and worldview assumptions in psychology and positive psychology in particular, and note some early steps in the development of positive psychology in the African context. In Sect. 1.3, we briefly describe the typical trajectory for the development of disciplines in general as proposed by philosophers of science, and then turn to developments in positive psychology in particular. The main part of this chapter then consists of the abstraction and description of main trends that we identify in the development of positive psychology as a scientific discipline. We identify and describe the characteristics of the three phases or waves of thought developments in positive psychology, with a specific focus on the newly emerging third wave. In Sect. 1.4 we note African value imprints that dovetail with assumptions of the third wave of PP. Lastly, we share some insights and thoughts about the way forward in Sect. 1.5.

1.2 Neglect of Culture, Context and Worldviews in Psychology and Positive Psychology

Research in psychology and in particular positive psychology, had thus far mainly been conducted from a Western perspective (Christopher & Hickinbottom, 2008; Henrich et al., 2010; Kim et al., 2018; Slife et al., 2017). In the last decade East Asian perspectives came more to the forefront and some differences in findings from those in the West were indicated (Kim et al., 2018; Uchida & Ogihara, 2012). Well-being studies had been neglected in the African context (Kim et al., 2018; Wilson-Fadiji & Wissing, 2021), but they are gaining momentum (e.g., Appiah et al., 2020; Chika Chukwuorji et al., 2019; Mahali et al., 2018; Wilson et al., 2018). Although increasingly more well-being studies are being conducted in Africa, it is often approached from a Western perspective and using measures developed in the West. The neglect is however not only at the level of culture fair measurement, but also mostly at the level of cultural applicability of constructs and assumptions about the world. Such assumptions speak to what is valued, and it is now increasingly explicitly recognized that values play a role in PP (Prinzing, 2020).

Christopher et al. (2008) welcomed the corrective brought by positive psychology to mainstream psychology, which had in the past primarily been focused on what is wrong with people, but also indicated the failures to explore well-being in diverse contexts and in plural societies. Christopher and Hickinbottom (2008) critically evaluated some of the key conceptual and moral underpinnings of PP and pointed out its shortcomings as neglecting cultural embeddedness of ideas, and using a one-sided individualist lens and an instrumentalist approach. In the same volume of papers on rethinking PP in the journal *Theory & Psychology*, Sundararajan (2008) also explored Asian conceptions of well-being relying on assumptions about the self that differ from assumptions in individualistic Western contexts. This volume, however, did not include any perspective from the African continent. Yet, it is not only PP that neglected the role of culture and context, but psychology as a discipline: Henrich et al. (2010) argued that psychology as discipline had been mainly driven as a science conducted from a Western, individualist perspective with educated and rich people from democratic societies as participants, while people with this profile comprise a small percentage of the world population. Although this picture is now changing, there is still a neglect of the role of worldviews in mainstream psychology as indicated by Slife and colleagues (2017) in their book titled *The hidden worldviews of psychology's theory, research and practice.* The same holds to a large extent for positive psychology. Alexandrova (2017) accentuated that philosophical assumptions (worldviews) influence our conceptualizations, the methods used in science, as well as the adopted confirmation processes and interpretations.

Worldviews are overarching philosophical beliefs about life and values, and are imbedded in cultural and social contexts (Slife et al., 2017; Onwuegbuzie & Frels, 2016). Worldviews can be seen as consisting of ontological, epistemological and axiological beliefs. Ontology refers to beliefs about the world and humans in particular. Epistemology refers to beliefs about how we develop and validate knowledge. Axiology/ethics/values refer to what we assume to be good and bad, or desirable and undesirable. Even if not recognized, worldviews will influence discipline- and topic-specific beliefs as well as preferred research methods. Unrecognized worldview assumptions are dangerous in research and practice as such "blind" scientists or practitioners will assume that all others share their assumptions, and that their own assumptions are the only correct ones. This had been the case with Western perspectives in psychology and positive psychology as mentioned in the critiques referred to above.

Embracing worldviews from diverse contexts, including African contexts, can enrich understandings of well-being and enhancement thereof in culture-sensitive and ethically appropriate ways. Therefore, the humble understanding of multiple perspectives, as also described by Nyamnjoh (2015/2017) and Nwoye (2018) from African perspectives, as well as by Guse et al. (2019) and Wissing et al. (2018), may contribute in future to a deeper understanding of well-being. Fortunately, development in science itself takes place and in recent years showed a trajectory towards embracing diverse perspectives.

Scholarly work in positive psychology started relatively late in the African context, but in South Africa some early voices could be noted such as those of Strümpfer (Wilson-Fadiji & Wissing, 2021). Strümpfer, Wissing, and Van Eeden conducted empirical work on well-being in the early nineties before the formal establishment of PP with a focus on salutogenesis and fortigenesis and signalled the emergence of a new subdiscipline they called "psychofortology" (Strümpfer, 1990, 1995, 2005; Strümpfer & Wissing, 1998; Wissing & Van Eeden, 1997, 2002) which became simultaneously known as positive psychology in America (cf. Seligman & Csikszentmihalyi, 2000). Contributions such as those by Eloff (2007) and the book *Well-being research in South Africa* (Wissing, 2013) marked the coming of a period of many well-being studies in South-Africa. Nowadays several large research teams in PP are active in South Africa, and well-being studies are emerging in many other African countries such as Ghana, Kenya, Tanzania, and Nigeria (for example, Appiah et al., 2020; Chika Chukwuorji et al., 2019; Dzokoto et al., 2019; Selvam & Collicutt, 2013) and across countries such as by Eloff et al. (2008). To a large extent these studies still lack reflection on the role of philosophical assumptions about the world and science and how these play out in the understanding and promotion of well-being. But voices from Africa are now starting to be recognized (Eloff, 2019; Nwoye, 2018; Nyamnjoh, 2015/2017) and pointing to the always shifting complexities of human being and becoming, taking worldviews into consideration.

1.3 Developments in Science: The Case of Positive Psychology

During the past two decades, positive psychology (PP) developed as a science similarly to other disciplines. Changes can be seen in assumptions, methods and focus. Old ideas are challenged and new perspectives put forward. It can, however, now also be seen that more is going on in PP than only accumulation of new knowledge: There are also gradual shifts in perspectives on metatheoretical, theoretical and empirical levels in line with tendencies previously identified in philosophy of science as paradigmatic shifts, as described below.

1.3.1 Developments in Science in General

Positive psychology (PP) developed similarly to most other scientific disciplines, with regard to accumulation of knowledge, but over time old assumptions, theories and methods were also challenged. Staats (1999) conceptualized the development of science in terms of accumulation of knowledge through a process of continuous differentiation and integration of information. There is, however, a difference between accumulation of knowledge and shifts in knowledge. Kuhn (1970, 1977), a philosopher of science, coined the idea of a "disciplinary matrix" which is a shared normative belief that includes ontological assumptions, values, and the assumed criteria for good scientific practice, and usually also a typical vocabulary and focus of research. Kuhn argued that periods of growth and accumulation of knowledge takes place in the phase of what he called "normal science". But sometimes researchers come across problems they cannot solve, and after various efforts without success, the so-called "revolutionary phase" emerges in which everything change. At this point researchers adopt new perspectives and assumptions, and they may resort to a completely new focus and theories, as well as new methods that are deemed appropriate. This is what Kuhn indicated as a "paradigm shift". The change thus includes the whole "scientific text" (Madsen, 1988), manifesting on a philosophical (worldview) level, a theoretical level, and an empirical level. In such a shift not only all components of the disciplinary matrix change, but also the direction of research.

Such paradigm shifts as described by Kuhn (1970, 1977) could be noticed to some extent in the natural sciences, but are not clearly demarcated in human and social sciences. Shifts do take place in the humanities and social sciences, but they develop more gradually, and old ideas may co-exist with new ideas (Madsen, 1988). Of course, there is also an integration of new knowledge and differentiation of aspects taking place over time in the growth of the discipline, but shifts and changes in assumptions, theories and methods do also occur. For example, old and new ways of understanding the nature of well-being, may continue to exist alongside each other. Of course, nowadays many other large scale changes and developments are taking place in science, including the science of PP, for example with regard to the use of new technologies, trends towards globalization, the emerging 4th Industrial Revolution, larger scope of projects (cf. Nicolescu, 2010, 2015), eResearch, large data bases from social media, and so forth. These aside for now, we will next move to a description of the noticed shifts in positive psychology as such, and how these developments manifest on metatheoretical, theoretical and empirical levels. We will also consider how some of the assumptions in the third wave of PP in particular resonate with African imprints from long ago—but which are also to some extent still at play in contemporary times.

1.3.2 Phases in the Development of Positive Psychology as a Science

In this chapter we argue that three waves or phases can be distinguished in the development of positive psychology across the previous two decades of its formal existence (1998/2000–2020). In summary, the first phase of PP (1998/2000–2010) focused strongly on advocating for the positive in human functioning in contrast to past perspectives that mostly focused on the negatives. Various facets of well-being were distinguished and received attention in empirical studies and theories. The second phase of PP (more or less 2010–2015) is marked by the recognition that negative facets of human life should also be taken into account in the dynamics of well-being. Cultural aspects were noted and some relatively more holistic and integrative theories were formulated. A third wave of PP (more or less 2015–2020 and continuing), with a strong focus on context and connections between people and among person and environment, can now be noticed to emerge (cf. Wissing et al., 2020). In this third phase, different disciplines focus on well-being which is explored in various domains of life. Multi- and transdisciplinary research and practice come to the forefront. This can be seen as an embracing of well-being in diverse contexts from multiple and transdisciplinary perspectives. New horizons for understanding and promoting well-being and health are opening up.

1.3.2.1 The First Phase/Wave of PP from 1998/2000–2010

It was initially debated whether PP was a new paradigm, a novel movement in psychology, or a new discipline, but these questions were soon put aside, and empirical research took off at an astounding pace—primarily from an individualist perspective. In 1998 Seligman announced in his presidential APA address that a new focus on what is well with people will be his main mission (Seligman, 1998). The first volume of publications on PP topics was published in 2000 in the *American Psychologist* (with Seligman and Csikszentmihalyi as guest editors). Soon many studies were conducted on positive traits, character strengths and processes. A flourishing area of well-being studies developed. In the early publications (e.g., the January issue of the *American Psychologist*, 2000) there was a strong call, in particular from Seligman (e.g., Seligman & Csikszentmihalyi, 2000) that "real scientific methods" should be used so that objective truths can be revealed similarly to how it is done in the natural sciences. It is noteworthy that, in this process, no attention was paid to the role of worldview assumptions.

Research in positive psychology aimed to understand and promote well-being and the quality of life by focusing on strengths and resources (Peterson & Seligman, 2004; Seligman & Csikszentmihalyi, 2000). Hart and Sasso (2011) indicated the exponential growth of PP in the first phase of its formal existence. In this phase of positive psychology's development, many constructs related to well-being came into focus, for example, positive emotions, satisfaction with life, creativity, gratitude, hope and many more—several of these already explored before the formal announcement of PP. Mainly the nature of well-being was explored in this phase, but later on also its dynamics as in Fredrickson's broaden and build model (Frederickson, 2001), and then also how well-being can be promoted and how the effects of interventions can be evaluated (e.g., Cohn & Fredrickson, 2010; Fredrickson et al., 2008; Lubbe & Eloff, 2004; Lyubomirsky, 2008; Seligman et al., 2005; Sheldon & Lyubomirsky, 2006; Wissing et al., 2008). Initially the focus was mostly on life satisfaction and subjective well-being known as *hedonic* (also named *feeling good*) happiness (e.g., Diener, 1984; Kahneman et al., 1999). Later the focus also shifted to perspectives on *eudaimonic* well-being (*functioning well*), including facets such as purpose, meaning, meaning-making and other well-being components (e.g., Emmons, 2005; Hicks & King, 2009; Lambert et al., 2009; Steger et al., 2011; Wong, 2011).

Apart from the focus on empirical and theoretical aspects of well-being, a quantitative methodological approach was advocated, with no attention to metatheoretical ontological assumptions and an implicit epistemological view that real knowledge can only be gained from quantitative, and preferably experimental designs. Some main characteristics typical of the first wave of PP can be abstracted.

Major characteristics of the first phase of PP as a science are as follows:

- Researchers explored what is best in people, their capacities and strengths, and how these can be enhanced, instead of focusing on how pathology can be remedied. There was thus an active advocating for a focus on the positives in human functioning (Ebersöhn, 2007; Ebersöhn & Eloff, 2006; Seligman & Csikszentmihalyi, 2000; Theron & Theron, 2010; Wissing & Van Eeden, 2002; Wissing & Temane, 2008).
- Researchers attempted to identify the more granular components of well-being. Increasingly more specific facets of well-being were explored, for example, apart from the initial focus on satisfaction with life and subjective well-being, more attention was paid to positive affect, optimism, flow, autonomy, meaning, mindfulness, grit and character strengths.
- As knowledge accumulated in PP, the similarities and differences among conceptualizations were analyzed, and higher order integrations emerged, for example, the clustering of constructs and assumptions in the so-called hedonic and eudaimonic perspectives (Deci & Ryan, 2008).
- The maturation of the field was shown in theory building by the development of the now well-known broaden and build model of positive emotions by Barbara Fredrickson (2001, 2006, 2009).
- Some existing theories in psychology were drawn into PP research, for example, flow (Csikszentmihalyi, 1997), the self-determination theory (SDT; Deci & Ryan, 1985), or Ryff's work which was actually conducted outside the formal PP movement, but focused on well-being and health (e.g., Ryff, 1989, 1995).
- Similar types of studies took place in mainstream PP, positive youth development, humanistic perspectives, quality of life perspectives, and asset-based approaches, conducted in a silo fashion without any interaction or recognition of each other's work.
- In the first phase of PP there was a neglect of attention to cultural contexts, ethics, and the multimodal nature of well-being.
- Quantitative methodologies prevailed, hypotheses were tested, efforts were made to establish causality, and generalizations of findings were made ignoring the role of contexts.
- Worldviews were not explicated but can be deducted to be individualist in orientation and based on the assumption that the reality can be known as it is, by applying objective methods. It was assumed that researchers were value-free.
- Main stream research in PP during the first phase can be described as WEIRD (cf. Henrich et al., 2010); that is, it was primarily conducted by and on participants from Western, Educated, Industrialized, Rich and Democratic countries

Table 1.1 Summary: first wave

Focus	Method	Worldviews Ontology, epistemology, values
Advocating for the positive—vs pathology—e.g. Seligman (1998) **Specific facets of well-being:** positive affect, differentiate more, subjective well-being **Clustering of constructs**—e.g., hedonic & eudaimonic **Theory development**—e.g., Fredrickson (2001) **Streams of similar research in silos**—e.g., main stream PP, humanistic perspectives, youth development, asset-based approaches—no interaction **Neglecting culture, ethics, & multimodal aspects of well-being** **WEIRD research**	Quantitative—controlled experiments & surveys Hypothesis verification Generalizations independent of contexts Causality quantitatively determined	Liberal **individualism** and naturalism Reality can be known by **objective methods** Positivist/Postpositivist Thinking based on assumptions of objectivism, **reductionism, linear causality** Researchers are **value-free**, objective, emotionally detached, should verify hypotheses empirically

(while the majority of people on earth are not WEIRD), although exceptions also existed as indicated by studies in the African continent.

See Table 1.1 for a summary of trends in the first wave of PP with regard to its focus, methods and metatheoretical assumptions.

1.3.2.2 The Second Phase/Wave of PP from More or Less 2010–2015

The major new contribution of the second wave of positive psychology was the explicit recognition that both the positives and negatives of life are important to understand well-being. Early in this phase the role of both the positives and negatives was highlighted in the rapid surge of research on resilience, showing that positive growth is sometimes possible even after severe stressors (e.g., Ebersöhn, 2012; Theron & Theron, 2010, 2014; Ryff, 2014; Uchida, 2011; Ungar, 2012; Wong, 2011). But formal recognition of the importance to also take note of the negatives of life for a deeper understanding of well-being, was only recognized later on in the second wave of PP. The second wave emerged while tendencies from the first wave of PP continued.

During the first phase of PP strong external critique was already launched at the underlying assumptions of PP from philosophical and other perspectives (e.g., Held, 2002, 2004, 2018; Lazarus, 2003; Norem & Chang, 2002; Ryff & Singer, 1998), but these were initially just ignored by most researchers in mainstream positive psychology. However, these critiques were gradually accepted and complemented with critique from internal voices in PP (cf. Guse, 2010; Lomas et al., 2015; McNulty & Fincham, 2012; Ryff, 2014; Wong, 2011). The core of these external and internal critiques was aimed at the idea that some phenomena (traits or events) were inherently positive (and thus also inherently desirable), and others inherently negative (and thus inherently undesirable), while ignoring context and culture. Researchers promoting the second wave of PP argued that the categorization of events or traits as positive or negative depends on context. For example, McNulty and Fincham (2012) pointed out that the meaning of supposedly positive constructs/behavior such as "forgiveness" depends on the context, illustrating this notion with the example of the consequences of forgiveness in a good versus an abusive relationship—forgiveness may build the relationship in the first instance, but may even lead to the possibility of death for the forgiver in the second case.

The inclusion of the positives as well as negatives of life in positive psychology research came into focus, amongst others, with the work of Wong (2011, 2012) and Lomas and Ivtzan (2015) who respectively referred to it as PP 2.0 and the "second wave" of PP. Apart from situational contexts as indicated by McNulty and Fincham (2012), cultural context was also indicated as highly important for the understanding of well-being constructs (Hitokoto & Uchida, 2015; Ogihara & Uchida, 2014; Schutte et al., 2013; Uchida & Ogihara, 2012). Lomas (2016) referred to many so-called untranslatable words in various languages, referring to aspects of well-being that may improve the understanding of the nuances well-being in cultural contexts. Lomas and Ivtzan (2015) highlighted the complex interplay and dynamics of the positives and negatives in human experiences, and that some constructs or phenomena can even contain both positive and negative connotations or feelings, for example the Portuguese word "saudade" which refers to a melancholic longing; or the German word "waldeinsamkeit" referring to a feeling of solitude and enchantment while being solitary in the woods; or the well-known "sehnsuht" which is a nice and painful romantic longing. The same word may have different connotations in different cultural contexts as argued by Shiah (2016). For example, from a Western perspective, a positive "self-esteem" is important for well-being, but from a Buddhist perspective, the self does not even exist. Self-esteem is also viewed as secondary to the importance of the group in interdependent or relatively collectivist cultural contexts (Shiah, 2016). Grant and Schwartz (2011) argued that too much of a good thing can be bad, for example extreme optimism may lead to dangerous risk taking, whereas something supposedly negative such as pessimism can have an upside in that it may lead to prudence. It is thus clear that the positives and negatives in human experiences are complexly intertwined and context-dependent. This phenomenon is not specifically related to constructs referring to the positives and negatives in life, but part of a universal linguistic manifestation of the important role of culture, history and geography in similar or more different meanings attached to words as recently indicated by Thompson et al. (2020).

Wong's (2011, 2012) dual-systems model of well-being integrates the positives and negatives as well as cultural contextual components in his meaning-centred eudaimonic perspective. He highlights the ethical and moral underpinnings of conceptualizations of well-being, implying the role of worldviews. Some multidimensional integrated theories of well-being were formulated in this phase of PP, such as the LIFE-model by Lomas et al. (2015). The multiplicity of

Table 1.2 Summary: second wave

Focus	Method	Worldviews Ontology, epistemology, values
Positives & negatives of life as facets of being • Intertwined • Meaning depend on context—situational and cultural • Construct/phenomenon contains in itself positive & negative facets **Culture as context** More holistic theories emerge **Increasingly more disciplines started to explore well-being**	Qualitative case studies, surveys, interviews Also small samples, in-depth studies—qualitative Mixed methods: QUAN & QUAL	**Post-formal; postmodern**—subject becomes predominant to the object **Constructivism**: radical & social Interpretivist **Research is value bound**, the researcher is part of what is being researched, cannot be separated and so will be **subjective** Integral—**Multiple worldviews**

metatheoretical perspectives assumed in perspectives on well-being became evident as was highlighted by Waterman (2013a, 2013b), and constructivist and qualitative interpretive perspectives emerged (e.g., Gergen, 2011; White & Jha, 2014). Various disciplines such as philosophy, sociology, human movement sciences, leisure studies, and more, started to explore facets and correlates of well-being (e.g., Haybron, 2011; Hefferon, 2013; Thin, 2014).

Major characteristics of the second phase of PP as a science are as follows:

- The main new trends in this wave of PP were the recognition that the positive and negative facets of life are interwoven, that the understanding of something as positive or negative depends on context (culture and situation), and that facets of human functioning may simultaneously reflect positive and negative connotations.
- The relevance and importance of cultural contexts for the understanding of well-being became increasingly strongly foregrounded.
- The multidimensional nature of well-being became captured in the development of relatively more holistic theories of well-being.
- Disciplines apart from psychology increasingly began to explore well-being topics.
- Mixed methods studies were more frequently used in this phase of PP, including in-depth qualitative studies; data were collected in interviews, focus groups, in small and large samples with surveys and other quantitative methods.
- On a metatheoretical level, multiple worldviews were recognized in PP during the second phase. Constructivist perspectives and interpretive approaches came into vogue; it was recognized that researchers are subjective and that research is not value-free—which of course influenced interpretations.

See Table 1.2 for a summary of trends in the second wave of PP with regard to its focus, methods and metatheoretical assumptions.

1.3.2.3 The Third Phase/Wave of PP from Around 2015–2020

In this phase, rigorous research and practice in PP were/are ongoing in line with the assumptions of the first and second waves, but a third wave is now also emerging. In this third wave (PP 3.0) more unequivocal emphasis is placed on contextualization, and interconnectedness (that includes spirituality/transcendence), and on multi-, inter-, and transdisciplinary research and practice with a view to the complexity of well-being issues (Wissing, 2018; Wissing et al., 2018, 2019). In this third wave of PP, "context" refers to countries, cultures, social and physical environments, life phases, gender categories, life domains, and other. The focus on interconnectedness facilitates post-disciplinary work in research and practice, with collaboration in multi-, inter-, and transdisciplinary teams (e.g., Delle Fave et al., 2017).

Ideas from the second wave are being taken forward during the third wave: Held (2018) accentuated that, in order to improve the understanding of well-being, PP should also explore the adaptive functioning of "negativity" just as it studies the adaptive functioning of "positivity". Lomas (2018) argued the normality of sadness in life which may also have inherent value, and foster growth and flourishing. In the third wave of PP, the positive and negative emotions are also further explored from a cultural perspective (e.g., Miyamoto et al., 2017). The intertwinedness of the positives and negatives accentuated in the second wave is explored in the third wave in evaluating of PP interventions aiming at targeting both enhancement of well-being and ameliorating negative symptoms showing their interwovenness (e.g., Geerling et al., 2020; Hendriks et al., 2019).

In the third wave of PP the unjustified assumptions of a value-free PP, as initially projected, are pointed out by O'Doherty (2016) as well as Di Martino et al. (2017). They highlight the neglect of context, social justice and values, and even contend that foci sometimes only conceal an egoist pursuit and personal satisfaction which ignore the possible negative effect of behaviors on others, the psychosocial environment and physical context. The accentuation of social justice indicates the importance of the wider society and political contexts. The third wave of PP in particular highlights the role of processes such as liberation, justice, and power, and the value of participation, mutuality, and the ethics of care in the understanding and promoting of well-being (cf. Di Martino et al., 2017).

Several authors thus indicated the importance of understanding well-being not only as an intra- and interpersonal phenomenon, but also as a quality of connectedness to the physical environment (e.g., Helne & Hirvilammi, 2015) and spiritual/religuous contexts (Sharma & Singh, 2019) which is in line with a strong relationality or cosmodernity assumptions (cf. Helne & Hirvilammi, 2015; Nicolescu, 2014a, 2015) on a methatheoretical level. The notion of taking various levels of well-being (e.g., individual, group, community, society, eco-system, and spiritual) into account, as well as links among levels, is argued by several researchers, for example Galderisi et al. (2015, 2017), Harrell (2018), Urata (2015), Warren and Donaldson (2018), and many more. A renewed interest in research on spirituality and religion on the one hand, and well-being on the other hand, can be noted amongst others, in the research of Chirico (2016), Lifshitz et al. (2019), Nicolescu (2014b), Van Cappellen et al. (2017), Sharma and Singh (2019), and Villani et al. (2019). This focus on spirituality and well-being resonates with longstanding contributions from Africa (cf. also Nwoye, 2017).

Studies by Delle Fave et al. (2017), Fowers et al. (2017), and Helne and Hirvilammi (2015) show the multimodal nature of well-being and the inextricable intertwinedness of the positives and negatives in human life in the context of frailty, suffering and illness, and also indicate the dependence of wellbeing on the health of the ecosystem. Delle Fave (2018) emphasizes the complex interplay between psychological and biological facets, and highlights the importance of understanding well-being within an interconnectedness approach. Such developments point to the importance of multi-, inter- and transdisciplinary research in the unraveling of the complexities inherent in well-being manifestations. The same is argued from a philosophical perspective by Finkenthal (2016).

On a metatheoretical level, the third wave of PP reflects multiple worldviews. An acceptance of the interconnectedness of everything can be seen in explicit strong relational ontological assumptions as by Helne and Hirvilammi (2015) and Nicolesco's (2014a, 2014b, 2015) metatheoretical ideas of cosmodernity and the hidden third. The implications of metatheoretical Aristotelian virtue ethics assumptions for theory and practice in well-being research is explored by various researchers (e.g., Berg, 2020; Fowers, 2016; Fowers & Anderson, 2018; Intelisano et al., 2020; Proctor, 2019). Epistemological assumptions on what proper methods are to produce trustworthy knowledge, make space for a variety of approaches.

The notion of the complex multimodalness of well-being, and the necessity of multi-, inter- and transdisciplinary research and practice for the understanding and promotion of well-being in increasingly complex contexts seems to be trickling through to the ground level of conversations and organization of PP conferences. Conferences are increasingly being advertised as multidisciplinary, for example, the third China International Conference on Positive Psychology 2015 was advertised as: "The conference is a multidisciplinary event where scholars who work on various aspects of positive psychology and human happiness can come together to present, discuss and exchange ideas and to foster interdisciplinary collaborative projects". The 2019 International Positive Psychology Association's Conference had "Nexus" as an overarching theme, referring to connectedness among people, ideas and disciplines. Signs of the third wave of PP can be noticed in research and practice, and with reference to the empirical and theoretical focus of studies, methods used and metatheoretical assumptions made.

The major characteristics of the third phase of PP as a science are as follows:

- There is a focus on contextualization, interconnectedness and complexity. Diverse meanings of "context" are taken into account, and efforts are made to understand the dynamics among individuals and the broader social, cultural and ecological contexts in well-being.
- There is an upsurge in attention to spirituality/transcendence as shown in references to worldviews as well as explorations on the empirical level.

Table 1.3 Summary: third wave—PP 3.0

Focus	Method	Worldviews Ontology, epistemology, values
Relatedness **Interconnectedness**—the in-between-quality, balancing opposites, harmonizing diversities **WB as multi-modal** holistic/ integral theories Human-environment balance **All contexts** important Multi-, inter-, & transdisciplinary **collaboration** **Spirituality**...	Multi-method research Transdisciplinary methodology Action research—intervention driven Data collection quantitative and qualitative—random and purposive Transdisciplinary hermeneutics	**Strong relationality/ cosmodernity**: every entity in the universe is defined by its relation to other entities **Humble co-existence of worldviews—plurality** **Transdisciplinary hermeneutics** **Reality of the included middle; knowledge is an emergent property, and is never fully or absolutely certain** **Pragmatism/critical dialectical pluralism/integrative research/ social justice approach** **Advocacy/participatory** **Virtues and values important**

- Recognition of complexity of well-being issues takes foreground, and includes attention to interconnectedness, context, and spirituality (complex: Latin roots *com* = "together", and *plex* = "woven"; = woven together) inviting post-disciplinary approaches for the understanding of well-being.
- Multi- and mixed-methods as well as more action research approaches are used. Quantitative and qualitative aspects are taken into account, with also specific focus on lay people's perspectives for a deeper understanding of well-being.
- A strong relational ontological perspective is emerging in worldviews. Values and ethical aspects are considered highly important in the understanding of well-being. Various worldviews now co-exist.
- A cosmodern metatheoretical view that assumes the relatedness of all things is promoting transdisciplinarity. Increasingly integration and cooperation among disciplines are developing. The most prominent characteristic of the third wave is the shift towards a post-disciplinary phase that can be seen in the strong advocacy for multi-, inter- and transdisciplinary research and practice for promotion of well-being. See Table 1.3 for a summary of trends in the third wave of PP with regard to its focus, methods and metatheoretical assumptions.

1.4 African Value Imprints and Positive Psychology

The linchpin of the third wave of PP as indicated above, is a transdisciplinary approach with a focus on the complexity of well-being, assuming the interwovenness of humans, nature, belief systems and contextual situatedness. The acceptance of the interconnectedness of things implies relational metatheoretical assumptions in ontology and epistemology such as found in the ideas of cosmodernity by Nicolescu (2014a, 2014b, 2015) and proposed by Nyamnjoh (2015/2017) in his perspectives about reality. The idea of multiplicity of systems, complexity and interconnectedness in life and reality is part of an old African imprint as expressed by Baloyi and Mokobe-Rabothata (2014, p. 265): "Africans understand their being-in-the-world as a qualitative tapestry of connected systems which deal with life issues collectively and collaboratively". The philosophical perspectives in which both the natural and supernatural worlds are seen as being intertwined, relevant and in need of being harmonized in order to ensure health and well-being was known long ago and assumed in African worldviews (cf. Eloff, 2008). Such complexities of being and relating are now also recognized in assumptions of the third wave of PP, although expressed differently.

Senghor (1970, p. 181) indicated that in an African context there is "a kind of knowledge that emerges from the harmonizing and fusing of things" (is this intuition, or what Michael [Polanyi, 1967]) long ago called "tacit knowledge" meaning we know more than we can tell?). Important here is the idea of harmonization. The importance of harmony in lay people's experiences of happiness and well-being has been shown in a multicultural mixed methods study by Delle Fave et al. (2016), but empirical evidence is lacking on the role of harmonizing as proposed by Senghor (1970) as an antecedent for well-being as an outcome. Igbokwe and Ndom (2008) indicated that good health in an African context means that the individual is in harmony with his/her cosmos (that includes the self, other people as well as the natural environment and spiritual forces). Disharmony manifests in physical, psychological and social illness. Igbokwe et al. (2015) developed a harmony-disharmony scale to evaluate in which areas of the individual's situatedness in the cosmos disharmony disrupts life, in order to ameliorate this, based on the principles of the harmony restoration theory. The perspective on the role of harmony and harmonization in health and well-being invites further empirical research, especially in instances where the environment and experienced spiritual forces are included.

The African notion that "people and things adopt different forms and manifest themselves differently according to context and necessity" as described by Nyamnjoh (2017, p. 258) also needs a deeper understanding and empirical exploration through a well-being lens. In Nyamnjoh's worldview, reality does not only consist of what can be observed or rationally accounted for—reality also includes the emotional, the intuitive, the invisible and the inexplicable. Nyamnjoh (2015/2017) proposes the idea of "conviviality" that refers to the processes of recognition and respect for the notion that reality is always in flux and people are always incomplete. This position is a metatheoretical stance (resonating with the acceptance of plurality of assumptions about the world), but also a theoretical perspective on human functioning. He argues that incompleteness is the normal way of being, and of life. Conviviality invites all people to reach out to others in their incompleteness—not in order to try to become complete in themselves, but to complement the other and make all of them more effective in their relationships and lives. Individual and collective interests are served if these are sought in acknowledgement and appreciation of the incompleteness of the self and others with whom they are connected. Conviviality means collaboration, dialogue, compassion and interdependence. It links people, build bridges, and consolidate the good life for all. Conviviality does not negate the existence of animosities, conflicts and tensions, but carefully seek a balance between intimacy and distance, knowing that there is a necessity for harmony which is an imperative for individual and collective success and well-being. As Nyamnjoh (2017, p. 263) indicates: "In a context where reality is more than meets the eye and matters are far from fixed, life becomes a process of negotiating and navigating possibilities of being and becoming". We need to further explore what such dynamics mean on empirical levels for experienced well-being in an African context, and for processes to enhance health and well-being.

Linking to the Nyamnjoh's ideas of incompleteness, Nwoye (2018) forwards the idea of the Madiban tradition referring to the incompleteness of either Western or African perspectives on science. He proposes that the inadequacies and incompleteness of Western psychology need to be complemented by the acknowledgement of supernatural forces and other invisible influences in people's lives. The term Madiban, comes from the word Madiba which refers to an African moral vision that emphasizes seeing the natural and supernatural as relevant realities (Nwoye, 2018). Such supernatural forces may not be measurable, but form part of metatheoretical assumptions about the world, and are reflected in lay people's experiences on which they can comment. The role of spirituality and environmental aspects in well-being, that are now coming into vogue in PP, had thus long ago already been known as important in an African belief system. What this means for the understanding and promotion of well-being and health in an African context, can now be further explored. Such studies had started as can be seen in the work of Ohajunwa and Mji (2018) who reviewed the literature on African indigenous conceptualizations of spirituality, and indicated the role thereof in notions of well-being.

A typical African strength (similar to the value in action character strengths described by Peterson & Seligman, 2004), is "hospitality" (cf. Kiige et al., 2019). Although the term "hospitality" is well known in general and is also specifically used in the context of the hospitality and tourism sector, it is a particularly valued practice in the African context—it is a basic moral, social and cultural value grounded in the worldview that no one exists alone. In a daily life context hospitality is a giving (of time, assistance, food, a place to stay, etc.) without expecting something back (Kiige et al., 2019; Olikenyi, 2001; Selvam & Collicutt, 2013). It is expressed in a generous, both hands-openness welcoming. Such a character strength resonates with qualities of positive relationships in PP, but exhibits more depth and unconditionality as typically practiced in a Western context. Hospitality, as an exceptional way of being welcoming, is in the African perspective rooted in views on morality and harmony (Matondo, 2012; Metz, 2016).

1.5 The Way Forward

The way forward for PP in general and in an African context in particular, requires: Firstly, in general, that researchers in PP self-reflect and make an effort—thus knowing own emotions, sensitivities, knowledge base, motivations, assumptions, values and worldviews, and respectfully making an effort to understand those of others. Secondly, in moving from me to us, multiple or cosmodern worldviews can be understood and embraced, leading to transcendence of binarity in worldviews and collaboration across cultures, as well as a search to work together in inter-, multi- and transdisciplinary research and practice in methodological endevours. Thirdly, with such a multi- and transdisciplinary approach and focus on interconnectedness, the nature and dynamics of the complexity of well-being can be explored and the lived experiences better understood. Such processes will engender multidisciplinary promotion of well-being as an outcome—on individual, group, societal, and ecological levels. Multi- and transdisciplinary efforts will enable researchers and practitioners to engage with complex well-being issues, such as well-being in times of pandemics, in contexts of inequality, violence, displacement of peoples, and climate change (cf. Dielman, 2015; Lueddeke, 2019), and may enhance the richness of resources, strengths and health for diverse people in diverse contexts. In a multi- and transdisciplinary approach there can be an integration of knowledge from a variety of groups, such as scientists, practitioners, policymakers, regulators, and the public. Fourthly, in moving forward, a renewed awareness of ethics need to be part of well-being research, because ethics is all about the quality of relations and responsibilities.

Considering the third wave of PP, and taking cognisance of the African psychological perspective that assumes the existence of natural and supernatural phenomena on both ontological and empirical levels, the question is: What can PP look like in an African context? It will amongst others imply the generation of dependable knowledge via a variety of methodological approaches as described by Nwoye (2018), and conducted in the third wave of PP research. The role of spirituality and interconnectedness that are now rising in importance in the focus of Western PP, had long been an imprint of African thought (e.g., Balcomb et al., 2017; Baloyi & Mokobe-Rabothata, 2014; Gyekye, 1995). The new challenge is to explore the harmonization of Western and African perspectives in PP on metatheoretical levels, with then also a specific focus on harmony and harmonization as manifestation of health and well-being on an empirical level. In both Western and African perspectives harmony, together with its concomitants of balance, peace, and equanimity, are taking foreground in the understanding of well-being and the dynamics involved. However, the manifestations thereof may differ in African contexts in comparison to the manifestation in Western contexts. More specifically, there is an important element of liveliness and vitality in direct perceptions and experiences in African contexts as described by Senghor that also manifests in a different quality of connectedness and "sunny" collectivism in Africa than for example in the Eastern more subdued collectivist contexts (Wissing & Temane, 2008; https://en.wikipedia.org/wiki/l%c3%a9opold_s%c3%a9dar_senghor).

Going forward, we suggest that "well-being studies" are used as the overarching umbrella term for studies on flourishing, positive traits, processes, behaviors, and interactions, to create space for the multi-modal nature and situational imbeddedness of well-being and multi- and transdisciplinary approaches to it, instead of the disciplinary restricted "positive psychology". The use of "well-being" as overarching umbrella term for phenomena reflecting optimal psychological function, or described as positive and life- and growth affirming, had already been used by Ryan and Deci (2001), Delle Fave et al. (2011), Wissing (2013) and others. The suggested use of "well-being studies" for multi- and transdisciplinary research and practice related to optimal health and well-being is also in line with the convergence of broad streams of research across disciplines that are noticed by others. For example, PP and quality of life studies (mainly from sociological and economical perspectives) are converging (Diener et al., 2018; Noll, 2018; Rojas, 2018; Veenhoven, 2018), and philosophical and psychological accounts of well-being are taking hands (Alexandrova, 2017; Intelisano et al., 2020). In this sense transdisciplinary studies on the multimodal and situatedness nature of well-being, is like a butterfly leaving a cocoon.

We further envisage that this butterfly may signal the emergence of a new multi- or transdisciplinary field of well-being research and practice in which different disciplines partake simultaneously and in close collaboration in the exploration and promotion of multimodal health and well-being in diverse contexts. Although these multi- and transdisciplinary well-being studies, with increasing sophistication and incorporation of modern technology and the fourth Industrial Revolution modes of operating, were born from PP, it may unfold as a new disciplinary endeavor, while the traditional PP studies within the confinement of psychology may also continue.

This envisaged transdisciplinary field of well-being studies may also transform the prevailing western individualistic/atomistic approach to open spaces for a more collaborative, contextually relevant and ecological perspective as reflected in typical African and more interdependent collectivist approaches—seeking harmonization not only in manifestations of well-being as subject matter, but also among disciplines and diverse metatheoretical assumptions, thus humbly recognizing the incompleteness of one perspective and approach. This new field of scientific endeavor can capitalize on developments of the fourth Industrial Revolution—with the humane heart still beating warmly. We need a lot of imagination, brave creativity and wise perspectives to deal with the many complexities, contradictions, and chaos that may arise when disciplines and professions come together to work on complex issues of life and well-being. But this is what we need to do to help shape the reality that we want. As imaginations and perspectives are imbedded in culture, we need many minds coming together from diverse contexts, transcending disciplines as well as academic, political and lay perspectives. Such an inclusive participatory model matters for authentic engagement—we all can contribute, and all have a stake in the outcome of the deliberations on how to understand and promote well-being in diverse contexts. The assumptions we make about reality, values, and the relative legitimacy of different forms of knowledge, will shape how we work together resulting in the eventual flourishing of a transdisciplinary field of well-being studies. See Diagram 1.1.

1.6 Summary and Conclusion

In this chapter we argued the problem and consequences of the previous neglect of attention to contextual and metatheoretical assumptions in positive psychology as discipline. After indicating development trajectories for disciplines as viewed from the philosophy of science, we traced noted developments in PP as science. We described the development of PP over time, highlighting changes in focus, methods and metatheoretical assumptions. We highlighted the emergence of the third wave of PP (third wave; PP 3.0) characterized by a focus on interconnectedness and complexities, multiple research methods and multi-and transdisciplinary approaches, and assumptions of plurality in worldview assumptions, and in particular strong relational or cosmodern perspectives. These developments reflect the shifts in thought processes that are linked to new integral and evolving knowledge patterns which are typical in the postdisciplinary discourses.

Many of the metatheoretical perspectives and assumptions about well-being and health, that are now part of the third wave, were already found in African perspectives long ago. It is suggested that harmonizing of Western and African perspectives is one way to ensure a deeper understanding of well-being, and that the latter can in particular be conceptualized in terms of harmony and related characteristics. From an African perspective good health and well-being means that a person is in harmony with his/her cosmos (that includes the self, other people as well as the natural environment and transcendental spiritual forces). The third wave of PP with acceptance of diverse worldviews, methods, and focus on interconnectedness and complexities of well-being as viewed from diverse disciplinary perspectives and its transdisciplinary outgrowth, is compared to a butterfly leaving its cocoon. However, we also think that this butterfly signals the development of an emerging new transdisciplinary domain of scientific endeavor. We think this domain will in future also develop apart from positive psychology which is discipline bound in name up until now. We suggest the new field of study pollinated by the third wave butterfly, can be named "Well-being studies" or "Transdisciplinary health and well-being studies".

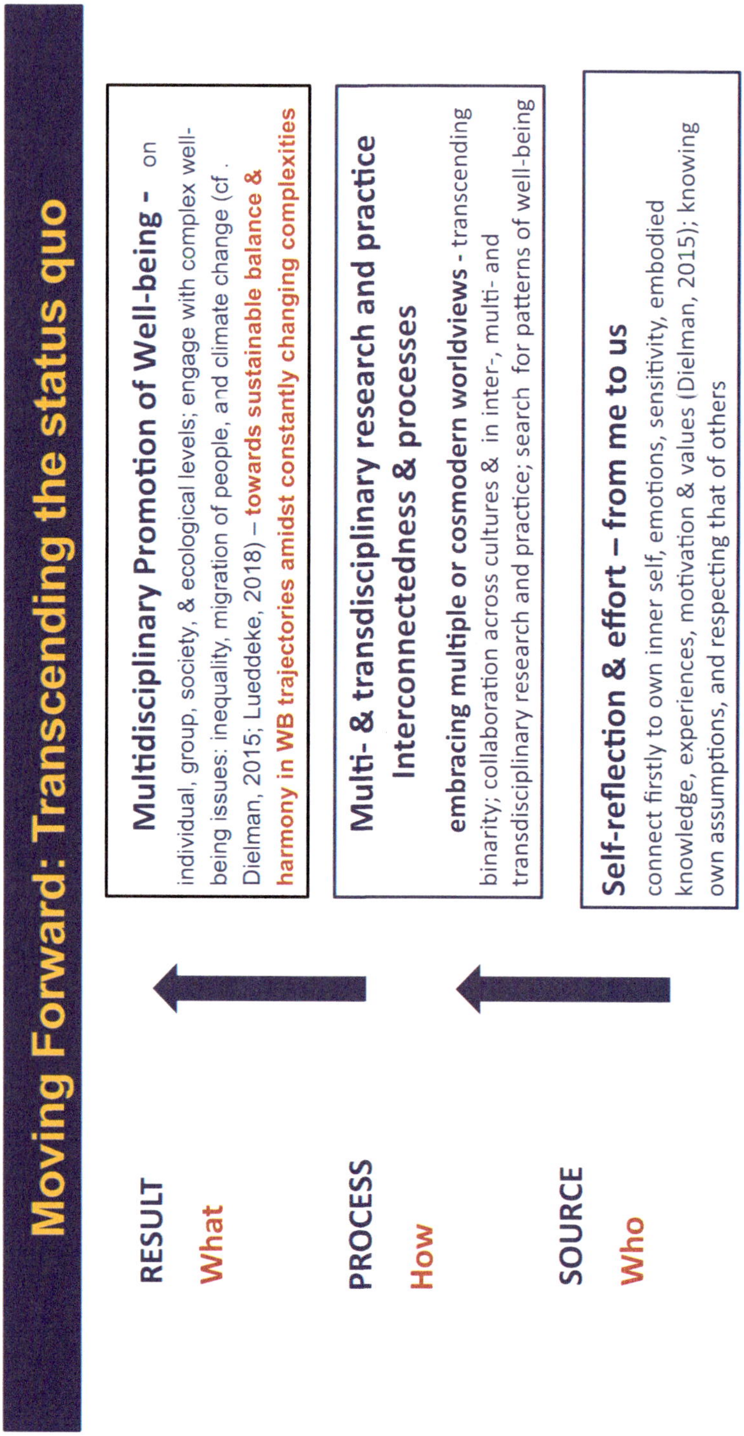

Diagram 1.1 Moving forward: transcending the status quo

Acknowledgement This work is based on the research supported in part by the National Research Foundation (NRF) of South Africa (grant numbers: 106050, 121948). We acknowledge that opinions, findings, conclusions and recommendations expressed are those of the authors and that the NRF accepts no liability whatsoever in this regard.

References

Alexandrova, A. (2017). *A philosophy for the science of well-being*. Oxford University Press.

Appiah, R., Wilson-Fadiji, A., Schutte, L., & Wissing, M. P. (2020). Effects of a community-based multicomponent positive psychology intervention on mental health of rural adults in Ghana. *Applied Psychology: Health and Well-Being (Online)*. https://doi.org/10.1111/aphw.12212

Balcomb, A., Chirongomas, S., Dah, I. D., Daniel, S., Deouyo, P., & Gaisie, R. K. (2017). Spirituality and hope in Africa: A study in five countries. *International Bulletin of Mission Research, 41*(5). https://doi.org/10.1177/2396939317730698

Baloyi, L., & Mokobe-Rabothata, M. (2014). The African conception of death: A cultural implication. In *Proceedings from the 21st International Congress of the International Association for Cross-Culural Psychology*, 232–243. Retrieved from https://scholarworks.gvsu.edu/iaccp_papers/119/

Berg, H. (2020). Virtue ethics and integration in evidence-based practice in psychology. *Frontiers in Psychology, 11*, 258. https://doi.org/10.3389/fpsyg.2020.00258

Chika Chukwuorji, J., Ekpedoho, E. A., Ifeagwazi, C. M., Iorfa, S. K., & Nwonyi, S. K. (2019). Psychometric properties of the Meaning in Life Questionnaire – Hausa version among internally displaced persons in Nigeria. *Transcultural Psychiatry, 56*(1), 103–122. https://doi.org/10.1177/1363461518794218

Chirico, F. (2016). Spiritual well-being in the 21st century: It is time to review the current WHO's health definition. *Journal of Health and Social Sciences, 1*(1), 11–16. https://doi.org/10.19204/2016/sprt2

Christopher, J. C., & Hickinbottom, S. (2008). Positive psychology, ethnocentrism, and the disguised ideology of individualism. *Theory & Psychology, 18*(5), 563–589. https://doi.org/10.1177/0959354308093396

Christopher, J. C., Richardson, F. C., & Slife, B. D. (2008). Thinking through positive psychology. *Theory & Psychology, 18*(5), 555–561. https://doi.org/10.1177/0959354308093395

Cohn, M. A., & Fredrickson, B. L. (2010). In search of durable positive psychology interventions: Predictors and consequences of long-term positive behavior change. *Journal of Positive Psychology, 5*(5), 355–366.

Csikszentmihalyi, M. (1997). *Finding flow: The psychology of engagement with everyday life*. Basic Books.

Deci, E. L., & Ryan, R. M. (1985). *Intrinsic motivation and self-determination in human behaviour*. Plenum Press.

Deci, E. L., & Ryan, R. M. (2008). Hedonia, eudaimonia, and well-being: An introduction. *Journal of Happiness Studies, 9*(1), 1–11. https://doi.org/10.1007/s10902-006-9018-1

Delle Fave, A. (2018, April 4–7). *The heuristic potential of interconnectedness models in well-being research*. Keynote presented at the First Africa Conference on Positive Psychology.

Delle Fave, A., Brdar, I., Freire, T., Vella-Brodrick, D., & Wissing, M. P. (2011). The eudaimonic and hedonic components of happiness: Qualitative and quantitative findings. *Social Indicators Research, 100*(2), 158–207.

Delle Fave, A., Brdar, I., Wissing, M. P., Araujo, U., Castro Solano, A., Freire, T., Hernandez-Pozo, M. D. R., Jose, P., Martos, T., Nafstad, H. E., Nakamura, J., Singh, K., & Soosai-Nathan, L. (2016). Lay definitions of happiness across nations: The primacy of inner harmony and relational connectedness. *Frontiers in Psychology, 7*, 30. https://doi.org/10.3389/fpsyg.2016.00030

Delle Fave, A., Bassi, M., Allegri, B., Cilia, S., Falautano, M., Goretti, B., Grobberio, M., Minacapelli, E., Marianna, P., Pietrolongo, E., Valsecchi, M., Pia Amato, M., Lugaresi, A., & Patti, F. (2017). Beyond disease: Happiness, goals, and meanings among persons with multiple sclerosis and their caregivers. *Frontiers in Psychology, 2216*. https://doi.org/10.3389/fpsyg.2017.02216

Di Martino, S., Eiroa-Orosa, F. J., & Arcidiacono, C. (2017). Community psychology's contributions on happiness and well-being: Including the role of context, social justice, and values in our understanding of the good life. In N. J. L. Brown, T. Lomas, & F. J. Eiroa-Orosa (Eds.), *The Routledge international handbook of critical positive psychology, Chapter 7* (18 pages in e-book). Routledge. https://doi.org/10.4324/9781315659794

Dielman, H. (2015). Transdisciplinary hermeneutics: Working from the inner self, creating ecologies of knowing. *Transdisciplinary Journal of Engineering & Science, 6*, 72–85.

Diener, E. (1984). Subjective well-being. *Psychological Bulletin, 95*(3), 542–575.

Diener, E., Oishi, S., & Tay, L. (2018). Advances in subjective well-being research. *Nature Human Behaviour, 2*, 253–260. https://doi.org/10.1038/s41562-018-0307-6

Dzokoto, V. A., Osei-Tutu, A., Scollon, C. N., Wallace, D., & Peters-Chitwood, L. (2019). Meaning and perceptions of the good life in Ghana. *Psychological Studies, 64*(1), 11–20. https://doi.org/10.1007/s12646-018-0475-5

Ebersöhn, L. (2007). Voicing perceptions of risk and protective factors in coping in a HIV & AIDS landscape reflecting on capacity for adaptiveness. *Gifted Education International, 23*(2), 149–159. https://doi.org/10.1177/026142940702300205

Ebersöhn, L. (2012). Adding 'flock' to 'fight and flight': A honeycomb of resilience where supply of relationships meets demand for support. *Journal of Psychology in Africa, 22*(1), 29–42. https://doi.org/10.1080/14330237.2012.10874518

Ebersöhn, L., & Eloff, I. (2006). Identifying asset-based trends in sustainable programmes which support vulnerable children. *South African Journal of Education, 26*(3), 457–472. Retrieved from https://www.ajol.info/index.php/saje/article/view/25082

Eloff, I. (2007). Finding the positives in psychology: What are we doing? *Journal of Psychology in Africa, 17*(1–2), 173–180. https://doi.org/10.1080/14330237.2007.10820164

Eloff, I. (2008). Editorial - Positive psychology: Celebrating strength and well-being in the cradle of humankind. *Journal of Psychology in Africa, 18*(1), 5–7. https://doi.org/10.1080/14330237.2008.10820166

Eloff, I. (Ed.). (2019). *Handbook of quality of life in African societies. In G. Tonon (Series Ed.), International handbooks of quality of life*. Springer. https://doi.org/10.1007/978-3-030-15367-0_1

Eloff, I., Achoui, M., Chireshe, R., Mutepfa, M., & Ofovwe, C. (2008). Views from Africa on positive psychology. *Journal of Psychology in Africa, 18*(1), 189–194. https://doi.org/10.1080/14330237.2008.10820185

Emmons, R. A. (2005). Striving for the sacred: Personal goals, life meaning, and religion. *Journal of Social Issues, 61*, 731–746.

Finkenthal, M. (2016). *Disciplinarian thinking, inter-disciplinarity and multi-disciplinarity revisited, with complexity in mind*. Trivent Publishing. Retrieved from http://trivent-publishing.eu/

Fowers, B. J. (2016). Aristotle on eudaimonia: On the virtue of returning to the source. In J. Vittersø (Ed.), *The handbook of eudaimonic well-being* (pp. 67–83). Springer.

Fowers, B. J., & Anderson, A. R. (2018). Aristotelian philia, contemporary friendship, and some resources for studying close relationships. In T. Harrison & D. I. Walker (Eds.), *The theory and practice of virtue education* (pp. 184–196). Routledge.

Fowers, B. J., Richardson, F. C., & Slife, B. D. (2017). *Frailty, suffering, and vice: Flourishing in the face of human limitations*. American Psychological Association. https://doi.org/10.1037/0000035-001

Frederickson, B. L. (2001). The role of positive emotions in positive psychology: The broaden-and-build theory of positive emotions. *American Psychologist, 56*, 218–226.

Fredrickson, B. L. (2006). Unpacking positive emotions: Investigating the seeds of human flourishing. *Journal of Positive Psychology, 1*(2), 57–59.

Fredrickson, B. L. (2009). *Positivity*. Random House.

Fredrickson, B. L., Cohn, M. A., Coffey, K. A., Pek, J., & Finkel, S. M. (2008). Open hearts build lives: Positive emotions, induced through loving-kindness meditation, build consequential personal resources. *Journal of Personality and Social Psychology, 95*(5), 1045–1062.

Galderisi, S., Heinz, A., Kastrup, M., Beezhold, J., & Sartorius, N. (2015). Toward a new definition of mental health. *World Psychiatry, 14*, 231–233.

Galderisi, S., Heinz, A., Kastrup, M., Beezhold, J., & Sartorius, N. (2017). A proposed new definition of mental health. *Psychiatria Polska, 51*(3), 407–411. https://doi.org/10.12740/PP/74145

Geerling, B., Kraiss, J. T., Kelders, S. M., Stevens, A. W. M. M., Kupka, R. W., & Bohlmeijer, E. T. (2020). The effect of positive psychology interventions on well-being and psychopathology in patients with severe mental illness: A systematic review and meta-analysis. *The Journal of Positive Psychology, 15*(5), 572–587. https://doi.org/10.1080/17439760.2020.1789695

Gergen, K. J. (2011). *Relational being: Beyond self and community*. Oxford University Press.

Grant, A. M., & Schwartz, B. (2011). Too much of a good thing: The challenge and opportunity of the inverted U. *Perspectives on Psychological Science, 6*(1), 61–76.

Guse, T. (2010). Positive psychology and the training of psychologists: Students' perspectives. *SA Journal of Industrial Psychology, 36*(2), 1–6. http://www.scielo.org.za/scielo.php?script=sci_arttext&pid=S2071-07632010000200004

Guse, T., Vescovelli, F., & Croxford, S.-A. (2019). Subjective well-being and gratitude among south African adolescents: Exploring gender and cultural differences. *Youth & Society, 51*(5), 591–615. https://doi.org/10.1177/0044118X17697237

Gyekye, K. (1995). *An essay on African philosophical thought: The Akan conceptual scheme*. Temple University Press.

Harrell, S. P. (2018). 'Being human together': Positive relationships in the context of diversity, culture, and collective well-being. In M. A. Warren & S. I. Donaldson (Eds.), *Toward a positive psychology of relationships: New directions in theory and research* (pp. 247–284). Praeger.

Hart, K. H., & Sasso, T. (2011). Mapping the contours of contemporary positive psychology. *Canadian Psychology, 52*, 82–92.

Haybron, D. M. (2011). Central Park: Nature, context, and human wellbeing. *International Journal of Wellbeing, 1*(2), 235–254. https://doi.org/10.5502/ijw.v1i2.6

Hefferon, K. (2013). *Positive psychology and the body: The somatopsychic side to flourishing*. McGraw Hill.

Held, B. S. (2002). The tyranny of the positive attitude in America: Observation and speculation. *Journal of Clinical Psychology, 58*, 965–992.

Held, B. S. (2004). The negative side of positive psychology. *Journal of Humanistic Psychology, 44*, 9–46.

Held, B. S. (2018). Positive psychology's a priori problem. *Journal of Humanistic Psychology, 58*(3), 313–342. https://doi.org/10.1177/0022167817739409

Helne, T., & Hirvilammi, T. (2015). Wellbeing and sustainability: A relational approach. *Sustainable Development, 23*(3), 167–175. https://doi.org/10.1002/sd.1581

Hendriks, T., Schotanus-Dijkstra, M., Hassankhan, A., de Jong, J., & Bohlmeijer, E. (2019). The efficacy of multi-component positive psychology interventions: A systematic review and metaanalysis of randomized controlled trials. *Journal of Happiness Studies, 21*, 357–390. https://doi.org/10.1007/s10902-019-00082-1

Henrich, J., Heine, S. J., & Norenzayan, A. (2010). The weirdest people in the world? *Behavioral and Brain Sciences, 33*, 6–83.

Hicks, J. A., & King, L. A. (2009). Meaning in life as a subjective judgment and a lived experience. *Social and Personality Psychology Compass, 3*(4), 638–653. https://doi.org/10.1111/j.1751-9004.2009.00193.x

Hitokoto, H., & Uchida, Y. (2015). Interdependent happiness: Theoretical importance and measurement validity. *Journal of Happiness Studies, 16*(1), 211–239.

Igbokwe, D. O., & Ndom, R. J. E. (2008). Harmony-disharmony therapy: A treatment method of African origin. *Nigerian Journal of Clinical Psychology, 6*(1–2), 61–77.

Igbokwe, D. O., Adeusi, S. O., Elegbeleye, A., & Agoha, B. C. E. (2015). Harmony-disharmony Scale: Development and initial factorial validation. *Covenant International Journal of Psychology, 1*(1), 33–49.

Intelisano, S., Krasko, J., & Luhmann, M. (2020). Integrating philosophical and psychological accounts of happiness and well-being. *Journal of Happiness Studies, 21*, 161–200. https://doi.org/10.1007/s10902-019-00078-x

Jaakkola, E. (2020). Designing conceptual articles: Four approaches. *Academy of Marketing Science Review, 10*(3), 18–26. https://doi.org/10.1007/s13162-020-00161-0

Kahneman, D., Diener, E., & Schwarz, N. (1999). *Well-being: The foundations of hedonic psychology*. Russell Sage Foundation.

Kiige, J. W., Selvam, S., & Njiru, L. (2019). Correlation between African hospitality and human flourishing among young African adults in Kenya. *International Journal of Scientific and Research Publications, 9*(9), 208–220.

Kim, H., Doiron, K., Warren, M. A., & Donaldson, S. I. (2018). The international landscape of positive psychology research: A systematic review. *International Journal of Wellbeing, 8*(1), 50–70. https://doi.org/10.5502/ijw.v8i1.651

Kosterec, M. (2016). Methods of conceptual analysis. *Filozofia, 71*(3), 220–230.

Kuhn, T. S. (1970). *The structure of scientific revolutions* (2nd ed.). University of Chicago Press.

Kuhn, T. S. (1977). Second thoughts on paradigms. In T. S. Kuhn (Ed.), *The essential tension: Selected studies in scientific tradition and change* (pp. 293–319). University of Chicago Press.

Lambert, N. M., Fincham, F. D., Stillman, T. F., & Dean, L. R. (2009). More gratitude, less materialism: The mediating role of life satisfaction. *The Journal of Positive Psychology, 4*(1), 32–42. https://doi.org/10.1080/17439760802216311

Lazarus, R. (2003). Does the positive psychology movement have legs? *Psychological Inquiry, 14*, 93–109.

Lifshitz, R., Nimrod, G., & Bachner, Y. G. (2019). Spirituality and wellbeing in later life: A multidimensional approach. *Aging & Mental Health, 23*(8), 984–991. https://doi.org/10.1080/13607863.2018.1460743

Lomas, T. (2016). Towards a positive cross-cultural lexicography: Enriching our emotional landscape through 216 'untranslatable' words pertaining to well-being. *The Journal of Positive Psychology, 11*(5), 546–558. https://doi.org/10.1080/17439760.2015.1127993

Lomas, T. (2018). The quiet virtues of sadness: A selective theoretical and interpretative appreciation of its potential contribution to wellbeing. *New Ideas in Psychology, 49*, 18–26. https://doi.org/10.1016/j.newideapsych.2018.01.002

Lomas, T., & Ivtzan, I. (2015). Second wave positive psychology: Exploring the positive-negative dialectics of wellbeing. *Journal of Happiness Studies, 2015*, 1–16. https://doi.org/10.1007/s10902-015-9668-y

Lomas, T., Hefferon, K., & Ivtzan, I. (2015). The LIFE model: A meta-theoretical conceptual map for applied positive psychology. *Journal of Happiness Studies, 16*(5), 1347–1364. https://doi.org/10.1007/s10902-014-9563-y

Lubbe, C., & Eloff, I. (2004). Asset-based assessment in educational psychology: Capturing perceptions during a paradigm shift. *Contemporary School Psychology, 9*, 29–38. https://doi.org/10.1007/BF03340905

Lueddeke, G. (2019). *Survival: One health, one planet, one future*. Routledge. https://doi.org/10.4324/9780429444081

Lyubomirsky, S. (2008). *The how of happiness: A scientific approach to getting the life you want*. Penguin Press.
Madsen, K. B. (1988). *A history of psychology in meta-scientific perspective*. North Holland.
Mahali, A., Lynch, I., Wilson-Fadiji, A., Tolla, T., Khumalo, S., & Naicker, S. (2018). Networks of well-being in the Global South: A critical review of current scholarship. *Journal of Developing Societies, 34*(3), 1–28.
Matondo, J.-P. (2012). Cross-cultural values comparison between Chinese and sub-Saharan Africans. *International Journal of Business and Social Science, 3*, 38–45.
McNulty, J. K., & Fincham, F. D. (2012). Beyond positive psychology? Toward a contextual view of psychological processes and well-being. *American Psychologist, 67*(2), 101–110.
Metz, T. (2016). Confucian harmony from an African perspective. *African and Asian Studies, 15*, 1–22.
Miyamoto, Y., Ma, X., & Wilken, B. (2017). Cultural variation in pro-positive versus balanced systems of emotions. *Current Opinion in Behavioral Sciences, 15*, 27–32. https://doi.org/10.1016/j.cobeha.2017.05.014
Nicolescu, B. (2010). Methodology of transdisciplinarity – Levels of reality, logic of the included middle and complexity. *Transdisciplinary Journal of Engineering & Science, 1*(1), 19–38.
Nicolescu, B. (2014a). Methodology of transdisciplinarity. *World Futures, 70*(3–4), 186–199. https://doi.org/10.1080/02604027.2014.934631
Nicolescu, B. (2014b). *From modernity to cosmodernity: Science, culture, and spirituality*. SUNY Press.
Nicolescu, B. (2015). The hidden third and the multiple splendor of being. In V. Bazhanov & R. W. Scholz (Eds.), *Transdisciplinarity in philosophy and science: Approaches, problems, prospects* (pp. 62–79). Navigator. Retrieved from http://basarab-nicolescu.fr/Docs_articles/TD_in_philosophy_Russia.pdf
Noll, H. H. (2018). Social monitoring and reporting: A success story in applied research on social indicators and quality of life. *Social Indicators Research, 135*(3), 951–964. https://doi.org/10.1007/s11205-016-1513-0
Norem, J. K., & Chang, E. C. (2002). The positive psychology of negative thinking. *Journal of Clinical Psychology, 58*, 993–1001.
Nwoye, A. (2017). An Africentric theory of human personhood. *Psychology in Society, 54*, 42–66.
Nwoye, A. (2018). African psychology and the emergence of the Madiban tradition. *Theory & Psychology, 28*(1), 38–64. https://doi.org/10.1177/0959354317742204
Nyamnjoh, F. B. (2015). Incompleteness: Frontier Africa and the currency of conviviality. *Journal of Asian and African Studies, 47*(2), 129–154. https://doi.org/10.1177/0021909615580867
Nyamnjoh, F. B. (2017). Incompleteness: Frontier Africa and the currency of conviviality. *Journal of Asian and African Studies, 52*(3), 253–270. https://doi.org/10.1177/0021909615580867
O'Doherty, K. C. (2016). Social justice, psychology, and outdated epistemologies: Commentary on Sugarman, Stam, Teo, and Walsh. *Journal of Theoretical and Philosophical Psychology, 35*(2), 135–139. https://doi.org/10.1037/teo0000017
Ogihara, Y., & Uchida, Y. (2014). Does individualism bring happiness? Negative effects of individualism on interpersonal relationships and happiness. *Frontiers in Psychology, 5*, 135. https://doi.org/10.3389/fpsyg.2014.00135
Ohajunwa, C., & Mji, G. (2018). The African indigenous lens of understanding spirituality: Reflection on key emerging concepts from a reviewed literature. *Journal of Religion and Health, 57*, 2523–2537. https://doi.org/10.1007/s10943-018-0652-9
Olikenyi, G. (2001). *African hospitality: A model for the communication of the gospel in the African cultural context*. Steyler Verlag.
Onwuegbuzie, A. J., & Frels, R. (2016). *Seven steps to a comprehensive literature review: A multimodal and cultural approach*. Sage.
Peterson, C., & Seligman, M. E. P. (2004). *Character strengths and virtues: A handbook and classification*. American Psychological Association.
Philips, R., & Wong, C. (2017). *Handbook of community well-being research*. Springer.

Polanyi, M. (1967). *The tacit dimension*. University of Chicago Press.
Prinzing, M. M. (2020). Positive psychology is value-laden—It's time to embrace it. *The Journal of Positive Psychology, 16*(2), 1–9. https://doi.org/10.1080/17439760.2020.1716049
Proctor, C. L. (2019). Virtue ethics in psychotherapy: A systematic review of the literature. *International Journal of Existential Positive Psychology, 8*(1), 1–22.
Rojas, M. (2018). Indicators of people's well-being. *Social Indicators Research, 135*(3), 941–950. https://doi.org/10.1007/s11205-016-1507-y
Ryan, R. M., & Deci, E. L. (2001). On happiness and human potentials: A review of research on hedonic and eudaimonic well-being. *Annual Review of Psychology, 52*(1), 141–166. https://doi.org/10.1146/annurev.psych.52.1.141
Ryff, C. D. (1989). Happiness is everything, or is it? Explorations on the meaning of psychological well-being. *Journal of Personality and Social Psychology, 57*(6), 1069–1081.
Ryff, C. D. (1995). Psychological well-being in adult life. *Current Directions in Psychological Science, 4*(4), 99–104.
Ryff, C. D. (2014). Self-realisation and meaning making in the face of adversity: A eudaimonic approach to human resilience. *Journal of Psychology in Africa, 24*(1), 1–12. https://doi.org/10.1080/14330237.2014.904098
Ryff, C. D., & Singer, B. (1998). The contours of positive human health. *Psychological Inquiry, 9* (1), 1–28.
Schutte, L., Wissing, M. P., & Khumalo, I. P. (2013). Further validation of the Questionnaire for Eudaimonic Well-being (QEWB). *Psychology of Well-being: Theory, Research and Practice, 3* (3), 1–22. Retrieved from http://www.psywb.com/content/3/3
Seligman, M. E. P. (1998). Building human strength: Psychology's forgotten mission. *APA Monitor, 29*(1). Retrieved from http://www.apa.org/monitor/jan98/pres.html
Seligman, M. E. P., & Csikszentmihalyi, M. (2000). Positive psychology: An introduction. *American Psychologist, 55*(1), 5–14.
Seligman, M. E. P., Steen, T. A., Park, N., & Peterson, C. (2005). Positive psychology progress: Empirical validation of interventions. *American Psychologist, 60*(5), 410–421.
Selvam, S. G., & Collicutt, J. (2013). The ubiquity of the character strengths in African traditional religion: A thematic analysis. In H. H. Knoop & A. Delle Fave (Eds.), *Well-being and cultures: A positive psychology perspective* (pp. 83–102). Springer.
Senghor, L. (1970). Negritude: A humanism of twentieth century. In M. Kilson & W. Cartey (Eds.), *The African reader: Independent Africa* (pp. 179–192). Vintage Books.
Sharma, S., & Singh, K. (2019). Religion and well-being: The mediating role of positive virtues. *Journal of Religion and Health, 58*(1), 119–131.
Sheldon, M., & Lyubomirsky, S. (2006). Achieving sustainable gains in happiness: Change your actions, not your circumstances. *Journal of Happiness Studies, 7*, 55–86.
Shiah, Y.-J. (2016). From self to nonself: The nonself theory. *Frontiers in Psychology, 7*, 124. https://doi.org/10.3389/fpsyg.2016.00124
Slife, B. D., O'Grady, K. A., & Kosits, R. D. (2017). *The hidden worldviews of psychology's theory, research, and practice*. Routledge.
Staats, A. W. (1999). Unifying psychology requires new infrastructure, theory, method, and a research agenda. *Review of General Psychology, 3*(1), 3–13. https://doi.org/10.1037//1089-2680.3.1.3
Steger, M. F., Oishi, S., & Kesebir, S. (2011). Is a life without meaning satisfying? The moderating role of the search for meaning in satisfaction with life judgments. *Journal of Positive Psychology, 6*(3), 173–180.
Strümpfer, D. J. W. (1990). Salutogenesis: A new paradigm. *South Africa Journal of Psychology, 20*(4), 265–276.
Strümpfer, D. J. W. (1995). The origins of health and strength: From salutogenesis to fortigenesis. *South Africa Journal of Psychology, 25*(2), 81–89.
Strümpfer, D. J. W. (2005). Standing on the shoulders of giants: Notes on early positive psychology (Psychofortology). *South Africa Journal of Psychology, 35*(1), 21–45.

Strümpfer, D. J. W. & Wissing, M. P. (1998, September). *Review of south African data on the sense of coherence scale as a measure of fortigenesis and salutogenesis*. In Paper presented at the Fourth Annual Congress of the Psychological Society of South Africa.

Sundararajan, L. (2008). Toward a reflexive positive psychology: Insights from the Chinese Buddhist notion of emptiness. *Theory & Psychology, 18*(5), 655–674. https://doi.org/10.1177/0959354308093400

Theron, L. C., & Theron, A. M. C. (2010). A critical review of studies of South African youth resilience, 1990–2008. *South African Journal of Science, 106*(7/8), 252, 8 pages. https://doi.org/10.4102/sajs.v106i7/8.252

Theron, L. C., & Theron, A. M. C. (2014). Meaning-making and resilience: Case studies of a multifaceted process. *Journal of Psychology in Africa, 24*(1), 24–32. https://doi.org/10.1080/14330237.2014.904099

Thin, N. (2014). Positive sociology and appreciative empathy: History and prospects. *Sociological Research Online, 19*(2), 1–14. https://doi.org/10.5153/sro.3230

Thompson, B., Roberts, S. G., & Lupyan, G. (2020). Cultural influences on word meanings revealed through large-scale semantic alignment. *Nature Human Behaviour, 4*, 1029–1038. https://doi.org/10.1038/s41562-020-0924-8

Uchida, Y. (2011). A holistic view of happiness: Belief in the negative side of happiness is more prevalent in Japan than in the United States. *Psychologia, 53*(4), 236–245.

Uchida, Y., & Ogihara, Y. (2012). Personal or interpersonal construal of happiness: A cultural psychological perspective. *International Journal of Wellbeing, 2*(4), 354–369. https://doi.org/10.5502/ijw.v2.i4.5

Ungar, M. (Ed.). (2012). *The social ecology of resilience*. Springer.

Urata, Y. (2015). A psychological model to determine meaning in life and meaning of life. In M. Morioka (Ed.), *Reconsidering meaning in life: A philosophical dialogue with Thaddeus Metz* (pp. 215–227). Waseda University.

Van Cappellen, P., Fredrickson, B. L., Saroglou, V., & Corneille, O. (2017). Religiosity and the motivation for social affiliation. *Personality and Individual Differences, 113*, 24–31. https://doi.org/10.1016/j.paid.2017.02.065

Veenhoven, R. (2018). Subjective well-being in nations. In E. Diener, S. Oishi, & L. Tay (Eds.), *Handbook of well-being*. DEF Publishers.

Villani, D., Sorgente, A., Iannello, P., & Antonietti, A. (2019). The role of spirituality and religiosity in subjective well-being of individuals with different religious status. *Frontiers in Psychology, 10*, 1525. https://doi.org/10.3389/fpsyg.2019.01525

Warren, M. A., & Donaldson, S. I. (2018). *Toward a positive psychology of relationships: New directions in theory and research*. Praeger.

Waterman, A. S. (2013a). The humanistic psychology–positive psychology divide contrasts in philosophical foundations. *American Psychologist, 68*(3), 124–133. https://doi.org/10.1037/a0032168

Waterman, A. S. (Ed.). (2013b). *The best within us: Positive psychology perspectives on eudaimonic functioning*. American Psychological Association.

White, S. C., & Jha, S. (2014). The ethical imperative of qualitative methods: Developing measures of subjective dimensions of well-being in Zambia and India. *Ethics and Social Welfare, 8*(3), 262–276. https://doi.org/10.1080/17496535.2014.932416

Wilson, A., Wissing, M. P., Ndima, L., & Somhlaba, N. Z. (2018). Representations of hope, goals, and meaning from lay person's perspectives in two African contexts. *Journal of Humanistic Psychology, 61*, 1–23. https://doi.org/10.1177/0022167818785070

Wilson-Fadiji, A., & Wissing, M. P. (2021). Positive psychology in sub-Saharan Africa. In E. C. Chang, C. A. Downey, H. Yang, I. Zettler, & M. Muyan (Eds.), *The international handbook of positive psychology: A global perspective on the science of positive human existence*. Springer.

Wissing, M. P. (Ed.). (2013). *Well-being research in South Africa. In A. Delle Fave (Series Ed.), Cross-cultural advancements in positive psychology (Vol. 4)*. Springer.

Wissing, M. P. (2018, April 4–7). *Embracing well-being in diverse contexts: The third wave of positive psychology*. In Invited address at the First Africa Positive Psychology Conference, Potchefstroom, South Africa.

Wissing, M. P., & Temane, Q. M. (2008). The structure of psychological well-being in cultural context: Towards a hierarchical model of psychological health. *Journal of Psychology in Africa, 18*(1), 45–55. https://doi.org/10.1080/14330237.2008.10820170

Wissing, M. P., & Van Eeden, C. (1997). Psychological well-being: A fortigenic conceptualisation and empirical clarification. In *Paper was presented at the 3rd Annual Congress of the Psychological Society of South Africa*, Durban, South Africa.

Wissing, M. P., & Van Eeden, C. (2002). Empirical clarification of the nature of psychological well-being. *South Africa Journal of Psychology, 32*(1), 32–44. https://doi.org/10.1177/008124630203200105

Wissing, J. A. B., Wissing, M. P., Du Toit, M. M., & Temane, Q. M. (2008). Psychometric properties of various scales measuring psychological well-being in a South African context: The FORT 1 Project. *Journal of Psychology in Africa, 18*(4), 511–520.

Wissing, M. P., Schutte, L., & Liversage, C. (2018, June 27–30). *Thought developments in positive psychology: The third wave and post-disciplinary move*. In Paper at the 9th European Conference on Positive Psychology, Budapest, Hungary.

Wissing, M. P., Schutte, L., & Wilson-Fadiji, A. (2019). Cultures of positivity: Interconnectedness as a way of being. In I. Eloff (Ed.), *Handbook of quality of life in African societies* (International handbooks of quality of life). Springer. https://doi.org/10.1007/978-3-030-15367

Wissing, M. P., Potgieter, J., Guse, T., Khumalo, T., & Nel, L. (Eds.). (2020). *Towards flourishing: Embracing Well-being in diverse contexts* (2nd ed.). Van Schaik.

Wong, P. T. P. (2011). Positive psychology 2.0: Towards a balanced interactive model of the good life. *Canadian Psychology, 52*(2), 69–81. https://doi.org/10.1037/a0022511

Wong, P. T. P. (2012). Toward a dual-systems model of what makes life worth living. In P. T. P. Wong (Ed.), *The human quest for meaning: Theories, research, and applications* (pp. 3–22). Taylor & Francis.

Chapter 2
Well-Being in Africa: Towards an Africa(n) Centred Positive Psychology

Angelina Wilson Fadiji, Itumeleng P. Khumalo, and Ncamisile Thumile Zulu

Abstract Psychology is concerned with human behaviour, therefore all psychologies are contextually-embedded and culturally informed. A movement towards globalising psychology would invariably diminish the localised socio-cultural situatedness of psychology, and instead seek to advance a dominant Euro-American centred psychology even in regions where such applications do not fit. The emergence of strong voices, and theoretically grounded and empirically supported positions from the global South in general and sub-Saharan Africa in particular, in studies of well-being allows for the opportunity to explore and describe an Africa (n) centred positive psychology. Acknowledging the limitations of cross-cultural psychological approaches, which have encouraged the uncritical transportation of Euro-American centred concepts and values, in this chapter we utilise assumptions from critical, cultural and African psychology to present our initial thoughts about a culturally embedded, socially relevant and responsive, and context respecting Africa (n) centred positive psychology. This challenge warrants consideration of early contributions to the study of well-being, its current data-driven positivist tendency, as well as African worldviews grounded in interdependence, collectivism, relatedness, harmony with nature, and spirituality. For an Africa(n) centred positive psychology, it is also essential to consider questions of epistemology, ways of knowing about the world and the human condition, context respecting knowledge, and theory building. Drawing on current scholarly evidence in sub-Saharan Africa, which emphasises relationality and societal values and norms shaping experiences of

A. Wilson Fadiji (✉)
Department of Educational Psychology, Faculty of Education, University of Pretoria, Pretoria, South Africa

Africa Unit for Transdisciplinary Health Research, Faculty of Health Sciences, North West University, Potchefstroom, South Africa

I. P. Khumalo
Department of Psychology, University of the Free State, Bloemfontein, South Africa

N. T. Zulu
University of KwaZulu-Natal, Durban, South Africa

L. Schutte et al. (eds.), *Embracing Well-Being in Diverse African Contexts: Research Perspectives*, Cross-Cultural Advancements in Positive Psychology 16,
https://doi.org/10.1007/978-3-030-85924-4_2

well-being, we propose future directions and discuss implications for empirical research and theory building within positive psychology which seeks to centre Africa and African experiences.

Keywords Well-being · African-centred · Positive psychology · Critical and African psychology

2.1 Introduction: Well-Being as Contextually and Culturally-Embedded

At the heart of the discipline of positive psychology is the need to explore, understand, and promote positive experiences and well-being (Seligman & Csikszentmihalyi, 2000). Established theoretical assumptions of well-being have distinguished between hedonic and eudaimonic well-being (Disabato et al., 2016; Ryan & Deci, 2001). Hedonic well-being, operationalised as subjective well-being, is expressed through the experience of positive affect, absence of negative affect and satisfactory evaluation of life (Diener, 2009; Diener et al., 2018). Notwithstanding the current lack of consensus on definitions of well-being (White, 2010). Waterman (2008, p. 236) concluded that Eudaimonia "includes a constellation of subjective experiences including feelings of rightness and centredness in one's actions, identity, strength of purpose, and competence". Eudaimonic well-being is related to the experience of personal growth, meaning and purpose in life (Diener et al., 2018).

The move towards the study of positive experiences served to introduce the positive psychology movement, partly in response to the earlier eminent focus on the prevention and treatment of psychological disorders (Seligman & Csikszentmihalyi, 2000). The current positive psychology body of knowledge is largely rooted in mainstream North American social psychology (Marecek & Christopher, 2018). Except for some pockets of excellence, especially in South Africa (see Eloff et al., 2008; Wilson Fadiji & Wissing, 2021), there is minimal evidence from other parts of Africa of efforts to develop ways of assessing subjective dimensions of well-being, which reflect the values and ideals of local people (Mahali et al., 2018). The argument for the need for more research reflecting local ideals is underscored in Clark (2003) who describes how ordinary people in rural and urban South Africa view human well-being based on the physical and social conditions they live in. Woodcock et al. (2008) highlighted that subjective quality of life should be conceived as "the outcome of the gap between people's goals and perceived resources in the context of their culture, values, and experiences of un/happiness" (p. 137).

White et al. (2016) observed the need to focus on what people feel and think they can be and do in the conceptualisation of well-being. This observation seems to support the notion of a bottom-up process of theory building informed by the views and experiences of those whom the knowledge is about. Further support for the need for well-being to reflect the ideals of the local people comes with research among children in Zambia that experienced relatively high levels of subjective well-being compared to Canadian counterparts despite their low-income status (Holder et al., 2016). In Nigeria, Agbo and Ome (2017) found that conceptions of happiness were centred on the self as compared to relational perspectives that were expected from communal/collectivistic contexts such as Africa. This finding was indicative of the multi-ethnic nature of Nigeria, and inherent intra-national differences in cultural beliefs and practices (Agbo & Ome, 2017). In other words, among this group in Nigeria, happiness was expressed as an independent self-construal (exemplified by the need for freedom, choice, creativity, and self-reliance), instead of the expected interdependent interpersonal self-construal, overlapping with collectivism (Agbo & Ome, 2017).

Perhaps as some may have argued that positive psychology is culture-bound (Marecek & Christopher, 2018), the same could be said for psychological measurement as it taps on participants' lived experiences (Lenz et al., 2018). From cross-cultural studies, it is known that not only is item content subject to cross-cultural variation, but response styles are also culture-dependent (Benítez et al., 2016) and influenced by cognitive ability associated with educational attainment (He & Van de Vijver, 2016). An example of this could be illustrated in the fact that although positive emotions are ubiquitous, it is in how and when they are experienced that cross-cultural variations emerge (Kitayama et al., 2000). This limitation becomes especially problematic in contexts where there is limited access to assessment tools for a particular culture. Working in Botswana, Chilisa and Tsheko (2014) advocate for mixed methods research approaches as being more adept to engaging with data and generating knowledge respecting of indigenous communities in Africa.

The universal conceptualisation and experience of positive psychology constructs can be adequately uncovered when consideration is given to the limitations of existing theories, empirical findings and assessment tools (see Hardin et al., 2014). The study of human behaviour including well-being are contextually-embedded and culturally informed (Christopher & Hickinbottom, 2008; Marecek & Christopher, 2018). Thus, the proposal of an Africa(n) centred positive psychology, also calls on the reconsideration of the attempt to universalise the Euro-American centric perspectives of experiences and understanding of well-being. However, our consideration of and proposal of an Africa(n) centred positive psychology does not serve as a reaction to global trends, rather it seeks to add to the existing body of knowledge. In doing this, we seek to make a case for what, how and why of (psychological) well-being studies which would centre Africa in their inquiry. An apt observation is made by Møller and Roberts (2017, pp. 161–162) that the "first written records on sub-Saharan well-being saw Africa through the lens of outsiders... who produced assessments... from their points of view".

2.2 Limitations of Cross-Cultural Psychology

In this chapter, while echoing voices on the need for contextually-embedded approaches to the study of well-being, we highlight the limitations of cross-cultural psychology as an approach to understanding well-being. Not only do we foreground cultural psychology studies, but we also illuminate the ontological and epistemological positions informed by a way of being in the world from an Africa(n) centred view (see Ratele, 2019). Although cross-cultural psychology studies have dominated the research approach to understanding well-being across groups, cultures, and nations; its limitations have been highlighted by Ellis and Stam (2015), among others. Ellis and Stam (2015) make a case for cultural psychology as a better way understanding individuals within their sociocultural context. There is an argument that cross-cultural psychology may be "perpetuating an individualist and Westernized psychology that ultimately adopts a veneer of culture but leaves deeper cultural questions outside of psychological research" (Ellis & Stam, 2015, p. 294). On the other hand, cultural psychologists oppose individualist assumptions that regard individuals separately from others and from the social and natural world. Notwithstanding such views from outside cross-cultural psychology, a prominent cross-cultural psychologist David Matsumoto (Matsumoto & Yoo, 2006) has traced the history of the field, and showed limitations of inter-group comparisons, and propagated for the advancements in the field.

In an attempt to make conceptualisations of well-being in the West more applicable to other cultures outside the West, there has been a wave of cross-cultural well-being research. Notable works include Cheng et al. (2011) exploring cultural models of independence, interdependence, conflict and integration among individualistic and collectivist countries in relation to subjective well-being, arguing that the sources of well-being may differ in strength among individuals due to distinct norms and values. In the sub-Saharan African region, there were mixed results regarding which models were applicable with the interdependency model being more applicable within this region. In the interdependency model, the major source of subjective well-being was the welfare of the group (Cheng et al., 2011; Uchida et al., 2004). The mixed results showed that it is not enough to do cross-cultural comparisons without the deep exploration of how existing norms and values manifest themselves in the experiences of well-being.

Further attempts at being context-specific in doing well-being research (through cross-cultural studies) showed that in non-western contexts with a higher Human Development Index (measure of average achievement in key dimensions of human development; HDI), generalised trust was strongly related to indices of health, well-being and health behaviours (Chan et al., 2017). Although the study took place in countries described mostly as collectivist (China, Ghana, India, and South Africa), the study showed that levels of socio-economic development were important in understanding the predictors of well-being. Indeed, the findings support the assumption of the moderating effect of HDI on the link between generalized trust and health, demonstrating that the likely health benefits of generalized trust might be stronger in more developed countries than less developed countries (Hamamura et al., 2017). A lesson drawn from this finding is that although the importance of HDI re-echoes findings from the West, it also shows that collectivist values that should foster trust might be hindered if the socio-economic context is not adequately considered in research and policy.

The preponderance of cross-cultural psychology work in well-being is not met with proportionate attention towards collating and consolidating empirical research in Africa. In essence, the ubiquity of research in the African context is not adequately grounded and synthesised with the aim of theory formulation and testing. In an analysis of American journals of psychology, Arnett (2008) and Webster et al. (2009) observed and concluded that publications in these journals reflect a neglect of the majority of the world, yet generalise their findings to the world, in what Webster et al. (2009) term American psychology becoming international. Similarly, with reference to positive psychology, Mahali et al. (2018) recognise the critique directed at the current conceptualisations of well-being, particularly for neglecting the role of cultural context, with most of the scholarship being generated in the global North. The idea that Euro-American notions of well-being frameworks and findings from empirical studies can be uncritically transported to the majority world disregards the fundamental differences in life circumstances and way of being (Mahali et al., 2018). Thus, the necessity for an Africa(n) centred positive psychology emerges. This emergence does not occur from a place of deficit or lack, nor does it become necessary because Africa is some exotic location. This need is apparent for the purpose of psychology's responsibility to centre Africa, the African, and her experience when considering the question of well-being from here.

Besides, in most cross-cultural psychology work, there is the tendency to make a conclusion regarding well-being in Africa by including one or two countries from the continent and several from the West (see Schimmack et al., 2002; Tamir et al., 2016). This means that the finding might be true of some African contexts but is not necessarily reflective of other African settings. This limitation is further compounded by the use of quantitative comparative tools of investigation rather than in-depth exploration in unearthing patterns and manifestations of well-being. This is because these studies are designed to confirm or disconfirm a-priori theories and do not leave much room for alternative ideas (Henrich et al., 2010). In the next section, we highlight three of the four "African psychologies" (psychology in Africa, critical, cultural African psychology, and psychological African Studies) towards contextually-relevant research in Africa. This discussion postulates the propositions we have about what Africa(n) centred positive psychology may look like. We then move on to discuss notable well-being research on the continent.

2.3 (Positive) Psychology in Africa, Critical (Positive) Psychology, Cultural (Positive) Psychology, and (Positive) Psychological African Studies

Using Ratele's (2016, 2017) framework for the idea and discipline of "African psychology", we explore how three of the four African psychologies are reflected in the current theoretical and empirical positive psychology research, so as to chart the way toward an Africa(n)-centred positive psychology. It is worth noting that the question of a situated and context respecting (positive) psychology is not new, nor is it unique to Africa (Ratele, 2016). In other settings (place of location and period in time), we have seen other scholars in the global South position and advocate for a psychology with relevance for their societies. Wong (2016), for example, has advocated for a Chinese Positive Psychology (CPP), which "calls for research programs that meet the needs of the Chinese people in their unique cultural and political context" (p. 1). In a related area of adolescence research, Raffaelli et al. (2013) recognise the injustice of Western-based research while 90% of the youth on earth live in the majority world. Back in Africa, the study by Mahali et al. (2018) makes the case for a global South oriented research interest; while Møller and Roberts (2017) dug up in the archives to explain well-being from the ancient roots of the African people. Nevertheless, the four African psychologies proposed by Ratele (2016, 2017) are Psychology in Africa, cultural African psychology, critical African psychology, and psychological African Studies.

First, we consider African psychology as "Psychology in Africa". The underlying assumption in this framework is that the discipline of psychology is universal and should be objective and value-free. It entails taking questions asked elsewhere and exploring it in Africa (Ratele, 2017). A major criticism raised against this orientation is that Africa is considered merely as a setting for questions and theories generated elsewhere to be tested rather than a critical outlook on human behaviour in this context. Much of positive psychology and well-being can be regarded as Psychology in Africa and for it to be more African-centred, well-being research must exist within prevailing political, social and economic realities while reformulating existing theories using a bottom-up approach. A noteworthy contribution in moving from research as "Psychology in Africa" within well-being is the work of White (2017), the author argued strongly to move away from current theorising on well-being when studying the African context and taking cognisance of the social and cultural milieu that affects an individual's experiences. Important to well-being from research conducted by White (2017) is the consideration of relational, material and subjective dimensions of well-being.

Second, cultural African psychology refers to prioritising the metaphysical, spiritual or cultural. This psychology is what Nwoye (2015), and others such as Edwards (2014) and Mkabela (2015), are talking about when articulating the notion of African psychology. Psychology is centred on the need to understand shared African language, values, beliefs and worldviews. Cultural African psychology attempts to resist cultural domination emerging from Western ideas and reaffirming the legitimacy of blackness (Ratele, 2017). Although useful, this orientation exalts some form of exceptionalism of the African culture. The advantage of this orientation for doing African-centred positive psychology is that culture is a lens that is constantly used to theorise and explain findings. In addition, the context in which such knowledge is generated is put at the forefront. An argument for African cultural psychology is evident in the work of Mahali et al. (2018) highlighting that understanding well-being in the global South (which includes Africa) must emerge from a relational perspective since relationships lie at the heart of the experience of well-being.

Third, Critical African psychology, goes beyond culture to focus on historical and modern contestations around culture (Painter et al., 2013). It aims for decolonising psychology and is to a large extent political in its agenda. Being critical also involves seeking social justice and emancipation while ensuring that we do perpetuate oppression and injustice. This is primarily achieved by an alertness to the circumstances of individuals by acknowledging their social or systemic context and without upholding the organisational status quo (Worth & Smith, 2017). Mkhize (2004) noted that critical African psychology should include research that furthers the needs of developing societies such as poverty, illiteracy and alienation. If African-centred positive psychology is to be critical, some hurdles will need to be overcome, including theorising and engaging in empirical work that considers the influence of political and economic power on psychological processes. Ratele (2017) argued that experts in psychology might need to combine more than one orientation in attempting to do African psychology. The boundaries of the different orientations are permeable and could serve as a way forward for African-centred positive psychology. In the next section, we review some empirical work permeating all the orientations but mostly as "Psychology in Africa".

Fourth, we consider psychological African studies. We begin this section with a caveat by acknowledging the complexity and perhaps the premature nature of the proposal of psychological African studies, to which Ratele (2019, p. 164) concedes to "not yet exist as a coherent enterprise". Nevertheless, this would be a transdisciplinary movement, finding expression in the linkages among disciplines, and concerned with the employment of tools from psychology to study Africa. Similarly, from a positive psychology perspective, we pose more questions, which the field should concern itself with. The first, which is central to the emergence of a field, is that when African psychology is "situated in practice" (Ratele, 2019, p. 151), what ought the positive psychology lens from here allow us to see and explore in the African condition? Typically, the consideration of well-being and quality of life should be extended to issues of peace, gender, use of space and time, as well as politics and the economy. Already, the subject of peace in Africa is a theme in the latest positive psychology teaching textbook by Wissing et al. (2020). Last, the possibility of (positive) psychological African studies challenges us to ask the question of how the theoretical resources and tools of positive psychology may be appropriated to study Africa. The inverse question of how knowledge found in African philosophy, literature, and history, among others, may be used to inform well-being promotion here and in other parts of the world, also becomes apparent.

2.4 Well-Being Research in Africa

Conceptualisations of well-being could be said to have been a concern in recent well-being research in Africa. In a systematic review of well-being research among young people in South Africa, there was a lack of consensus on the definition of well-being partly because of the tendency to treat this construct as unidimensional rather than considering its multifaceted nature (Govender et al., 2019). Common among the studies reviewed was the shift towards a strengths and assets-based approach from the approach to well-being as the absence of mental disorders. However, there was inconsistency in the measurement tools employed, most of these been developed and imported from the West without necessary adaption. A further limitation with current well-being research is the minimal use of qualitative research approaches aimed at providing bottom-up perspectives on the construct (Govender et al., 2019).

In addressing the lack and importance of qualitative approaches in explaining well-being, Wilson Fadiji et al. (2019) found that based on data from employed adults in Ghana, theoretical distinctions between eudaimonia and hedonia could not be ascertained. Moreover, conceptualisations of well-being extended beyond traditional psychological notions to include material and relational dimensions. These material dimensions include health status and household finances (Ngamaba, 2016). The intertwined nature of these dimensions points to the essence of a holistic exploration of well-being as well as the need for more in-depth studies.

A study conducted among Igbos of Eastern Nigeria revealed that some Nigerians defined happiness with words reflecting both emotion and cognitive assessment of life. Words pointing to positive emotions were predominant followed by words reflecting subjective assessment of satisfaction with life (Agbo & Ome, 2017). Interestingly, participants were more likely to look inwards when defining happiness. This is conflicting with suggestions in the literature that indicate that non-Western societies view happiness from communalistic perspectives.

Recent researches have attempted to test existing theoretical notions of well-being. Emerging evidence points to the interdependent nature of happiness and meaning among Ghanaians. In determining notions of a good life, Dzokoto et al. (2019) noted that work-related meaning and happiness were intertwined among individuals scoring high on well-being. Similar findings come with Wilson Fadiji et al. (2019) where qualitative responses to conceptualisations of well-being reflected that meaning and happiness could not be clearly distinguished. The findings suggest that while some factors may consistently predict the good life across diverse cultural settings, adequate consideration of culturally-constructed meaning and well-being systems, in general, is needed.

There has been extant empirical work on well-being that we can categorise as Psychology in Africa (see Ratele, 2017). This existing body of work has capitalised on western measurement instruments and accompanying theories as a basis for well-being research in Africa. For instance, the question of the predictors of hedonic and eudaimonic well-being has been explored, these theoretical dimensions being grounded in western models of thought. Evidence from South Africa and Ghana has shown that several contextual variables do emerge as important predictors of hedonic well-being (Guse et al., 2019; Wilson & Somhlaba, 2017). Guse et al. (2019) intimated that female South African adolescents had higher levels of satisfaction with school, self, and friends. A divergent view emerged among male adolescents in Ghana who had higher levels of emotional well-being whereas females did better on hope. Of noteworthy, is the finding on females doing better on eudaimonic well-being (Wilson & Somhlaba, 2017). In a multivariate analysis among older adults in South Africa, wealth, status, health, activity limitation, race and age were significantly associated with happiness among men and women (Chirinda & Phaswana-Mafuya, 2019) with higher levels of happiness among men. In line with these findings, further evidence demonstrated the ability to plan financial futures and having sustainable income sources as important predictors of happiness in South Africa (Van Aardt et al., 2019). The findings on gender and age differences reinforce the need to consider how the context influences well-being. In the case of older South African females, it is possible that lowered happiness was due to socio-economic limitations and other forms of disempowerment that might culturally-driven (Chirinda & Phaswana-Mafuya, 2019).

Intrinsic life goals of adolescents have also been explored as a background characteristic predicting well-being. Among adolescents in South Africa, a sense of community (as a life goal) predicted positive affect (Davids et al., 2017). This finding differed from previous studies that indicated that adolescents from less affluent backgrounds aspired for extrinsic goals (Brdar et al., 2009; Davids & Roman, 2013). However, Brdar et al. (2009) argued that it is not just about what an individual aspires for but the reasons for those aspirations. Moreover, the intrinsic life goals of a sense of community are linked to the collectivist nature of most South African communities. Similar to background characteristics of collectivism and contextual variables, Wilson and Somhlaba (2017) argued that self-reports of psychological well-being needs to be understood in the context of socio-developmental variables. In South Africa, the debilitating effects of apartheid had rippled effects on the psychological well-being of young South African adults because the early years of child development did not provide an environment for healthy development (Savahl et al., 2015).

A number of themes have dominated well-being research in Africa; we will discuss some prominent ones in the following paragraphs. Salient in well-being research is the notion of spirituality. Western research has classified spirituality as one of the characters strengths (Park et al., 2006). Spirituality also predicts the experience of meaning in life (Steger et al., 2008). Spirituality has been explored in several African contexts. For instance, Temane and Wissing (2006) tested the mediated role of spirituality in the relationship between context and psychological well-being, their findings indicated that in the Mafikeng group, the variance explained for hedonic well-being was greater than among the Potchefstroom group. This is because the Mafikeng group comprised of black South Africans who tend to place greater value on spirituality.

Other studies in South Africa have pointed to the salient role that spirituality plays in psychological well-being (Nell, 2014; Wissing et al., 2014). Spirituality fosters a sense of identity, purpose and vertical connectedness. Moreover, spirituality is important for well-being in this context because of the interconnected worldview that affects the different spheres of life.

To further illustrate on the importance of spirituality, Wilson et al. (2018) highlighted that harmony and a sense of identity through connections with divinity shape relational well-being among older adults in rural parts of South Africa. Related to this, spirituality was identified as both a source of hope for Ghanaian adolescents but also a source of meaning linked to goals among South Africans (Wilson et al., 2018). Spirituality provides a source of support and a sense of belonging with a larger group as well as with divine forces beyond the individual (Wilson & Somhlaba, 2016). On hedonic well-being, spirituality and religiosity are linked to the experience of life satisfaction among Ghanaians (Addai et al., 2014).

Closely tied to spirituality, relationships and social bonds have formed an important topic of exploration. In Rwanda, the importance of friends, weekly religious attendance, and national pride positively predicted happiness (Ngamaba, 2016). The main reference for natural and cultural property is not a single individual, but the community as a whole. Members of indigenous communities promote harmonious relationships through principles of equality and respect for all, particularly women and elders given that they are the main source of traditional knowledge (Magni, 2017). Emphasising the importance of relationships, previous studies on the notions of a good life point to social status and ability to command respect. However, these were embedded in the need to maintain social connections and provide for the need of younger generations (van der Geest, 1998).

In the attempt to further understand well-being in other contexts outside the West, values as a precedent for emotions have been explored. Values are argued to be the way we want to experience life, while emotions are our actual experiences. In African contexts such as Ghana, values of transcendence were related to empathy and compassion while in more western samples, when values of self-enhancement were highly endorsed, it was linked to emotions of pride and anger (Tamir et al., 2016). Tamir et al. (2016) argued that endorsement of values was associated with a stronger need for emotional expressions that embody value consistent themes. For instance, in collectivist contexts, the more individuals endorsed self-transcendent values such as caring, the more they desired to experience relational emotions of love. This study showed that cultures have the potential to evoke different sets of emotions that are in congruence with desired values and beliefs.

A major critique of well-being research in Africa is the use of tools from the West without determining its ecological validity (Wilson Fadiji et al., 2019). In order to address this limitation, a number of studies have tested the validity of measures developed in the West. Recent among them include the Satisfaction with Life Scale (Lenz et al., 2018; Wilson Fadiji et al., 2019); Mental Health Continuum-Short Form (Schutte & Wissing, 2017), multidimensional perceived social support scale (Wilson et al., 2017), Personal Well-being Index (Żemojtel-Piotrowska et al., 2017) and meaning in life scale (Temane et al., 2014). Compared to the validation of instruments, evidence on tools generated in Africa for well-being assessment is almost non-existent. A reflection of the current state of affairs for well-being research in

Africa requires that scholars begin to think and make strides towards a more relevant positive psychology.

2.5 The Way Forward for an African-Centred Positive Psychology

White's (2010) definition of well-being resonates with the Africa(n) centred positive psychology in that it offers well-being to be a *social process* with material, relational and subjective dimensions. Similarly, King et al. (2014), in demonstrating the evolution of the concept of well-being, position it as an ecologically embedded concept which is multidimensional, dynamic, person-specific, and culture-specific. Dovetailing with the ideas of ecologically embedded well-being, and well-being as a social process, is the concept of contextualism proposed and tested in 37 countries by Owe et al. (2013). Contextualism, which is an important part of cultural collectivism, refers to the importance of contexts to understand people. It includes reference to contextual and relational features in how people describe and explain themselves (Owe et al., 2013). The features of contextualism comprise social and relational contexts such as family, social groups, social positions and physical environments. This orientation does not mean that an individual is understood as a de-traited (disregard of disposition) being, but rather that they believe that their context also forms part of the core of their being (Owe et al., 2013). As a natural extension of their description of content and location of well-being, King et al. (2014) propose that there be appropriate methodological approaches to assess well-being in socioecological contexts. An example would be the mixed methods approaches advocated for by Chilisa and Tsheko (2014), which are more adept to engaging with generating knowledge of indigenous communities in Africa.

Before we can begin the way forward towards generating ideas on African-centred positive psychology, there is a need to engage with the questions scholars such as Ratele have raised on the roots of African psychology. Ratele (2017) suggests engaging with what African psychology is and what kinds of scholarly formulations can be regarded as such. Nwoye (2015) put forward that there is a need to delineate African psychology as work from, for, and within African countries, suggesting a separation from work done by other African American scholars outside the continent. Within the field of positive psychology, one would wonder whether such a distinction would be useful. According to Nwoye, "African psychology can be taken to refer to the systematic and informed study of the complexities of human mental life, culture and experience in the pre- and post-colonial African world" (Nwoye, 2015, p. 104), which Ratele (2017) argues only forms part of his thoughts on African Psychology.

The Africentric paradigm according to Nwoye (2015) is built on the assumption that visible and invisible worlds greatly affect each other and are intertwined. The core argument is that western psychology is prone to defining a person only in terms of body and behaviour and in some instances does not account for the role of spirituality in human well-being. In this paradigm, there is also the need to consider meanings attached to "what is" rather than accepting reality without questioning (Nwoye, 2015).

Macleod (2018) suggests that an important way forward in ensuring African-centred psychology is by engaging in research and literature collation of the theoretical, empirical and epistemological knowledge generated within South Africa and other Global Southern contexts. This is because a grounded praxis of integrating knowledge around well-being will allow for new insights and the transference of knowledge that is generated in context. The consolidation process must involve grounded techniques of research to generate texts based on Global Southern research with work done in the Global North being minimal (Macleod, 2018).

In a sense, what we are calling for is the need to "go back" to existing work not only in the form of systematic reviews but generating conceptual knowledge on well-being that can inform theoretical work both on the continent and beyond. This approach is necessary because critical scholarship should not only challenge the status quo in a project of deconstruction but also reconstruction and construction by attempting to contest power and produce social change through effective interventions (Teo, 1999).

In a relatively old study, Neff and Olsen (2007) argue against a utilitarian inquiry into subjective well-being research. A critical-realist perspective that avoids a mix up between data and reality is suggested. Specifically, instead of relying on the numbers being used in a theoretical vacuum, a method of triangulation with rich qualitative analysis will unearth both the subjective and objective dimensions of well-being. In exploring happiness, it is important to find out what the dimensions of happiness are in each milieu, with reference to specific dimensions of life, and to integrate that knowledge into policy. This is because individual persons are always in dynamic interaction with institutions, norms, cultures and structures that can be adequately studied using a depth ontology that views human existence as multi-layered (Neff & Olsen, 2007). Well-being can be fully explored only when the subjectivity and reflexivity of both the respondent and researcher are combined.

In addition to consolidation and engaging in a qualitative enquiry into well-being, well-being research in Africa must begin to move towards theorising and testing these theories. The consolidation and integration of existing work on various aspects of well-being should move to a point where theories of well-being can be tested and evaluated using quantitative data. Such theories can also inform the adaptation and creation of instruments.

Moving from theory testing, Prilleltensky (2017) argued for the need to interrogate the interiorisation of well-being in empirical research and practice. From a critical psychology standpoint, positive psychology is noted as tending to locate the source, signs and strategies of well-being in the individual. This notion builds on the work of Davies (2015) that indicates that positive psychology as a science runs the risk of blaming individuals for their misery and giving less attention to the context that has contributed to it. This oversight has epistemic, moral and political consequences. A proper understanding of well-being is hindered when we do not take into account the cultural and environmental landscape surrounding the experience of well-being. Morally speaking, this leads to a case of victim-blaming of individuals for their lack or experience of low well-being (Prilleltensky, 2017).

Furthermore, Prilleltensky (2017) argues for a redefinition of wellness that bridges the gap between critical perspectives and positive psychology. In the context of research on well-being in Africa, a redefinition of well-being, we recommend, will tap into scholarly work on the good life and quality of life. Such definitions are likely to include the supply of material goods to maintain social connections and respect. It could also include the experience of harmony at different levels-intrapersonal and interpersonal. Such connectedness will be both horizontal and vertical with each having differing influences on the individual's experience of well-being. The idea of fairness in relationships, at work, school and in community (Biglan, 2015; Marmot, 2015) as a definition of well-being may also hold some relevance for this context. Although it is not an easy answer as one would ask "what would you call fair", it still holds promise because it considers environmental, social and political players in the creation and experience of well-being.

In critical positive psychology, some researchers have questioned positivistic orientations in establishing knowledge (Hefferon et al., 2017) noting that science is not founded only on quantitatively-based research. As a way forward for African-centred positive psychology, there is the need to incorporate more qualitative and participatory methods, which offer insights into specific groups and allow for transformative change. The social constructions of our understandings of well-being will offer deeper and relevant insights necessary for social change (Chamberlain & Murray, 2009). In doing this, there is also the need not to forget that a balance is needed in complimenting qualitative strategies of enquiries with numerical methods that tell us the extent of a certain occurrence and the nature and experience of such occurrences.

2.6 Concluding Remarks

In concluding, we postulate that an Africa(n) centred positive psychology ought to not only centre the African and her experience of being in the world, as an object (i.e., the researched), but also as an active subject (i.e., the knower and inquirer) participating in well-being knowledge generation. The pluralistic nature of this research also means that the location and direction of the lens through which well-being is examined is multifocal. It ought to simultaneously embrace a view of culture as having many forms and a variety of textures and contours (see Cohen, 1999).

This chapter highlights the intertwined thread which binds people's experiences, the intellectual traditions of critical (positive) psychology, and bottom-up cultural psychology methodologies in the context informed and culture respecting well-being frameworks. We are of the school of thought that cross-cultural work is not adequate for deeply exploring well-being in context. There are social, political, economic and historical factors that must all be considered as we rethink this move towards an

African-centred positive psychology. In a nutshell, what would an African-centred positive psychology look like? This outlook on positive psychology will be critical, theory-driven, empirically supported with appropriate tools of research while taking into cognisance the social and political milieu in which well-being is experienced. Forward-looking, we argue for an African-centred positive psychology that considers meanings attached to an experience rather than accepting established epistemologies on face-value. Building on this is the integration of existing knowledge to enable us to move on to uncovering meta-theoretical underpinnings of well-being experiences in context. The next steps can include critical-realist approaches to knowledge generation that locates the source and strategies both in the individual and beyond. All of these pointers require a great deal of conscious effort and will be no small feat; however, raising the awareness of the need for African cultural models of well-being will allow current scholars to go beyond confirming Western theories to exploring divergent views and consolidating these into broader parsimonious frameworks for explaining human behaviour. We are in no way suggesting that no strides have been made in the study of well-being in Africa. Wilson Fadiji and Wissing (2021) acknowledge the late development of positive psychology in Africa, as much as they show the depth of its development and influence. It may, however, be observed in their continental review, that most of the studies conducted here are situated in what Ratele (2017, p. 313) refers to "Psychology *in* Africa". As tempting as it may be to not water-down our proposal for a trajectory towards an Africa (n) centred positive psychology, the following qualifier is important for the future development of the field/ discipline: "*African* in the phrase African psychology has to be in parentheses as a signal to the fact that the objective is to contribute towards all psychological knowledge produced in Africa or about "African" and Africans; and more specifically, to produce Africa(n)-centred knowledge that is at home in Africa as well as within global psychology" (Ratele, 2016, p. 4).

References

Addai, I., Opoku-Agyeman, C., & Amanfu, S. K. (2014). Exploring predictors of subjective well-being in Ghana: A micro-level study. *Journal of Happiness Studies, 15*(4), 869–890. https://doi.org/10.1007/s10902-013-9454-7

Agbo, A. A., & Ome, B. (2017). Happiness: Meaning and determinants among young adults of the Igbos of eastern Nigeria. *Journal of Happiness Studies, 18*(1), 151–175. https://doi.org/10.1007/s10902-016-9722-4

Arnett, J. J. (2008). The neglected 95%: Why American psychology needs to become less American. *American Psychologist, 63*(7), 602–614.

Benítez, I., He, J., Van de Vijver, F. J., & Padilla, J. L. (2016). Linking extreme response style to response processes: A cross-cultural mixed methods approach. *International Journal of Psychology, 51*(6), 464–473.

Biglan, A. (2015). *The nurture effect: How the science of human behavior can improve our lives and our world*. New Harbinger.

Brdar, I., Rijavec, M., & Miljković, D. (2009). Life goals and Well-being: Are extrinsic aspirations always detrimental to Well-being? *Psihologijske Teme, 18*(2), 317–334.

Chamberlain, K., & Murray, M. (2009). Critical health psychology. *Critical Psychology: An Introduction, 2*, 144–158.

Chan, D., Hamamura, T., Li, L. M. W., & Zhang, X. (2017). Is trusting others related to better health? An investigation of older adults across six non-western countries. *Journal of Cross-Cultural Psychology, 48*(8), 1288–1301. https://doi.org/10.1177/0022022117722632

Cheng, C., Jose, P. E., Sheldon, K. M., Singelis, T. M., Cheung, M. W. L., Tiliouine, H., et al. (2011). Sociocultural differences in self-construal and subjective well-being: A test of four cultural models. *Journal of Cross-Cultural Psychology, 42*, 832–855. https://doi.org/10.1177/0022022110381117

Chilisa, B., & Tsheko, G. N. (2014). Mixed methods in indigenous research: Building relationships for sustainable intervention outcomes. *Journal of Mixed Methods Research, 8*(3), 222–233.

Chirinda, W., & Phaswana-Mafuya, N. (2019). Happy life expectancy and correlates of happiness among older adults in South Africa. *Aging & Mental Health, 23*(8), 1000–1007.

Christopher, J. C., & Hickinbottom, S. (2008). Positive psychology, ethnocentrism, and the disguised ideology of individualism. *Theory & Psychology, 18*(5), 563–589. https://doi.org/10.1177/0959354308093396

Clark, D. A. (2003). Concepts and perceptions of human well-being: Some evidence from South Africa. *Oxford Development Studies, 31*(2), 173–196. https://doi.org/10.1080/1360081030742 8

Cohen, R. J. (1999). What qualitative research can be. *Psychology & Marketing, 16*(4), 351–367.

Davids, E. L., & Roman, N. V. (2013). Does family structure matter? Comparing the life goals and aspirations of learners in secondary schools. *South African Journal of Education, 33*(3), 1–12.

Davids, E. L., Roman, N. V., & Kerchhoff, L. J. (2017). Adolescent goals and aspirations in search of psychological well-being: From the perspective of self-determination theory. *South Africa Journal of Psychology, 47*(1), 121–132. https://doi.org/10.1177/0081246316653744

Davies, W. (2015). *The happiness industry: How the government and big business sold us well-being*. Verso Books.

Diener, E. (2009). Positive psychology: Past, present and future. In S. J. Lopez & C. R. Snyder (Eds.), *Oxford handbook of positive psychology* (pp. 7–11). Oxford University Press.

Diener, E., Oishi, S., & Tay, L. (2018). Advances in subjective well-being research. *Nature Human Behaviour, 2*(4), 253–260. https://doi.org/10.1038/s41562-018-0307-6

Disabato, D. J., Goodman, F. R., Kashdan, T. B., Short, J. L., & Jarden, A. (2016). Different types of well-being? A cross-cultural examination of hedonic and eudaimonic well-being. *Psychological Assessment, 28*(5), 471–482. https://doi.org/10.1037/pas0000209

Dzokoto, V. A., Osei-Tutu, A., Scollon, C. N., Wallace, D., & Peters-Chitwood, L. (2019). Meaning and perceptions of the good life in Ghana. *Psychological Studies, 64*(1), 11–20. https://doi.org/10.1007/s12646-018-0475-5

Edwards, S. D. (2014). Integral approach to South African psychology with special reference to indigenous knowledge. *Journal of Psychology in Africa, 24*(6), 526–532. https://doi.org/10.1080/14330237.2014.997044

Ellis, B. D., & Stam, H. J. (2015). Crisis? What crisis? Cross-cultural psychology's appropriation of cultural psychology. *Culture & Psychology, 21*(3), 293–317.

Eloff, I., Achoui, M., Chireshe, R., Mutepfa, M., & Ofovwe, C. (2008). Views from Africa on positive psychology. *Journal of Psychology in Africa, 18*(1), 189–194. https://doi.org/10.1080/14330237.2008.10820185

Govender, K., Bhana, A., McMurray, K., Kelly, J., Theron, L., Meyer-Weitz, A., . . . Tomlinson, M. (2019). A systematic review of the South African work on the well-being of young people (2000–2016). *South Africa Journal of Psychology, 49*(1), 52–69. https://doi.org/10.1177/0081246318757932

Guse, T., Vescovelli, F., & Croxford, S.-A. (2019). Subjective well-being and gratitude among South African adolescents: Exploring gender and cultural differences. *Youth & Society, 51*(5), 591–615. https://doi.org/10.1177/0044118X17697237

Hamamura, T., Li, L. M. W., & Chan, D. (2017). The association between generalized trust and physical and psychological health across societies. *Social Indicators Research, 134*(1), 277–286. https://doi.org/10.1007/s11205-016-1428-9

Hardin, E. E., Robitschek, C., Flores, L. Y., Navarro, R. L., & Ashton, M. W. (2014). The cultural lens approach to evaluating cultural validity of psychological theory. *American Psychologist, 69*(7), 656–668.

He, J., & Van de Vijver, F. J. (2016). The motivation-achievement paradox in international educational achievement tests: Toward a better understanding. In *The psychology of Asian learners* (pp. 253–268). Springer.

Hefferon, K., Ashfield, A., Waters, L., & Synard, J. (2017). Understanding optimal human functioning – The 'call for qual' in exploring human flourishing and well-being. *The Journal of Positive Psychology, 12*(3), 211–219. https://doi.org/10.1080/17439760.2016.1225120

Henrich, J., Heine, S. J., & Norenzayan, A. (2010). Most people are not WEIRD. *Nature, 466*(7302), 29–29.

Holder, M. D., Coleman, B., Krupa, T., & Krupa, E. (2016). Well-being's relation to religiosity and spirituality in children and adolescents in Zambia. *Journal of Happiness Studies, 17*(3), 1235–1253. https://doi.org/10.1007/s10902-015-9640-x

King, M. F., Renó, V. F., & Novo, E. M. (2014). The concept, dimensions and methods of assessment of human well-being within a socioecological context: A literature review. *Social Indicators Research, 116*(3), 681–698.

Kitayama, S. H., Markus, H. R., & Kurokawa, M. (2000). Culture, emotion, and well-being: Good feelings in Japan and the United States. *Cognition and Emotion, 14*(1), 93–124.

Lenz, A., Watson, J. C., Luo, Y., Norris, C., & Nkyi, A. (2018). Cross-cultural validation of four positive psychology assessments for use with a Ghanaian population. *International Journal for the Advancement of Counselling, 40*(2), 148–161. https://doi.org/10.1007/s10447-017-9317-8

Macleod, C. I. (2018). The case for collation to inform debate and transform practice in decolonising psychology. *South Africa Journal of Psychology, 48*(3), 372–378. https://doi.org/10.1177/0081246318784508

Magni, G. (2017). Indigenous knowledge and implications for the sustainable development agenda. *European Journal of Education, 52*(4), 437–447.

Mahali, A., Lynch, I., Fadiji, A. W., Tolla, T., Khumalo, S., & Naicker, S. (2018). Networks of well-being in the global south: A critical review of current scholarship. *Journal of Developing Societies, 34*(4), 373–400. https://doi.org/10.1177/0169796X18786137

Marecek, J., & Christopher, J. C. (2018). Is positive psychology an indigenous psychology? In N. J. L. Brown, T. Lomas, & F. J. Eiroa-Orosa (Eds.), *The Routledge international handbook of critical positive psychology*. Routledge.

Marmot, M. (2015). The health gap: The challenge of an unequal world. *The Lancet, 386*(10011), 2442–2444. https://doi.org/10.1016/S0140-6736(15)00150-6

Matsumoto, D., & Yoo, S. H. (2006). Towards a new generation of cross-cultural research. *Perspectives on Psychological Science, 1*(3), 234–250.

Mkabela, Q. N. (2015). Ubuntu as a foundation for researching African indigenous psychology. *African Journal of Indigenous Knowledge Systems, 14*(2), 284–291.

Mkhize, N. (2004). Sociocultural approaches to psychology: Dialogism and African conceptions of the self. In K. Ratele, D. Norman, N. Mkhize, P. Kiguwa, & A. Collins (Eds.), *Self, community and psychology*. UCT Press.

Møller, V., & Roberts, B. (2017). New beginnings in an ancient region: Well-being in sub-Saharan Africa. In R. J. Estes & M. J. Sirgy (Eds.), *The pursuit of human well-being: The untold global history* (pp. 161–215). Springer Nature.

Neff, D. F., & Olsen, W. K. (2007). Measuring subjective well-being from a realist viewpoint. *Methodological Innovations Online, 2*(2), 44–66. https://doi.org/10.4256/mio.2007.0011

Nell, W. (2014). Exploring the relationship between religious fundamentalism, life satisfaction, and meaning in life. *Journal of Psychology in Africa, 24*(2), 159–166. https://doi.org/10.1080/14330237.2014.903074

Ngamaba, K. H. (2016). Happiness and life satisfaction in Rwanda. *Journal of Psychology in Africa, 26*(5), 407–414. https://doi.org/10.1080/14330237.2016.1208930

Nwoye, A. (2015). What is African psychology the psychology of? *Theory & Psychology, 25*(1), 96–116. https://doi.org/10.1177/0959354314565116

Owe, E., Vignoles, V. L., Becker, M., Brown, R., Smith, P. B., Lee, S. W., . . . Baguma, P. (2013). Contextualism as an important facet of individualism-collectivism: Personhood beliefs across 37 national groups. *Journal of Cross-Cultural Psychology, 44*(1), 24–45.

Painter, D., Kiguwa, P., & Böhmke, W. (2013). Contexts and continuities of critique: Reflections on the current state of critical psychology in South Africa. *Annual Review of Critical Psychology, 13*, 849–869.

Park, N., Peterson, C., & Seligman, M. E. P. (2006). Character strengths in fifty-four nations and the fifty US states. *The Journal of Positive Psychology, 1*(3), 118–129. https://doi.org/10.1080/17439760600619567

Prilleltensky, I. (2017). Foreword: Interiorizing and interrogating well-being. In N. J. Brown, T. Lomas, & F. J. Eiroa-Orosa (Eds.), *The Routledge international handbook of critical positive psychology*. Routledge.

Raffaelli, M., Lazarevic, V., Koller, S. H., Nsamenang, A. B., & Sharma, D. (2013). Introduction: Special issue on adolescents in the majority world. *Journal of Research on Adolescence, 23*(1), 1–8.

Ratele, K. (2016). *Who needs African psychology when we are happy with psychology in Africa*? Paper presented at the Rhodes University, Dept of Psychology's Social Change Awards.

Ratele, K. (2017). Four (African) psychologies. *Theory & Psychology, 27*(3), 313–327. https://doi.org/10.1177/0959354316684215

Ratele, K. (2019). *The world looks like this from here: Thoughts on African psychology*. Wits University Press.

Ryan, R. M., & Deci, E. L. (2001). On happiness and human potential: A review of research on hedonic and eudaimonic well-being. *Annual Review of Psychology, 52*, 141–166.

Savahl, S., Adams, S., Isaacs, S., September, R., Hendricks, G., & Noordien, Z. (2015). Subjective well-being amongst a sample of South African children: A descriptive study. *Child Indicators Research, 8*(1), 211–226.

Schimmack, U., Radhakrishnan, P., Oishi, S., Dzokoto, V., & Ahadi, S. (2002). Culture, personality, and subjective well-being: Integrating process models of life satisfaction. *Journal of Personality and Social Psychology, 82*(4), 582–593.

Schutte, L., & Wissing, M. P. (2017). Clarifying the factor structure of the mental health continuum short form in three languages: A bifactor exploratory structural equation modeling approach. *Society and Mental Health, 7*(3), 142–158. https://doi.org/10.1177/2156869317707793

Seligman, M. E. P., & Csikszentmihalyi, M. (2000). Positive psychology: An introduction. *American Psychologist, 55*, 5–14.

Steger, M. F., Kashdan, T. B., Sullivan, B. A., & Lorentz, D. (2008). Understanding the search for meaning in life: Personality, cognitive style, and the dynamic between seeking and experiencing meaning. *Journal of Personality, 76*(2), 199–228. https://doi.org/10.1111/j.1467-6494.2007.00484.x

Tamir, M., Schwartz, S. H., Cieciuch, J., Riediger, M., Torres, C., Scollon, C., Dzokoto, V., Zhou, X., & Vishkin, A. (2016). Desired emotions across cultures: A value-based account. *Journal of Personality and Social Psychology, 111*(1), 67–82. https://doi.org/10.1037/pspp0000072

Temane, L., Khumalo, I. P., & Wissing, M. P. (2014). Validation of the meaning in life questionnaire in a South African context. *Journal of Psychology in Africa, 24*(1), 51–60. https://doi.org/10.1080/14330237.2014.904088

Temane, Q. M., & Wissing, M. P. (2006). The role of spirituality as a mediator for psychological well-being across different contexts. *South Africa Journal of Psychology, 36*(3), 582–597. https://doi.org/10.1177/008124630603600309

Teo, T. (1999). Methodologies of critical psychology: Illustrations from the field of racism. *Annual Review of Critical Psychology, 1*, 119–134.

Uchida, Y., Norasakkunkit, V., & Kitayama, S. (2004). Cultural constructions of happiness: Theory and empirical evidence. *Journal of Happiness Studies, 5*(3), 223–239.

Van Aardt, C. J., de Clercq, B., & Meiring, J. (2019). The stochastic determinants of happiness in South Africa: A micro-economic modelling approach. *Journal of Economic and Financial Sciences, 12*(1), 1–14.

Van der Geest, S. (1998). Yebisa Wo Fie: Growing old and building a house in the Akan culture of Ghana. *Journal of Cross-Cultural Gerontology, 13*(4), 333–359. https://doi.org/10.1023/A:1006563032706

Waterman, A. S. (2008). Reconsidering happiness: A eudaimonist's perspective. *Journal of Positive Psychology, 3*(4), 234–252.

Webster, G. D., Nichols, A. E., & Schember, T. O. (2009). American psychology is becoming more international. *American Psychologist, 64*, 566–568. https://doi.org/10.1037/a0016193

White, S. C. (2010). Analysing wellbeing: A framework for development practice. *Development in Practice, 20*(2), 158–172. https://doi.org/10.1080/09614520903564199

White, S. C. (2017). Relational wellbeing: Re-centring the politics of happiness, policy and the self. *Policy & Politics, 45*(2), 121–136.

White, S. C., Fernandez, A., & Jha, S. (2016). Beyond the grumpy rich man and the happy peasant: Mixed methods and the impact of food security on subjective dimensions of wellbeing in India. *Oxford Development Studies, 44*(3), 332–348. https://doi.org/10.1080/13600818.2015.1120278

Wilson Fadiji, A., Meiring, L., & Wissing, M. P. (2019). Understanding well-being in the Ghanaian context: Linkages between lay conceptions of well-being and measures of hedonic and eudaimonic well-being. *Applied Research Quality Life, 16*, 649–677. https://doi.org/10.1007/s11482-019-09777-2

Wilson Fadiji, A., & Wissing, M. P. (2021). Region of sub-Saharan Africa. In E. C. Chang, C. Downey, H. Yang, I. Zetler, & M. Muyan (Eds.), *International handbook of positive psychology: A global perspective on the science of positive human existence*. Springer.

Wilson, A., & Somhlaba, N. Z. (2016). Psychological well-being in a context of adversity: Ghanaian adolescents' experiences of hope and life satisfaction. *Africa Today, 63*(1), 85–103. https://doi.org/10.2979/africatoday.63.1.0085

Wilson, A., & Somhlaba, N. Z. (2017). Gender, age, religion and positive mental health among adolescents in a Ghanaian socio-cultural context. *Child Indicators Research*, 1–28. https://doi.org/10.1007/s12187-017-9495-2

Wilson, A., Wissing, M. P., Ndima, L., & Somhlaba, N. Z. (2018). Representations of hope, goals, and meaning from lay person's perspectives in two African contexts. *Journal of Humanistic Psychology*. https://doi.org/10.1177/0022167818785070

Wilson, A., Wissing, M. P., & Schutte, L. (2018). "We help each other": Relational patterns among older individuals in South African samples. *Applied Research in Quality of Life*. https://doi.org/10.1007/s11482-018-9657-5

Wilson, A., Yendork, J. S., & Somhlaba, N. Z. (2017). Psychometric properties of multidimensional scale of perceived social support among Ghanaian adolescents. *Child Indicators Research, 10*(1), 101–115. https://doi.org/10.1007/s12187-016-9367-1

Wissing, M. P., Khumalo, I. P., & Chigeza, S. C. (2014). Meaning as perceived and experienced by an African student group. *Journal of Psychology in Africa, 24*(1), 92–101. https://doi.org/10.1080/14330237.2014.904101

Wissing, M. P., Potgieter, J. C., Guse, T., Khumalo, I. P., & Nel, L. (2020). *Towards flourishing: Embracing wellbeing in diverse contexts* (2nd ed.). Van Schaik Publishers.

Wong, P. T. (2016). Chinese positive psychology revisited. *International Journal of Existential Positive Psychology, 6*(1), 1–7.

Woodcock, A., Camfield, L., McGregor, J. A., & Martin, F. (2008). Validation of the WeDQoL-goals-Thailand measure: Culture-specific individualised quality of life. *Social Indicators Research, 94*(1), 135. https://doi.org/10.1007/s11205-008-9357-x

Worth, P., & Smith, M. (2017). Critical positive psychology: A creative convergence of two disciplines. In J. L. Brown, T. Lomas, & F. J. Eiroa-Orosa (Eds.), *The Routledge international handbook of critical positive psychology* (pp. 3–10). Routledge.

Żemojtel-Piotrowska, M., Piotrowski, J. P., Cieciuch, J., Adams, B. G., Osin, E. N., Ardi, R., … Maltby, J. (2017). Measurement invariance of personal well-being index (PWI-8) across 26 countries. *Journal of Happiness Studies, 18*(6), 1697–1711. https://doi.org/10.1007/s10902-016-9795-0

Chapter 3
Socially Influenced Health Norms: Their Construction and Enactment in African Culture Settings

Elias Mpofu and Elias Machina

Abstract People understand their health and well-being from a both a physical and social perspective. For that reason, socio-cultural affiliations influence community health norms. This is particularly important in low resource settings of Africa, where marginal public health service infrastructure necessitates collective health actions at the community level. This chapter proposes the view that socially influenced health norms explain the ways through which African culture followers make health support choices. African culture followers identify with traditionalist, transitional or modern orientations, and aligned health norms. Although the typical African culture followers may not be consciously aware of how their social affiliation influences their health norms, they nonetheless would know and engage in health practices consistent with their cultural orientation. In this chapter, we (a) describe social affiliation influences on health practices of African culture followers; (b) briefly characterize the ontology of health norms in African culture communities; (c) consider diversity in social affiliation among African culture followers and their implications for health promotion interventions; (d) evaluate the relative importance of alternative social affiliations to health norms among African culture followers; and (e) propose a research protocol useful for studying African culture followers' health norm orientations important to public health interventions with them.

Keywords Social affiliation · Identities · Health equity · Health access and promotion · Traditionalist · Public health · Social · Social policy · Transitional · Modern

---

E. Mpofu (✉)
University of North Texas, Denton, TX, USA

University of the Witwatersrand, South Africa

University of Sydney, Sydney, NSW, Australia
e-mail: Elias.Mpofu@unt.edu; Elias.Mpofu@sydney.edu.au

E. Machina
Western Sydney University, Sydney, NSW, Australia

L. Schutte et al. (eds.), *Embracing Well-Being in Diverse African Contexts: Research Perspectives*, Cross-Cultural Advancements in Positive Psychology 16,
https://doi.org/10.1007/978-3-030-85924-4_3

3.1 Introduction

People's social affiliations influence their health outcomes in myriad ways. A well-documented social affiliation influence is that people's health status is closer to that of others with whom they share a social world, primarily defined by the physical community habitat (Cramm et al., 2012; MacQueen et al., 2001; Mpofu, 2015). The physical or geographical community habitat is a reliable proxy indicator of the public health services members of a community could access (Polo et al., 2015). However, social affiliations drive the actual use of public health services (Cramm et al., 2012; Mpofu, 2015). Social affiliation is about a sense of connectedness and belonging to others with whom one shares a world-view (Nsamenang, 2006; Stetsenko & Arievitch, 2004). Social affiliations are in part a product of the "dynamic, irreducible tension" between individual functioning and the sociocultural context (Penuel & Wertsch, 1995, p. 84; see also Wertsch, 1991) as individuals self-define in their lives (Holland et al., 2001). Social affiliations influence health beliefs and practices (Cohen, 2004; Luke & Munshi, 2007; Mpofu, 2018). We propose social affiliation influences on health norms of African culture followers, and a prospective research protocol to gather the evidence on socially influenced health norms in African culture settings.

Health is a state of wellbeing for coping with normal stresses of life, while being productively engaged with the community (Galderisi et al., 2015). Social affiliations have a controlling effect on people's health practices, priming them to adopt particular health practices rather than alternative or competing ones (Brenner, 2001; Luke & Munshi, 2007; Mpofu, 2018). For that reason, social community members share a health identity with networked others. These shared health identities result from the interplay between personal factors (e.g., knowledge of, beliefs and values towards health practices), relationship factors (health practice approval by significant others, family acceptance, etc.), and health care provider perceptions (social attitudes, trust in providers, et cetera).

Traditionalist African culture communities are collectivistic in orientation (Mbiti, 1991; Mpofu, 2010; Nsamenang, 2008). Communities are groups of people who live in a geographic area, have some level of social interaction, share a sense of belonging, or share common political and social responsibilities (MacQueen et al., 2001). In collectivistic African culture, people are concerned with norm conformity and interdependence, and tend to make use of their social affiliations to achieve the social outcomes they aspire. This collectivistic cultural orientation would be the primary lens through which African culture followers perceive their social worlds for health and wellbeing (Agulanna, 2010). For instance, traditionalist African culture epistemology combines constructs of mind and body, and spirit (Levers, 2006a), and practices grounded in the metaphysical (Agulanna, 2010; Cramm et al., 2012). As discussed later in the chapter, a traditionalist African culture affiliation influences predisposition to utilize complementary or alternative medicine rather than modern medicine, while a modern culture affiliation is associated with use of modern rather than complementary or alternative medicine (Makgahlela & Sodi, 2017; Mpofu et al., 2010).

This chapter explores health norms among African culture communities. First, we briefly explore the historical and cultural foundations of social affiliations important for health norms development among African culture followers. Second, we discuss the significance of social affiliations to health norms in African culture community settings, including cultural rule, role, and value orientations. This discussion also considers how social affiliations are contingent in their influence on likelihood to adopt new health practices in the face of prevailing historical traditionalist belief systems. Finally, we propose some ways by which some Africa culture followers may achieve health norms aligned to their social affiliations, while others may experience significant acculturative stress from navigating competing health norms across social affiliations. In doing so, we present a research protocol to guide investigations to understand socially contingent health norms by African culture followers.

3.2 Historical Foundations of Health Norms in African Communities

Africa comprises 56 nation states with huge diversity in health and wellbeing statuses. The North-Eastern African countries of the Sudan and Somalia as well as from the Central African countries of Democratic Republic of the Congo, Rwanda, and Uganda have a history of protracted civil wars and forced displacements. Their health care systems seek to address war-related pandemics with the public health infrastructure underdevelopment (Gough et al., 2004; Kalipeni & Oppong, 1998; Van Leeuwen et al., 2016). The population health needs of the politically stable African countries such as Botswana, Ghana, South Africa, Tanzania, and Zambia would be explained by national differences in public health resource allocation priorities (Asante et al., 2006; Gough et al., 2004; Mutale et al., 2013). Moreover, the health and wellbeing of citizens with marginal economies such as Malawi, Mozambique, and Zimbabwe would be fragile, compared to that of citizens of Botswana, Namibia, Rwanda, and South Africa (Deaton, 2008). Moreover, the relative neglect of public health systems in leading countries like Nigeria and other North and West African nations is well-documented (United Nations High Commission on Refugees, UNHCR, 2019). This is an important caveat to ensuing discussion on health identities of African communities, given the fact that Africa is a huge continent with diversity of human habitats as well as health and wellbeing support systems.

Africa also is a continent with thousands of subcultures. As examples, the predominantly Arab culture of North and North Eastern Africa presents a distinctly different cultural orientation compared to the "abantu" culture of sub-Saharan Africa (Idang, 2015; Patai, 1973). Moreover, numerous subethnic groupings are prevalent within the Arab and Bantu culture regions. Many of the countries of Africa include ethnic communities with distinct cultural identities, each with its own cultural mores. Often these ethnic identities determine social affiliations, perhaps more than their African continental affiliation. Nonetheless, the Arab and sub-Saharan communities are collectivist in cultural orientation in placing a higher value of the needs of the social collective over those of the individual, caring for each other materially and socially (Idang, 2015).

The entire African continent shares a history of colonization by Western countries, with the exception of Ethiopia. As a result, African communities adopted Western and indigenous cultural ethos to an extent, and which would be important to their public health services.

African culture adherents are in three types: traditionalist, transitional, and modern (Van der Merwe et al., 2016). As previously noted, those with traditionalist culture orientation have a metaphysical health belief orientation in which mind, body and soul are intricately bound (Makgahlela & Sodi, 2017; Mpofu et al., 2010; Levers, 2006a, 2006b; Van der Merwe et al., 2016). Those with modern culture orientation identify with public health services following scientific medicine. Those in transitional culture orientation straddle both metaphysical and public health belief orientations, contingent on prevailing health needs. Those with a modern culture orientation tend to be with higher levels of formal education compared to those with a traditionalist cultural orientation (Gyasi et al., 2016), whereas those in transitional culture orientation seek to benefit from both their traditionalist culture beliefs and also those based on modern science (Mpofu et al., 2010; Van der Merwe et al., 2016).

For the typical African culture followers, their social affiliations include age-based seniority, clan identity, subsistence economy partnerships and perhaps, a formal occupation. Among traditionalist African culture followers, their predominantly subsistence economies encourage collective inter-dependency or reciprocity in roles and responsibilities. However, the majority African communities have marginal access to public health care services from historical and contemporary socio-economic deprivation (Tanser et al., 2006), and their communal social affiliation identities are major pathways by which they transact health and wellbeing (Bojuwoye, 2005; Levers, 2006b; Mpofu et al., 2011).

3.3 Health Identities: Their Cultural Mediation and Transmission

Health identities, defined by a shared understanding with social affiliation others of what it is like being with wellness or ill-being (Cramm et al., 2012; Mpofu, 2010). One's social affiliation serves an adaptive function, in part because "life structures are in constant motion, changing with time and evolving as new life circumstances unfold" (Hutchison, 2015, p. 277). Social affiliations influence health identifies, and individuals may change their health norms from exploring and adopting those of their new affiliation (Märtsin, 2008; Penuel & Wertsch, 1995). That being the case, social health behavior rules, roles and value orientations of the affiliation community define an individual's health norms (Kelman, 2006; Mpofu, 2018; Mpofu et al., 2011).

The evolution, transmission and sustenance of health norms within communities occur through a process of social mediation (Brenner, 2001; Mpofu, 2018; Mumby, 1987). For instance, Cultural-historical activity theory (CHAT; Engeström, 1999; Vygotsky, 1978) would posit that a health community's norms influence the wellbeing of the followers, by which the followers are active learners in a socio-cultural process foregrounded by historical learning experiences (Cole & Engeström, 2007; Leont'ev, 1978; Vygotsky, 1978). African culture followers acquire their health norms through the social mediation of networked others (e.g., family, community leaders) who are committed to translating those community's core health they believe to ensure the survival of the community (Kabagenyi et al., 2016; Makgahlela & Sodi, 2017; Mpofu et al., 2010).

CHAT makes a distinction between activities and actions (Leont'ev, 1978; Vygotsky, 1978). From a CHAT perspective, health *activities* are those social affiliates enact to ensure the existence of the collective social entity while health *actions* are what the members do to achieve an activity. For instance, in traditionalist African culture followers share a keen interest in activities for collective wellbeing through actions (e.g., inter-dependent or mutually beneficial roles: Afolabi & Dennis, 2019; Lew-Levy et al., 2019; Owuse, 2019) believed to achieve the purpose or object of an activity (i.e., community health and wellbeing: Brenner, 2001; Mpofu et al., 2010). Following a CHAT perspective, actions on their own (e.g., inter-dependent, reciprocal actions) cannot be explained outside the motives for which they are enacted (e.g., collective community health and wellbeing) (see also Mpofu et al., 2011). In traditionalist African culture, an implicit cultural-historical transmission process is at play, through invisible (or taken for granted or assumed knowledge) action for everyday living, premised on reciprocity in rules, roles and values (Mpofu et al., 2010; Sodi & Phethi, 2017). These knowledge heritages, passed on by oral culture transmission as well as participatory learning experiences in everyday settings, have the medical oversight of traditional healers (Mpofu et al., 2010).

Traditional Healers (*Dingaka*, *Izangoma*, *Lituela*, *Nyanga*, *Ondudu*, and *Sangoma*) are a group of persons recognized by the community in which they live as being competent to provide health care by using vegetable, animal and mineral substances and other methods (Chavunduka, 1986; Levers, 2006a, 2006b; Mpofu et al., 2010). These health practices are based on the "prevalent beliefs in the community regarding physical, mental and social well-being and the causation of disease and disability" (World Health Organization, 1978, p. 41). A majority of African culture followers perceive traditional healers as credible in their health service practices.

However, in the enactment of an action (e.g., traditional healer sharing knowledge on a potent herbal extraction treatment) to achieve an activity (collective wellbeing), a contradiction may arise (e.g., a traditional healers need to protect privileged herbal specialist knowledge from being widely disseminated in the community) and the general health promotion good (collective wellbeing) (Mpofu et al., 2010). The traditional healer may perceive to risk losing his or her privileged herbal knowledge if more members of the community social affiliates also knew of the herbal plants' extraction for self-medication, despite his or her belief in the common good from wider dissemination (a contradiction). In resolving the contradiction, the herbal specialist may train apprentices for a controlled dissemination of the specialist treatments for the community good, while protecting their "patent" rights.

To achieve aspired health norms, African culture community members must build on their present and prospective social affiliations to best navigate rule, roles, and values for both their individual and collective wellbeing. We briefly discuss prospective rule, role, and value orientation among African culture followers.

Rule, Role, and Value Orientation Rule orientation refers to understanding the affordances and penalties for quality of participation in a particular environment (Kelman, 2006). In Africanist culture settings, followers adopt health norms grounded in social rule following to guide their collective wellbeing activities (Mbiti, 1991; Mpofu, 1994). Role orientation is about understanding what it takes to carry out obligatory tasks for a social role (Brenner, 2001; Karmon, 2007). In this regard, African culture followers must acquire a dependable knowledge of essential role functions for collective health and wellbeing (Edwards, 2016). The typical African culture follower may not have the luxury of self-determination in their social affiliation, as they are born into collective culture responsibility, obviating the searching for ways to achieve personal wellbeing independent of the collective. As previously noted, typical African culture followers base their wellbeing on that of the collective.

Value orientation refers to the extent to which an individual identifies with the underlying beliefs behind the workings of a social system (Holland et al., 2001; Kelman, 2006). In this regard, the collectivist value orientation is protective of personal health and that of social collective. Nonetheless, some African culture followers grapple with the tensions from navigating both the collectivistic origin culture and influences of modern cultures on their health practices (Gyasi et al., 2016). A common theme among identity theories is that of exploration and integration of multiple cultural perspectives, with greater exploration and integration leading to a more balanced and cohesive self-concept (Kunst et al., 2015; Märtsin, 2008). However, African culture followers in transitional value orientation may not sufficiently self-explore from fear to the uncertainties of risk for social exclusion and discrimination by the collective. Moreover, they also may have mental health ill-being from a sense of disavowal or self-estrangement from culture of origin beliefs in conflict with those of modern cultures they may not have fully internalized (Mpofu et al., in press).

Health norms of African culture followers are gendered, and highly contingent on religious belief following. As previously noted, predispositions to use traditional (complementary and alternative medicine) and/or modern medicine influence African culture health norms. The next section explores how social affiliations of gender and religion following influence health norms of African culture followers.

Gendered Affiliations African culture communities are patriarchal and males have a greater say on defining activities for collective health and wellbeing while the views of women and children may be unrecognized or discounted (Agadjanian, 2005; Mbiti, 1991). This is despite the fact that women and children carry the greater burden implementing the practice actions for health and wellbeing (e.g., nutrition and housekeeping) for "spectator" male community members. For example, girls are less likely than boys to be provided with health care, food, or education in many parts of the world (Johnson et al., 2009; Mcommh et al., 2015; World Health Organization, 2018), including in Africa (Francis et al., 2011), while women are often malnourished due to the priority of feeding other family members first. Women congregates of a traditionalist indigenous church community were treated to a different and gendered standard than their male peers (Mpofu et al., 2011; Hallfors et al., 2016; see also Box 3.1 below).

The community collective generally does not question the male leadership in community health and well-being activities. This gendered social more generates "undiscussable" contradictions (Engeström, 1999), which may harm the health and wellbeing of women and children by neglect (Mpofu et al., 2011). This does not rule out the possibility of social more enactment "anomalies" by which women and children can question undiscussable practices (e.g., female circumcision: Shell-Duncan, 2008), preferring to achieve sexual health outcomes differently than the historical, traditional way. Thus, the interrogation of historical "non-discussables" has the capacity to self-transform collective wellbeing through the adoption of new health norms.

Religious Affiliation Religious affiliation is the most dominant community social influence in African culture settings (Haddad, 2013; Hallfors et al., 2016; Mbiti, 1991). For that reason, religious beliefs are potent conduits for access and utilization of health services by African culture followers (Mpofu et al., 2010, 2011). This is, in part, because religious affiliation influences health norms through moral directives, spiritual experiences (which solidify moral commitments), role models, and community and leadership skills (e.g., participation in faith believe rites). Furthermore, religious affiliations also influence coping skills (e.g., prayer, confession, forgiveness, religious funeral rites), provides socio-cultural capital (e.g., participation in a sacred music program; access to respected elders) and social network (dense networks of religion adherents; contact with respected faith belief leaders) (Mpofu et al., 2011; Smith et al., 2002).

Constructs from moral and ethical theory (Haidt et al., 1993; Shweder et al., 1997, 2008) also provide additional rationale for the significance of religion to the social affiliation among African culture followers. Moral and ethical theory, distinguishes among broad cultural-behavioral templates of an Ethic of Autonomy, Ethic of Community and Ethic of Divinity. The Ethic of Autonomy places an emphasis an individual's liberty and independence while safeguarding the rights of others. The

Ethic of Autonomy is aligned to Western individualistic culture in which religion beliefs are a specific area of life, having little impact on interpersonal or societal issues (Haidt et al., 1993; Shweder et al., 2008). The Ethic of Community is strongly aligned to collectivistic cultural orientation, and places emphasis on group norms like loyalty, honor, conformity and chastity (Shweder et al., 2008). The Ethic of Divinity is prevalent in African collectivistic societies and postulates that humans as well as animals contain divine elements to be protected by special rites and customs. As an example, traditionalist Africans believe that plants, animals and humans exist in a symbiotic relationship so that the well-being of plants and animals explains health in humans (Levers, 2006a). The Ethic of Divinity is premised on the belief that religiosity permeates all spheres of life, and explains health statuses of populations (Shweder et al., 1997, 2008). Box 3.1 presents case examples of an African indigenous church group follower observations for Ethnic of Divinity (see also Hallfors et al., 2016; Mpofu et al., 2011).

Box 3.1 African Culture Ethic of Divinity Illustration-Spiritually Endowed Community Abilities

As members grow in spiritual strength, they become specialized in various attributes of community work. For example, spiritual leaders can become exceptionally gifted spiritual medical physicians specializing in diseases that can afflict the baby's soft spot on the head. Others can specialize in the ability to drive away demons that sometimes inhabit members of the public that are not members of the sect. The overall idea is that the main spiritual leader allocates various conditions to different specialized spiritual physicians.

Box 3.2 African Culture Ethic of Divinity Illustration-Spiritually Sanctioned Womanhood

The church elders will be monitoring your movements to establish whether you have repented from your sins. When they are satisfied that you are now walking in the right way then they will pray for you and you will start doing the church activities again. There are certain times when women are asked not to wear the church garments. When a woman is menstruating or when she has given birth, she is not allowed to wear the church garments. If she gives birth to a baby boy, she has to wait until one month and a week and if it is a girl, she has to wait for two months two weeks.

(Author Original, unpublished interview material with African indigenous church followers)

African culture followers may perceive religion beliefs and personal preferences to influence their health norms (Mpofu, 2016). These personal preferences may arise from ongoing adaptive learning to manage health promotion opportunities with modern medicine. With modernity or acquisition of global culture orientation, identities have "to be created and recreated on a more active basis than before" (Giddens, 2000, p. 65). The greater the cultural distance between their culture of origin and the host culture, the more adaptive learning people have to engage to function in the host culture (Berry, 1997).

3.4 Traditional and Alternative Medicine Adherence

An estimated 80% of African culture people seek treatment from traditional healers (United Nations Programme on HIV/AIDS, 2000; World Health Organization, 2004). African traditional healers are not a homogeneous group; rather, they represent various types of practitioners, including Herbalists, Spiritual Healers, Traditional Doctors, Spirit Mediums, and Traditional Healer Practitioners (THPs). The scope of practice of traditional healing spans all aspects of human living and that of animals and other living organisms (Levers, 2006a). In many African cultural settings, the state of being healthy entails a harmonious relationship between the humans, their physical environment and spiritual world of the ancestors and the gods who sustain them (Mbiti, 1991; Mpofu et al., 2010; Rugira et al., 2013).

While transitional culture Africans would seek treatment from both traditional healers and Western medical professionals, depending upon the nature of the problem (Gyasi et al., 2016; Mpofu, 2006), traditionalist culture Africans would prioritize the services of indigenous healers (Levers, 2006a; Mpofu et al., 2010). They would only seek the services of Western-trained medical practitioners if traditional healing practices fail to improve the condition (Gyasi et al., 2016; Mpofu, 2003). Those of a modern cultural orientation likely would seek health consultation primarily with public health services. African culture adherents increasingly adopt Western forms of health care. However, Western biomedical approaches tend to marginalize indigenous healing knowledge, which would disadvantage traditionalist African culture adherents (Levers, 2006a, 2006b).

Despite the fact that traditional healers are highly visible as healthcare providers to millions of indigenous Africans, their collaboration with public health services is marginal (Elujoba et al., 2005; Levers, 2006b; Mpofu et al., 2010). Increasingly, some traditional healers have incorporated biomedical practices into their healing activities, thereby identifying with both traditional and allopathic medical procedures (Marsland, 2007). Traditional healer referrals to public health services are also on the increase (Harper et al., 2004; Marsland, 2007; Sorsdahl et al., 2010), portending greater health benefit to African culture followers consulting with traditional healers than hitherto. Moreover, traditional healing practice is professionalizing across the continent, and the Traditional Healers Organization of Africa represents the entire continent and has local chapters in various countries (Chavunduka, 1986; Levers, 2006b). The World Health Organization (WHO, 1978, 2001) is for collaboration between biomedical and indigenous healing communities, which would allow African culture adherents choice of health services to access. However, for the most part, Western medicine in Africa has remained reluctant to collaborate with the healers (Bateman, 2010; Levers, 2006a, 2006b), presenting a barrier to inclusive health care practices for the benefit of the general population. On the one hand, traditionalist culture Africans are at risk from "charlatan" or "renegade" healing practices from untrained healer practitioners seeking economic gains (Levers, 2006b). On the other hand, charlatan practices also swell the ranks for modern medicine, with serious health risks to unsuspecting African culture followers (Attaran et al., 2004; Pepper & Slabbert, 2011).

3.5 Health Norm Identity Development in African Culture Communities: A Research Protocol Proposal

To create interventions to improve the health and wellbeing of African culture communities, research needs to ask if an intervention will benefit only those with a particular cultural orientation (traditionalist, transitional or modern). Without that knowledge, otherwise promising health care interventions run the risk of poor adoption, perpetuating health care disparities across communities. Conversely, to the extent that research identifies interventions aligned to African culture value orientations in their diversity, the interventions would be easy to disseminate and use with the culture followers. Yet, there is limited research health norms development among African culture community followers on the spectrum of social affiliations from traditionalist to modern (Abdullahi, 2011; Mpofu et al., 2010). Moreover, African culture adherents self-identifying with the same social affiliations might vary in their health norms, depending on their personal preferences. In fact, it might not be the "Africanness" that determines an individual's health norms; rather, an African culture follower's health norms might be from the personal experiences with and rewards from accessing various health system services. Thus, there is need for research on the varied pathways to adoption of health practices between and within cultural value orientations.

As previous discussion clearly shows, African culture affiliation statuses may influence health norms adoption through the activities and actions the followers would engage. That being the case, research on health norms development in African culture settings should examine the salient health activities and actions across the three orientations: traditionalist, transitional or modern (see also Gyasi et al., 2016). Within culture orientations, prospective health norms development interventions should take regard of the gendered and religion social affiliation identities as well as preference for modern medicine and traditional or complementary medicine. The ensuing discussion considers a prospective research protocol to advance health norms development among African culture followers.

As previously noted, African culture, followers construct their health norms within social affiliations, which the followers perceive to be binding on their health

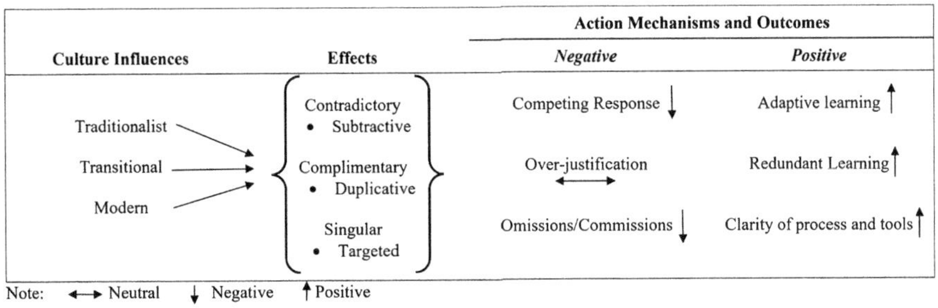

Fig. 3.1 Prospective research protocol on influences on African Culture follower health norms development

activities and actions. African culture followers would engage in health activities they interpret to give expression to their social affiliations, the context of personal values (Chipeta et al., 2010; Mpofu et al., 2011). African culture followers would develop interpretive heath norms, in the absence of explicit guidelines (as is typically the case with oral tradition, participatory learning cultures: Lew-Levy et al., 2019). Adoption of interpretive health norms by African culture followers presents a window of opportunity for public health promotion initiatives with them. This opportunity is from the fact that interpretive health norms are flexible or adaptable, allowing for uptake of public health promotion interventions not previously considered (Mpofu, 2018).

As observed previously, African culture followers differ in the extent to which they allow scope for interpretive health norms. For instance, the more traditionalist African culture has a strongly homogenizing effect against social action innovation by the followers, narrowing the scope for interpretative health norms by the individual members for collaboration with public health services (Chipeta et al., 2010; Kabagenyi et al., 2016). The more liberal African culture adherents (e.g., modern) would allow wider scope to the members to adopt interpretive health norms, enhancing their participation of public health services (Gyasi et al., 2016). Three processes could explain resultant health norms with traditionalist modern culture or transitional culture influences with personal choice: prioritization, negotiation, and complementarity (see Fig. 3.1).

Prioritization Traditionalist African culture followers prioritize health norms premised on metaphysical beliefs only (Chavunduka, 1986; Gyasi et al., 2016; Levers et al., 2006; Mpofu et al., 2010). In this case, a traditionalist culture value orientation singularly explains the health norms of the followers. As an example, belief in the omni-presence of ancestors (the living-dead) in daily life provides ongoing interpretive context for prevalent chronic health conditions (Masuku & Khoza-Shangase, 2018) and including resilient living (Van Leeuwen et al., 2016; Mpofu et al., 2010). Those with traditionalist culture adherence prefer traditional or alternative complementary medicine (Mpofu et al., 2010; Peltzer, 2009), grounded in strong religion beliefs (Bojuwoye, 2005; Levers, 2006a, 2006b; Mpofu, 2010). Adherence to traditionalist culture values only, would carry the strength of clarity of health norms, inclusive of the processes and tools for promoting personal health (Makgahlela & Sodi, 2017).

Similarly, beliefs in the public health services rather than traditional or complementary medicine practices would explain health norms among African modern culture followers. For instance, modern culture adherence was associated with universal uptake of preventive health interventions than would be the case with traditionalist culture values, even when adherents had misgivings about its claims (Smith, 2003; WHO, 2000; Williams & Calnan, 1996).

Adherence to a singular health norms identity carries health risks from disvaluing other valid ways to health. For instance, some adulthood initiation ceremonies may overlook the health needs of the vulnerable youths who may benefit from options to learning adulthood roles differently (Bojuwoye, 2005; Meissner & Buso, 2007; Mogotlane et al., 2004). In this case, the traditionalist culture rites of passage may be harmful to some children from not implementing collaboratively with public health care facilities. African culture followers with a modern orientation only may miss the benefits of traditional or alternative medicine, where it may be a best choice for some health conditions. For instance, typical African culture followers held to the belief that traditional or complementary medicines are of incremental value to treatment care beyond outcomes with modern medicine alone (Nuwaha & Musinguzi, 2013).

Prospectively, unlike transitional culture or modern culture adherents, *transitional culture* followers with their emerging health identities, may adopt a bicultural or hybrid health norms. However, bicultural or hybrid health norms may carry risk of suboptimal health norms for navigating the tensions of competing African traditionalist culture and modern public health practices.

Negotiation African culture followers perceiving competing traditionalist culture and modern culture influences may seek for negotiated health norms to resolve the costs to health outcomes from conflicting values. The health norms cost would arise from the *subtractive effect* of the traditionalist and modern culture orientations resulting in weaker health norms. This would be the case with transitional culture followers conflicted to accept both traditional and modern medicine, whilst also wanting the benefits of both medical systems (Chipeta et al., 2010; Mpofu et al., 2010). Business management studies reported a similar subtractive effect from counter-interference between externally and internally focused change interventions (Hartnell et al., 2011). This subtractive effect could result from contrasting values generating competing responses (active vs. passive health norms) with weaker resultant health norms than would be the case if with adherence to a singular influence value system (i.e., traditionalist or modern culture).

There is evidence from public health studies to suggest lower commitment and motivation to engage public health services by traditionalist African culture followers perceiving to be processing two potentially competing health norms (Gyasi et al., 2016; Mpofu et al., 2010; Nuwaha & Musinguzi, 2013). The fact is that the risk for mortality from preventable and treatable health conditions is higher among traditionalist African culture followers whose health norms are weakened by what they perceive to be competing knowledge systems (Chipeta et al., 2010; Mogotlane et al., 2004; Shweder, 2000). Thus, weaker health norms resulting from competing value systems may lower commitment and motive to engage in healthy behaviors.

However, competing influences on personal health norms also may have the beneficial effect of *adaptive learning* from attempts to resolve contradictions with reflection (Hofer et al., 2007; Volet, 1997). Emergent health values may result from successful resolution of contradictory health norm with adaptive learning. This effect may result from the higher personal investment in adaptive learning resulting in a stronger commitment to the negotiated health norms (Hofer et al., 2009).

Complementarity Traditionalist culture and modern culture influences may augment or complement each other resulting in an *additive effect* on health norms among African culture followers. For instance, across the spectrum of African culture value orientations (traditionalist, transitional and modern), people would value the benefits of healthy life styles. A traditionalist culture interpretation would consider adherence to a healthy life style consistent with participatory health with the community, including the living-dead in one's health choices whereas a modern culture would foreground public health access and services (Mpofu et al., 2010; Mpofu et al., 2011). A modern culture health norms orientation may benchmark health behaviors against objective epidemiological evidence rather than on anecdotal local community evidence as would be the case with a traditionalist culture orientation. Conceivably, strong health norms may result from the mutual reinforcement of health behaviors supported across culture orientations. Multiple cultural pathways to the same health norms would make for more reliable translation into related health behaviors than with a single cultural pathway.

However, redundancy in health values may not necessarily result in stronger health norms than with adherence to singular value system. A redundancy loss effect (Mayer et al., 2001) or over-justification effect (Ryan & Deci, 2000, 2002) may result in weaker overall health norms. A *redundancy loss effect* may result from split attention to seemingly disparate cultural orientation system influences than otherwise would be the case if attending to a single cultural influence system (i.e., traditionalist or modern). In the latter case, attending to more of the same is less beneficial than attending to one stimuli of a type (Mayer et al., 2001; Ryan & Deci, 2000, 2002). Ryan and Deci (2000, 2002) proposed a self-determination motivational response by which if actions over-justified, they take away from their self-direction. Applied to health norms acquisition with African culture adherents, the joint or overlapping effect of traditionalist, transitional and modern cultural orientations mediated by personal choice could result in non-committal or neutral strength health norms. In other words, neutral strength health norms would result with dualism, in which people straddled between modern and traditionalist health norms, with no commitment to either (Chipeta et al., 2010; Thwala et al., 2012). Moreover, people may be driven in their choices by what they believe to self-determine their social outcomes (inclusive of health) (Ng et al., 2012) so that their health norms ultimately derive from personal choice alone. Regardless, with traditionalist African culture following, volition in health norms would be aspirational, due to the controlling effects of affiliation beliefs (Gyasi et al., 2016; Mpofu et al., 2010).

3.6 Summary and Conclusion

Social affiliation lies at the core of who a person is and shapes the ways by which the individual perceives and engages with the world. In collectivistic African culture communities, social affiliation would explain the health norms people practice. While there are various shades of adherence to African cultural values, followers likely adopt those health norms they perceive to work for them in the context of prevailing health needs. The typical African culture follower likely holds to health norms aligned with traditionalist beliefs, even with access to modern public health services. Similarly, African culture followers with a knowledge of public health services may still consult traditional or complementary medicine with social affiliation others who valued traditional medicine more.

Those African culture followers who perceive benefit from both traditional and modern health services would be with health norms that overlap across culture orientations. They may derive superior health outcomes from the mutual reinforcement of their health beliefs and practices. African culture followers who held either traditionalist or modern health service preferences may optimize on the health benefits of the particular care orientation they hold, while potentially losing out on the benefits of the care practices of alternative affiliation system. There is evidence to suggest that African culture followers would adopt dual health norms, which they implement in parallel fashion. Research needs to provide guidance on health norms development among African culture followers across the spectrum of social affiliations: prioritization, negotiation and complementarity. The evidence for health service utilization by African culture followers with these competing health norms is still preliminary, and yet to be competitively tested. However, findings would inform public health policy for best practices in health norms development with African culture followers. Moreover, a health norms development framework to result from the research would guide evolving partnerships between African traditional and modern medicine practices.

References

Abdullahi, A. A. (2011). Trends and challenges of traditional medicine in Africa. *African Journal of Traditional, Complementary and Alternative Medicines, 8*(5S), 115–123.

Afolabi, O. A., & Dennis, U. (2019). Reciprocal altruism: It's relationship to locus of control and dispositional optimism among Nigerian undergraduates. *Journal of Psychology in Africa, 29*(2), 155–158. https://doi.org/10.1080/14330237.2019.1594652

Agadjanian, V. (2005). Fraught with ambivalence: Reproductive intentions and contraceptive choices in a sub-Saharan fertility transition. *Population Research and Policy Review, 24*(6), 617–645.

Agulanna, C. (2010). Community and human well-being in an African culture. *Trames, 14*(3), 282–297.

Asante, A. D., Zwi, A. B., & Ho, M. T. (2006). Equity in resource allocation for health: A comparative study of the Ashanti and northern regions of Ghana. *Health Policy, 78*(2–3), 135–148.

Attaran, A., Barnes, K. I., Curtis, C., d'Alessandro, U., Fanello, C. I., Galinski, M. R., ... Talisuna, A. (2004). WHO, the Global Fund, and medical malpractice in malaria treatment. *The Lancet, 363*(9404), 237–240.

Bateman, C. (2010). Bridging the divide: Anthropologist/sangoma challenges delegates. *South African Medical Journal, 100*(2), 80–81.

Berry, J. W. (1997). Immigration, acculturation and adaptation. *International Journal of Applied Psychology, 46*(5), 5–34.

Bojuwoye, O. (2005). Traditional healing practices in southern Africa: Ancestral spirits, ritual ceremonies and holistic healing. In R. Moodley & W. West (Eds.), *Integrating traditional healing practices into counseling and psychotherapy* (pp. 61–72). Sage.

Brenner, L. (2001). *Controlling knowledge: Religion, power and schooling in a west African Muslim society*. Indiana University Press.

Chavunduka, G. L. (1986). The organisation of traditional medicine in Zimbabwe. In M. Last & G. L. Chavunduka (Eds.), *The professionalisation of African medicine* (International African Seminars New Series, no. 1) (pp. 29–49). Manchester University Press in association with the International African Institute.

Chipeta, E. K., Chimwaza, W., & Kalilani-Phiri, L. (2010). Contraceptive knowledge, beliefs and attitudes in rural Malawi: Misinformation, misbeliefs and misperceptions. *Malawi Medical Journal, 22*(2), 38–41. https://doi.org/10.4314/mmj.v22i2.58790

Cohen, S. (2004). Social relationships and health. *American Psychologist, 59*(8), 676.

Cole, M., & Engeström, Y. (2007). Cultural-historical approaches to designing for development. In J. Valsiner & A. Rosa (Eds.), *The Cambridge handbook of sociocultural psychology* (pp. 484–507). Cambridge University Press. https://doi.org/10.1017/CBO9780511611162.026

Cramm, J. M., Møller, V., & Nieboer, A. P. (2012). Individual-and neighbourhood-level indicators of subjective well-being in a small and poor Eastern Cape township: The effect of health, social capital, marital status, and income. *Social Indicators Research, 105*(3), 581–593.

Deaton, A. (2008). Income, health, and well-being around the world: Evidence from the Gallup World Poll. *Journal of Economic Perspectives, 22*(2), 53–72.

Edwards, S. D. (2016). The global coherence initiative: A global psychological paradigm for health promotion. *Journal of Psychology in Africa, 26*(2), 194–198. https://doi.org/10.1080/14330237.2016.1163915

Elujoba, A. A., Odeleye, O. M., & Ogunyemi, C. M. (2005). Traditional medicine development for medical and dental primary health care delivery system in Africa. *African Journal of Traditional, Complementary, and Alternative Medicines, 2*(1), 46–61.

Engeström, Y. (1999). *Learning, working and imagining: Twelve studies in activity theory*. Orienta-Konsultit.

Francis, S. A., Battle-Fisher, M., Liverpool, J., Hipple, L., Mosavel, M., Soogun, S., & Mofammere, N. (2011). A qualitative analysis of South African women's knowledge, attitudes, and beliefs about HPV and cervical cancer prevention, vaccine awareness and acceptance, and maternal-child communication about sexual health. *Vaccine, 29*(47), 8760–8765.

Galderisi, S., Heinz, A., Kastrup, M., Beezhold, J., & Sartorius, N. (2015). Toward a new definition of mental health. *World Psychiatry, 14*(2), 231–233.

Giddens, A. (2000). *Runaway world: How globalization is reshaping our lives*. Routledge.

Gough, I., Wood, G., Barrientos, A., Bevan, P., Room, G., & Davis, P. (2004). *Insecurity and welfare regimes in Asia, Africa and Latin America: Social policy in development contexts*. Cambridge University Press.
Gyasi, R. M., Asante, F., Abass, K., Yeboah, J. Y., Adu-Gyamfi, S., & Amoah, P. A. (2016). Do health beliefs explain traditional medical therapies utilisation? Evidence from Ghana. *Cogent Social Sciences, 2*(1). https://doi.org/10.1080/23311886.2016.1209995
Haddad, B. (2013). Religion & AIDS in Africa. *Population Studies, 67*(2), 252–254. https://doi.org/10.1080/00324728.2013.790604
Haidt, J., Koller, S. H., & Dias, M. G. (1993). Affect, culture, and morality, or is it wrong to eat your dog? *Journal of Personality and Social Psychology, 65*(4), 613–628.
Hallfors, D., Iritani, B., Cho, Y., Lusano, W., Mpofu, E., & Rusakaniko, S. (2016). "I thought if I marry the prophet I would not die": Religion as context for marriage, HIV prevention, and reproductive health among young orphaned wives in Zimbabwe. *Journal of the Psychosocial Aspects of HIV and AIDS, 13*(1), 178–187.
Harper, M. E., Hill, P. C., Bah, A. H., Manneh, K., McAdam, K. P. W. J., & Lienhardt, C. (2004). Traditional healers participate in tuberculosis control in The Gambia. *The International Journal of Tuberculosis and Lung Disease, 8*(10), 1266–1268.
Hartnell, C. A., Ou, A. Y., & Kinicki, A. (2011). Organizational culture and organizational effectiveness: A meta-analytic investigation of the competing values framework's theoretical suppositions. *Journal of Applied Psychology, 96*(4), 677–694.
Hofer, M., Schmid, S., Fries, S., Dietz, F., Clausen, M., & Reinders, H. (2007). Individual values, motivational conflicts and learning for school. *Learning and Instruction, 17*(1), 17–28.
Hofer, M., Schmid, S., Fries, S., Zivkovic, I., & Dietz, F. (2009). Value orientations and studying in school–leisure conflict: A study with samples from five countries. *Learning and Individual Differences, 19*(1), 101–112.
Holland, D., Lachicotte, W. S., Skinner, D., & Cain, C. (2001). *Identity and agency in cultural worlds*. Harvard University Press.
Hutchison, E. D. (2015). *Dimensions of human behavior: The changing life course* (5th ed.). Sage.
Idang, G. E. (2015). African culture and values. *Phronimon, 16*(2), 97–111.
Johnson, J. L., Greaves, L., & Repta, R. (2009). Better science with sex and gender: Facilitating the use of a sex and gender-based analysis in health research. *International Journal for Equity in Health, 8*(1), 14. https://doi.org/10.1186/1475-9276-8-14
Kabagenyi, A., Reid, A., Ntozi, J., & Atuyambe, L. (2016). Socio-cultural inhibitors to use of modern contraceptive techniques in rural Uganda: A qualitative study. *The Pan African Medical Journal, 25*, 78. https://doi.org/10.11604/pamj.2016.25.78.6613
Kalipeni, E., & Oppong, J. (1998). The refugee crisis in Africa and implications for health and disease: A political ecology approach. *Social Science & Medicine, 46*(12), 1637–1653.
Karmon, A. (2007). Institution organization of knowledge: The missing link in educational discourse. *Teacher's College Record, 109*, 603–634.
Kelman, H. C. (2006). Interests, relationships, identities: Three central issues for individuals and groups in negotiating their social environment. *Annual Review of Psychology, 57*, 1–26.
Kunst, J. R., Thomsen, L., Sam, D. L., & Berry, J. W. (2015). "We are in this together": Common group identity predicts majority members' active acculturation efforts to integrate immigrants. *Personality and Social Psychology Bulletin, 41*(10), 1438–1453.
Leont'ev, A. N. (1978). *Activity, consciousness, and personality*. Prentice-Hall.
Levers, L. L. (2006a). Samples of indigenous healing: The path of good medicine. *International Journal of Disability, Development, and Education, 54*, 479–488.
Levers, L. L. (2006b). Traditional healing as indigenous knowledge: Its relevance to HIV/AIDS in Southern Africa and the implications for counselors. *Journal of Psychology in Africa, 16*, 87–100.
Levers, L. L., Kamanzi, D., Mukamana, D., Pells, K., & Bhusumane, D.-B. (2006). Addressing urgent community mental health needs in Rwanda: Culturally sensitive training interventions. *Journal of Psychology in Africa, 16*, 261–272.

Lew-Levy, S., Crittenden, A. N., Boyette, A. H., Mabulla, I. A., Hewlett, B. S., & Lamb, M. E. (2019). Inter- and intra-cultural variation in learning-through-participation among Hadza and BaYaka forager children and adolescents from Tanzania and the Republic of Congo. *Journal of Psychology in Africa, 29*(4), 309–318. https://doi.org/10.1080/14330237.2019.1647957

Luke, N., & Munshi, K. (2007). Social affiliation and the demand for health services: Caste and child health in South India. *Journal of Development Economics, 83*(2), 256–279.

MacQueen, K., McLellan, E., Metzger, D., Kegeles, S., Strauss, R., Scotti, R., et al. (2001). What is community? An evidence-based definition for participatory public health. *American Journal of Public Health, 91*(12), 1929–1938.

Makgahlela, M. W., & Sodi, T. (2017). Cultural conceptions of a bereavement-related illness in a South African indigenous community. *Journal of Psychology in Africa, 26*(6), 541–545. https://doi.org/10.1080/14330237.2016.1250407

Marsland, R. (2007). The modern traditional healer: Locating 'hybridity' in modern traditional medicine, southern Tanzania. *Journal of Southern African Studies, 33*, 751–765.

Märtsin, M. (2008). *Identity construction as a personal sense-making process: A case study of Estonian students in the United Kingdom* (Doctoral thesis). University of Bath. Retrieved from http://opus.bath.ac.uk/

Masuku, K. P., & Khoza-Shangase, K. (2018). Spirituality as a coping mechanism for family caregivers of persons with aphasia. *Journal of Psychology in Africa, 28*(3), 245–248. https://doi.org/10.1080/14330237.2018.1475518

Mayer, R. E., Heiser, J., & Lonn, S. (2001). Cognitive constraints on multimedia learning: When presenting more material results in less understanding. *Journal of Educational Psychology, 93*(1), 187.

Mbiti, J. S. (1991). *An introduction to African religion* (2nd ed.). Heinemann.

Mcommh, A. S. S., Crawshaw, P., & Oakley, A. (2015). "Men behaving badly": Patriarchy, public policy and health inequalities. *International Journal of Men's Health, 14*(3), 250.

Meissner, O., & Buso, D. L. (2007). Traditional male circumcision in the eastern cape – Scourge or blessing? *South African Medical Journal, 97*(5), 371–373.

Mogotlane, S. M., Ntlangulela, J. T., & Ogunbanjo, B. G. A. (2004). Mortality and morbidity among traditionally circumcised Xhosa boys in the eastern Cape Province, South Africa. *Curationis, 27*(2), 57–62.

Mpofu, E. (1994). Exploring the self-concept in an African culture. *Journal of Genetic Psychology, 155*, 341–354.

Mpofu, E. (2003). Conduct disorder: Presentation, treatment options and cultural efficacyin an African setting. *International Journal of Disability, Community and Rehabilitation, 2*, 1. Retrieved December 22, 2005, from http://www.ijdcr.ca/VOL02_01_CAN/articles/mpofu.shtml

Mpofu, E. (2006). Majority world health care traditions intersect indigenous and complementary and alternative medicine (Editorial for special issue on indigenous healing practices). *International Journal of Disability, Development and Education, 53*, 375–379.

Mpofu, E. (Ed.). (2010). *Counseling people of African ancestry*. Cambridge University Press.

Mpofu, E. (Ed.). (2015). *Community-oriented health services: Practices across disciplines*. Springer.

Mpofu, E. (2016). Follower-centric influences on sexual decision making in a Pentecostal church faith community. *Religions, 7*, 66. https://doi.org/10.3390/rel7060066

Mpofu, E. (2018). How religion frames health norms: A structural theory approach. *Religions, 9*(4), 119. https://doi.org/10.3390/rel9040119

Mpofu, E., Dune, T. M., Hallfors, D. D., Mapfumo, J., Mutepha, M. M., & January, J. (2011). Apostolic faith organization contexts for health and well-being in women and children. *Ethnicity and Health, 16*(6), 551–566.

Mpofu, E., Hadjida, H., & Levers, L. L. (in press). Identity development among African youth refugee immigrants to Australia. In S. S. Chuang, D. J. Johnson, S. Rasmi, & J. Glozman (Eds).

Formation and identity: The intersectionality of development, culture, and immigration. Springer.

Mpofu, E., Peltzer, K., & Bojuwoye, O. (2010). Indigenous healing practices in sub-Saharan Africa. In E. Mpofu (Ed.), *Counseling people of African ancestry* (pp. 3–21). Cambridge University Press.

Mumby, D. K. (1987). The political function of narrative in organizations. *Communication Monographs, 54*, 113–127.

Mutale, W., Chintu, N., Amoroso, C., Awoonor-Williams, K., Phillips, J., Baynes, C., Michel, C., Taylor, A., & Sherr, K. (2013). Improving health information systems for decision making across five sub-Saharan African countries: Implementation strategies from the African Health Initiative. *BMC Health Services Research, 13*(2), S9. https://doi.org/10.1186/1472-6963-13-S2-S95

Ng, J. Y. Y., Ntoumanis, N., Thogersen-Ntoumani, C., Deci, E. L., Ryan, R. M., Dudd, J. L., & Williams, G. C. (2012). Self-determination theory applied to health contexts: A meta-analysis. *Perspectives on Psychological Science, 7*(4), 325–340.

Nsamenang, A. B. (2006). Human ontogenesis: An indigenous African view on development and intelligence. *International Journal of Psychology, 41*, 293–297.

Nsamenang, A. B. (2008). Culture and human development. *International Journal of Psychology, 43*(2), 73–77.

Nuwaha, F., & Musinguzi, G. (2013). Use of alternative medicine for hypertension in Buikwe and Mukono districts of Uganda: A cross sectional study. *BMC Complementary and Alternative Medicine, 13*(1), 301. https://doi.org/10.1186/1472-6882-13-301

Owuse, S. A. (2019). "Do unto others what you want. . .": Reciprocity and childcare in the Kumasi metropolis of Ghana. *Journal of Psychology in Africa, 29*(5), 466–473.

Patai, R. (1973). *The Arab mind*. Charles Scribner's Sons.

Peltzer, K. (2009). Utilization and practice of traditional/complementary/alternative medicine (TM/CAM) in South Africa. *African Journal of Traditional, Complementary, and Alternative Medicines, 6*(2), 175–185.

Penuel, W. R., & Wertsch, J. V. (1995). Vygotsky and identity formation: A sociocultural approach. *Educational Psychologist, 30*(2), 83–92.

Pepper, M. S., & Slabbert, M. N. (2011). Is South Africa on the verge of a medical malpractice litigation storm? *South African Journal of Bioethics and Law, 4*(1), 29–35.

Polo, G., Acosta, C. M., Ferreira, F., & Dias, R. A. (2015). Location-allocation and accessibility models for improving the spatial planning of public health services. *PLoS One, 10*(3), e0119190.

Rugira, J., Nienaber, A. W., & Wissing, M. P. (2013). Psychological well-being among Tanzanian University students. *Journal of Psychology in Africa, 23*(3), 425–430.

Ryan, R. M., & Deci, E. L. (2000). Self-determination theory and the facilitation of intrinsic motivation, social development, and well-being. *American Psychologist, 55*, 68–78.

Ryan, R. M., & Deci, E. L. (2002). An overview of self-determination theory: An organismic-dialectical perspective. In E. L. Deci & R. M. Ryan (Eds.), *Handbook of self-determination research* (pp. 3–33). University of Rochester Press.

Shell-Duncan, B. (2008). From health to human rights: Female genital cutting and the politics of intervention. *American Anthropologist, 110*(2), 225–236.

Shweder, R. A. (2000). What about "female genital mutilation"? And why understanding culture matters in the first place. *Daedalus, 129*(4), 209–232.

Shweder, R. A., Haidt, J., Horton, R., & Joseph, C. (2008). The cultural psychology of the emotions: Ancient and renewed. In M. Lewis, J. M. Haviland-Jones, & L. F. Barrett (Eds.), *Handbook of emotions* (pp. 409–427). The Guilford Press.

Shweder, R. A., Much, N. C., Mahapatra, M., & Park, L. (1997). The "big three" of morality (autonomy, community, divinity) and the "big three" explanations of suffering. In A. M. Brandt & P. Rozin (Eds.), *Morality and health* (pp. 119–169). Taylor & Frances/Routledge.

Smith, R. (2003). Limits to medicine. Medical nemesis: The expropriation of health. *Journal of Epidemiology & Community Health, 57*(12), 928–928.

Smith, C., Denton, M. L., Faris, R., & Regnerus, M. (2002). Mapping American adolescent religious participation. *Journal for the Scientific Study of Religion, 41*(4), 597–612.

Sodi, T., & Phethi, T. (2017). Influences on help-seeking pathways among people with chronic illness and disease in a rural South African community. *Journal of Psychology in Africa, 27*(3), 286–289.

Sorsdahl, K., Stein, D. J., & Flisher, A. J. (2010). Traditional healer attitudes and beliefs regarding referral of the mentally ill to Western doctors in South Africa. *Transcultural Psychiatry, 47*(4), 591–609.

Stetsenko, A., & Arievitch, I. (2004). The self in cultural-historical activity theory: Reclaiming the unity of social and individual dimensions of human development. *Theory and Psychology, 14*(4), 475–503.

Tanser, F., Gijsbertsen, B., & Herbst, K. (2006). Modelling and understanding primary health care accessibility and utilization in rural South Africa: An exploration using a geographical information system. *Social Science & Medicine, 63*(3), 691–705.

Thwala, S. B., Holroyd, E., & Jones, L. K. (2012). Health belief dualism in the postnatal practices of rural Swazi women: An ethnographic account. *Women and Birth, 25*(4), e68–e74.

United Nations High Commissioner for Refugees. (2019). *Handbook and guidelines on procedures and criteria for determining refugee status under the 1951 Convention and the 1967 Protocol Relating to the Status of Refugees*. Retrieved on May 1, 2021 from http://www.refworld.org/docid/4f33c8d92.html

United Nations Programme on HIV/AIDS. (2000). *Collaboration with traditional healers in HIV/AIDS prevention and care in sub-Saharan Africa: A literature review*. Joint United Nations Programme on HIV/AIDS.

Van der Merwe, K., Ntinda, K., & Mpofu, E. (2016). African perspective of personality psychology. In L. Nicholas (Ed.), *Personality psychology* (pp. 53–69). Oxford University Press Southern Africa.

Van Leeuwen, J. M., Adkins, S., Mirassou-Wolf, T., Schweiger, W. K., & Grundy, R. (2016). An evaluation of the mental health facilitator programme in rural Uganda: Successes and recommendations for future implementation. *Journal of Psychology in Africa, 26*(3), 288–299.

Volet, S. E. (1997). Cognitive and affective variables in academic learning: The significance of direction and effort in students' goals. *Learning and Instruction, 7*(3), 235–254.

Vygotsky, L. S. (1978). *Mind in society: The development of higher psychological processes*. Harvard University Press.

Wertsch, J. V. (1991). A sociocultural approach to socially shared cognition. In L. B. Resnick, J. M. Levine, & S. D. Teasley (Eds.), *Perspectives on socially shared cognition* (pp. 85–100). American Psychological Association. https://doi.org/10.1037/10096-004

Williams, S. J., & Calnan, M. (1996). The 'limits' of medicalization?: Modern medicine and the lay populace in 'late'modernity. *Social Science & Medicine, 42*(12), 1609–1620.

World Health Organization. (1978). *The promotion and development of traditional medicine. Technical reports services, 666*. Author.

World Health Organization. (2000). *The world health report 2000: Health systems: Improving performance*. Author.

World Health Organization. (2001). *Legal status of traditional medicine and complimentary/alternative medicine: A worldwide review*. Retrieved May 22, 2008, from http://www.who.int/medicinedocs/index.fcgi?sid=Q10rVtjd9ee80ca7000000004742e93f&a=d&c=medicinedocs&d=Jh2943e.10#Jh2943e.10

World Health Organization. (2004). *Preamble to the constitution of the World Health Organization as adopted by the International Health Conference, New York, 1948*. Retrieved September 28, 2020, from http://www.who.int/about

World Health Organization. (2018). *Gender, equity and human rights: General Information.* Retrieved on June 6, 2020 from: http://www.who.int/gender-equity-rights/understanding/gender-definition/en/

Part II
Measuring Well-Being in Africa

Chapter 4
Factorial Validity of the Twi Version of the Mental Health Continuum-Short Form and Prevalence of Mental Health in a Rural Ghanaian Sample

Richard Appiah, Marié P. Wissing, Angelina Wilson Fadiji, and Lusilda Schutte

Abstract Positive mental health, and the validity of its assessment instruments, are largely unexplored in the Ghanaian context. This study examined the factor structure of the Twi version of the Mental Health Continuum-Short Form and explored the prevalence of positive mental health in a sample of rural Ghanaian adults ($N = 444$). A bifactor exploratory structural equation modelling (ESEM) model fit the data better than competing models (confirmatory factor analysis [CFA], bifactor CFA, and ESEM models). We found a high omega reliability coefficient for the general positive mental health factor ($\omega = .97$) and marginal reliability scores for the emotional ($\omega = .51$) and social well-being ($\omega = .57$) subscales, but a low reliability score for the psychological well-being subscale ($\omega = .41$). Findings support the existence of a general mental health factor, and confirm the underlying three-dimensional structure of mental health, but suggest that caution should be applied when interpreting subscale scores, especially for the psychological well-being subscale. Based on Keyes's criteria for the categorical diagnosis of the presence of positive mental health, 25.5% of the sample were flourishing, with 74.5%

R. Appiah (✉)
Africa Unit for Transdisciplinary Health Research, Faculty of Health Sciences, North-West University, Potchefstroom, South Africa

College of Health Sciences, University of Ghana, Accra, Ghana
e-mail: riappiah@ug.edu.gh

M. P. Wissing · L. Schutte
Africa Unit for Transdisciplinary Health Research, Faculty of Health Sciences, North-West University, Potchefstroom, South Africa

A. Wilson Fadiji
Africa Unit for Transdisciplinary Health Research, Faculty of Health Sciences, North-West University, Potchefstroom, South Africa

Department of Educational Psychology, Faculty of Education, University of Pretoria, Pretoria, South Africa

L. Schutte et al. (eds.), *Embracing Well-Being in Diverse African Contexts: Research Perspectives*, Cross-Cultural Advancements in Positive Psychology 16,
https://doi.org/10.1007/978-3-030-85924-4_4

functioning at suboptimal levels (31.1% languishing, 41.4% with moderate mental health) and may benefit from contextually relevant positive psychological interventions, which may also buffer against psychopathology.

Keywords Mental health continuum-short form · Translation of measurement instrument · Psychological well-being · Structural validity · Rural poor · Twi · Ghana

4.1 Introduction

There is an increasing trend towards exploring constructs and factors that promote human flourishing and positive mental health. Over the past decade, researchers have made considerable efforts to formulate, pilot-test, and implement strengths-based interventions to optimise positive human experiences and functioning of individuals, families, communities, and organisations (Appiah, Wilson Fadiji et al., 2020; Bolier et al., 2013; Wellenzohn et al., 2018; Woodworth et al., 2016). Until recently, mental health was equated to the absence of mental illness (Keyes, 2005; Keyes & Martin, 2017). However, presently, researchers, clinicians, and public health practitioners acknowledge that a complete state of health is not only the absence of disease (Keyes, 2014; Kühn & Rieger, 2017). Mental health is now understood as a multidimensional construct, where individuals manifest the characteristics of positive mental health as well as the absence of mental illness (Keyes, 2002, 2014; Weiss et al., 2016), rather than just the absence of psychopathological symptoms. Mental health is operationalised and defined as a state of *well-being* (Galderisi et al., 2015). In its simplest term, well-being refers to appropriate psychological functioning (Heintzelman, 2018; Keyes, 2006) and can be understood as a positive attribute which consists of objective (e.g., possession of material resources such as having a home, education, or health care) and subjective (an individual's perception about his or her own life) well-being (Diener et al., 2018; Diener & Ryan, 2009).

4.1.1 Operationalisation of Well-Being

Two main conceptual perspectives on well-being have been postulated: hedonic and eudaimonic (Delle Fave et al., 2011; Kahneman et al., 1999). Whereas the hedonic perspective associates subjective well-being with the experience of positive emotions, higher life satisfaction, and reduction of negative emotions (Diener & Ryan, 2009; Kahneman et al., 1999), the eudaimonic view of well-being refers to an individual's realisation of his or her highest potential that results in optimal positive functioning in life (Ryff & Keyes, 1995; Waterman, 2013). Eudaimonic well-being comprises two dimensions: psychological well-being (PWB; Ryff, 1989), which emphasises an individual's expression of optimal functioning, and social well-being

(SWB; Keyes, 1998), which reflects how well individuals function in their interactions with significant others.

Keyes (2002) conceptualised and proffered a tripartite model of mental health that describes three dimensions of mental health: emotional well-being (EWB), psychological well-being (PWB), and social well-being (SWB). While EWB describes the presence of positive affect and satisfaction with life, PWB reflects an individual's intrapersonal and close interpersonal functioning. SWB encompasses a sense of welfare and happiness, experiences of an individual's well-being in society, as well as individuals' satisfaction with their social structure and function (Keyes, 1998). A high level of positive mental health, called *flourishing*, requires the presence of a high level of subjective well-being (i.e., high levels of positive affect and life satisfaction; with low levels of negative affect) and an optimal level of psychological and social functioning. Similarly, an experience of low levels of subjective well-being and psychological and social functioning is termed *languishing*. Individuals whose scores do not fit the classification of flourishing or languishing are considered to be in *moderate mental health*. This tripartite model, together with empirical evidence from Ryff's (1989) model of psychological well-being, became the conceptual foundation that guided the development of the 40-item self-administered Mental Health Continuum-Long Form (MHC-LF; Keyes, 2002, 2005). An abridged 14-item version, the Mental Health Continuum-Short Form (MHC-SF, Keyes, 2005; Keyes et al., 2008) was later compiled to assess the three dimensions of well-being (psychological, emotional, and social well-being), and for the categorical diagnosis of positive mental health.

Keyes (2005) also distinguished between positive mental health and mental illness as existing on two continua. Keyes's dual-continua model assumes that positive mental health is related to, but is distinguishable from, mental illness (Keyes, 2005, 2014). Accordingly, an individual can present with symptoms of mental illness, such as a depressive episode, and simultaneously exhibit a high level of positive mental health (flourishing).

4.1.2 Instrument Validation in Well-Being Research: Language and Translation Issues

The need for consideration of the cultural context in assessing attributes of mental health has long been emphasised (Greenaway et al., 2018; Woody et al., 2015). Owing to vast cultural differences, for instance between Western and African societies, it is important that measures that were developed and normed in one cultural context are validated in other cultural contexts before their scores are interpreted (De Kock et al., 2013; Woody et al., 2015). For instance, most existing mental health measures in use for research and clinical practice in Ghana originate from Western countries, were developed from Western perspectives, standardised with predominantly Western samples, and assumed individualistic cultural orientation and value systems (Bermant et al., 2011). That there are cultural differences in the understanding and expression of mental health has been well established (Diener et al., 2018; Oishi, 2010). While research evidence has differentiated between East Asian (collectivistic) and Western (individualistic) expressions of well-being (e.g., Schimmack et al., 2002; Uchida & Kitayama, 2009), there is limited evidence from Africa, particularly from the Ghanaian context. Although a number of measurement instruments are currently used to assess mental health and well-being in various population groups in Ghana, only a few of these assessment tools (e.g., Multidimensional Scale of Perceived Social Support, General Health Questionnaire, Perceived Social Support from Family and the Friends Scale) have been validated in their original English versions by Wilson et al. (2016) and Glozah and Pevalin (2015, 2017), respectively. To our knowledge, only one study reports the process and findings from translating and validating the Twi versions of five selected measures of mental health and well-being in Ghana (Appiah, Schutte, et al., 2020).

There exist several questionnaires that assess various dimensions of mental well-being across the lifespan. However, most are either limited to assessing one dimension (e.g., Satisfaction with Life Scale [Diener et al., 1985]) or a few dimensions of well-being (e.g., Positive and Negative Affect Schedule [Watson et al., 1988]). Others are lengthy (e.g., World Health Organization Quality of Life-100 [WHOQOL Group, 1998]) or are bifocal, assessing both well-being and psychopathology (e.g., Affectometer 2 [Kammann & Flett, 1983]). A valid and reliable measure is needed that provides a complete assessment of mental health by considering all dimensions of well-being. The MHC-SF is a well-established multidimensional measure that assesses the dimensions of emotional, social, and psychological well-being. The MHC-SF has been translated and validated in several cultural contexts, including Dutch (Franken et al., 2018), Argentinean (Perugini et al., 2017), Iranian (Rafiey et al., 2017), Vietnamese (Rogoza et al., 2018), Serbian (Jovanovic, 2015), Italian (Petrillo et al., 2015), Polish (Karaś et al., 2014), and Afrikaans, English and Setswana samples from South Africa (Schutte & Wissing, 2017). However, at present, the MHC-SF has not been validated in its English version or in any local dialect for research in Ghana. Furthermore, although the validity of the MHC-SF has been widely explored, there is limited literature on its psychometric properties among rural samples (e.g., Keyes et al., 2008; Rogoza et al., 2018).

4.1.3 Factor Structure of the MHC-SF

Previous studies provide support for a three-factor structure of the MHC-SF, distinguishing EWB, SWB, and PWB (e.g., Kennes et al., 2020; Lamers et al., 2011; Perugini et al., 2017; Rafiey et al., 2017; Rogoza et al., 2018). In all cases, a correlated three-factor model produced a better fit than competing one- and two-factor models (with the latter distinguishing hedonic and eudaimonic factors, where the eudaimonic factor comprises social and psychological well-being items). The three-factor model has also demonstrated strict measurement invariance across gender and educational level (Joshanloo et al., 2013), as well as metric and partial scalar invariance across gender and educational groups (Karaś et al., 2014). Many studies examining the structure of the MHC-SF applied confirmatory factor analysis (CFA; e.g., Bower, 2017; Guo et al., 2018; Perugini et al., 2017; Rafiey et al., 2017).

However, CFA relies on the restrictive independent cluster model which does not account for two noteworthy sources of construct-relevant multidimensionality (Morin et al., 2016). First, CFA does not account for the hierarchical nature of psychological constructs where items can be expected to be associated with the intended specific factors (e.g., EWB, SWB, or PWB) as well as hierarchically-superior constructs (e.g., overall positive mental health; Morin et al., 2016). Second, in CFA, the cross-loadings of items on nontarget factors are assumed to be zero. This assumption does not account for the imperfect nature of items that operationalise psychological constructs where cross-loadings are often present, particularly in the case of conceptually overlapping constructs (Morin et al., 2016). This presents a potential risk for overly inflated factor loadings as a result of the absence of specified cross-loadings on the nontarget specific factors, which may also lead to an overestimation of factor correlations in situations when the nontarget loadings are not close to zero (Morin et al., 2016).

The first and second limitations of CFA are addressed by bifactor CFA (Reise, 2012) and exploratory structural equation modelling (ESEM; Asparouhov & Muthén, 2009), respectively. A bifactor CFA model separates the variance explained by the specific factors from the variance explained by the general factor. It determines whether there is a general underlying factor that directly affects the items in addition to the role the specific factors play (Marsh et al., 2014; Morin et al., 2016). ESEM incorporates exploratory factor analysis (EFA) within the framework of structural equation modelling and allows for the inclusion of cross-loadings (Marsh et al., 2014).

Nonetheless, researchers report that when testing bifactor models within a CFA structure, the strength of the general factor may become inflated when cross-loadings are not specified on the specific factors of the multidimensional constructs (Asparouhov & Muthén, 2009; Marsh et al., 2014; Rogoza et al., 2018). The bifactor ESEM model resolves this limitation by simultaneously allowing items to load on both general and specific factors as well as on all nontarget factors where cross-loadings are set as close to zero as possible (Lamborn et al., 2018; Longo et al., 2020; Morin et al., 2016). Recent empirical research that examined the factor structure of the MHC-SF using competing models for diverse populations found the three-factor bifactor ESEM model to best fit the data (see Lamborn et al., 2018; Longo et al., 2020; Schutte & Wissing, 2017; Silverman et al., 2018).

4.1.4 Prevalence of Positive Mental Health

The MHC-SF has been widely used to estimate the prevalence of positive mental health of adolescents and adults in various contexts. Comprehensive epidemiological surveillances focusing on optimal functioning of individuals and groups using the MHC-SF have associated high levels of mental health (flourishing) with superior physical and psychosocial functioning (Keyes, 2005), whereas, by contrast, negative outcomes such as poor emotional health, more missed days of work, and frequent limitations of daily living were related to low levels of well-being (languishing) (Keyes, 2002, 2005). Researchers found, for instance, a prevalence of 54.4% of flourishers among a sample of adolescents from West of Scotland (Bower, 2017), 51.8% among American college students (Keyes et al., 2012), 37.9% among American youth (Keyes, 2006), and 11.7% among Korean high school students (Lim, 2014). Comparatively, lower levels of flourishing have been reported for adults, including 28.5% among Italian adults (Petrillo et al., 2015). In a 2012 national survey of Canadians aged 15 or older, Gilmour (2014) reported a high prevalence of flourishing of 76.9%. All studies mentioned here based their rates of flourishing on scores on the MHC-SF.

A limited amount of research has explored the prevalence of positive mental health in Africa, with existing research focusing mostly on South African samples. For instance, Keyes et al. (2008) reported a rate of 20% flourishing, 67.8% moderate mental health, and 12.2% languishing for a sample of Setswana-speaking adults in the North West province of South Africa. Van Schalkwyk and Wissing (2010) also reported a rate of 5% languishing, 53% moderate mental health, and 42% flourishing for multicultural secondary school adolescents in the Western Cape Province of South Africa. Wissing and Temane (2013) also examined the proportion and correlates of positive mental health among various groups of South Africans and found flourishing rates ranging from 28% for a sample of teachers to 61.7% among rural Setswana-speaking adults, and languishing rates ranging from 1.5% among teachers to 9% among urban Setswana-speaking adults. Rugiera et al. (2013) found relatively high levels of flourishing for samples of undergraduate students from three Tanzanian universities (80.7%, 70.6%, and 68.3%, with an average of 72.7% flourishing). On average, 3.5% of participants languished and 23.6% reported moderate mental health. Salama-Younes (2011) also reported a 20% flourishing rate for a sample of Egyptian adolescents. Table 4.1 presents examples of percentages of positive mental health (flourishing and languishing) in different countries from previous studies.

In Ghana, studies that explore the concept and prevalence of positive mental health are limited. Consistently, the prevalence of mental health has been conceptualised and measured in terms of mental disorders. Most available studies employed proxies in their measurement of the presence of positive mental well-being. For instance, Pokimica et al. (2012) and Addai and Pokimica (2010) assessed subjective well-being by measuring individuals' standard of living rather than how they feel about their overall life. Previous research has explored the construct of well-being among various Ghanaian samples (see Asante, 2012; Doe, 2016; Glozah, 2015; Wilson & Somhlaba, 2016). However, as far as could be established, presently, there is a dearth of research that examines the prevalence of positive mental health in Ghana. Only two studies were retrieved that assessed the prevalence of mental health using the MHC-SF in a sample of rural adults (Appiah, Schutte, et al., 2020) and individuals with sickle cell disease (Appiah, Tutu, et al., 2020). Data on the positive mental health of a population could provide contextual understanding of

Table 4.1 Prevalence of positive mental health assessed by MHC-SF in previous studies

Author(s), year	Target group	Age span	Sample size	Flourishing; Languishing	Country
Bower, 2017	Adolescents	13–16	790	54.4%; 7.4%	Scotland
Dyrbye et al., 2012	College students	Not applicable	4400	51.6%; 29.2%	United States
Gilmour, 2014	Adolescents and adults	15–75 or older	25,113	76.9%; 1.5%	Canada
Góngora & Solano, 2017	Adults	18–85	627	39.7%; 5.7%	Argentina
Guo et al., 2018	Middle school students	Not applicable	5399	57.4%; 5.2%	China
Karaś et al., 2014	Aged above 16	16–81	2115	26.0%;15.5%	Poland
Keyes et al., 2012	College students	18 or older	5689	51.8%; 3.6%	United States
Keyes et al., 2008	Adults	30–80 or older	1050	20.0%; 12.2%	South Africa
Keyes, 2006	Adolescents	12–18	1234	37.9%; 6%	United States
Keyes, 2005	Adults	25–74	3032	18%; 17%	United States
Lim, 2014	Adolescents	10th grade, mean 16.08	547	11.7%; 13.0%	South Korea
Petrillo et al., 2015	Adults	18–89	1438	28.5%; 10.5%	Italy
Rugiera et al., 2013	Undergraduate students	19–40	279	72.7%; 3.5%	Tanzania
Salama-Younes, 2011	Adolescents	12–18	339	23.5%; 11.56%	Egypt
Singh & Junnarkar, 2015	Adolescents	13–18	539	46.4%; 2.4%	India
Van Schalkwyk & Wissing, 2010	Adolescents	15–17	665	42%; 5.0%	South Africa
Wissing & Temane, 2013	Adults	16–35	694	61.7%; 5.9%	South Africa
Yin et al., 2013	Adults	20–60 or older	2021	43.4%; 7.1%	China

the nature, structure, and manifestations of well-being in that population which could contribute to developing and evaluating contextually appropriate interventions to promote positive mental health and well-being, which may also protect against psychopathology (Keyes, 2005, 2014).

4.1.5 The Present Study

The MHC-SF constitutes a useful measure of positive mental health in clinical and nonclinical epidemiological samples because of its comprehensiveness and brevity (Lamers et al., 2011; Silverman et al., 2018). Although the MHC-SF has been used extensively to assess the levels of positive mental health in various contexts, the evidence for its factorial validity and prevalence of positive mental health based on its scores have not been explored in any Ghanaian sample. An examination of the factorial validity of the MHC-SF in a rural, resource-limited sample is necessary to determine its utility as a measure of positive mental health in this population. Therefore, in this study, we first sought to explore and compare various psychometric models (i.e., CFA, bifactor CFA, ESEM, and bifactor ESEM) to determine the best fitting model and the reliability of the MHC-SF in a Twi-speaking rural Ghanaian sample. The second aim was to establish the prevalence of levels of positive mental health in the sample.

4.2 Method

4.2.1 Design and Context

This study employed a cross-sectional field-survey design to collect primary data from participants. The setting for this study was the Sunyani West District (SWD), one of 27 districts of the Brong Ahafo region of Ghana, which has a population of 85,272 with a total of 10,715 households (Ghana Statistical Service, 2013). The district has several clusters of small (about 150 households or less) rural poor (average income less than US$1.90 per day per head) or ultra-poor (average income less than US$1.25 per day per head) communities (Ghana Statistical Service, Ghana Health Service, and ICF International, 2015; World Bank Group, 2018). Most communities have basic (primary) schools but have no access to electricity or safe drinking water. Often, communities are scattered far apart and connected by poor road networks. The majority of residents are small-scale farmers who trade in food crops. Residents share comparable socioeconomic and cultural profiles (Ghana Statistical Service, 2013).

4.2.2 Setting and Participants

Participants were recruited from four rural poor, highly collective communities in the SWD of the Brong Ahafo region of Ghana. Using a computer-generated number sequence, communities were randomly selected from a list of 18 provided by the District Assembly. The majority of residents of these communities are poor with

Table 4.2 Demographic profile of participants

Variable	*n*	%
Gender		
Male	240	54.1
Female	204	45.9
Age	*Mean* = 37.9 (*SD* = 11.4; Range = 18–76)	
Marital Status		
Single	55	12.4
Married	326	73.4
Cohabiting	14	3.2
Divorced/Separated	25	5.6
Widowed	24	5.4
Education		
None	205	46.2
Primary	78	17.6
Junior High	85	19.1
Senior High	41	9.2
Tertiary	8	1.8
Other	2	6.1

individual daily income of less than US$ 1.25 (categorised as ultra-poor) to US$1.90 (categorised as poor; Cooke et al., 2016; Ghana Statistical Service et al., 2015). The majority of residents in the four communities share similar sociodemographic characteristics: are middle-aged, are Christians, have primary school level of education, and are small-scale farmers (Ghana Statistical Service et al., 2015).

Participants were of both genders, aged from 18 to 76 years, have resided in the communities for at least 24 months, and were fluent in the Twi language. Initially, 38 purposively selected participants from the target population were recruited to evaluate the translated version of the MHC-SF (together with five other measures) for comprehensibility and to assess the response format. We then recruited adult participants ($N = 444$) from the four selected communities into this study. The majority of participants were male, married, and had little or no formal education. The mean age was 37.9 ($SD = 11.2$, ranging from 18 to 76). The sociodemographic characteristics of the participants are shown in Table 4.2.

4.2.3 Measure

The MHC-SF (Keyes, 2005) consists of 14 items that measure various facets of well-being. The MHC-SF has three subscales: Emotional Well-Being (MHC-EWB; also called hedonic well-being: Items 1–3); Social Well-Being (MHC-SWB; part of the positive functioning domain: Items 4–8); and Psychological Well-Being (MHC-PWB; part of the positive functioning domain: Items 9–14). The MHC-SF allows for two kinds of assessment: the three levels of positive mental health, including flourishing, languishing, and moderate mental health, and three dimensions of well-being (social, psychological, and emotional). Statements are rated on a Likert scale, which ranges from 0 (*Never*) to 5 (*Every day*), with a higher score indicating a higher prevalence of positive mental health. A categorical diagnosis of *flourishing* is made when an individual reports experiences as "*Every day*" or "*Almost every day*" for at least one of the three hedonic well-being items and six of the 11 positive functioning items. A diagnosis of *languishing* requires a report of experience as "*Never*" or "*Once or twice*" for at least one of the three hedonic well-being symptoms and six of the 11 positive functioning symptoms. Individuals are categorised as *moderately mentally healthy* if their scores do not fit the criteria for flourishing or languishing. The MHC-SF total score has demonstrated good internal consistency ($\alpha > .80$) and discriminant validity in many samples (e.g., Keyes et al., 2008; Lamers et al., 2011). Keyes et al. (2008) found Cronbach's alpha values of .74 for the overall MHC–SF scale, .67 for the MHC-PWB subscale, .73 for the MHC-EWB subscale, and .59 for the MHC-SWB subscale in a sample of Setswana-speaking adults from the North West province of South Africa.

4.2.3.1 Preparation of Scale

We followed the research-committee approach (Brislin, 1970; Van de Vijver & Leung, 1997) in the scale translation. First, the scale was translated into Twi by a bilingual translator and back-translated into English by another. Thereafter, the English versions (original and the back-translated) were compared by a research committee which comprised the two bilingual translators (one has significant experience in psychological assessment), a professor of English (who is also fluent in Twi), the lead author (who is a native Twi-speaker and a clinical psychologist), and a local collaborator (an academic and fluent in Twi) to evaluate the synthesis of the two independent translations. To ensure culture-sensitive appropriateness of the Twi version, we pilot-tested the Twi-translated version with 38 individuals recruited from the target population to cognitively appraise the items on the questionnaire. Participants were asked to rate the instructions, each item, and the response format as "clear" or "unclear", share what they thought the items were asking, repeat the items in their own words, tell what came to mind when they heard a particular phrase or word, explain how they chose their answers, and indicate which phrases or words they misunderstood or found unacceptable or offensive (Rafiey et al., 2017; Sousa & Rojjanasrirat, 2011). Participants who rated instructions, questions, or the response formats as unclear were asked to give suggestions for revision. The evaluation of the English back-translation of the Twi version showed one difference in meaning in the wording for item 9. This was resolved by the research committee by evaluating the difference, taking a consensus decision, and applying the necessary revision. A copy of the Twi version can be obtained from the corresponding author.

4.2.4 Ethical Considerations and Procedure

Ethical approval for this study was granted by the Health Research Ethics Committee (HREC) of the North-West University (NWU-00109-17-S1), South Africa, and the Noguchi Memorial Institute for Medical Research Institutional Review Board (NMIMR-IRB) of the University of Ghana (NMIMR.IRB CPN 007/17-18), Ghana. Permission was also sought from the Regional and District Health Directorates of the SWD. The chiefs and community leaders of the communities involved were presented with copies of the ethical approval and permission letters, and then provided goodwill permission for the research team to conduct the study. Together with the community leaders, the team recruited and trained an individual in each community who acted as an independent mediator. The independent mediator led the research team to introduce the study to members of selected households in the week preceding the data gathering. Four individuals with psychology and research backgrounds who were also fluent in Twi were recruited and given extensive training on research ethics, relevant field protocols, and the procedure for administration of measures. A fifth surveyor acted as an auditor and conducted random spot-checks and back-checks.

Before recruitment and the data gathering interviews, each selected individual was assured of confidentiality and anonymity of data, and the process to ensure these ethical principles were well explained and clarified. All participants were informed about their right to withdraw from participating in the study until the data analysis stage, without any consequences. The independent mediator and surveyors obtained informed consent (thumbprints) from individuals who agreed to participate. The MHC-SF, together with other questionnaires, were interviewer-administered because many participants could not read or write. Interviews lasted for about an hour and were conducted at a time and place that provided privacy. Data were collated within 1 month.

4.2.5 Data Analysis

The SurveyCTO software (version 2.41), an electronic mobile technology web-based survey data-collection platform, was used to collect data (Dobility Inc., 2018). The data was cleaned in the Statistical Package for the Social Sciences (SPSS) version 25 (IBM Corporation, 2017) before the analyses. There were no missing data. We conducted factor analysis using Mplus 8.3 (Muthén & Muthén, 1998–2018). CFA and bifactor CFA models were parameterised by fixing the variances of the latent factors to one (Van de Schoot et al., 2012). For the ESEM and bifactor ESEM models, oblique target rotation and orthogonal bifactor target rotation were respectively applied (Morin et al., 2016). For target rotation in the ESEM and bifactor ESEM models, the cross-loadings (i.e., loadings on nontarget factors) were set to approximately, but not constrained to, zero (Asparouhov & Muthén, 2009).

We tested and compared the following models to examine the factor structure of the MHC-SF: a one-factor CFA model, where all items of the MHC-SF loaded onto a single factor (Model 1); a three-factor CFA model with three correlated factors, namely EWB, SWB, and PWB (Model 2); a three-factor bifactor CFA model, with three orthogonal specific factors (EWB, SWB, and PWB) and an orthogonal general factor (Model 3); a three-factor ESEM model that allowed cross-loadings on non-target factors (Model 4); and a three-factor bifactor ESEM model with three orthogonal specific factors, where cross-loadings were allowed, and an orthogonal general factor (Model 5). Graphical representations of the models are presented in Fig. 4.1.

Consistent with recommended practices (see Byrne, 2016), the following fit indices were considered to determine how well each model fit the data: the comparative fit index (CFI) and Tucker-Lewis index (TLI) where values greater than .90 indicate reasonable fit, while values greater than .95 indicate good fit. For both the standardised root mean square residual (SRMR) and the root mean square error of approximation (RMSEA), values below .08 suggest reasonable fit and values below .05 indicate good fit. Results of the chi-square test are also reported (p-value larger than 0.05 would indicate good fit), but were not the primary indicators for decision making due to its sensitivity to sample size. The factor loadings were also examined to detect well-defined factors, where factor loadings of $\pm.40$ and above, but $\pm.30$ at minimum, are considered indicative of good fit, provided that the sample size is greater than 350 (Hair et al., 2010). Additionally, we inspected the size and significance of the target and nontarget loadings. Finally, R^2-values (i.e., the percentage of the item's variance explained by the model) were considered, with small values revealing possible local misfit.

We followed the formula and principles stipulated by Sánchez-Oliva et al. (2017) to calculate the model-based omega coefficients of composite reliability (McDonald, 1970), which is $\omega = (\Sigma|\lambda_i|)^2 / ([\Sigma|\lambda_i|]^2 + \Sigma\delta_{ii})$, with λ_i representing the factor loadings and δ_{ii} the error variances. For a discussion on the application of ω to bifactor models, see Perreira et al. (2018); for an application of the formula to a bifactor ESEM model of the MHC-SF, see Schutte and Wissing (2017). We utilised the SPSS to compute the categorisation and prevalence of positive mental health by applying Keyes's criteria for the categorisation of mental health (Keyes, 2005; Robitschek & Keyes, 2009).

4.3 Results

4.3.1 Best Model Fit for MHC-SF

Fit statistics for all five models are presented in Table 4.3. The single-factor CFA model showed poorest fit to the data (Model 1). Except for the bifactor CFA model (Model 3), which failed to converge, all remaining models (Models 2, 4, 5) displayed acceptable model fit. The interfactor correlations of the three-factor CFA model (Model 2) were large (.85 for EWB with SWB; .83 for EWB with PWB; and .94 for

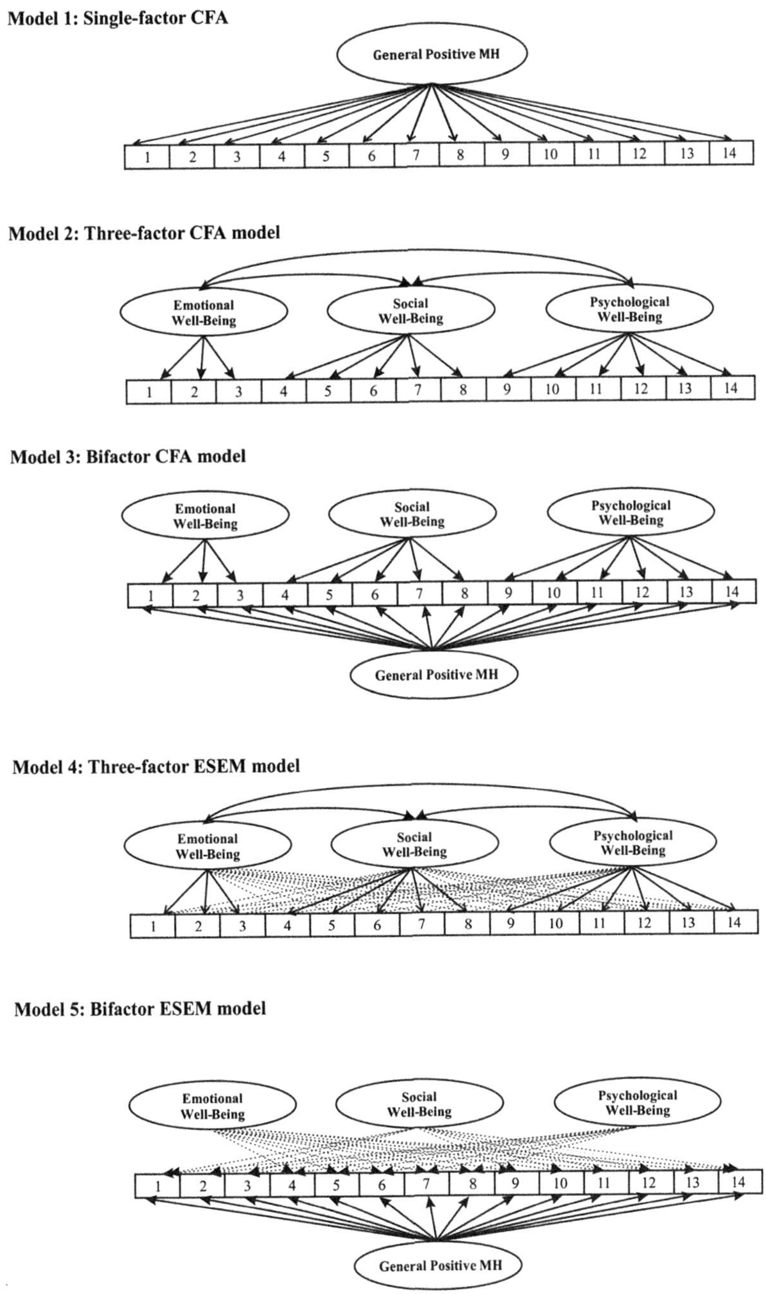

Fig. 4.1 Statistical models tested for the Mental Health Continuum-Short Form (MHC-SF). *CFA* confirmatory factor analysis; *ESEM* exploratory structural equation modelling; *MH* mental health

Table 4.3 Fit statistics of MHC-SF Models

Model	χ^2	*df*	*p*	CFI	TLI	RMSEA	90% CI	SRMR
Model 1	300	77	<.001	.929	.916	.083	.073, .093	.038
Model 2	177.06	74	<.001	.967	.960	.057	.047, .068	.029
Model 3	No convergence							
Model 4	75.21	52	.019	.993	.987	.033	.014, .048	.015
Model 5	51.05	41	.135	.997	.993	.024	.000, .043	.024

Note: χ^2 = chi-square test statistic; *df* = degrees of freedom; *p* = probability value; CFI = comparative fit index; TLI = Tucker-Lewis index; RMSEA = root mean square error of approximation; 90% CI = 90 percent confidence interval of the RMSEA; SRMR = standardised root mean square residual; Model 1 = single-factor CFA (confirmatory factory analysis) model; Model 2 = three-factor CFA model; Model 3 = bifactor CFA model; Model 4 = ESEM (exploratory structural equation modelling) model; Model 5 = bifactor ESEM model

SWB with PWB). These large correlations may be suggestive of the presence of a general positive mental health factor. The interfactor correlations of the three-factor ESEM model (Model 4) were also large (.77 for EWB with SWB; .76 for EWB with SWB; and .83 for SWB with PWB), which again suggested the possible presence of a general positive mental health factor. A bifactor ESEM model (Model 5) presented with superior fit compared to the other models.

4.3.2 *Factor Loadings*

Following its superior model fit, we display the standardised factor loadings for the bifactor ESEM model (Model 5) in Table 4.4. All items presented with strong and statistically significant loadings on the general positive mental health factor (factor loadings: .32 to .90). Notably, item 2 ("In the past month, how often did you feel that you were interested in life?") exhibited a comparatively low but statistically significant factor loading of .32 on the general factor. All three items intended to measure EWB had statistically significant loadings on the target factor, but the loading for item 2 was relatively small. For the SWB factor, item 6 exhibited a high and significant loading on its intended factor, item 8 a moderate and statistically significant loading, and item 5 a weak but statistically significant loading. Items 4 and 7 had low and nonsignificant loadings on the intended SWB factor, while item 4 had small but statistically significant cross-loadings on the EWB and the PWB factors. None of the PWB items loaded significantly on the PWB factor or attained significant cross-loadings on any other specific factor, except item 11, which exhibited a weak, statistically nonsignificant cross-loading on the EWB factor. Item 2 had an exceptionally small R^2-value (0.18), which means that only 18% of the item's variance is explained by the model. All other items presented with high R^2-values, ranging from 0.69 to 0.88.

Table 4.4 Standardised factor loadings for the bifactor ESEM model

Item and intended subscale	MH	EWB	SWB	PWB	R^2
1. Happiness, EWB	**.75****	**.40****	.03	.12	.72
2. Interested in life, EWB	**.32****	**.21***	.05	−.18	.18
3. Satisfaction with life, EWB	**.72****	**.52****	.03	−.01	.87
4 Social contribution, SWB	**.76****	.24**	**.13**	.21**	.69
5. Social integration, SWB	**.86****	.00	**.18****	.09	.77
6. Social actualization, SWB	**.82****	.12	**.46****	−.02	.88
7. Social acceptance, SWB	**.82****	−.08	**.15**	−.12	.71
8. Social coherence, SWB	**.78****	.04	**.34****	−.09	.74
9. Self-acceptance, PWB	**.86****	.02	.04	**−.10**	.76
10. Environmental mastery, PWB	**.89****	.02	.03	**.08**	.80
11. Positive relations with others, PWB	**.89****	−.07	−.09	**−.01**	.76
12. Personal growth, PWB	**.82****	−.02	.03	**.22**	.72
13. Autonomy, PWB	**.86****	−.08	−.07	**.31**	.85
14. Purpose in life, PWB	**.90****	−.01	.00	**.25**	.85

Note: Target factor loadings are presented in bold. *ESEM* exploratory structural equation modelling; *MH* general positive mental health; *EWB* emotional well-being; *SWB* social well-being; *PWB* psychological well-being; R^2 percentage variance of the item explained by the factors
$^*p < .05$. $^{**}p < .01$

4.3.3 Reliability

The omega coefficient of composite reliability for the general positive mental health factor of the bifactor ESEM model was .97, which support this factor's reliability. For the specific factors, the reliability coefficients were $\omega = .51$ (EWB); $\omega = .57$ (SWB); and $\omega = .41$ (PWB). When considering the guideline suggested by Perreira et al. (2018) that omega coefficients of $\omega > .50$ represent satisfactory reliability for bifactor models, one would conclude that the MHC-EWB and MHC-SWB subscales demonstrated satisfactory reliability, but not the MHC-PWB subscale. However, considering the common guideline that reliability coefficients larger than .70 suggest sufficient reliability (e.g., Kline, 2000; Nunnally & Berstein, 1995), we suggest that, while the current results support the use of a general positive mental health factor score in the current sample, caution should be applied when using subscale scores, especially for the PWB subscale.

4.3.4 Prevalence of Positive Mental Health

We applied Keyes's criteria for the assessment and categorisation of positive mental health to determine the prevalence of levels of mental health, using participants' scores on the MHC-SF. The results showed that, from the total sample, a third

(33.1%) was languishing, a quarter (25.5%) was flourishing, and the majority (41.4%) experienced moderate mental health.

4.4 Discussion

In the present study, we tested and compared various psychometric models (i.e., CFA, bifactor CFA, ESEM, and bifactor ESEM) to determine the best fitting model for the MHC-SF and to establish the prevalence of positive mental health in a rural poor Twi-speaking Ghanaian adult sample. A three-factor bifactor ESEM model better fit the data than competing models. The model yielded strong and significant target loadings for the general positive mental health factor and partially for the EWB and SWB target factors, but not for the PWB target factor. The total scale, and the MHC-EWB and MHC-SWB subscales, but not the MHC-PWB subscale, attained satisfactory reliability. The majority of participants experienced moderate mental health, a third was languishing, while a quarter was flourishing.

Consistent with previous research that evaluated competing models of the MHC-SF structure (e.g., Lamborn et al., 2018; Longo et al., 2020; Schutte & Wissing, 2017), our results supported the superiority of the three-factor bifactor ESEM model with excellent global fit indexes. The EWB and SWB specific factors attained marginal reliability, while reliability of the PWB specific factor was weak. The reliability scores in the present study are consistent with previous studies that reported high reliability for the general positive mental health factor, but moderate and low reliability estimates for the specific factors. For instance, Schutte and Wissing (2017) reported high omega reliability scores (.86. to .90) for the general mental health factor for their three samples and scores ranging from .36 to .62 for the subscales. Our results are comparable to recent research that reported strong and statistically significant factor loadings for all 14 items and a high reliability coefficient for the general factor, but lower reliability coefficients for the three subscales (Lamborn et al., 2018; Longo et al., 2020; Silverman et al., 2018). Similar to findings from previous research that examined the MHC-SF using bifactor ESEM (e.g., Lamborn et al., 2018; Longo et al., 2020; Rogoza et al., 2018; Schutte & Wissing, 2017; Silverman et al., 2018), our findings support the use of the overall MHC-SF scale score, but suggest that subscales score be interpreted with caution. Given the low reliability score and low factor loadings on the target PWB factor, the MHC-PWB subscale should especially not be used in this population.

Items 4 ("That you had something important to contribute to society") and 7 ("That people are basically good") failed to load on their target SWB factor—suggesting that our sample (rural adults in a collectivistic society) perceived the evaluation of their contribution to society and their views and judgment of society as part of their overall positive mental health, but not as part of a clearly distinguished social well-being factor. A possible explanation for the weak loading of item 4 could be attributed to the intrapsychic conflict and the psychological burden that may be experienced when one is tasked to evaluate oneself in a collectivistic, rural community or society, such as in the context of this study. In the Ghanaian cultural context, it is not expected of an individual to talk about his or her achievements (or personal attributes) in the public space. Often, such self-evaluations are considered as pride or boasting (e.g., Appiah et al., 2007; Gyekye, 2010). Several Ghanaian proverbs exist to succinctly teach about reticent, "*Showing off made the hyrax lose its tail*" and "*If you boast in every way and you are in want, things will be difficult for you*".

Theoretically, item 4 requires an evaluation of one's abilities in relation to others. Indeed, item 4 loaded significantly, instead, on both the EWB and PWB factors, but not onto its targeted SWB factor. Another possible explanation is that individuals' views about the contributions they make to society may be more aligned with the psychological and emotional dimensions of well-being than the social dimension, given the cultural norms of the participants of this study. Similar patterns of behaviour of item 4 have been reported in previous studies (Joshanloo, 2016; Silverman et al., 2018). A recent study where multidimensional scaling was applied to data on the MHC-SF from a large American sample revealed that items 4 and 5 are closer to hedonic and psychological well-being and are more personal than social (Joshanloo, 2018). In the context of the current study, it is possible that participants viewed item 7 in the same light (as for item 4) when tasked to evaluate whether or not other people are good. It is noteworthy that item 7 did not cross-load on any nontarget factor, although it exhibited a high and statistically significant loading on the overall positive mental health factor.

A remarkable finding in this current study was that none of the items that were intended to measure PWB loaded significantly on the PWB specific factor. Except for item 11, which showed a weak loading on the EWB factor, none of the six items under PWB demonstrated significant cross-loadings on any other specific factor. This suggests that the items intended to measure PWB are mostly representative of a general positive mental health factor rather than a specific PWB factor for the current sample. Previous studies reported similar findings where most (if not all) items of the PWB factor failed to load significantly on this factor (Longo et al., 2020; Schutte & Wissing, 2017; Silverman et al., 2018). A possible explanation for this finding in the current sample may be attributed to the collectivistic cultural orientation of participants. Participants reside and function in a highly collectivistic society and may have perceived and interpreted items in the MHC-PWB subscale (which primarily assess an individual's evaluation of intra-personal aspects of the self) as an evaluation of one's abilities and contributions to society rather than solely as psychological well-being. In most small, unified, rural, and collectivistic communities in Ghana, individuals refrain from self-evaluation of their attributes and contributions to society for fear of being misconstrued for pride and self-centeredness (see Gyekye, 2010, 2013). Similar cultural influence on the expression of well-being, particularly PWB, was also reported in a South African study. Schutte and Wissing (2017) found significant factor loadings on PWB for an Afrikaans sample in their study (who were more likely to have a Western heritage, and more individualistic), but not for their Setswana and English samples (who were more likely to have an African heritage, and more collectivistic). These findings suggest that positive psychological experiences and functioning on an intrapsychic level are more situated and distinguished in Western (individualistic) cultures than in non-Western (collectivistic) cultures. Further comparative research is needed, for instance, with urban elite samples from Ghana who may be a bit more individualistic, to confirm this assertion and to further understand the impact of cultural heritage on the experience and expression of psychological well-being in African and other collectivistic contexts.

Compared with previous research, our results on the prevalence of positive mental health differ in many ways, probably due to the differences in the sociodemographic profile of participants and the context of the studies. The majority of participants in the present study were experiencing moderate mental health (41.4%), a third (33.1%) was languishing, and a quarter (25.5%) was flourishing. The percentage of flourishers found in the present study is relatively higher than the 20% (12.2% languishing) reported among South African Setswana-speaking adults (Keyes et al., 2008), the 18% (17% languishing) reported among a large sample of a nationally representative American adults (Keyes, 2002), and the 14% (7% languishing) reported for a Setswana-speaking adult sample in a relatively similar remote rural setting of South Africa (Wissing & Temane, 2013). A likely explanation for the relatively higher percentage of flourishers in our study, compared with other studies, could be the general optimism and positive outlook which are typical of the Ghanaian peoples. There is evidence indicating that Ghanaians are generally resilient (Abukari, 2018), optimistic (Moyer et al., 2009), and happy (Dzokoto, 2012), despite life's difficulties. These characteristics, fostered in the Ghanaian collectivistic cultural values (Gyekye, 1995) and high religiosity (Ghana Statistical Service, 2013), might have contributed to the high proportion of flourishers in spite of the economic difficulties. Nonetheless, a higher proportion of flourishers than found in this study has been reported among United States college students (51.8% and 3.6% languishing; Keyes et al., 2012), Chinese adult teacher trainees (44% and 7% languishing; Yin et al., 2013), and Setswana-speaking adults in a remote rural setting of South Africa in 2010 (62% and 6% languishing; Wissing & Temane, 2013). Our findings present a high prevalence of flourishing in this rural poor Ghanaian adult sample compared to results from other countries with adult samples (e.g., Egypt, Poland, South Africa, and South Korean), but also lower than results from few other countries (e.g., China and United States).

A surprising yet concerning finding of the current study was the high proportion of languishers (33%), which appears to be one of the highest reported among a nonclinical sample. This proportion is twice as much as the 17% reported among a large sample of a nationally representative American adults (Keyes, 2002) and much higher than the 7% reported by Wissing and Temane (2013) for a South African adult sample within a relatively similar remote rural context in 2005. This high level of languishers may probably be as a result of the severe economic and resource constraints faced by this group. It is well established that individuals living in rural poor and resourced-limited communities report higher levels of stress, are more susceptible to diseases, poverty, and poor mental well-being, and do not have the same level of access to medical care, education, and social resources as do their urban counterparts (Kelly et al., 2011; Lewis et al., 2013). These restraints lessen their ability to aspire and thrive well amidst life's difficulties and adversities, with adverse consequences for their mental health (Nepomuceno et al., 2016). Languishing has been associated with significant psychosocial deficiencies at levels similar to an episode of depression, which in turn leads to poor emotional health, and consequently blunts people's ability to flourish or to be productive (Keyes, 2002, 2014).

A possible explanation for the differences between findings of the present study and those of Wissing and Temane (2013; data collated in 2010) may, perhaps, be the low socio-economic status, educational levels, and geographic settings of the sample in this present study. A wealth of research demonstrates that low socio-economic status (as well as living in extreme poverty in rural and low-resourced communities) increases the susceptibility to poor mental health and lower psychological well-being (Kelly et al., 2011; Lewis et al., 2013; Nepomuceno et al., 2016). Whereas samples from these two studies were drawn from rural communities, participants in the present study were members of clusters of poor and ultra-poor communities whose members were categorised as living below 50% of the poverty line (Ghana Districts League Table, 2018; Ghana Statistical Service, 2013). Between South Africa and Ghana, the former is well advanced with a far higher Gross Domestic Product and other stronger economic indicators (World Bank Group, 2019). Furthermore, in the present study, only 1.8% of the sample had attained tertiary education, while 46% had no formal education—sociodemographic variables were not reported for the Setswana-speaking sample. In essence, more individuals in the South African sample were experiencing optimal mental health than those in this present study: 14% and 79% were flourishing and experiencing moderate mental health, respectively, as against 25.5% flourishing and 41.1% moderate mental health in this Ghanaian sample. Wissing and Temane (2013) partially associated the level of flourishers in their study with the World Cup Soccer which was held in 2010 in South Africa around the period of data collection.

The findings from this study should be considered in light of a few limitations. First, all the participants in this study were drawn from communities within one district in Ghana. A representative sample is needed to make meaningful generalisation of results to the broader Ghanaian context. Second, the cross-sectional study design did not permit the establishment of a causal association between positive mental health (or the protective factors of mental health) and its potential risk factors. Future studies should consider a longitudinal design with samples drawn from various backgrounds, including English-speaking adults.

4.5 Conclusions

As far as could be established, this is the first study to validate the Twi version of the MHC-SF and to assess the prevalence of positive mental health in a rural poor Ghanaian adult sample. A bifactor ESEM model displayed superior fit, and findings supported the reliability of the overall MHC-SF scale, but marginal reliability scores for the MHC-EWB and MHC-SWB subscales, and a weak reliability score for the MHC-PWB subscale. Although our results supported an underlying three-factor structure of the MHC-SF, convincing support was only established for use of scores on the general positive mental health factor, with caution suggested for using and interpreting subscale scores. On the basis of the low reliability score of the PWB subscale, it is recommended that the global score, rather than the subscale scores, should be used and interpreted for the current group. We postulate that the collectivistic cultural practices of our sample may have contributed to their failure to clearly distinguish the PWB-specific factor. Future research should focus on exploring and improving the item content for the MHC-PWB subscale in this particular Ghanaian population and/or understanding the nature and dynamics of PWB in collectivistic contexts. Although a quarter of participants were flourishing, put together, a larger proportion (languishers and moderate mentally healthy individuals) were not functioning optimally and could benefit from context-appropriate positive psychology interventions designed specifically to promote mental health and build resilience of this and other groups with with similar geographic and socioeconomic characteristics.

Acknowledgements The authors remain thankful to all participants, chiefs and elders of the communities, and research assistants involved in this study. The authors also thank Amanda Cromhout for her assistance with analysing the data. The first author is thankful to the National Institute for the Humanities and Social Sciences (South Africa) for the award of the African Pathways NIHSS-CODESRIA Doctoral Scholarship towards his doctoral studies at the North-West University (NWU). The scholarship source did not have any influence on the design of the study, data collection, and analysis or writing of the manuscript. The first author is also grateful to the NWU for the receipt of Doctoral and International Students' bursaries during the period of his studentship.

References

Abukari, Z. (2018). "Not giving up": Ghanaian students' perspectives on resilience, risk, and academic achievement. *SAGE Open*. https://doi.org/10.1177/2158244018820378

Addai, I., & Pokimica, J. (2010). Ethnicity and economic well-being: The case of Ghana. *Social Indicators Research, 99*(3), 487–510.

Appiah, P., Appiah, K. A., & Agyeman-Dua, I. (2007). *Bu me be: Proverbs of the Akans*. Lynne Reinner Publishers.

Appiah, R., Schutte, L., Wilson Fadiji, A., Wissing, M. P., & Cromhout, A. (2020). Factorial validity of the Twi versions of five measures of mental health and well-being in Ghana. *PLoS One, 15*(8), e0236707. https://doi.org/10.1371/journal.pone.0236707

Appiah, R., Tutu, B., Oman, M., & Ndaa, P. (2020). Prevalence of positive mental health and functioning among adults with sickle cell disease in Ghana. *Ghana Medical Journal, 54*(4), 245–252. https://doi.org/10.4314/gmj.v54i4.7

Appiah, R., Wilson Fadiji, A., Wissing, M. P., & Schutte, L. (2020). Effects of a community-based multicomponent positive psychology intervention on mental health of rural adults in Ghana. *Applied Psychology: Health and Well-Being, 12*(3), 828–862. https://doi.org/10.1111/aphw.12212

Asante, K. O. (2012). Social support and the psychological wellbeing of people living with HIV/AIDS in Ghana. *African Journal of Psychiatry, 15*(5), 340–345.

Asparouhov, T., & Muthén, B. (2009). Exploratory structural equation modeling. *Structural Equation Modeling: A Multidisciplinary Journal, 16*(3), 397–438.

Bermant, G., Talwar, C., & Rozin, P. (2011). To celebrate positive psychology and extend its horizons. In K. M. Sheldon, T. B. Kashdan, & M. F. Steger (Eds.), *Designing positive psychology: Taking stock and moving forward* (pp. 430–438). Oxford University Press.

Bolier, L., Haverman, M., Kramer, J., Westerhof, G. J., Riper, H., Smit, F., & Bohlmeijer, E. (2013). Positive psychology interventions: A meta-analysis of randomized controlled studies. *BMC Public Health, 13*(119). https://doi.org/10.1186/1471-2458-13-119

Bower, R. (2017). *Psychometric evaluation of the Mental Health Continuum-Short Form (MHC-SF) with adolescents living in the West of Scotland* (Doctoral dissertation). Retrieved from http://theses.gla.ac.uk/8438

Brislin, R. W. (1970). Back-translation for cross-cultural research. *Journal of Cross-Cultural Psychology, 1*(3), 185–216.

Byrne, B. M. (2016). *Structural equation modelling with AMOS: Basic concepts, applications, and programming* (3rd ed.). Routledge.

Cooke, E., Hague, S., & McKay A. (2016). *The Ghana poverty and inequality report: Using the 6th Ghana living standards survey*. Retrieved May 02, 2019, from http://africainequalities.org/wp-content/uploads/2016/07/Ghana_Poverty_and_Inequality_Analysis_FINAL_Match_20161.pdf

De Kock, F., Kanjee, A., & Roodt, G. (2013). Cross cultural test adaptation and translation. In C. Foxcroft & G. Roodt (Eds.), *Introduction to psychological assessment in the South African context* (4th ed., pp. 83–106). Oxford University Press.

Delle Fave, A., Brdar, I., Freire, T., Vella-Brodrick, D., & Wissing, M. P. (2011). The eudaimonic and hedonic components of happiness: Qualitative and quantitative findings. *Social Indicators Research, 100*(2), 185–207.

Diener, E., Emmons, R. A., Larsen, R. J., & Griffin, S. (1985). The satisfaction with life scale. *Journal of Personality Assessment, 49*(1), 71–75.

Diener, E., Oishi, S., & Tay, L. (2018). Advances in subjective well-being research. *Nature Human Behavior, 2*(4), 253–260. https://doi.org/10.1038/s41562-018-0307-6

Diener, E., & Ryan, K. (2009). Subjective well-being: A general overview. *South Africa Journal of Psychology, 39*(4), 391–406. https://doi.org/10.1177/008124630903900402

Dobility Inc. (2018). *SurveyCTO*. Retrieved February 18, 2019, from https://www.surveycto.com/about/

Doe, F. (2016). The impact of workplace bullying on workers' psychological and emotional well-being: A study of 139 University staff in Ghana. *International Journal of Innovative Research & Development, 5*(3), 18–23.

Dyrbye, L. N., Harper, W., Moutier, C., Durning, S. J., Power, D. V., Massie, F. S., Eacker, A., Thomas, M. R., Satele, D., Sloan, J. A., & Shanafelt, T. D. (2012). A multi-institutional study exploring the impact of positive mental health on medical students' professionalism in an era of high burnout. *Academic Medicine, 87*(8), 1024–1031.

Dzokoto, V. A. (2012). Ghanaian happiness: Global, cultural, and phenomenological perspectives. In H. Selin & G. Davey (Eds.), *Happiness across cultures* (pp. 311–327). Springer.

Franken, K., Lamers, S. M. A., Ten Klooster, P. M., Bohlmeijer, E. T., & Westerhof, G. J. (2018). Validation of the mental health continuum-short form and the dual continua model of well-being and psychopathology in an adult mental health setting. *Journal of Clinical Psychology, 74*(12), 2187–2202. https://doi.org/10.1002/jclp.22659

Galderisi, S., Heinz, A., Kastrup, M., Beezhold, J., & Sartorius, N. (2015). Toward a new definition of mental health. *World psychiatry: Official Journal of the World Psychiatric Association (WPA), 14*(2), 231–233. https://doi.org/10.1002/wps.20231

Ghana Statistical Service. (2013). *2010 population and housing census: National analytical report*. Ghana statistical service. Retrieved August 18, 2019, from http://www.statsghana.gov.gh/docfiles/2010phc/National_Analytical_Report.pdf

Ghana Statistical Service (GSS), Ghana Health Service (GHS), & ICF International. (2015). *Ghana demographic and health survey 2014*. GSS, GHS, and ICF International.

Ghana's District League Table. (2018). *2018/19 District league table II with new perspectives and modified methodology*. Retrieved from https://www.unicef.org/ghana/media/2131/file/2018-2019-The-District-League-Table-II.pdf

Gilmour, H. (2014). Positive mental health and mental illness. *Health Reports, 25*(9), 3–9.

Glozah, F. N. (2015). Exploring Ghanaian adolescents' meaning of health and wellbeing: A psychosocial perspective. *International Journal of Qualitative Studies on Health and Wellbeing, 10*(1), 26370. https://doi.org/10.3402/qhw.v10.26370

Glozah, F. N., & Pevalin, D. J. (2015). Factor structure and psychometric properties of the general health questionnaire (GHQ-12) among Ghanaian adolescents. *Journal of Child and Adolescent Mental Health, 27*(1), 53–57. https://doi.org/10.2989/17280583.2015.1007867

Glozah, F. N., & Pevalin, D. J. (2017). Psychometric properties of the perceived social support from family and friends scale: Data from an adolescent sample in Ghana. *Journal of Child and Family Studies, 26*(1), 88–100.

Góngora, V. C., & Solano, A. C. (2017). Assessment of the mental health continuum in a sample of Argentinean adults. *Psychology, 8*, 303–318.

Greenaway, K. H., Kalokerinos, E. K., & Williams, L. A. (2018). Context is everything (in emotion research). *Social and Personality Psychology Compass*. https://doi.org/10.1111/spc3.12393

Guo, C., Tomson, G., Keller, C., & Söderqvist, F. (2018). Prevalence and correlates of positive mental health in Chinese adolescents. *BMC Public Health, 18*(1), 1–11. https://doi.org/10.1186/s12889-018-5133-2

Gyekye, K. (1995). African philosophy. In R. Audi (Ed.), *The Cambridge dictionary of philosophy* (pp. 11–12). Cambridge University Press.

Gyekye, K. (2010). African ethics. In E. Zalta (Ed.), *Stanford encyclopedia of philosophy*. Retrieved from https://plato.stanford.edu/entries/african-ethics/

Gyekye, K. (2013). *Philosophy culture and vision: African perspectives. Selected essays*. Sub-Saharan Publishers.

Hair, J., Black, W. C., Babin, B. J., & Anderson, R. E. (2010). *Multivariate data analysis*. Pearson Education International.

Heintzelman, S. J. (2018). Eudaimonia in the contemporary science of subjective well-being: Psychological well-being, self-determination, and meaning in life. In E. Diener, S. Oishi, & L. Tay (Eds.), *Handbook of well-being*. DEF Publishers.

IBM Corporation. (2017). *IBM SPSS statistics for Windows, version 25.0*. IBM Corp.

Joshanloo, M. (2016). Revisiting the empirical distinction between hedonic and eudaimonic aspects of well-being using exploratory structural equation modeling. *Journal of Happiness Studies, 17*(5), 2023–2036.

Joshanloo, M. (2018). Optimal human functioning around the world: A new index of eudaimonic well-being in 166 nations. *British Journal of Psychology, 109*(4), 637–655. https://doi.org/10.1111/bjop.12316

Joshanloo, M., Wissing, M. P., Khumalo, I. P., & Lamers, S. M. A. (2013). Measurement invariance of the mental health continuum-short form (MHC-SF) across three cultural groups. *Personality and Individual Differences, 55*(7), 755–759. https://doi.org/10.1016/j.paid.2013.06.002

Jovanovic, V. (2015). Structural validity of the Mental Health Continuum-Short Form: The bifactor model of emotional, social and psychological well-being. *Personality and Individual Differences, 75*, 154–159. https://doi.org/10.1016/j.paid.2014.11.026

Kahneman, D., Diener, E., & Schwarz, N. (1999). *Well-being: The foundations of hedonic psychology*. Russell Sage Foundation.

Kammann, N. R., & Flett, R. (1983). Affectometer 2: A scale to measure current level of general happiness. *Australian Journal of Psychology, 35*(2), 259–265.

Karaś, D., Cieciuch, J., & Keyes, C. L. M. (2014). The Polish adaptation of the Mental Health Continuum-Short Form (MHC-SF). *Personality and Individual Differences, 69*, 104–109. https://doi.org/10.1016/j.paid.2014.05.011

Kelly, B. J., Lewin, T. J., Stain, H. J., Coleman, C., Fitzgerald, M., Perkins, D., Carr, V. J., Fragar, L., Fuller, J., Lyle, D., & Beard, J. R. (2011). Determinants of mental health and well-being within rural and remote communities. *Social Psychiatry and Psychiatric Epidemiology, 46*(12), 1331–1342. https://doi.org/10.1007/s00127-010-0305-0

Kennes, A., Peeters, S., Janssens, M., Reijnders, J., Lataster, J., & Jacobs, N. (2020). Psychometric evaluation of the mental health continuum-short form (MHC-SF) for Dutch adolescents. *Journal of Child and Family Studies, 29*(11), 3276–3286. https://doi.org/10.1007/s10826-020-01803-4

Keyes, C. L. M. (1998). Social well-being. *Social Psychology Quarterly, 6*, 121–140.

Keyes, C. L. M. (2002). The mental health continuum: From languishing to flourishing in life. *Journal of Health and Social Behavior, 43*(2), 207–222. https://doi.org/10.2307/3090197

Keyes, C. L. M. (2005). Mental illness and/or mental health? Investigating axioms of the complete state model of health. *Journal of Consulting and Clinical Psychology, 73*(3), 539–548. https://doi.org/10.1037/0022-006X.73.3.539

Keyes, C. L. M. (2006). Mental health in adolescence: Is America's youth flourishing? *American Journal of Orthopsychiatry, 76*(3), 395–402. https://doi.org/10.1037/0002-9432.76.3.395

Keyes, C. L. M. (2014). Mental health as a complete state: How the salutogenic perspective completes the picture. In G. F. Bauer & O. Hämmig (Eds.), *Bridging occupational, organizational and public health: A transdisciplinary approach* (pp. 179–192). Springer.

Keyes, C. L. M., Eisenberg, D., Perry, G. S., Dube, S. R., Kroenke, K., & Dhingra, S. S. (2012). The relationship of level of positive mental health with current mental disorders in predicting suicidal behavior and academic impairment in college students. *Journal of American College Health, 60*(2), 126–133. https://doi.org/10.1080/07448481.2011.608393

Keyes, C. L. M., & Martin, C. C. (2017). The complete state model of mental health. In M. Slade, L. Oades, & A. Jarden (Eds.), *Wellbeing, recovery and mental health* (pp. 86–97). Cambridge University Press.

Keyes, C. L. M., Wissing, M. P., Potgieter, J., Temane, Q. M., Kruger, A., & Van Rooy, S. (2008). Evaluation of the mental health continuum-short form (MHC-SF) in Setswana speaking south Africans. *Clinical Psychology and Psychotherapy: An International Journal of Theory and Practice, 15*(3), 181–192. https://doi.org/10.1002/cpp.572

Kline, P. (2000). *Handbook of psychological testing*. Routledge.

Kühn, S., & Rieger, U. M. (2017). Health is a state of complete physical, mental and social well-being and not merely absence of disease or infirmity. *Surgery for Obesity and Related Diseases, 13*(5), 887.

Lamborn, P., Cramer, K. M., & Riberdy, A. (2018). The structural validity and measurement invariance of the mental health continuum-short form (MHC-SF) in a large Canadian sample. *Journal of Well-Being Assessment, 2*(1), 1–19.

Lamers, S. M. A., Westerhof, G. J., Bohlmeijer, E. T., Ten Klooster, P. M., & Keyes, C. L. M. (2011). Evaluating the psychometric properties of the mental health continuum-short form (MHC-SF). *Journal of Clinical Psychology, 67*(1), 99–110. https://doi.org/10.1002/jclp.20741

Lewis, M. L., Scott, D. L., & Calfee, C. (2013). Rural social service disparities and creative social work solutions for rural families across the life span. *Journal of Family Social Work, 16*(1), 101–115.

Lim, Y. J. (2014). Psychometric characteristics of the Korean mental health continuum–short form in an adolescent sample. *Journal of Psychoeducational Assessment, 32*(4), 356–364. https://doi.org/10.1177/0734282913511431

Longo, Y., Jovanović, V., Sampaio de Carvalho, J., & Karaś, D. (2020). The general factor of well-being: Multinational evidence using Bifactor ESEM on the mental health continuum– Form. *Assessment, 27*(3), 596–606. https://doi.org/10.1177/1073191117748394

Marsh, H. W., Morin, A. J. S., Parker, P. D., & Kaur, G. (2014). Exploratory structural equation modeling: An integration of the best features of exploratory and confirmatory factor analysis. *Annual Review of Clinical Psychology, 10*, 85–110. https://doi.org/10.1146/annurev-clinpsy-032813-153700

McDonald, R. P. (1970). The theoretical foundations of principal factor analysis, canonical factor analysis, and alpha factor analysis. *British Journal of Mathematical and Statistical Psychology, 23*(1), 1–21.

Morin, A. J. S., Arens, A. K., & Marsh, H. W. (2016). A bifactor exploratory structural equation modeling framework for the identification of distinct sources of construct-relevant psychometric multidimensionality. *Structural Equation Modeling, 23*(1), 116–139. https://doi.org/10.1080/10705511.2014.961800

Moyer, C. A., Yang, H., Kwawukume, Y., Gupta, A., Zhu, Y., Koranteng, I., Yasmin, E., Wei, Y. M., Greene, J., Calhoun, C., Ekpo, G., Beems, M., Ryan, M., Adanu, R., & Anderson, F. (2009). Optimism/pessimism and health-related quality of life during pregnancy across three continents: A matched cohort study in China, Ghana, and the United States. *BMC Pregnancy and Childbirth, 9*, 39. https://doi.org/10.1186/1471-2393-9-39

Muthén, L. K., & Muthén, B. O. (1998–2018). *Mplus (Version 8.3)*. Muthén & Muthén.

Nepomuceno, B. B., Cardoso, A. A. V., Ximenes, V. M., Barros, J. P. P., & Leite, J. F. (2016). Mental health, wellbeing, and poverty: A study in urban and rural communities in northeastern Brazil. *Journal of Prevention & Intervention in the Community, 44*(1), 63–75.

Nunnally, J., & Berstein, I. (1995). *Psychometric theory*. Mcgraw-Hill.

Oishi, S. (2010). Culture and well-being: Conceptual and methodological issues. In E. Diener, J. F. Helliwell, & D. Kahneman (Eds.), *International differences in well-being* (pp. 34–69). Oxford University Press.

Perreira, T. A., Morin, A. J. S., Hebert, M., Gillet, N., Houle, S. A., & Berta, W. (2018). The short form of the workplace affective commitment multidimensional questionnaire (WACMQ-S): A bifactor-ESEM approach among healthcare professionals. *Journal of Vocational Behavior, 106*, 62–83. https://doi.org/10.1016/j.jvb.2017.12.004

Perugini, M. L. L., Iglesiaa, G., Solano, A. C., & Keyes, C. L. (2017). The mental health continuum–short form (MHC–SF) in the Argentinean context: Confirmatory factor analysis and measurement invariance. *Europe's Journal of Psychology, 13*(1), 93–108.

Petrillo, G., Capone, V., Caso, D., & Keyes, C. L. M. (2015). The mental health continuum–short form (MHC–SF) as a measure of well-being in the Italian context. *Social Indicators Research, 121*(1), 291–312. https://doi.org/10.1007/s11205-014-0629-3

Pokimica, J., Addai, I., & Takyi, B. K. (2012). Religion and subjective well-being in Ghana. *Social Indicators Research, 106*(1), 61–79.

Rafiey, H., Alipour, F., LeBeau, R., Amini Rarani, M., Salimi, Y., & Ahmadi, S. (2017). Evaluating the psychometric properties of the mental health continuum-short form (MHC-SF) in Iranian earthquake survivors. *International Journal of Mental Health, 46*(3), 243–251. https://doi.org/10.1080/00207411.2017.1308295

Reise, S. P. (2012). The rediscovery of bifactor measurement models. *Multivariate Behavioral Research, 47*(5), 667–696. https://doi.org/10.1080/00273171.2012.715555

Robitschek, C., & Keyes, C. L. M. (2009). Keyes' model of mental health and the role of personal growth initiative as a parsimonious predictor. *Journal of Counseling Psychology, 56*(2), 321–329.

Rogoza, R., Truong Thi, K. H., Różycka-Tran, J., Piotrowski, J., & Żemojtel-Piotrowska, M. (2018). Psychometric properties of the MHC-SF: An integration of the existing measurement approaches. *Journal of Clinical Psychology, 74*(10), 1742–1758.

Rugiera, J., Nienaber, A. W., & Wissing, M. P. (2013). Psychological well-being among Tanzanian students. *Journal of Psychology in Africa, 23*(3), 49–53.

Ryff, C. D. (1989). Happiness is everything, or is it? Explorations on the meaning of psychological well-being. *Journal of Personality and Social Psychology, 57*, 1069–1081.

Ryff, C. D., & Keyes, C. L. M. (1995). The structure of eudaimonic well-being revisited. *Journal of Personality and Social Psychology, 69*(4), 719–727. https://doi.org/10.1037//0022-3514.69.4.719

Salama-Younes, M. (2011). Validation of the mental health continuum-short form and subjective vitality scale with Egyptian adolescent athletes. In I. Brdar (Ed.), *The human pursuit of well-*

being: A cultural approach (pp. 221–234). Springer. https://doi.org/10.1007/978-94-007-1375-8_19

Sánchez-Oliva, D., Morin, A. J., Teixeira, P. J., Carraça, E. V., Palmeira, A. L., & Silva, M. N. (2017). A bifactor exploratory structural equation modeling representation of the structure of the basic psychological needs at work scale. *Journal of Vocational Behavior, 98*, 173–187.

Schimmack, U., Diener, E., & Oishi, S. (2002). Life-satisfaction is a momentary judgment and a stable personality characteristic: The use of chronically accessible and stable sources. *Journal of Personality, 70*(3), 345–384.

Schutte, L., & Wissing, M. P. (2017). Clarifying the factor structure of the mental health continuum-short form in three languages: A bifactor exploratory structural equation modeling approach. *Society and Mental Health, 7*(3), 142–158. https://doi.org/10.1177/2156869317707793

Silverman, A. L., Forgeard, M., Beard, C., & Björgvinsson, T. (2018). Psychometric properties of the mental health continuum–short form in a psychiatric sample. *Journal of Well-Being Assessment, 2*(1), 57–73.

Singh, K., & Junnarkar, M. (2015). Correlates and predictors of positive mental health for school going children. *Personality and Individual Differences, 76*, 82–87.

Sousa, V., & Rojjanasrirat, W. (2011). Translation, adaptation and validation of instruments or scales for use in cross-cultural health care research: A clear and user friendly guideline. *Journal of Evaluation in Clinical Practice, 17*, 268–274. https://doi.org/10.1111/j.1365-2753.2010.01434.x

Uchida, Y., & Kitayama, S. (2009). Happiness and unhappiness in east and west: Themes and variations. *Emotion, 9*, 441–456. https://doi.org/10.1037/a0015634

Van de Schoot, R., Lugtig, P., & Hox, J. (2012). A checklist for testing measurement invariance. *European Journal of Developmental Psychology, 9*(4), 486–492. https://doi.org/10.1080/17405629.2012.686740

Van de Vijver, F. J. R., & Leung, K. (1997). *Methods and data analysis for cross-cultural research.* Sage.

Van Schalkwyk, I., & Wissing, M. P. (2010). Psychosocial well-being in a group of South African adolescents. *Journal of Psychology in Africa, 20*(1), 53–60.

Waterman, A. (2013). *The best within us. Positive psychology perspectives on eudaimonia.* American Psychological Association.

Watson, D., Clark, L. A., & Tellegen, A. (1988). Development and validation of brief measures of positive and negative affect: The PANAS scales. *Journal of Personality and Social Psychology, 54*(6), 1063–1070. https://doi.org/10.1037/0022-3514.54.6.1063

Weiss, L. A., Westerhof, G. J., & Bohlmeijer, E. T. (2016). Can we increase psychological well-being? The effects of interventions on psychological well-being: A meta-analysis of randomised controlled trials. *PLoS One, 11*(6), e0158092. https://doi.org/10.1371/journal.pone.0158092

Wellenzohn, S., Proyer, R. T., & Ruch, W. (2018). Who benefits from humor-based positive psychology interventions? The moderating effects of personality traits and sense of humor. *Frontiers in Psychology, 9*, 821. https://doi.org/10.3389/fpsyg.2018.00821

Wilson, A., & Somhlaba, N. Z. (2016). Psychological well-being in a context of adversity: Ghanaian adolescents' experiences of hope and life satisfaction. *Africa Today, 63*(1), 85–103. Retrieved from https://muse.jhu.edu/article/629573

Wilson, A., Yendork, J. S., & Somhlaba, N. Z. (2016). Psychometric properties of multidimensional scale of perceived social support among Ghanaian adolescents. *Child Indicators Research, 10*(1), 101–115.

Wissing, M. P., & Temane, Q. M. (2013). The prevalence of levels of wellbeing revisited in an African context. In C. L. M. Keyes (Ed.), *Mental well-being: International contributions to the study of positive mental health* (pp. 71–90). Springer.

Woodworth, R. J., O'Brien-Malone, A., Diamond, M. R., & Schüz, B. (2016). Happy days: Positive psychology interventions effects on affect in an N-of-1 trial. *International Journal of Clinical and Health Psychology, 16*(1), 21–29. https://doi.org/10.1016/j.ijchp.2015.07.006

Woody, S. R., Miao, S., & Kellman-McFarlane, K. (2015). Cultural differences in social anxiety: A meta-analysis of Asian and European heritage samples. *Asian American Journal of Psychology, 6*(1), 47–55. https://doi.org/10.1037/a0036548

World Bank Group. (2018). *3rd Ghana economic update – Agriculture as an engine of growth and jobs creation*. World Bank.

World Bank Group. (2019). *World Bank World Development Indicators, 1960–2018*. [data collection]. 27th Edition. UK Data Service. SN: 4814. https://doi.org/10.5257/wb/wdi/2019-02

World Health Organization Quality of Life-100 (WHOQOL Group). (1998). Development of the World Health Organization WHOQOL-BREF quality of life assessment. *Psychological Medicine, 28*(3), 551–558. https://doi.org/10.1017/s0033291798006667

Yin, K. L., He, J. M., & Fu, Y. F. (2013). Positive mental health: Measurement, prevalence, and correlates in a Chinese cultural context. In C. L. M. Keyes (Ed.), *Mental well-being: International contributions to the study of positive mental health* (pp. 111–132). Springer.

Chapter 5
Conceptualising and Measuring Hospitality in Relation to Wellbeing in Kenya: Is Hospitality a Character Strength?

Sahaya G. Selvam, Joyce Wanjiru Kiige, and Jeketule Soko

Abstract Hospitality is recognised as a salient value across most cultures, including in Africa. Yet, empirical research is narrowly focused on the hospitality industry. Psychological studies on hospitality are lacking. Therefore, the present research, consisting of three studies, explored hospitality within the theoretical framework of character strengths and wellbeing. Study 1 examined the perception of hospitality among several ethnic groups in Kenya and identified dimensions that define hospitality: spending time with guests, enjoying their presence, having long conversations, not being disturbed when guests arrive unannounced, welcoming them in one's residence, providing good food, making sacrifices to make them feel at home, and providing comfortable accommodation. Based on the qualitative data, in Study 2, a 9-item scale of hospitality was developed and validated. Factor analysis identified two factors: logistical and dispositional hospitality. The scale showed high internal consistency reliability and satisfied criteria of validity. Study 3 tested the association between hospitality and wellbeing using the Tangaza Hospitality Scale and the Mental Health Continuum-Short Form. Findings showed that dispositional hospitality predicts mental health: $R = .428$, $R^2 = .183$, $p < .01$. It is hoped that hospitality will gain more currency within positive psychology, and eventually be listed as a character strength.

Keywords Hospitality · African hospitality · Hospitality and wellbeing · Africa and positive psychology · Tangaza Hospitality Scale

S. G. Selvam (✉) · J. W. Kiige · J. Soko
Tangaza University College, Nairobi, Kenya

L. Schutte et al. (eds.), *Embracing Well-Being in Diverse African Contexts: Research Perspectives*, Cross-Cultural Advancements in Positive Psychology 16,
https://doi.org/10.1007/978-3-030-85924-4_5

5.1 Introduction

Hospitality is recognised as a salient value across most cultures, even if expressions of it could take different forms. Most religious traditions require their adherents to offer hospitality even to strangers (Sharpley, 2009). From the story of Abraham welcoming three strangers in the middle of the day found in the Hebrew Scriptures to Paul thanking the churches for their hospitality in the Christian scriptures, the Judeo-Christian tradition is awash with hospitality (Bolin, 2004). Offering hospitality, even to strangers, is also at the heart of the Hindu culture. Even today, the distribution of food and goods to strangers is literally practised even in modern city streets by adherents of Hinduism and Sikhism (George, 2009). Islam has enshrined within itself the Arabic desert dwellers' virtue of hospitality and generosity (*karam*, Sobh et al., 2013). Heal (1990) points out that in ancient Rome as well as in early modern England, hospitality was considered a value among good citizens; this included not only hosting friends and relatives for dinners but also welcoming strangers.

Literature in cultural anthropology highlights the important role of hospitality in the social life of the peoples of Africa. African homesteads are open spaces, ever ready to welcome familiar and unfamiliar guests. In urban Africa, it might have mutated itself to a different form, but the value of hospitality with food and fun is never lost. Healey (1981), a Christian missionary, appreciates the hospitality of the people of Africa as a concrete expression of openness and presence. According to Moila (2002), African hospitality is simply a practical expression of African cultural and moral value. Hospitality is a way of life. It is an extension of the unconditional African generosity (Echema, 1995). According to Odera Oruka, a Kenyan philosopher, in his African sagacity, happiness itself is defined as being open to all people (Oruka, 1990).

Despite these traditions—global and African—contemporary research on hospitality tends to narrowly focus on hotel and tourism industries. The main difference between "hospitality as a cultural value" and "hospitality as an industry" is that in the latter, the relationship between the host and guest lasts only as long as the guest can pay (Ashness & Lashley, 1995). Lashley (2015) further makes a distinction between "hospitality" which is related to welcoming and hosting of tourists with direct monetary benefits, and "hospitableness" which refers to altruistic hospitality that is carried out as an end in itself. Hospitableness is "offered merely for the pleasure of giving other people pleasure" (Lashley, 2015, p. 1). Research on hospitality needs to further explore its cultural and private aspects and its association with collective and individual affective and cognitive dimensions. Insights gained from studies on hospitableness would, without doubt, enhance research in the hospitality industry as well. Despite this distinction, in this chapter the term "hospitality" is used to connote the cultural value and individual trait-like disposition of hospitableness.

In the editorial of the launching issue of the journal *Hospitality and Society*, Lynch et al. (2011) point out several other factors currently affecting research around hospitality. One of these is the lack of interdisciplinarity in the field. Therefore, they advocate for an "intellectual hospitality" in which different academic disciplines can enrich each other on the understanding of hospitality. Inspired by this clarion call, the scope of the present research project was to provide some insights on hospitality from the perspective of positive psychology.

Thus far, studies on hospitality from a psychology perspective, particularly examining the association between hospitality and wellbeing, are meagre. Selvam and Collicutt (2013), while examining the ubiquity of character strengths within the African traditional religions and cultures, realised that hospitality emerged spontaneously in their data as a possible entrant into the catalogue of character strengths, Values in Action (Peterson & Seligman, 2004). This is justifiable given that Peterson (2006) agrees that the list of character strengths is still a work in progress. Selvam and Collicutt recommended further exploration of this. The current research was undertaken in response to that recommendation. Even as this research project was underway, Biswas-Diener et al. (2019) attempted to conceptualise and measure hospitality within the framework of positive psychology by developing the Brief Hospitality Scale. The scale, which has 4 items, is shown to have very robust psychometric properties. They have also examined the association among hospitality, wellbeing, and the dimensions of the Big Five model of personality. A few years prior to the work of Biswas-Diener and colleagues, Blain and Lashley (2014) had developed a flexible questionnaire that measures three dimensions of what they termed "hospitableness": (a) Desire to put guests before yourself—4 items; (b) Desire to make guests happy—5 items; (c) Desire to make guests feel special—4 items. Thus, the questionnaire had 13 items in all.

While the questionnaire of Blain and Lashley (2014) was developed in British and European contexts, the Brief Hospitality Scale (Biswas-Diener et al., 2019) was initially conceptualised in the American context and later validated across 12 nations. None of these countries are from the African continent. Therefore, the need still remains for exploring hospitality as a character strength within the African context, by conceptualising and developing an instrument to measure the construct. Therefore, this research project aimed at contributing to the study of hospitality by conceptualising and measuring hospitality in the Kenyan/African context from the perspective of positive psychology focusing on character strengths and wellbeing. In so doing, the study aims to examine the possibility for hospitality being considered a character strength.

5.2 The Current Research

The current research consisted of three studies in fulfilling the above aim:

Study 1: A qualitative study aimed to identify the dimensions of hospitality by examining the perception and experience of hospitality among several ethnic groups in Kenya. The envisaged output of this study was a list of dimensions that conceptualise hospitality in the African context, and the outcome was a scale that could be used to measure hospitality.

Study 2: Based on the emerging themes of the qualitative data, the second study aimed to validate a 9-item scale of hospitality—the Tangaza Hospitality Scale.

Study 3: The final study aimed to test the association between hospitality and wellbeing using the Tangaza Hospitality Scale and Mental Health Continuum Scale—Short Form (Keyes, 2009). This phase of the project also aimed to verify which of the dimensions of hospitality (dispositional or logistical) had a stronger association with wellbeing. Taken together, if hospitality as a construct is distinctly measurable and correlates positively to different dimensions of wellbeing, then this study would contribute to the discussion on considering hospitality as a candidate character strength (Peterson & Seligman, 2004).

Ethical clearance for the project was granted by the Kenya National Commission for Science, Technology, and Innovation (NACOSTI) after it was locally cleared by the Tangaza University College. Data was collected in all phases of the project with due respect to the norms of research ethics, including informed consent from the participants. This was ensured through signed forms from the participants. Data collection was partly led by the second author as part of her dissertation work. The rest of the data was collected with the help of research assistants who were post-graduate students, after due training that included a call to cultural sensitivity. The whole process was designed and overseen by the first author. The third author was involved in data analysis. Participation in the study was voluntary and participants did not receive incentives.

5.3 Study 1: Qualitative Study on Perceived Concept of Hospitality

5.3.1 Purpose

Brotherton (1999) provides a detailed account of the difficulty experienced in hospitality research in defining hospitality itself. According to him, hospitality as a product, a process, and an experience are often confused. If we want to measure hospitality to ascertain its correlation to wellbeing, we first need to define it. Therefore, the purpose of this study was to explore how people conceptualise hospitality in their ordinary lives.

For this purpose, a qualitative method of data collection and analysis was considered most suitable. Besides, it was envisaged that the emerging themes from this study could form the basis of items for the development of a scale to measure hospitality in the African context. It is a common practice to use qualitative studies to inform development of scales (Rowan & Wulff, 2007). Besides, qualitative research designs demonstrate a sensitivity to linguistic and sociocultural contexts (Yardley, 2017). Therefore, qualitative studies are ideal to be used in positive psychology in scale development, particularly when cultural content is explored (Delle Fave & Bassi, 2009). Moreover, as Robbins (2008, p. 96) argues: "Eudaimonic happiness cannot be purely value-free, nor can it be completely studied without using both nomothetic and idiographic (i.e., quantitative and qualitative) methods in addressing problems of value". Therefore, a qualitative research design served the purpose of Study 1 in the current 3-phase research project which used a sequential mixed-method design.

5.3.2 Method

With the help of 12 research assistants who were postgraduate students of counselling psychology, semi-structured in-depth interviews were conducted in English and Swahili. All interviews were transcribed and those in Swahili were also translated by a person who was not a research assistant. The authenticity of the translations was verified by the first two authors together. This phase of the study included 148 participants across Kenya. Of these, 53% were male. The mean age of participants was 41.1 years (*SD* = 17.2), the youngest being 18 and the oldest being 73 years old. The participants represented 12 ethnic communities of Kenya; there were also about 20 participants from other countries of Africa who were living in Kenya at the time of the study. The following questions served as the tentative set of key questions for the in-depth interviews; other probing questions were added in response to the emerging conversation:

1. What are the best experiences of hospitality that you have had when you have visited other people or families?
2. Could you describe how you generally welcome guests at your home?
3. What are the components of the ideal expression of hospitality in your culture?
4. What words, phrases, and sayings are used to describe African hospitality in your culture?
5. What changes do you see in the way hospitality is practised nowadays as compared to olden days?

The interviews lasted an average of 25–30 min and were audio-recorded, transcribed, translated, and coded for thematic analysis. "Thematic analysis is a method of identifying, analysing and reporting patterns (themes) within data" (Braun & Clarke, 2006, p. 79). Themes are more than just phrases and expressions found in the data; hence, thematic analysis implies a certain level of interpretation of the mind of the participants (Boyatzis, 1998), and to give voice to them. The coding process was carried out by the first two authors, initially independently. In the second stage, the coders compared their themes and if differences arose between them, a dialogue was carried out between the two coders. Finally, the themes reported below were selected from the transcribed text on the basis of frequency and distribution among participants.

As described above, the reliability of the study was ensured by more than one person carrying out the coding of the data, and by maintaining a paper trail. The validity of the findings was ensured by a triangulation process among the data, identified themes, and existing literature (Jonsen & Jehn, 2009). The themes reported here are corroborated by the literature in the discussion section that follows the findings.

5.3.3 *Findings*

5.3.3.1 Hospitality Is Welcoming Guests

Almost all participants acknowledged that hospitality is considered a virtue across African cultures. If one is not hospitable then one is frowned upon by society. Guests are a blessing, as one 20-year-old male participant from the Nandi ethnic group in Kenya put it, "In our culture, we like a guest as a blessing from God. We need to honour him and make him happy."[1]

Most of the participants understood hospitality as an act of welcoming visitors, and sometimes even strangers. Some of the participants were more specific and described hospitality as being kind to, paying attention to, and taking time with others to make them feel at home. For instance, a 39-year-old female participant said, "It is an art of welcoming somebody and making somebody feel at home, free and relaxed." This was also echoed by a male participant aged 24, who said hospitality "is an act of welcoming anybody any time to enable him/her feel at home without necessarily looking at their financial status."

Some participants acknowledged that there is a difference between welcoming guests casually at home and for family functions such as weddings and funerals—these tend to be formal and entail a lot of prior preparation and could take place outside the actual home of the host. For the sake of handling a large number of guests at a family function, the event could be held at a common hall or a hotel. On these occasions, there may not be personal interaction with everyone. These formal functions are now on the increase. However, if the visit is casual and routine-like, then the guest is hosted at home. Sometimes the visitor might just walk in unannounced. The way they are welcomed is informal with a lot of personal attention.

Welcoming guests has its set of rituals. It always begins with a greeting, and enquiry about the situation of where they come from (about the family, animals, and other aspects). This is followed by offering a drink. A female participant said, "When the person arrives, first of all, you offer him or her a seat, then you give them water to drink... Then later on, you greet the person and tell the person: 'Feel at home'." In the Kenyan context, the drink could be alcoholic, or non-alcoholic, or tea, or a type of milk. For example, the members of the Kalenjin ethnic group in Kenya frequently spoke of *amursik*—a type of sour milk that is offered to guests.

[1]The sexist language is part of the verbatim data from interviews. The authors do not subscribe to such language. However, this is maintained here to demonstrate authenticity.

5.3.3.2 Being with and Spending Time with Guests

In the Kenyan context and, by extension, in Africa, when a guest is at home the hosts make sure that someone is sitting with the guest all the time, engaging them in conversation. The guest is not to be left alone. Usually, as some members of the family engage in such conversations, others would busy themselves preparing the meal. The meal becomes urgent especially when the guest is in a hurry and is not planning to spend the night with the hosts.

There is an expression of "being with" the guest. In the African context, when the arrival of the guest is known in advance, they are waited for and received as far from the home as possible and accompanied to the home of the host. Similarly, the guest is accompanied as they bid farewell as far as the host can physically go. "To be escorted" is a common expression in Eastern Africa. There is a nuance to the accompanying, as a 55-year-old male participant states, "usually visitors are escorted with gifts especially if a visitor comes with some gifts, which is usually in the form of foodstuff. The time that visitor will be leaving there is a need to give them something in return. Sometimes some visitors are escorted with songs especially if they are in-laws. They are treated in a very special way." In most of the East African cultures, the basket or the bag that the guest brought their gift in is never returned empty. The guests' gifts are thus reciprocated with gifts from the host.

5.3.3.3 Having Savouring Conversation

Speaking "nicely" to a visitor is as important as offering food to the guest to make them comfortable. A 49-year-old participant reiterated this as she said, "Hospitality is of two types: there is hospitality of receiving someone... And you make them feel at home just by your conversation, and there is no need for even a big meal, and another way of being hospitable is you occupy yourself by preparing for the guest something to eat. But this depends on how they come." Another participant seconded this opinion, saying, "although food is important, speaking nicely to a person is more important. The way you will receive them they will be very comfortable and feel at home. And they would like to visit you another day. Yes, so hospitality is not just about food." The same participant also acknowledged that nice conversation can occur at least after the meal, especially if the host was busy preparing the meal.

One way of beginning a conversation and engaging in a conversation with the guest, especially if the guest is only a friend and not a relative, is to start showing the family photo albums. The photos give good background information about the host to the guest and further tighten the ties between the two. Another way of keeping the guest busy is to take them around the village or the field for a walk. In any case, the guest should not feel bored at the home of the guest. They must feel good.

5.3.3.4 Preparing and Providing Good Food and Drinks

Food and drinks are part of hospitality. If the guest is really in a hurry, they should at least drink some water at the home of the guest. Especially female participants in the interviews invariably alluded to the aspect of food in hospitality. For instance, one middle-aged woman said rather excitedly, "for me cooking food and serving others makes me feel good. I feel proud of the food I have cooked especially when they eat well. Remember, this includes cooking special meals and showing to the guests I am overjoyed about their presence when you serve them by interacting with the guests makes me feel happy. I feel satisfied that I have shown them good hospitality."

Food and drinks are important aspects of welcoming guests because we do not know what they have endured during the journey. Most guests are too shy to request for a drink or something to eat; therefore, it is the duty of the host to offer it to them even if they do not request it. The people of the Kikuyu ethnic group say, "Hunger is not to be interrogated. You just give food." A 63-year-old member of the Kalenjin ethnic community said, "If you know in advance that the guest is arriving, you prepare in advance. You prepare special dishes, such as *amursik*—fermented milk; and *red ugali*—a stiff porridge made from millet. Sometimes even a goat is slaughtered in honour of the guest."

5.3.3.5 Preparation of Place and Accommodation

One way of showing a spirit of welcome to the guest is to have prepared the physical environment: by cleaning the environment, arranging the furniture in order, and changing covers and decorations. Usually, the whole family helps with the preparations. While speaking about their understanding of hospitality, most of the participants described hospitality as creating room/space for others. Some went ahead to explain that a room prepared with a lot of attention would make the guest feel cared for and respected. For instance, a 20-year-old male participant expressed his understanding of hospitality purely in terms of the accommodation: "For me, it is so important to put up a guest in a comfortable place, because they are coming to an unfamiliar environment." This was echoed by a female participant, aged 30, who said: "hospitality has to do with accommodating people and being generous and kind-hearted."

Other participants acknowledged that sometimes this entails a certain degree of self-sacrifice, not only in terms of the time spent and extra work done, but also giving up one's own comfort for the sake of the guest. This implies sometimes giving up your cosy bed for the guest and sleeping on the couch for the night. The presence of the guest may intrude on your privacy, but you are ready for this in order to express genuine hospitality.

5.3.3.6 No Problem Even If They Came Unannounced

Many participants acknowledged that guests, especially those who come from far, usually send a message about their coming, sometimes weeks before their travel. Nowadays, people might give short notice through mobile phones. Even though it is preferred that guests inform the host before they visit, they cannot be sent away if they just turned up. In rural areas, they are likely to find someone around the homestead; however, in urban settings, the host family members could be away, leaving the guest stranded. Participants acknowledged this range of dynamics in welcoming guests who come uninvited and unannounced. However, everyone who delved into this topic acknowledged that it is important to be polite to guests. This might entail changing one's own programme to welcome guests, or sharing the food that is already prepared with the guests, or enduring extra work and fatigue to express hospitality.

5.3.4 *Discussion*

Study 1 set out to explore how ordinary Kenyans conceptualise hospitality. The findings of this study informed the items for the development of a hospitality scale. From the above findings, the following dimensions of hospitality could be identified: generally, Africans welcome guests at home; hospitality is expressed by being with and spending time with guests; being with the guests is accompanied by having savouring conversations; true hospitality implies not being upset even if guests turned up unannounced; hospitality also includes providing good food, drinks, and accommodation.

In this brief discussion section, two tasks are aimed at. First, the reported themes are corroborated with existing literature (Jonsen & Jehn, 2009). Second, the themes are further discussed in reference to the two existing scales of hospitality (Biswas-Diener et al., 2019; Blain & Lashley, 2014).

There is ample literature on hospitality in Africa. Most of this literature discusses hospitality from anthropological, philosophical, and theological perspectives. These types of sources have provided the content for previous discussions on character strengths (Dahlsgaard et al., 2005). What emerges from the literature regarding hospitality in Africa largely corresponds to the emerging themes of the present study. To begin with, hospitality to strangers and unannounced guests is something that stands out in the literature as typical of African hospitality (Magesa, 1998; Mugambi, 1989). Welcoming guests into the homes and even offering a readymade space for them to stay is further highlighted in the literature (Kiaziku, 2007, 2009). Kiaziku (2007, p. 139) points out that "Africans consider it right and important that each house has some rooms for guests." Furthermore, the spirit of hospitality consists of sharing what a family has (Kiaziku, 2007). It is expressed by not only offering food and drinks, but also in availing one's time and presence to the guests

(Mulandi, 2003). In general, guests are considered to be a blessing because they bring gifts, information, and news from far, and they provide a reason for a good meal that will be enjoyed by everyone (Healey & Sybertz, 1996). These selected authors provide support for what this study concluded as findings from the interviews with the participants.

These dimensions are also similar to those included in the questionnaire developed by Blain and Lashley (2014). Their instrument measures three dimensions of hospitableness: (a) desire to put guests before yourself; (b) desire to make guests happy; (c) desire to make guests feel special. These dimensions are further divided into 13 items, which include statements such as: "I put guests' enjoyment before my own"; "The comfort of guests is most important to me"; "I get a natural high when I make my guests feel special"; and "When hosting I try to feel at one with the guests". These items are similar to those concepts expressed by the African participants. Again, what these participants have expressed resonates well with the items in the Brief Hospitality Scale (Biswas-Diener et al., 2019): "I enjoy hosting others"; "When I host others, I feel good about myself"; "Being hospitable is something that comes easily to me"; "I am a very hospitable person". Interestingly, these two measures remain more at the affective level, and do not integrate the logistical aspects of hospitality, such as preparing food and accommodation. Therefore, there is a need for a scale that would capture the specificities of the African expression of hospitality and that would capture the inner processes as well as the external expressions.

5.4 Study 2: Validation of the Tangaza Hospitality Scale

5.4.1 *Purpose*

The purpose of the second study was to validate the Tangaza Hospitality Scale which was developed with the items drawn from the emerging themes of Study 1. This phase of the project aimed at testing the psychometric properties of the scale by means of inter-item correlation and factor analyses, among other statistical tests. It also attempted to validate the scale by measuring the association of the dimensions of hospitality against constructs such as subjective happiness and extraversion.

5.4.2 *Method*

5.4.2.1 Participants

In an attempt to verify the psychometric properties of the scale and to validate it, Study 2 included 216 participants (52.3% male) in Nairobi, conveniently sampled. Their mean age was 36.3 (SD = 12.0), the youngest being 18 and the oldest being

74 years old. The participants represented a range of religious, educational, and economic backgrounds.

5.4.2.2 Instruments

Tangaza Hospitality Scale Initially, a 10-item scale was created from the emerging themes of Study 1. The items were scored on a 5-point Likert scale, from 1 (*very much unlike me*) to 5 (*very much like me*). The participants were asked to indicate the degree to which each statement was true of them personally. One of the reversed items did not consistently correlate with the rest of the items and hence was excluded from the rest of the analysis. The item reads: “I expect my guests to accept whatever I offer them, and I do not work hard to offer them what they prefer.” See Appendix for the 9-item scale.

Subjective Happiness Scale This scale, developed by Lyubomirsky and Lepper (1999), consists of 4 items that measure global subjective happiness on a 7-point Likert scale. One of the items is reversed. By 1999, it was validated in 14 studies with a total of 2732 participants. As of now, it has been used in over 3000 other studies (Lyubomirsky & Lepper, 1999).

Measure of Extraversion Hospitality entails a certain level of sociability; hence, it was hypothesised in the present study that there would be a positive correlation between levels of hospitality and the personality trait of extraversion. Therefore, only the 8 items measuring extraversion from the 44-item Big Five Inventory (BFI-44; John & Srivastava, 1999) were used. Items of extraversion measure different facets including gregariousness, assertiveness, energy, excitement-seeking, enthusiasm, and warmth. A meta-analysis of studies conducted over 24 years (1991–2014) that used the BFI-44 showed Cronbach’s coefficient alpha of each dimension to be nearly 0.8 (Li et al., 2015).

5.4.3 Findings

Descriptive statistics of the individual items of the Tangaza Hospitality Scale (Table 5.1) showed that among the studied population, “welcoming guests in the residence” attained the highest mean score, suggesting that the sample often welcomes their guests at home and does not meet up with them at a common place. Preparing better food and drinks than usual for the guests may not be a concern as suggested by the relatively low mean score of item 9. Nonetheless, on all items the sample scored well above the scale midpoint of 3.

There was no significant effect of demographic variables on levels of hospitality: gender, age, education, and religious backgrounds. Comparing the level of hospitality on the basis of gender, the mean of the total scores of hospitality suggested that women are likely to be more hospitable than men (Male = 31.79, SD = 6.6;

Table 5.1 Mean score of items

	Mean	*SD*
1. Welcoming guests in the residence	3.95	1.04
2. Enjoying spending time with guests	3.92	0.99
3. Not disturbed when they come unannounced	3.71	1.23
4. Having long conversations with guests	3.58	1.15
5. Alright when a family member brings guests (R)	3.34	1.20
6. Effort in preparing good food	3.75	1.16
7. Ensuring that guests have a good place to sleep	3.59	1.28
8. Enjoying being with guests (R)	3.50	1.16
9. Better food and drinks than usual	3.33	1.30

$N = 216$; Range: 1 to 5

Female = 33.46, SD = 6.2); however, this fell short of statistical significance, $t\,(210) = -1.877, p = .062$.

Initially, a correlation analysis was carried out among all 10 items, using Pearson's r. As said earlier, one of the items was not correlating consistently with the rest of the items; therefore, it was eliminated from the rest of the analysis. The correlation between other items was significant, except for item 9 which did not correlate significantly with 2 items, namely "Having long conversation with guests" and "Enjoying being with guests" (see Table 5.2). This result, however, must be considered together with that of the factor analysis.

Factor analysis, using principal component analysis with varimax rotation, suggested the emergence of a two-factor model (Table 5.3). The factors have been named: Dispositional Hospitality (with 6 items) that explains 38.6% of the variance (Eigenvalue = 3.483), and Logistical Hospitality (with 3 items) explaining 13.44% of the variance (Eigenvalue = 1.999). The correlation between the scores of Dispositional Hospitality and Logistical Hospitality was significant, but not too high, suggesting that they are indeed distinct but related constructs, $r = .460, p < .01$.

The internal consistency reliability test using Cronbach's α for the grouping of items into two subscales yielded levels that are generally good (see Table 5.4). Therefore, the scale was considered reliable to be used among the Kenyan population.

In order to test the construct validity of the Tangaza Hospitality Scale, a correlational analysis was carried out among the three variables of the study (Hospitality, Subjective Happiness, and Extraversion) and the two dimensions of hospitality, using Pearson's r (Table 5.5). There was a significant correlation among almost all the variables. It is interesting to note that Dispositional Hospitality and Logistical Hospitality correlate quite differently with other variables. Dispositional Hospitality has a stronger correlation than the latter with other variables. For instance, Logistical Hospitality did not significantly correlate with Extraversion. Although the correlation between Hospitality Total and Extraversion was rather weak, it was significant; it also correlated strongly with Subjective Happiness (Pearson's $r = .304, p < .01$).

Table 5.2 Correlation between items of the Tangaza Hospitality Scale

	Item1	Item2	Item3	Item4	Item5	Item6	Item7	Item8	Item9
1. Welcoming guests in the residence	1								
2. Enjoying spending time with guests	.572**	1							
3. Not disturbed when they come unannounced	.451**	.403**	1						
4. Having long conversations with guests	.307**	.423**	.321**	1					
5. Alright when a family member brings guests	.263**	.308**	.391**	.228**	1				
6. Effort in preparing good food	.314**	.302**	.312**	.298**	.223**	1			
7. Ensuring that guests have a good place to sleep	.304**	.353**	.397**	.260**	.301**	.333**	1		
8. Enjoying being with guests	.341**	.462**	.237**	.316**	.393**	.170*	.232**	1	
9. Better food and drinks than usual	.206**	.268**	.158*	.121	.144*	.354**	.447**	.060	1

$^{*}p < .05$; $^{**}p < .01$

Table 5.3 Results of factor analysis on Tangaza Hospitality Scale

	Dispositional Hospitality	Logistical Hospitality
1. Welcoming guests in the residence	**.661**	.278
2. Enjoying spending time with guests	**.726**	.282
3. Not disturbed when they come unannounced	**.596**	.317
4. Having long conversations with guests	**.599**	.156
5. Alright when a family member brings guests (R)	**.603**	.137
8. Enjoying being with guests (R)	**.747**	−.081
6. Effort in preparing good food	.255	**.647**
7. Ensuring that guests have a good place to sleep	.306	**.694**
9. Better food and drinks than usual	−.020	**.848**

Bold indicates the loading of items to the respective factors

Table 5.4 Results of Reliability Test

Dimensions	No. of items	Possible score range	Mean	*SD*	Cronbach's α
Dispositional Hospitality	6	6 to 30	21.96	4.61	.765
Logistical Hospitality	3	3 to 15	10.64	2.84	.646
Hospitality Scale	9	9 to 45	41.969	6.47	.791

Table 5.5 Correlation between hospitality and subjective happiness & extraversion

	Dispositional Hospitality	Logistical Hospitality	Hospitality total	Subjective happiness	Extraversion
Dispositional Hospitality	1				
Logistical Hospitality	.460**	1			
Hospitality Total	.919**	.773**	1		
Subjective Happiness	.347**	.135*	.304**	1	
Extraversion	.268**	.005	.190**	.164*	1

$^{*}p < .05$; $^{**}p < .01$

5.4.4 Discussion

In the factor-analysis, the 9-item scale yielded a two-factor model. The two factors are named Dispositional Hospitality and Logistical Hospitality. Dispositional Hospitality includes items that delve into an individual's attitudes and preferences as regards hospitality. These items could build up to one's character trait. On the other hand, logistical hospitality would include items that refer to how an individual goes about expressing their dispositional hospitality in terms of preparing the environment, including food and sleep, to make the guest comfortable. Dispositional hospitality could be considered similar to "hospitableness", and logistical hospitality to "hospitality" (Lashley, 2015). Biswas-Diener et al. (2019) make no such distinctions in their Brief Hospitality Scale, which has items with a single factor. Their items focus on the positive affective states of hospitality. Therefore, the Tangaza Hospitality Scale, due to its inclusion of the logistical aspects of hospitality, could be a good alternative to the Brief Hospitality Scale.

The mean scores of all the items were above average. The overall mean score of hospitality was negatively skewed (−727), suggesting that participants are generally optimistic about themselves. Demographic variables did not show any significant association with the scores of hospitality. However, in the study by Biswas-Diener et al. (2019), women scored significantly higher in hospitality as compared to men. In the present study, the results were tending towards such a situation, but it fell short of statistical significance. The patterns in correlations (Table 5.5) suggest that hospitality is inherently a positive variable, supporting one of the characteristics of character strengths (Peterson & Seligman, 2004). Moreover, it is significantly correlated to subjective wellbeing. These are useful arguments for the inclusion of hospitality in the catalogue of character strengths. We will revisit them in the general conclusion to this chapter.

5.5 Study 3: Hospitality and Mental Health

5.5.1 Purpose

The third study had two major objectives: (1) to further verify the psychometric properties of the Tangaza Hospitality Scale; (2) to test the correlation between hospitality and mental health.

5.5.2 Method

5.5.2.1 Participants

The present study included 283 young adults (45.2% male), aged between 18 and 35, from four locations in Kenya. They represented a great variety, including those from rural and urban areas, married and unmarried, and employed and unemployed.

5.5.2.2 Instruments

Study 3 had two main variables: hospitality and mental health. Hospitality was measured using the Tangaza Hospitality Scale as evolved from Study 2 above. The second variable was measured using the Mental Health Continuum Scale—

Short Form (Keyes, 2009). Keyes' scale comprehensively measures the degree of positive mental health, understood as flourishing (Keyes, 2002). Laid out in a 6-point Likert scale, the 14 items represent three dimensions of flourishing: 3 items for emotional (hedonic) wellbeing, 5 items for social wellbeing, and 6 items for psychological wellbeing. Social wellbeing and psychological wellbeing add up to eudemonic wellbeing. The scale is recognised as having excellent psychometric properties (Lamers et al., 2011), and has been previously validated among the African population (Keyes et al., 2008).

5.5.3 *Findings*

As for the first objective of Study 3, in verifying the psychometric properties of the Tangaza Hospitality Scale, the results were very similar to those of Study 2. Factor analysis again yielded two factors: Dispositional Hospitality, with 6 items explaining 30.33% of the total variation (Eigenvalue = 2.73); and Logistical Hospitality, with 3 items explaining 15.03% of the total variation (Eigenvalue = 1.353). Cronbach's α for the two sub-dimensions and the overall hospitality scale was above .60.

The second objective was to test the correlation between hospitality and mental health as understood as human flourishing. Pearson's correlation was employed, and the results are summarised in Table 5.6. The data shows a significant positive correlation between the overall hospitality score and scores on the Mental Health Continuum—Short Form ($r = .417, p < .01$). The data also reveals that hospitality had a significant correlation with the threedimensions of human flourishing. Interestingly, Dispositional Hospitality had higher levels of correlation with all the dimensions of Mental Health, as compared with Logistical Hospitality.

Table 5.7 presents the outcome of the hierarchical multiple regression testing two models, using mental health as measured by the Mental Health Continuum—Short Form as the dependent variable. Model 1, with Dispositional Hospitality as the single predictor, yielded a significant result, $R = .428$, $R^2 = .183, p < .01$. However,

Table 5.6 Correlation between hospitality and mental health

	HT	DH	LH	MHC	EWB	SWB	PWB
Hospitality Total (HT)	1						
Dispositional Hospitality (DH)	.919**	1					
Logistical Hospitality (LH)	.785**	.476**	1				
Mental Health Continuum (MHC)	.417**	.428**	.258**	1			
Emotional Wellbeing (EWB)	.417**	.422**	.266**	.750**	1		
Social Wellbeing (SWB)	.278**	.307**	.137*	.809**	.531**	1	
Psychological Wellbeing (PWB)	.341**	.334**	.284**	.838**	.447**	.439**	1

Note: N = 283; *$p < .05$; **$p < .01$

Table 5.7 Model summary

					Change statistics				
Model	R	R^2	Adjusted R^2	Std. Error	R^2	F	df1	df2	Sig.
1	.428[a]	.183	.180	.84675662	.183	62.895	1	281	.000
2	.432[b]	.187	.181	.84629481	.004	1.307	1	280	.254

[a] Predictors: (constant), dispositional hospitality
[b] Predictors: (constant), dispositional hospitality, logistical hospitality

when Logistical Hospitality was introduced as a second predictor in model 2, the relationship of the variables increased minimally, but not significantly, $R = .432$, $R^2 = .187$, $p = .254$. This means that Dispositional Hospitality contributes 18.3% while Logistical Hospitality contributes only .4% to the model. Furthermore, while the effect of Dispositional Hospitality is significant, that of Logistical Hospitality is not significant at p-value .05.

5.5.4 *Discussion*

The general finding of Study 3 is that there is a significant positive correlation between hospitality and human flourishing ($r = .417$, $p < .01$). This implies that variation in hospitality was accompanied by variation in human flourishing among this sample of young African adults in Kenya. These findings are consistent with those of the study by Biswas-Diener et al. (2019) which showed that hospitality was significantly correlated with life satisfaction, positive affect, optimism, and flourishing, as measured by the New Well-being Measures of Diener et al. (2010).

Overall, the findings of this study support the premise that character strengths are significantly associated with dimensions of wellbeing (Table 5.6). However, as Table 5.7 suggests, not all dimensions of character strengths have equal predictive value on happiness and life satisfaction (Peterson et al., 2007). It would also be interesting to verify the predictive value of hospitality on wellbeing as compared to other character strengths.

5.6 General Discussion

Study 1, as per its aim, explored the perception of the African/Kenyan population on hospitality. This provided a viable framework for the development of the Tangaza Hospitality Scale in Study 2. In Study 3, the correlations between hospitality and well-being was explored.

In Study 2 and Study 3, hospitality was found to be positively correlated to wellbeing. More specifically, Study 2 focused on subjective happiness as measured by the Subjective Happiness Scale (Lyubomirsky & Lepper, 1999), and Study 3 on mental health as measured by the Mental Health Continuum—Short From, which considers the dimensions of emotional wellbeing, social wellbeing, and psychological wellbeing. This suggests that hospitality as a practice has a significant association with individual and collective wellbeing. This is consistent with the claim of Peterson and Park (2006) that character strengths have a robust association with wellbeing at the individual and collective levels, even though sometimes the link to the collective level may be more robust than to the individual level.

One of the major contributions of the present research was the identification of Dispositional and Logistical Hospitality as distinct constructs which are measurable as such. Moreover, the data indicated that Dispositional Hospitality has higher levels of correlation with all the dimensions of mental health, as compared with Logistical Hospitality. This might suggest that "disposition", which is more closely related to character strengths, may have a stronger association with wellbeing, and the logistical aspects of hospitality that are extraneous to the individual may be less associated with wellbeing. In a similar vein, it emerged in Study 2 that Dispositional Hospitality rather than Logistical Hospitality was more strongly correlated with extraversion which is a personality trait. This once again suggests that Dispositional Hospitality could be considered to be trait-like. Relating this to literature, we might consider dispositional hospitality being close to what Lashley (2015) has called "hospitableness", which is a cultural value, and logistical hospitality being related to "hospitality", which often is the focus of the hospitality industry. After all, the aim of the hospitality industry is mainly to provide efficiently the three logistical aspects: food, drinks, and accommodation. Lashley contrasts this with the cultural domains of hospitality which include the social values and contexts in which hospitality takes place. The present study has shed further light on the cultural domains of hospitality which are related to individual disposition.

5.7 Conclusion

The present research project set out to contribute to the study of hospitality within the framework of positive psychology focusing on character strengths and wellbeing, specifically by conceptualising and measuring hospitality in the African context. This large aim was realised through a three-tier project. It was our hope that the evidence emerging from these studies could be used to make a tentative case for considering hospitality to be a character strength.

The project commenced with a qualitative study (Study 1) which explored the experience and perception of hospitality among participants drawn from Kenya. Out of this study, the following themes were identified as dimensions that define hospitality in the Kenyan or, by extension, the African sociocultural context: Africans welcome guests at home; hospitality is expressed in being with and spending time with guests; being with the guests is carried out together with savouring conversations; true hospitality implies not being upset even if guests turned up unannounced; and hospitality also includes providing good food, drinks, and accommodation. Thus, Study 1 fulfilled the first clause of the aim of the present research project, namely, to conceptualise hospitality within the African context.

The list of dimensions that emerged from Study 1 informed the items for the development of a scale of hospitality. In the quantitative study that followed (Study 2), the psychometric properties of the proposed scale were evaluated. Factor analysis identified dispositional and logistical hospitality as two dimensions of hospitality. While the internal consistency reliability indices of the two sub-scales were at acceptable levels, Cronbach's alpha for the whole scale was .791. In a test for construct validity, the scores of hospitality and its sub-dimensions positively correlated with subjective wellbeing and extraversion. In this way, Study 2 satisfied the second clause of the general aim of the research project; that is, to measure hospitality in the African context. The Tangaza Hospitality Scale is a contribution of the present project to the study of hospitality within the framework of positive psychology.

Finally, Study 3 considered the relationship between hospitality and wellbeing employing the Tangaza Hospitality Scale and Mental Health Continuum Scale—Short Form (Keyes, 2009). The findings and their implications have been discussed above. Taken together, the three mentioned studies have unpacked the focus of investigating hospitality from a positive psychology perspective in a logical manner.

As for its methodology, in line with the suggestion of Ong and van Dulman (2007), this study integrated qualitative and quantitative approaches in a sequential mixed method design. However, one of the limitations of this study could be that since the study was carried out in Kenya, most of the participants were Kenyans. We want to maintain that since the understanding of hospitality among Kenyans corroborates well with the literature from elsewhere in Africa (Echema, 1995; Healey, 1981; Moila, 2002), the dimensions of hospitality identified in this research may be extended well beyond Kenya. In future research, the Tangaza Hospitality Scale should be validated across cultures within Africa and elsewhere. Moreover, in the studies reported above, test-retest reliability was not verified; this too remains one of the tasks ahead. The two-factor model and the internal consistency reliability need to be further ascertained across cultures. In general, hospitality research must be explored within the framework of positive psychology, using the scales now available, stretching it outside the confines of the hospitality industry.

Based on the findings emerging from the above studies, could the desire of Selvam and Collicutt (2013) be fulfilled? Would hospitality qualify to be a candidate character strength? Peterson and Seligman (2004) in their catalogue of character strengths and virtues furnish ten criteria that a new entrant should satisfy. Since all these criteria were not directly tested in the present study, we suggest a future project specifically examining hospitality within the framework of the ten criteria.

Nonetheless, the present project has added some evidence for hospitality to be considered as a character strength. For instance, the present study provided preliminary support for the notion that hospitality contributes to various fulfilments that constitute good life, for oneself and for others, as measured in terms of subjective wellbeing and mental health. Remarkably, similar outcomes have also been furnished by Biswas-Diener et al. (2019), even though they used different sets of scales to measure life satisfaction (Diener et al., 1985) and positive affect (Diener et al., 2010). Secondly, it has also emerged in the present research and other studies (Biswas-Diener et al., 2019; Blain & Lashley, 2014) that hospitality is measurable. These scales have measured hospitality in terms of thoughts (desire to provide the best for the guest), feeling (enjoying hosting guests), and behaviour (preparing food and accommodation).

Finally, as Biswas-Diener et al. (2019) have discussed in detail, hospitality seems distinct from other prosocial strengths. Hospitality carries with it the following characteristics: empathy, cordiality, warmth, congeniality, sociability, and generosity. While empathy and generosity are closely related to kindness, and warmth and congeniality are related to love (Peterson & Seligman, 2004), hospitality is a unique prosocial behaviour and attitude that entails a transaction between the guest and host in which the former shares personal time and other resources just because they enjoy doing so. Moreover, kindness and love may not have a dimension of welcome. "Purchasing a theatre ticket for a friend who forgot her wallet, for instance, is generous but not—by definition—hospitable" (Biswas-Diener et al., 2019, p. 15). Hospitality is more nuanced than love and kindness, and, therefore, can be considered a distinct construct.

Based on these indications, together with Biswas-Diener et al. (2019), we tentatively suggest that hospitality deserves the status of a character strength within the framework of positive psychology. Future studies, we hope, will strengthen this proposal.

Appendix: Tangaza Hospitality Scale

To what degree are the following statements true of you personally. Answer bluntly as you know you are at the present, and not what you wish to be. Circle the number applicable.

1.	I like to welcome guests at my residence.	1 Very much unlike me	2 Unlike me	3 Neither like me nor unlike me	4 Like me	5 Very much like me
2.	I enjoy spending ample time with my guests.	1 Very much unlike me	2 Unlike me	3 Neither like me nor unlike me	4 Like me	5 Very much like me
3.	Even if guests come unannounced, I can welcome them without a sour face.	1 Very much unlike me	2 Unlike me	3 Neither like me nor unlike me	4 Like me	5 Very much like me

(continued)

4.	Having taken care of the logistics, I sit and have long conversations with my guests.	1 Very much unlike me	2 Unlike me	3 Neither like me nor unlike me	4 Like me	5 Very much like me
5.	I get disturbed when a family/community member walks in with a guest for a meal.	1 Very much unlike me	2 Unlike me	3 Neither like me nor unlike me	4 Like me	5 Very much like me
6	I go out of my way to prepare good food and drinks for guests.	1 Very much unlike me	2 Unlike me	3 Neither like me nor unlike me	4 Like me	5 Very much like me
7.	Even if I sleep on a couch, I make sure that my guests have a good place to sleep in.	1 Very much unlike me	2 Unlike me	3 Neither like me nor unlike me	4 Like me	5 Very much like me
8.	I just welcome guests out of politeness, not because I enjoy being with them.	1 Very much unlike me	2 Unlike me	3 Neither like me nor unlike me	4 Like me	5 Very much like me
9.	I make sure that my guests have better food and drinks than I would normally have.	1 Very much unlike me	2 Unlike me	3 Neither like me nor unlike me	4 Like me	5 Very much like me

Note:
The following items are reversed: 5 & 8
Logistical Hospitality = 6, 7, 9
Dispositional Hospitality = 1, 2, 3, 4, 5, 8

References

Ashness, D., & Lashley, C. (1995). Empowering service workers at Harvester Restaurants. *Personnel Review, 24*(8), 17–32.

Biswas-Diener, R., Kushlev, K., Su, R., Goodman, F., Kashdan, T., & Diener, E. (2019). Assessing and understanding hospitality: The Brief Hospitality Scale. *International Journal of Wellbeing, 9*(2), 14–26.

Blain, M., & Lashley, C. (2014). Hospitableness: The new service metaphor? Developing an instrument for measuring hosting. *Research in Hospitality Management, 4*(1 & 2), 1–8.

Bolin, T. M. (2004). The role of exchange in ancient Mediterranean religion and its implications for reading Genesis 18-19. *Journal for the Study of the Old Testament, 29*(1), 37–56.

Boyatzis, R. E. (1998). *Transforming qualitative information: Thematic analysis and code development*. Sage.

Braun, V., & Clarke, V. (2006). Using thematic analysis in psychology. *Qualitative Research in Psychology, 3*(2), 77–101.

Brotherton, B. (1999). Towards a definitive view of the nature of hospitality and hospitality management. *International Journal of Contemporary Hospitality Management, 11*(4), 165–173.

Dahlsgaard, K., Peterson, C., & Seligman, M. E. P. (2005). Shared virtue: The convergence of valued human strengths across culture and history. *Review of General Psychology, 9*, 203–213.

Delle Fave, A., & Bassi, M. (2009). Sharing optimal experiences and promoting good community life in a multicultural society. *Journal of Positive Psychology, 4*, 280–289.

Diener, E. D., Emmons, R. A., Larsen, R. J., & Griffin, S. (1985). The satisfaction with life scale. *Journal of Personality Assessment, 49*(1), 71–75.

Diener, E. D., Wirtz, D., Tov, W., Kim-Prieto, C., Choi, D. W., Oishi, S., & Biswas-Diener, R. (2010). New well-being measures: Short scales to assess flourishing and positive and negative feelings. *Social Indicators Research, 97*(2), 143–156.

Echema, A. (1995). *Corporate personality in traditional Igbo society and the sacrament of reconciliation* (Vol. 538). Peter Lang.

George, S. K. (2009). Hospitality as openness to the other: Levinas, Derrida and the Indian hospitality ethos. *Journal of Human Values, 15*(1), 29–47.

Heal, F. (1990). *Hospitality in early modern England*. Clarendon Press.

Healey, J. G. (1981). *The fifth gospel: In search of black Christian values*. SCM Press.

Healey, J., & Sybertz, D. (1996). *Towards an African narrative theology*. Paulines Africa.

John, O. P., & Srivastava, S. (1999). The Big-Five trait taxonomy: History, measurement, and theoretical perspectives. In L. A. Pervin & O. P. John (Eds.), *Handbook of personality: Theory and research* (Vol. 2, pp. 102–138). Guilford Press.

Jonsen, K., & Jehn, K. A. (2009). Using triangulation to validate themes in qualitative studies. *Qualitative Research in Organizations and Management: An International Journal, 4*(2), 123–150.

Keyes, C. L. M. (2002). The mental health continuum: From languishing to flourishing in life. *Journal of Health and Social Behavior, 43*, 207–222.

Keyes, C. L. M. (2009). *Atlanta: Brief description of the mental health continuum short form (MHC-SF)*. Retrieved May 3, 2021, from https://www.aacu.org/sites/default/files/MHC-SFEnglish.pdf

Keyes, C. L., Wissing, M., Potgieter, J. P., Temane, M., Kruger, A., & van Rooy, S. (2008). Evaluation of the mental health continuum–short form (MHC–SF) in Setswana-speaking South Africans. *Clinical Psychology & Psychotherapy, 15*(3), 181–192.

Kiaziku, P. A. (2007). *Consecrated life in Bantu Africa*. Paulines Africa.

Kiaziku, P. A. (2009). *Culture and inculturation: A bantu viewpoint*. Paulines Africa.

Lamers, S. M., Westerhof, G. J., Bohlmeijer, E. T., ten Klooster, P. M., & Keyes, C. L. (2011). Evaluating the psychometric properties of the Mental Health Continuum-Short Form (MHC-SF). *Journal of Clinical Psychology, 67*(1), 99–110.

Lashley, C. (2015). Hospitality and hospitableness. *Research in Hospitality Management, 5*(1), 1–7.

Li, H., Xu, J., Chen, J., & Fan, Y. (2015). A reliability meta-analysis for 44 items big five inventory: Based on the reliability generalization methodology. *Advances in Psychological Science, 23*(5), 755–765.

Lynch, P., Molz, J. G., Mcintosh, A., Lugosi, P., & Lashley, C. (2011). Theorizing hospitality. *Hospitality & Society, 1*(1), 3–24.

Lyubomirsky, S., & Lepper, H. S. (1999). A measure of subjective happiness: Preliminary reliability and construct validation. *Social Indicators Research, 46*(2), 137–155.

Magesa, L. (1998). *African religion: The moral traditions of abundant life*. Paulines Africa.

Moila, M. P. (2002). *Challenging issues in African Christianity*. Powell Bible Centre.

Mugambi, J. N. K. (1989). *Christianity and African culture*. Acton Publishers.

Mulandi, J. (2003). Religious formation from the African perspective. *African Ecclesial Review, 45*(1), 47–70.

Ong, A. D., & van Dulman, M. H. M. (2007). *Oxford handbook of methods in positive psychology*. Oxford University Press.

Oruka, H. O. (1990). *Sage philosophy: Indigenous thinkers and modern debate on African philosophy*. E. J. Brill.

Peterson, C. (2006). Values in action (VIA): Classification of strengths. In M. Csikszentmihalyi & I. S. Csikszentmihalyi (Eds.), *A life worth living: Contributions to positive psychology* (pp. 29–48). Oxford University Press.

Peterson, C., & Park, N. (2006). Character strengths in organizations. *Journal of Organizational Behavior, 27*(8), 1149–1154.

Peterson, C., Ruch, W., Beermann, U., Park, N., & Seligman, M. E. (2007). Strengths of character, orientations to happiness, and life satisfaction. *The Journal of Positive Psychology, 2*(3), 149–156.

Peterson, C., & Seligman, M. E. P. (2004). *Character strengths and virtues: A handbook and classification*. Oxford University Press.

Robbins, B. (2008). What is the good life? Positive psychology and the renaissance of humanistic psychology. *Humanistic Psychologist, 36*, 96–112.

Rowan, N., & Wulff, D. (2007). Using qualitative methods to inform scale development. *The Qualitative Report, 12*(3), 450–466.

Selvam, S. G., & Collicutt, J. (2013). The ubiquity of the character strengths in African traditional religion: A thematic analysis. In H. H. Knoop & A. Delle Fave (Eds.), *Well-being and cultures: A positive psychology perspective* (pp. 83–102). Springer.

Sharpley, R. (2009). Tourism, religion and spirituality. In T. Jamal & M. Robinson (Eds.), *The SAGE handbook of tourism studies* (pp. 237–253). Sage.

Sobh, R., Belk, R. W., & Wilson, J. A. (2013). Islamic Arab hospitality and multiculturalism. *Marketing Theory, 13*(4), 443–463.

Yardley, L. (2017). Demonstrating the validity of qualitative research. *The Journal of Positive Psychology, 12*(3), 295–296.

Chapter 6
The Factor Structure of the Peer and Community Relational Health Indices in Two South African Samples: A Bifactor Exploratory Structural Equation Modelling Approach

Amanda Cromhout, Lusilda Schutte, and Marié P. Wissing

Abstract The Peer and Community Relational Health Indices (RHIP and RHIC), with subscales Engagement, Zest/Empowerment, and Authenticity, have been validated in (non-African) studies, but conflicting results were obtained regarding their factor structure. Therefore, and in view of the importance of relationships in the African context, the aim of this study was to investigate the factor structure of the RHIP and RHIC in two South African adult samples. Sample 1 ($n = 286$) completed the RHIC and RHIP in English. Sample 2 ($n = 400$) completed the RHIC in Setswana. Confirmatory factor analysis (CFA), bifactor CFA, exploratory structural equation modelling (ESEM) and bifactor ESEM were applied to the data. Reduced three-factor bifactor ESEM models displayed good fit for all scales. Problematic scale items were removed based on statistical and substantive grounds. Reliability scores were acceptable for the global factor of all scales. The reliability scores for some specific factors of the RHIP-English and the RHIC-English were acceptable, but unacceptable for all specific factors of the RHIC-Setswana. The study provides preliminary support for use of total scale scores, but not all subscale scores. The importance of considering culture and context when developing and applying measures of relational well-being is emphasised.

Keywords Relational health · Peer relationships · Community relationships · Psychometric properties · Bifactor exploratory structural equation modelling

---

A. Cromhout (✉) · L. Schutte · M. P. Wissing
Africa Unit for Transdisciplinary Health Research (AUTHeR), Faculty of Health Sciences, North-West University, Potchefstroom, South Africa
e-mail: 11792833@nwu.ac.za

L. Schutte et al. (eds.), *Embracing Well-Being in Diverse African Contexts: Research Perspectives*, Cross-Cultural Advancements in Positive Psychology 16,
https://doi.org/10.1007/978-3-030-85924-4_6

6.1 Introduction

Interconnectedness and being in relationship with others and a Higher Power, are widely recognised as core to being well, particularly in African communities (Wissing et al., 2019). The current study will investigate the phenomenon of relational well-being in South African samples by examining the psychometric properties of scales measuring peer and community relational health using recently developed psychometric techniques.

6.1.1 *Relatedness as a Core Facet of Being Well, Especially in African Contexts*

The belongingness hypothesis postulates that humans have a drive to form and maintain significant and enduring interpersonal relationships. This drive is satisfied when individuals have frequent and affectively pleasant interactions with others within the context of a stable and lasting framework of mutual concern for each other (see Baumeister & Leary, 1995). The need to belong is therefore satisfied within the context of close (intimate) relationships. When asked, the majority of people are likely to agree that positive connections with others are important contributors to both individual and community well-being. There is ample research to support this. Attachment theory (Bowlby, 1973) stresses the important role of early relational experiences in forming attachment behaviours which, in turn, influence relational experiences and behaviour in later life (e.g., Goodboy & Bolkan, 2011; McDermott et al., 2017; Merz & Jak, 2013). Many recent theories and models of well-being continue to emphasise the important role of positive relationships for well-being. Feeney and Collins (2015) proposed that relationships contribute towards thriving through different social support mechanisms that not only serve to protect the individual against the negative consequences of stress in adverse conditions, but also serve as a catalyst for engagement in activities that promote growth and thriving in the absence of adversity. According to basic psychological needs theory, a subtheory of self-determination theory (Deci & Ryan, 2000), relatedness (i.e., the need to belong and to feel connected to others) is one of three basic psychological needs (together with autonomy and competence) that must be satisfied in order for growth and psychological well-being to ensue (Deci & Ryan, 2000; Rigby & Ryan, 2018). When any one or more of these needs are not satisfied, maladaptive behaviour patterns may develop, resulting in reduced levels of well-being (Deci & Ryan, 2000; Olafsen et al., 2017). Keyes's (2002, 2005, 2007) mental health continuum model discerns psychological, social, and emotional well-being as the constituents of well-being, with relationships and relational aspects as important facets of psychological and social well-being. The relationality-meaning model (Wissing, 2014; Wissing & Delle Fave, 2013) emphasises that relationships and connections are core to experiencing meaning in life and that relationships and meaning are essential for well-being. Jordan (2017), a proponent of relational-cultural theory (Miller, 1976), indicated that humans are "wired to connect" (p. 231) and that "we grow through and towards connection throughout our lives" (p. 231).

The importance of relationships is particularly prominent in African research. In contrast to individualistic cultures that stress aspects such as autonomy, self-sufficiency, and individuality (e.g., Hofstede, 2011), collectivistic (African) cultures deem relationships an essential component of personhood (e.g., Ezenweke & Nwadialor, 2013) and emphasis is placed on community and interdependence, rather than on individuality (e.g., Ezenweke & Nwadialor, 2013; Hofstede, 2011; Mbiti, 1990). The African philosophy of Ubuntu, meaning "I am because we are, and since we are, therefore, I am" (Mbiti, 1970, p. 141) expresses the centrality of interconnectedness and relatedness in African contexts. As illustration of the importance of relationships and relatedness in African contexts, Wissing et al. (2020) found that adult and older adult samples from rural and urban areas in Ghana and South Africa valued family, interpersonal (nonfamily), spirituality/religion, and community/society relationships as important sources of meaning. Motivations for why these relationships were important included reasons such as the giving and receiving of love and support; experiencing a sense of sharing and reciprocity (family); experiencing a sense of belonging and integration; experiencing harmony or balance in interpersonal relationships; sharing experiences and contributing to the lives of others (interpersonal); cultivating faith; experiencing personal identity and a sense of harmony (spirituality/religion); and contribution to the community (community/society).

Roos et al. (2019) found that social contact with others, participating in sociocultural and spiritual rituals, and keeping busy (either alone or with others) mitigated loneliness in a South African cohort of older black women who reported ruptured intergenerational relationships and lack of connection to the rural township they were relocated to during the Apartheid years in South Africa. Despite the importance of connectedness for well-being, Wissing (2014) indicated that more research that focuses on relationships as human bonds and connections, as well as on the dynamics of relational processes, is needed to understand the role of relationships in well-being. Feeney and Collins (2015) also pointed out that more is to be learned about the specific mechanisms through which relationships work to promote well-being. One theory that emphasises relational well-being and the importance of interconnectedness is the relational-cultural theory (Miller, 1976). Relational-cultural theory forms the basis of this study and will therefore be introduced in the next paragraph.

6.1.2 Relational-Cultural Theory

Relational-cultural theory (Miller, 1976) is a developmental theory which assumes that happiness and well-being are the result of the extent to which individuals are involved in growth-fostering relationships. According to relational-cultural theory, we grow when we build growth-fostering connections with others, as well as through community (Jordan, 2008). This theory was originally developed to better understand the relational experiences of women and marginalised minority groups whose relational experiences, according to Miller (1976), were misrepresented by traditional developmental theories that emphasised separation-individuation as the ultimate developmental outcome (Miller & Striver, 1997). Whereas traditional developmental theories highlight aspects such as autonomy, separation, and self-sufficiency as important outcomes of human development, relational-cultural theory accentuates increasing relational competence and the ability to form meaningful and growth-fostering connections with others as an essential outcome of human development (Frey et al., 2005; Jordan, 2000, 2001). Although research on the relational-cultural theory mainly focused on women in line with the feminist roots of the theory (Jordan, 2017; Liang et al., 2002), the theory is now also applied to the relational experiences of men, with culture as an important consideration in the understanding of relationships (Alvarez & Lazzari, 2016; Jordan, 2017; Liang et al., 2007).

The core tenets of relational-cultural theory include notions such as that individuals grow through their connections with others throughout the lifespan, psychological growth is characterised by increasing relational competence, mature functioning is characterised by mutuality rather than separation, authenticity is essential for genuine engagement, and that mutual empathy and mutual empowerment are key components of growth-fostering relationships (Jordan, 2000). As such, growth-fostering relationships are characterised by four components according to relational-cultural theory (Jordan, 2010; Miller & Striver, 1997), namely *authenticity,* the individual's capacity to engage genuinely with others by bringing his or her real self to the relationship, while being aware of the impact of one's actions on the other; *mutual engagement,* the individual's commitment and attunement to the relationship, and the ability to maintain a sense of self, while also being open to the change experiences within the relational context; *differences/conflict,* the ability to deal with differences/conflict in such a way that differences can be expressed and dealt with, and to accept these differences; and *empowerment/zest,* a sense of personal strength, and feeling encouraged and inspired to take action (Jordan, 1986, 1997, 2010; Miller & Striver, 1997).

The outcomes associated with the presence of growth-fostering relationships are referred to as the "five good things", namely an increased sense of zest; clarity about the self, others and the relationship; a sense of self-worth; increased capacity for creativity and productivity; and a desire to connect more with others (Jordan, 2008, 2010; Miller, 1986). However, even within the context of growth-fostering relationships, disconnection will sometimes be experienced and result in feeling misunderstood and disappointed (Jordan, 2010). Although constant feelings of disconnection may result in isolation or withdrawal, people can also experience growth when dealing with disconnections (Jordan, 2008).

While the significance of relationships in African cultural contexts is widely recognised, it is not known whether theories developed elsewhere in the world, such as relational-cultural theory, will fit in African contexts. Relational well-being may be conceptualised or manifest differently in different cultural contexts, which may make the theory inappropriate in cultural contexts that differ from the context where it was developed. One way to examine the appropriateness of a theory or model in a given context, is to investigate the psychometric properties of an instrument that was developed based on the theory or model. If the instrument fails to display good psychometric properties, it may indicate that the theory or model is not merely transferrable to the new context (of course, there may also be other explanations, such as translation issues). Such findings will imply that applying the instrument in research or practice may produce skewed and invalid findings, and uncritical use of scale scores can be very detrimental to individuals and groups. On the other hand, if the instrument displays good psychometric properties, further investigations can be done using the scale's scores which can give a fuller picture of the extent to which the theory applies in the new context. The Relational Health Indices were developed to operationalise relational-cultural theory, and the appropriateness of these instruments in selected African samples will be a first step towards exploring the applicability of the theory in these contexts. In the next paragraph, the Relational Health Indices (Liang et al., 2002) will be introduced.

6.1.3 Measuring Relational Well-Being: The Relational Health Indices

The Relational Health Indices (RHI, Liang et al., 2002) are based upon the relational-cultural theory (Miller, 1976) and measure relational health in three types of relationships, namely peer (RHIP), community (RHIC), and mentor relationships (RHIM, Liang et al., 2002). Initially, each scale was developed to consist of four subscales that measured authenticity, mutual engagement, conflict/differences, and empowerment/zest, respectively (Liang et al., 2002). For both the RHIP and the RHIM, data showed that the conflict/differences factor was not well identified, and therefore this subscale was dropped in each case. For the RHIC, modification indices showed cross-loadings for items measuring authenticity and items measuring conflict/differences, and therefore these subscales were merged and labelled "authenticity" for the RHIC. Hence, each scale finally consisted of three subscales (Engagement, Zest/Empowerment, Authenticity; Liang et al., 2002). More details on the scales' composition are provided in the Method section of this chapter.

Inconsistent results were obtained across studies regarding the factor structure of the RHI scales. Liang et al. (2002) found support for the postulated three-factor structure in a multicultural female student sample (White = 58%, Asian/Pacific Islander = 28%, Black = 4.3%, Hispanic = 4.3%, Native American = 1%, Other = 4%). However, in a subsequent study Liang et al. (2007) found support for a unidimensional factor structure for each of the scales in a multicultural student sample (White = 85%, Asian = 6%, Hispanic 4%, Black = 3%, Other = 2%) that also included male participants. Frey et al. (2005) found evidence for a unidimensional structure for the RHIP and the RHIM, but a two-factor structure for the RHIC in an American student sample (European American/White = 73%, Hispanic American = 11%, Asian American = 6%, international students = 4%, African American = 2%, Native American/Alascan = 1%, unidentified = 3%) that included male and female participants. Lenz et al. (2016) reported a three-factor structure for the Spanish version of each of the scales in a Spanish-speaking young adult sample who reported Spanish/Latin identities and who lived in Spanish/Latin communities (Lima, Peru, and the Mexican American border of the United States). The sample consisted of male and female participants. As far as we could establish, the psychometric properties of the Relational Health Indices were not yet explored in any African samples.

In all studies that did investigate the psychometric properties of the Relational Health Indices, the factor structure of the scales was explored using confirmatory factor analysis (CFA), except for the study by Frey et al. (2005) that applied principal component analysis with oblimin rotation. Principal component analysis aims for parsimony by extracting the essence of a dataset through the creation of linear combinations of the variables (components) rather than identifying latent factors that explains the maximum variance of the variables which is done in exploratory factor analysis, which is built on the common factor model (Alavi et al., 2020). Since principal component analysis may not have been ideal for the purpose it was used in Frey et al. (2005), results should be interpreted with caution. In addition, CFA, which was used in all other validation studies of the Relational Health Indices, is based upon statistical assumptions that may lead to biased parameter estimates, and hence inaccurate conclusions from those estimates (Morin, Arens, & Marsh, 2016). These limitations will be addressed in the next paragraph. The RHIP and the RHIC are relevant to this study.

6.1.4 Determining Factorial Validity: Traditional and Recent Approaches

Testing factorial validity (or dimensionality) involves examining whether the hypothetical factor structure, that is, the interrelationships between the items and their latent structure, applies to a dataset (Boateng et al., 2018). Once the factor structure has been confirmed/established, scale scores can be calculated that can be used in subsequent analyses, including tests of reliability and evaluation of criterion and construct validity (Boateng et al., 2018). Traditionally, factorial validity is determined by applying either exploratory factor analysis (EFA) when the relationship between the observed and unobserved variables are uncertain, or confirmatory factor analysis (CFA) when there is some *a priori* hypothesis about the relationship between the observed and latent variables (Byrne, 2012). In the case of EFA, all associations between the latent and observed variables are freely estimated (Howard et al., 2018), thus each observed variable is regressed on each latent variable (Kline, 2013). Unlike EFA, the cross-loadings of indicators (observed variables) on nontarget factors (latent variables) are constrained to zero in CFA, which means that each indicator is regressed only on the target factor (Howard et al., 2018). This is because

CFA is based upon the independent cluster model (ICM) where the cross-loadings of indicators on nontarget factors are assumed to be zero (Howard et al., 2018). However, imposing these constraints may result in biased parameter estimates as two sources of construct-relevant multidimensionality are not accounted for (Morin, Arens, & Marsh, 2016).

The first source of construct-relevant multidimensionality relates to the nature of the indicators used to measure the constructs. When constructs are conceptually-related, the indicators will rarely be uniquely associated with the target factor but will mostly have some construct-relevant association with nontarget factors too (Howard et al., 2018; Morin, Arens, & Marsh, 2016). These cross-loadings should be accounted for to ensure that potential true influence of the nontarget factor on the indicator is not ignored. If these cross-loadings remain unmodelled, sources of misspecification are concealed, which in turn might be expressed as model misfits and impact the goodness-of-fit indices. Also, the discriminant validity of factors can be affected if biased parameter estimates of factor correlations generate artificial multicollinearity when the factors are used for prediction (Howard et al., 2018).

The second source of construct-relevant multidimensionality relates to hierarchically-ordered constructs (Howard et al., 2018; Morin, Arens, & Marsh, 2016). In higher-order factor models it is hypothesised that multiple factors can combine into a single or multiple higher-order factors (Howard et al., 2018), and that the association between the indicators and the higher-order factor is fully mediated by the first-order factor (Morin, Arens, Tran, & Caci, 2016). The first-order factor therefore reflects the variance explained by the higher-order factor, and the unique variance that is explained by each first-order factor (Morin, Arens, Tran, & Caci, 2016). Therefore, no unique variance is explained by the higher-order factor, as its variance is completely explained by the first-order factors.

These two sources of construct-relevant multidimensionality are psychometrically accounted for in exploratory structural equation modelling (ESEM, Asparouhov & Muthén, 2009) and bifactor modelling (Howard et al., 2018; Morin, Arens, Tran, & Caci, 2016) respectively. ESEM models the associations that indicators have with nontarget factors (cross-loadings), over and above their associations with the target factor (Howard et al., 2018; Morin, Arens, & Marsh, 2016). When cross-loadings are small and in line with theoretical expectations, they can be interpreted as the influence of the nontarget factor on the construct-relevant part of the indicator. However, alternative models should be considered if the cross-loadings are unexplainable, or larger than the target factor loadings (Morin, Arens, & Marsh, 2016).

Bifactor modelling, as opposed to hierarchical models, hypothesises that a unitary global factor coexists with some specific factors, and that the global factor influences all the indicators directly. The global factor represents the variance that is shared by all the indicators (i.e., the common variance), and the variance that is shared by a specific subset of indicators is represented by the specific factors (Howard et al., 2018; Morin, Arens, Tran, & Caci, 2016). The variance that is attributable to the global factor can therefore be separated from the variance that is attributable to the specific factors, while the direct relations between the indicators and the global and specific factors are estimated simultaneously (Howard et al., 2018; Morin, Arens,

Tran, & Caci, 2016). Bifactor modelling can be applied to standard CFA models, called a bifactor CFA model; or ESEM models, called a bifactor ESEM model.

When constructs are conceptually-related and/or hierarchically-ordered, use of models that allow for the incorporation of cross-loadings and/or a general factor, such as bifactor CFA, ESEM (Asparouhov & Muthén, 2009), and bifactor ESEM (Jennrich & Bentler, 2011) may represent the data better (Morin, Arens, Tran, & Caci, 2016). The particular model specifications are important as cross-loadings that are not accounted for may result in inflated estimates of the global factor in bifactor CFA models, and a global factor that is not accounted for in an EFA model may result in inflated estimates of the cross-loadings (Howard et al., 2018).

6.1.5 The Present Study

Close connections are important for well-being, particularly in African contexts. Research on relational well-being partly depends on psychometrically and substantively sound measurement instruments of important relational constructs. As the psychometric properties of measures may be impacted by the statistical techniques used to analyse the data, especially when these techniques are based upon statistical assumptions that may not hold, the application of statistical techniques that overcome these limitations becomes important. As far as could be established, the psychometric properties of the Relational Health Indices have not yet been studied in any African contexts. Investigation of the psychometric properties of the scales in African contexts will provide insight into the extent to which the scale and underlying theory can be transferred to the current contexts. More generally, it may provide some insight into the nature and manifestations of relational well-being in the African samples under study. In addition, conflicting results were obtained regarding the factor structure of the scales in other contexts where traditional CFA and principal component analysis were applied, and further investigation of the factor structure may contribute to a better understanding of the constructs and their operationalisations. Finally, statistical analyses (such as bifactor CFA, ESEM, and bifactor ESEM), that address the limitations inherent to CFA, have not yet been applied to these scales. In the present study, these statistical techniques were applied to the data on the RHIP and RHIC from two South African adult samples to determine the factor structure of the RHIP and the RHIC in these samples, and determine the potential applicability of the scales in these contexts.

6.2 Method

6.2.1 Research Design and Participants

A quantitative, cross-sectional survey design was implemented. The samples formed part of the FORT3 research project (The prevalence of levels of psychosocial health:

dynamics and relationships with biomarkers of (ill) health in South African social contexts; Wissing 2008/2012), and the South African leg of the Prospective Urban and Rural Epidemiological study (PURE-SA, Teo et al., 2009). Participants from the FORT3 research project (Sample 1) were an adult sample (n = 286, male = 97, female = 185, unspecified gender = 4, M_{age} = 36.72, SD_{age} = 13.25) with a grade 12 level of education as minimum. Sample 1 completed the RHIC and the RHIP in English. Participants indicated their home language as English (25.8%), Setswana (4.5%), Afrikaans (47.4%), Other (18.8%), or missing (3.5%), suggesting that this was a multicultural sample.

Participants from the PURE-SA/FORT3 overlap research project (Sample 2) were an adult subsample (n = 400, male = 116, female = 282, unspecified gender = 2, M_{age} = 61.57, SD_{age} = 8.87) consisting of 200 participants from a rural/deep rural area and 200 participants from an urban area in South Africa. Participants had a grade 12 level of education or less. Sample 2 completed the RHIC in Setswana. Participants reported their home language as Setswana (82.5%), or Other (17.3%), with 0.3% not indicating their home language. Participants who indicated "Other" as their home language specified another of the 11 official languages of South Africa as their home language, with the majority naming Xhosa or Sesotho. Participants' reported home language suggests that Sample 2 was a mainly African sample.

6.2.2 *Measures*

6.2.2.1 Socio-Demographic Questionnaire

Socio-demographic data, such as age, gender, and home language were collected.

6.2.2.2 The Relational Health Indices

The Relational Health Indices (Liang et al., 2002) measure relational health in three separate types of relationships, namely peer relationships (RHIP), community relationships (RHIC), and mentor relationships (RHIM) on a 5-point Likert-type scale ranging from 1 (*never*) to 5 (*always*). The RHIP and RHIC are relevant for the current study. The RHIP (Liang et al., 2002) consists of 12 items and three subscales, namely Engagement (RHIP-E, 4 items), Zest/Empowerment (RHIP-Z, 4 items), and Authenticity (RHIP-A, 4 items). Liang et al. (2002) reported Cronbach's alpha values of .74 (RHIP-E), .73 (RHIP-Z), .69 (RHIP-A), and .85 (RHIP composite score).

The RHIC (Liang et al., 2002) consists of 14 items and has three subscales, namely Engagement (RHIC-E, 5 items), Zest/Empowerment (RHIC-Z, 5 items), and Authenticity (RHIC-A, 4 items). Liang et al. (2002) reported Cronbach's alpha values of .86 (RHIC-E), .87 (RHIC-Z), .75 (RHIC-A), and .90 (RHIC composite score).

6.2.3 *Ethical Considerations and Procedure*

The FORT3 and PURE-SA research projects obtained ethics approval from the Health Research Ethics Committee of the North-West University, South Africa, with ethics approval numbers NWU 00002-07-A2 and NWU-00016-10-A1, respectively. Additionally, the PURE-SA research project obtained ethics approval from the provincial Department of Health. Participants gave written informed consent. Participation was voluntary. Sample 1 completed the questionnaires on their own time and at a place of their convenience, while trained fieldworkers administered the questionnaires for Sample 2. Sample 1 did not receive incentives for participation, but Sample 2 received a small token of appreciation. Data was handled confidentially. Minimal risk was associated with the study. For Sample 1, debriefing was offered if needed, but no participant indicated such need. For Sample 2, participants with high scores on a measure of depression were referred for mental health screening at the nearest clinic or hospital. Referral letters were handed and explained to the participants in person, and they were encouraged to take the letter to the nearest clinic or hospital for mental health screening. The nearby health care centres were informed about the study and the possibility that participants may be referred for screening. The contact details of a registered clinical psychologist who was part of the research team was provided on the referral letter, should the health care provider have any questions pertaining to the study and the referral. Data for Sample 1 was collected from 2011 to 2014 and for Sample 2 from 2017 to 2019.

The RHIC was translated from English into Setswana by a professional translator. Scale items were adapted to reflect their meaning in a culturally appropriate manner. An independent translator back-translated the scales into English (Brislin, 1980). A research committee, consisting of academics of whom some were native speakers of Setswana and were fluent in English, as well as community members fluent in English and Setswana, compared the back-translated versions with the original English versions and made adaptations to the Setswana translation where needed (Van de Vijver & Hambleton, 1996; Van de Vijver & Leung, 1997).

6.2.4 *Data Analysis*

6.2.4.1 Stage 1: Descriptive Statistics

IBM SPSS Statistics 25 were used to calculate the means, standard deviations, skewness, and kurtosis for each scale item of the RHIP and RHIC.

6.2.4.2 Stage 2: Factorial Validity

Mplus 8.3 (Muthén & Muthén, 1998–2019) were used to apply CFA, bifactor-CFA, ESEM, and bifactor-ESEM to determine the factor structure of the RHIP and RHIC.

Full information maximum likelihood estimation was used to handle missing data. The weighted least square mean and variance adjusted (WLSMV) estimator for categorical data was applied. Cross-loadings were fixed to zero for CFA and bifactor CFA models. For ESEM and bifactor ESEM models target rotation was applied and cross-loadings were estimated to be close to, but not exactly zero (Asparouhov & Muthén, 2009). Model fit was evaluated by considering global fit indexes, standardised factor loadings, expected parameter change values, and modification indices (Byrne, 2012). In terms of global model fit indices, the chi-square statistic (χ^2), comparative fit index (CFI), Tucker-Lewis index (TLI), root mean square error of approximation (RMSEA), and the standardised root mean square residual (SRMR) are reported. Note that the CFI, TLI, RMSEA, and SRMR received more emphasis than the chi-square statistic when interpreting model fit as the χ^2-statistic is sensitive to sample size. In terms of general interpretation guidelines, CFI and TLI values larger than .90 have previously been considered to indicate good model fit, but more recently values larger than .95 are advised as indication of good model fit (Byrne, 2012; Hu & Bentler, 1999). RMSEA and SRMR values smaller than 0.08 represent reasonable model fit and values smaller than 0.05 may be considered to indicate good model fit (Byrne, 2012). However, caution must be applied when interpreting global fit indices, since recent research has shown that global fit indices are largely influenced by measurement quality, and uncritical use of cutoff values is not advised (McNeish et al., 2018). In addition, these guideline values may not be simply transferrable to the WLSMV estimator, and caution should be used when applying them in this case (Xia, 2016, Xia & Yang, 2018).

6.2.4.3 Stage 3: Internal Consistency Reliability

Omega hierarchical coefficients were calculated by applying the formula used by Sánchez-Oliva et al. (2017). Omega coefficients larger than .50 represent sufficient reliability for bifactor models (Perreira et al., 2018).

6.3 Results

6.3.1 Stage 1: Descriptive Statistics

For Sample 1 item mean scores for the RHIP-English ranged between 3.50 (*SD* = 1.24, item 8) and 4.36 (*SD* = 0.85, item 5), skewness values between −1.43 (item 5) and − 0.40 (item 7), and kurtosis values between −0.88 (item 7) and 1.83 (item 5). For the RHIC-English item mean scores ranged between 2.74 (*SD* = 1.19, item 3) and 3.49 (*SD* = 0.91, item 8), skewness values between −0.45 (item 8) and 0.23 (item 3), and kurtosis values between −0.97 (item 9) and 0.90 (item 8).

For Sample 2 the mean scores of the RHIC-Setswana items ranged between 2.52 ($SD = 1.05$, item 10) and 3.88 ($SD = 1.02$, item 1), skewness values between −1.23 (item 1) and 0.36 (item 10), and kurtosis values between −1.29 (item 9) and 1.49 (item 1). The descriptive statistics for the individual scale items are presented in Table 6.4 in Appendix.

6.3.2 Stage 2A: Factorial Validity of the RHIP-English, RHIC-English, and RHIC-Setswana

Table 6.1 shows the fit indices of the models tested, namely a one-factor CFA model (Model 1), a three-factor CFA model (Model 2), a three-factor bifactor CFA model (Model 3), a three-factor ESEM model (Model 4), and a three-factor bifactor ESEM model (Model 5). The models tested for the RHIP-English are presented in Fig. 6.1, and those for the RHIC-English and RHIC-Setswana in Fig. 6.2.

For Sample 1, Model 1 of the RHIP-English did not fit the data. Model 2 yielded a model with reasonable model fit. Model 3 did not converge. Model fit improved when cross-loadings (Model 4) and, in addition, a general factor (Model 5) were modelled. Model 5 best fitted the data after Zest/Empowerment item 9 ("I have a greater sense of self-worth through my relationship with my friend") and Authenticity item 11 ("I can tell my friend when he/she has hurt my feelings"), that had negative residual variances, were removed from the scale.[1]

After consideration of substantive reasons for model modification, such as whether the item is correctly placed in the assigned subscale and whether the item measures the intended construct, we concluded that there was no clear substantive justification for model modifications. However, as the items posed statistical challenges in the current sample, the items were removed. Future research may focus on whether this result will replicate in other samples. Model 5, with items 9 and 11 removed, displayed good model fit (CFI = .999, RMSEA = 0.027).

For Samples 1 and 2 the one-factor structure (Model 1) revealed poor model fit for the RHIC. For Sample 1, the residual covariance matrix of Model 2 was not positive definite. Model 3 for Sample 1 and Models 2 and 3 for Sample 2 yielded models with psi-matrices that were not positive definite. Model fit improved when cross-loadings were modelled (Model 4) and when a general factor was modelled in addition to cross-loadings (Model 5). Model 5 revealed the best fit for Samples 1 and 2 with CFI and TLI values larger than .95 and RMSEA and SRMR values smaller than 0.05 after item 9, which had a negative residual variance for both versions of the RHIC, was removed. Item 9 ("There is a lot of backbiting and gossiping in this community") likely does not capture the intended meaning of the Authenticity factor that refers to the capacity for genuine engagement with others and bringing one's real self

[1] Before removal of items 9 and 11, the residual variances were specified to be larger than zero but this resulted in an unidentified model.

Table 6.1 Fit indices for the one-factor and three-factor structure models

Latent model	χ^2	*df*	*p*	CFI	TLI	RMSEA	90%CI	SRMR
Sample 1: RHIP-English								
Model 1	407.780	54	<.001	.917	.898	0.151	(0.138; 0.165)	0.055
Model 2	289.066	51	<.001	.944	.927	0.128	(0.114; 0.142)	0.046
Model 3	No convergence							
Model 4	130.106	33	<.001	.977	.954	0.101	(0.083; 0.120)	0.030
Model 5[a]	13.352	11	0.270	.999	.997	0.027	(0.000; 0.071)	0.011
Sample 1: RHIC-English								
Model 1	1566.263	77	<.001	.772	.731	0.261	(0.250; 0.272)	0.106
Model 2[b]	308.093	74	<.001	.964	.956	0.106	(0.093; 0.118)	0.054
Model 3[c]	362.879	63	<.001	.954	.934	0.129	(0.117; 0.143)	0.048
Model 4	200.775	52	<.001	.977	.960	0.100	(0.086; 0.115)	0.030
Model 5[d]	53.581	32	0.0098	.997	.992	0.049	(0.024; 0.071)	0.013
Sample 2: RHIC-Setswana								
Model 1	665.781	77	<.001	.863	.837	0.138	(0.129; 0.148)	0.066
Model 2[c]	651.283	74	<.001	.865	.834	0.140	(0.130; 0.150)	0.066
Model 3[c]	No fit indices produced							
Model 4	223.995	52	<.001	.960	.930	0.091	(0.079; 0.103)	0.035
Model 5[d]	58.232	32	0.0031	.994	.985	0.045	(0.026; 0.064)	0.018

Note. RHIC = Relational Health Indices – Community Scale; RHIP = Relational Health Indices – Peer Scale; Model 1 = one-factor confirmatory factor analysis (CFA) model; Model 2 = three-factor CFA model; Model 3 = three-factor bifactor-CFA model; Model 4 = three-factor exploratory structural equation modelling (ESEM) model; Model 5 = three-factor bifactor-ESEM model; χ^2 = Chi-square; *df* = degrees of freedom; *p* = probability value; CFI = Comparative fit index; TLI = Tucker-Lewis Index; RMSEA = Root mean square error of approximation; 90% CI = 90% confidence interval of the RMSEA; SRMR = Standardised root-mean square residual

[a]Items 9 and 11 removed due to a negative residual variance

[b]Residual covariance matrix not positive definite

[c]Psi matrix not positive definite

[d]Item 9 removed due to a negative residual variance

to relationships. The item seems rather to capture negative relational interaction than authenticity *per se*. Item 9 was therefore removed.

Our results point towards the multidimensionality of the RHIP and the RHIC, while the existence of a global factor in each case is also supported, with the three-factor, bifactor ESEM model yielding the best fit for both scales. Next, we investigated the factor loadings of the bifactor ESEM model.

6.3.3 Stage 2B: Standardised Factor Loadings

The standardised factor loadings of the RHIP-English, RHIC-English, and RHIC-Setswana are presented in Tables 6.2 and 6.3, respectively. For the RHIP-English all items, except item 4 loaded significantly on the general factor. Items 4 and 12 loaded

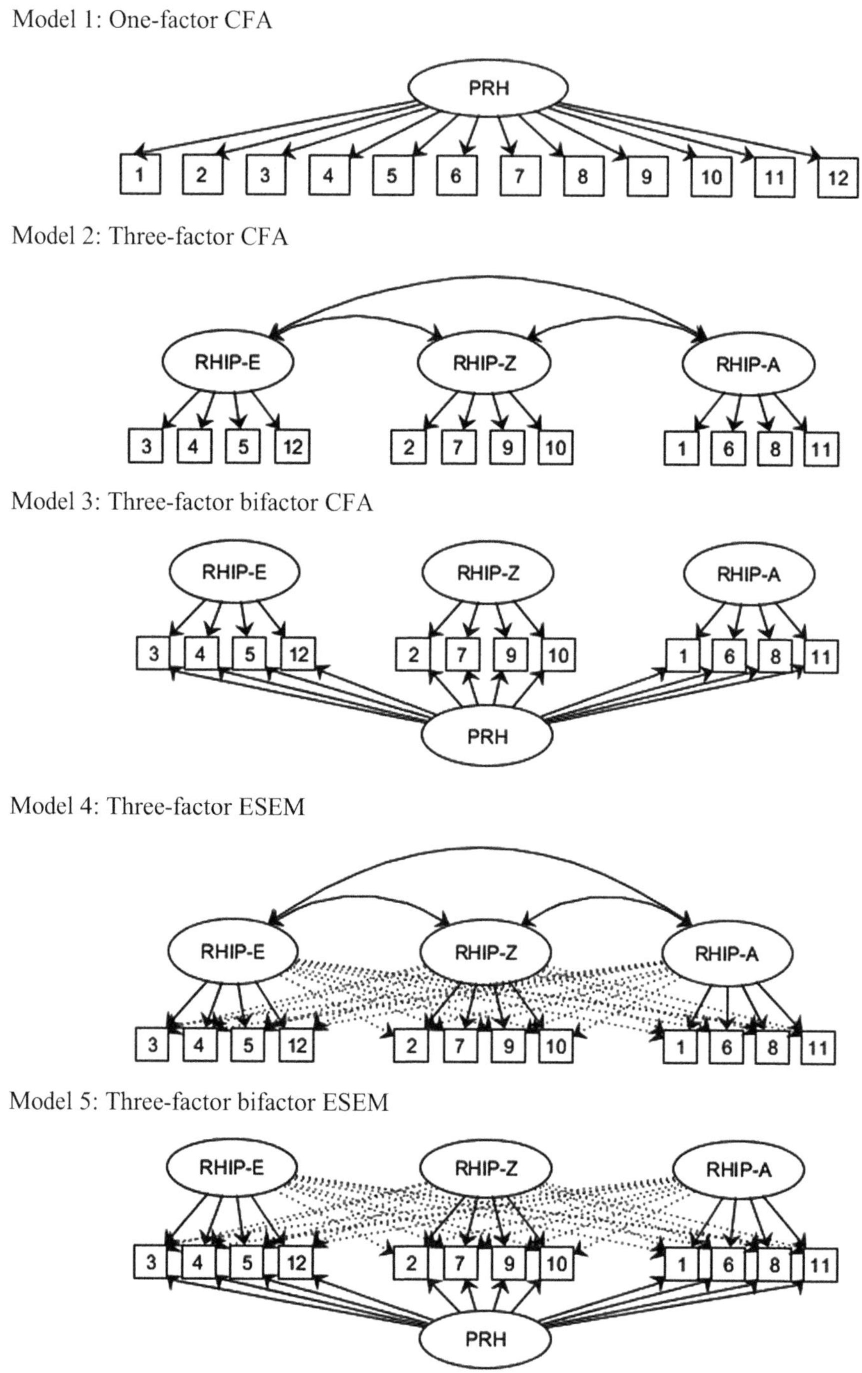

Fig. 6.1 Representation of the various models tested for the RHIP-English. RHIP = Relational Health Indices – Peer Scale; PRH = Peer Relational Health factor; RHIP-E = Engagement subscale; RHIP-Z = Zest/Empowerment subscale; RHIP-A = Authenticity subscale

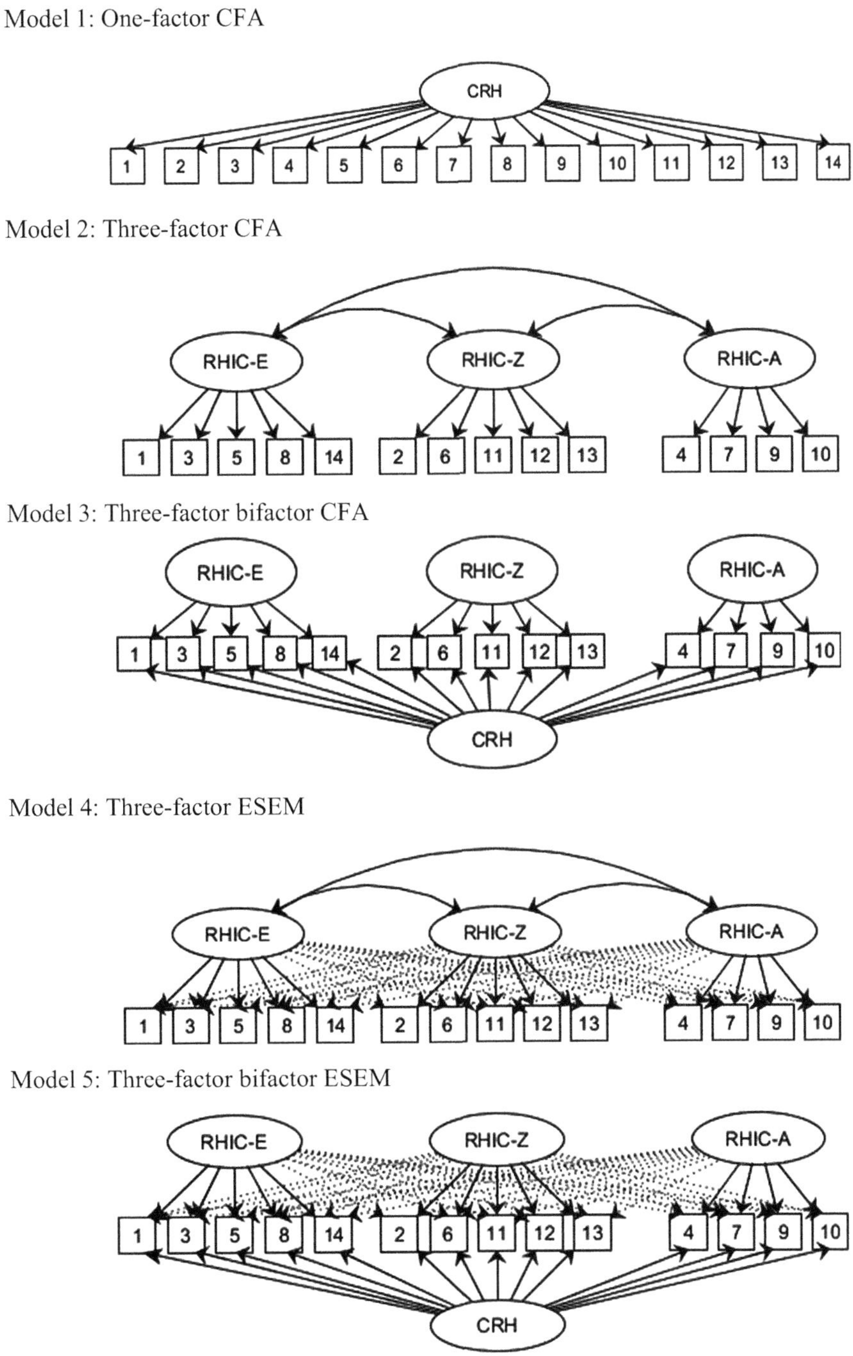

Fig. 6.2 Representation of the various models tested for the RHIC-English and RHIC-Setswana. RHIC = Relational Health Indices – Community Scale; CRH = Community Relational Health factor; RHIC-E = Engagement subscale; RHIC-Z = Zest/Empowerment subscale; RHIC-A = Authenticity subscale

Table 6.2 Standardised Factor Loadings and Omega Coefficients for the Three-factor Bifactor ESEM Model (item 9 and 11 removed) of the RHIP-English

	RHIP-English				
Item	GF	RHIP-E	RHIP-Z	RHIP-A	RV
Engagement					
3	**0.86***	**0.26**	−0.01	−0.11*	0.18*
4	**0.80***	**0.33***	0.03	0.09	0.24*
5	**0.86***	**−0.05**	−0.15	−0.05	0.23*
12	**0.88***	**−0.35***	0.05	−0.03	0.09*
Zest/empowerment					
2	**0.82***	0.24*	**0.22***	0.07*	0.21*
7	**0.53***	−0.17*	**0.18**	0.00	0.65*
9[a]	–	–	–	–	–
10	**0.68***	−0.13*	**0.18**	0.05	0.49*
Authenticity					
1	**0.67***	0.05	0.00	**0.66***	0.11*
6	**0.66***	−0.12*	0.18*	**0.38***	0.38*
8 (R)	**0.23***	0.12	−0.18	**0.22***	0.85*
11[a]	–	–	–	–	–
Omega coefficients	*0.93*	*0.57*	*0.20*	*0.54*	

Note. Target factor loadings are represented in bold. GF = general factor; RHIP: Relational health indices – Peer scale; RHIP-E = engagement factor; RHIP-Z = zest/empowerment factor; RHIP-A = authenticity factor; RV = residual variance. (R) = reverse scored items
[a]Items 9 and 11 removed due to negative residual variances
*$p < 0.05$

significantly on the Engagement target factor, only item 2 loaded significantly on the Zest/Empowerment target factor, and all Authenticity items loaded significantly on the target factor. Target factor loadings were mostly higher than cross-loadings, except for Zest/Empowerment item 2 that had a larger statistically significant cross-loading on the Engagement factor. Scale items loaded stronger on the general factor than on the specific (target) factors.

For the RHIC-English all items, except item 4 loaded significantly on the general factor. Items 3, 8, and 14 loaded significantly on the Engagement factor. All Zest/Empowerment items, except item 2, loaded significantly on the target factor. The Authenticity factor had no statistically significant target factor loadings. Target factor loadings were generally larger than cross-loadings, with some exceptions (e.g., Engagement items 1 and 14 cross-loaded on the Zest/Empowerment factor, Engagement item 5 cross-loaded on the Authenticity factor, Zest/Empowerment item 6 cross-loaded on the Engagement factor). All items loaded stronger on the general factor than on their specific (target) factors, except for the Authenticity items that loaded stronger on the specific factor, suggesting that the items are more representative of the Authenticity factor than the general factor.

Table 6.3 Standardised Factor Loadings and Omega Coefficients for the Three-factor, Bifactor ESEM Models (item 9 removed) of the RHIC-English and RHIC-Setswana

	RHIC-English					RHIC-Setswana				
Item	GF	RHIC-E	RHIC-Z	RHIC-A	RV	GF	RHIC-E	RHIC-Z	RHIC-A	RV
Engagement										
1	**0.84***	**−0.04**	−0.29*	−0.02	0.20*	**0.63***	**0.64***	−0.11	0.18	0.15*
3	**0.75***	**0.30***	0.02	0.02	0.34*	**0.62***	**−0.13**	−0.17*	0.01	0.57*
5	**0.88***	**0.13**	−0.06*	0.18*	0.18*	**0.72***	**−0.10**	−0.01	0.01	0.48*
8	**0.66***	**−0.26***	0.07	0.18*	0.46*	**0.60***	**0.07**	−0.04	0.03	0.63*
14	**0.82***	**0.15***	0.31*	0.06*	0.21*	**0.75***	**0.13**	0.36*	−0.24	0.22*
Zest/empowerment										
2	**0.88***	−0.11	**−0.14**	−0.19	0.17*	**0.66***	0.36*	**−0.14**	0.12	0.40*
6	**0.80***	0.12*	**0.09***	0.04	0.34*	**0.64***	−0.21*	**−0.12**	−0.16	0.51*
11	**0.78***	−0.12*	**0.40***	−0.08*	0.20*	**0.64***	−0.08	**0.35***	0.25*	0.41*
12	**0.77***	0.01	**0.39***	−0.05	0.26*	**0.70***	0.05	**0.36***	0.13	0.36*
13	**0.65***	0.12*	**0.46***	−0.13*	0.34*	**0.74***	0.09	**0.35***	−0.27*	0.25*
Authenticity										
4 (R)	**0.01**	−0.05	−0.05	**0.65**	0.58*	**−0.37***	0.16*	0.06	**−0.01**	0.83*
7 (R)	**0.20***	−0.01	0.00	**0.61**	0.59*	**−0.34***	0.25*	0.10	**0.30**	0.70*
9 (R)[a]	**–**	–	–	–	–	–	–	–	–	–
10 (R)	**0.13***	0.08	−0.11	**0.43**	0.78*	**0.05**	−0.09	−0.10	**−0.15**	0.96
Omega coefficients	*0.93*	*0.35*	*0.62*	*0.59*		*0.90*	*0.36*	*0.47*	*0.08*	

Note. Target factor loadings are represented in bold. RHIC = relational health indices – Community scale; GF = general factor; RHIC-E = engagement factor; RHIC-Z = zest/empowerment factor; RHIC-A = authenticity factor; RV = residual variance. (R) = reverse scored items.

[a]Item 9 removed due to a negative residual variance

*$p < 0.05$

Except for item 10 of the RHIC-Setswana, all items loaded significantly on the general factor of the RHIC-Setswana. Item 1 loaded significantly on the intended Engagement factor, and items 11, 12, and 13 loaded significantly on the intended Zest/Empowerment factor. There were no statistically significant target factor loadings on the Authenticity factor. Target factor loadings were larger than cross-loadings, except for a few items that had larger statistically significant cross-loadings on nontarget factors (e.g., Engagement items 3 and 14 cross-loaded on the Zest/Empowerment factor, Zest/Empowerment items 2 and 6 cross-loaded on the Engagement factor, and Authenticity item 4 cross-loaded on the Engagement factor). Overall, the Engagement and Zest/Empowerment items loaded stronger on the general factor than on their specific (target) factors. The Authenticity items, that are all negatively worded, had negative or small loadings on the general factor, and small negative loadings on the Authenticity factor, except for item 7 that had a target factor loading of 0.30. Together, these results are suggestive of the factorial validity of the RHIP-English, RHIC-English, and RHIC-Setswana. Next, we considered the internal consistency reliabilities.

6.3.4 *Stage 3: Internal Consistency Reliability*

The omega coefficients for the RHIP-English, RHIC-English, and RHIC-Setswana are presented in Tables 6.2 and 6.3 respectively. The general factor of the RHIP-English, RHIC-English, and RHIC-Setswana had sufficient reliability scores with ω-values larger than .90. The Engagement and Authenticity factors obtained sufficient reliability scores for the RHIP-English. For the RHIC-English the Zest/Empowerment and Authenticity factors had sufficient reliability scores, but reliability scores for the specific factors of the RHIC-Setswana were insufficient with ω-values smaller than .50 for all specific factors.

6.4 Discussion

The aim of this study was to investigate the factorial validity of the RHIP and the RHIC in South African adult samples by applying advanced methods of statistical analysis (bifactor CFA, ESEM, and bifactor ESEM) that address the limitations inherent to the ICM on which CFA is based. To the best of our knowledge, this study is the first to explore the psychometric properties of these scales in South African contexts and to apply bifactor CFA, ESEM, and bifactor ESEM to the RHIP and the RHIC. The three-factor, bifactor ESEM models (items with negative residual variances removed) displayed a good fit for the RHIP-English, RHIC-English, and the RHIC-Setswana. The general relational health factor obtained sufficient reliability scores in all instances. Subscale reliability scores were acceptable for two of the three factors for the RHIP-English and the RHIC-English, but insufficient for the RHIC-Setswana. Some specific findings are discussed in the next paragraphs.

6.4.1 Dimensionality of the RHIP and RHIC

The proposed three-factor structure of the RHIP and the RHIC has been supported to some extent in the current samples. Reliability scores indicate that a general peer relational health factor can be interpreted reliably for the RHIP-English, but the scores on the Zest/Empowerment subscale should be interpreted with caution. For the RHIC-English and the RHIC-Setswana a general community relational health factor can be interpreted, but caution should be applied when interpreting the scores on the Engagement subscale of the RHIC-English and the subscale scores for the RHIC-Setswana. When internal consistency reliability scores are low, it means that items in the scale do not co-vary to a sufficient extent with their summated score (Boateng et al., 2018), implying that the summed score is not a reliable representation of the individual item scores and should be used with caution. Our results point towards the multidimensionality of relational health in peer and community contexts, while supporting the existence of a general factor in each case, as indicated by the improvement in model fit when the two sources of construct-relevant multidimensionality were accounted for. Firstly, cross-loadings of items on nontarget factors indicate that the specific factors are interrelated and that the scale items of the RHIP-English, RHIC-English, and RHIC-Setswana were also influenced by the nontarget factors, in addition to the influence of the target factor (cf. Howard et al., 2018; Morin, Arens, & Marsh, 2016). As these cross-loadings were mostly smaller than target factor loadings for the RHIP-English, RHIC-English, and RHIC-Setswana they can be regarded as the influence of the nontarget factor on the construct-relevant part of the item (Morin, Arens, & Marsh, 2016). A few statistically significant cross-loadings that were larger than target factor loadings may indicate a need to consider alternative models (see Morin, Arens, & Marsh, 2016). However, after considering these cross-loadings, we concluded that there was no substantive justification for such modifications in the current samples as the items appeared to be stronger indicators of their target factors than the nontarget factors.

Secondly, a general peer relational health and a general community relational health factor underlie the RHIP-English, RHIC-English and RHIC-Setswana, respectively, as indicated by the improvement in model fit when a general factor was included in the analysis. The general peer and community relational health factors influence all the scale items of the RHIP-English, RHIC-English, and the RHIC-Setswana respectively, and coexist with the specific relational health factors.

6.4.2 Problematic Scale Items

For Sample 1, the Zest/Empowerment item 9 ("I have a greater sense of self-worth through my relationship with my friend") and Authenticity item 11 ("I can tell my friend when he/she has hurt my feelings") of the RHIP-English had negative residual variances. When measures are modified, it is desirable that modifications are made on both statistical and substantive grounds (Byrne, 2012). After considering the placement of these items in their respective subscales and the extent to which they measure their intended factors, we concluded that model modification was not substantively justified and the items were removed on statistical grounds only. Future research should explore whether this result will replicate in other samples.

Authenticity item 9 ("There is a lot of backbiting and gossiping in this community") of the RHIC had a negative residual variance for both samples. Upon closer inspection of the item we concluded that the item might not have captured the intended (opposite) meaning of the Authenticity factor that refers to genuineness in interpersonal interaction and being one's real self. Although "backbiting" and "gossiping" may be linked to nonauthentic relational interaction, it refers more to negative relational behaviour than to the opposite of authenticity *per se*. The item was therefore removed. Considering that this item was problematic in both language groups, it may indicate that the problem may be with the specific item, but the possible influence of context or even methodological issues also need to be kept in mind. In the next paragraph, we make suggestions for the possible further development of the RHI.

6.4.3 Possible Further Development of the RHI

When the psychometric properties of the RHI scales were evaluated for the first time the Conflict/Differences factor of the RHIP was excluded from the scale because it was defined by only a few items (Liang et al., 2002). For the RHIC the items measuring the Authenticity and Conflict/Differences factors cross-loaded, suggesting that the Conflict/Differences factor was not well-identified, and the factors were then modelled as a single factor. As such, a separate Conflict/Differences factor was not included in the original scales, resulting in scales that measure only three of the four characteristics of growth-fostering relationships as discerned by relational-cultural theory (Miller, 1976). As the ability to deal with differences and resolve conflict plays an integral role in growth-fostering relationships (e.g., Miller, 1976), future research may focus on developing scale items that measure this factor, or a new Constructive Problem-solving factor. Such developments can also in particular take into account findings with regard to constructive communication and constructive conflict resolution. Furthermore, an emic approach is suggested as conflict resolution may differ cross-culturally. For example, LeFebvre and Franke (2013) indicated that people from individualistic cultures tended to have a more rational decision-making style (i.e., following a logic and structured approach to making decisions) in conflict decision-making and people from collectivistic cultures tended to have a more dependent decision-making style (i.e., being reliant on support and guidance from others). These cultural differences should be considered when scale items are constructed.

Another possible consideration is the inclusion of positively-worded items in the Authenticity subscale of the RHIC that currently consists of only reverse phrased items. Although the inclusion of reverse phrased items has psychometric merit, such as that it can help to prevent acquiescence bias (e.g., Böckenholt, 2019), the practice is often criticised as the positively-worded and reverse phrased items often load on two separate factors when unidimensional constructs are measured (e.g., Suárez-Alvarez et al., 2018). The reverse phrased items can therefore measure the absence of authenticity rather than the presence thereof. We further propose that item 10 ("Members of this community are very competitive with each other") of the RHIC, like item 9, does not tap the intended meaning of the Authenticity factor and may be revised or replaced with a more suitable item, for example, "Members of this community can be themselves when they are with each other". We suggest that scale developers should be mindful that, when two factors are combined to form a single factor, the items may no longer be clear indicators of the intended target factor. Items for the intended target factor should therefore be selected on both statistical and substantive grounds.

6.4.4 *The Role of Culture*

Considering the cultural background of our current samples, one should be cognisant that the relational experiences and expectations of people from individualistic and collectivistic cultures may differ. Whereas people are expected to look after themselves and their immediate family in individualistic cultures, people from collectivistic cultures are integrated into interconnected in-groups (e.g., extended families) that provide continuous protection and loyalty (Hofstede, 2011). In this regard Wilson et al. (2019) found that older participants (60 years or older) from rural and deep rural communities in South Africa (both collectivistic African contexts) indicated the giving and receiving of continued support, having a sense of security and identity, the need to experience interpersonal harmony, and dependability and trust as some of the reasons why relationships were important to them. Although the same relational facets may be important to a variety of cultures, these facets may manifest differently across cultures, and it is important that measures are sensitive to these differences. More research is needed to determine if our findings will replicate in other, larger samples. Should the results repeat, researchers may consider an emic approach to scale development to ensure that the cultural meaning of the constructs is captured in the scale items.

6.5 Limitations and Recommendations

Although this study contributed to the understanding of the dimensionality of relational health in peer and community contexts, there were also limitations. Firstly, the sample sizes in this study were relatively small, especially considering that the WLSMV estimator usually requires large sample sizes, which needs to be kept in mind as a limitation when interpreting the results. Secondly, the RHI scales do not measure the Conflict/Differences factor of growth-fostering relationships and future research may focus on developing a Constructive Problem-solving subscale that also consider findings on constructive communication and constructive problem-solving. These items should be sensitive to cultural differences in conflict resolution. Thirdly, the Authenticity factor of the RHIC may be adapted to include positively-worded items that capture the intended meaning of the factor. Fourthly, our groups were too small to test for gender invariance. Considering the initial development of relational-cultural theory to understand the relational experiences of women, and the later application of the theory to men also, future research may explore the gender invariance of the RHI scales.

6.6 Conclusion

A general relational health factor coexists with the specific factors of the RHIP-English, RHIC-English, and the RHIC-Setswana. The RHIP-English, RHIC-English, and RHIC-Setswana show potential for use in the current samples provided that the problematic scale items are removed. Specifically, in all instances the general factor can be used and interpreted. The scores of the Zest/Empowerment subscale of the RHIP-English; the scores of the Engagement subscale of the RHIC-English; and all subscale scores of the RHIC-Setswana should be interpreted with caution. The RHI scales could be further developed to include a Constructive Problem-solving factor as an important facet of growth-fostering relationships. Findings highlight that scale developers should be mindful that items indeed measure the (new) target factor when two factors are combined to form a single factor. Furthermore, the advantages and disadvantages of including reverse phrased items in scales should be considered when scales are developed. Culture and context are important considerations in the development and application of measures of relational well-being.

Funding This work is based on research supported in part by the National Research Foundation of South Africa (Grant Number: 106050, 91557, 123266, 120060, 121948). The Grantholders acknowledge that opinions, findings and conclusions or recommendations expressed in any publication generated by the NRF-supported research are those of the authors, and that the NRF accepts no liability whatsoever in this regard.

Funding to the first author was provided in the form of a Doctoral degree scholarship and a bursary from the Faculty of Health Sciences of the North-West University, South Africa.

This chapter is based on an earlier draft in the PhD of the first author.

Declaration of Interest The authors do not have any conflicts of interest to declare.

Appendix

Table 6.4 Descriptive statistics of the individual items of the RHIP-English, RHIC-English, and RHIC-Setswana

	RHIP-English				RHIC-English				RHIC-Setswana			
Item	*M*	*SD*	Skewness	Kurtosis	*M*	*SD*	Skewness	Kurtosis	*M*	*SD*	Skewness	Kurtosis
1	4.24	0.87	−1.10	1.04	3.41	0.98	−0.31	−0.13	3.88	1.02	−1.23	1.49
2	4.20	0.86	−1.03	1.00	3.27	0.97	−0.10	−0.38	3.58	0.98	−0.83	0.40
3	4.19	0.85	−1.07	1.41	2.74	1.19	0.23	−0.69	3.05	1.22	−0.20	−1.00
4	4.09	0.85	−0.80	0.65	3.42	1.09	−0.31	−0.56	3.06	1.16	0.18	−0.80
5	4.36	0.85	−1.43	1.83	3.06	1.04	−0.15	−0.50	3.61	1.02	−0.88	0.44
6	3.98	1.01	−0.87	0.22	2.96	1.07	−0.16	−0.57	3.31	1.08	−0.52	−0.50
7	3.51	1.24	−0.40	−0.88	3.29	1.18	−0.21	−0.81	3.08	1.20	0.20	−1.10
8	3.50	1.24	−0.56	−0.58	3.49	0.91	−0.45	0.09	3.52	1.04	−0.73	−0.04
9	3.86	1.02	−0.88	0.41	3.12	1.24	−0.20	−0.97	2.85	1.38	0.05	−1.29
10	3.80	0.96	−0.65	0.24	2.90	1.21	0.04	−0.87	2.52	1.05	0.36	−0.34
11	3.86	1.03	−0.70	−0.09	3.02	1.11	−0.22	−0.72	3.62	0.92	−0.92	0.95
12	4.05	0.91	−1.00	1.20	2.76	1.10	0.09	−0.68	3.54	1.03	−0.78	0.14
13					2.78	1.19	0.01	−0.95	3.53	0.99	−0.92	0.58
14					2.75	1.14	0.13	−0.74	3.53	1.09	−0.74	−0.12

Note. RHIP = Relational Health Indices – Peer Scale; RHIC = Relational Health Indices – Community Scale; *M* = mean; *SD* = standard deviation

References

Alavi, M., Visentin, D. C., Thapa, D. K., Hunt, G. E., Watson, R., & Cleary, M. (2020). Exploratory factor analysis and principal component analysis in clinical studies: Which one to use? *Journal of Advanced Nursing, 76*(8), 1886–1889. https://doi.org/10.1111/jan.14377

Alvarez, A. R., & Lazzari, M. M. (2016). Feminist mentoring and relational cultural theory: A case example and implications. *Journal of Women and Social Work, 31*(1), 41–54. https://doi.org/10.1177/0886109915612512

Asparouhov, T., & Muthén, B. O. (2009). Exploratory structural equation modeling. *Structural Equation Modeling, 16*(3), 397–438. https://doi.org/10.1080/10705510903008204

Baumeister, R. F., & Leary, M. R. (1995). The need to belong: Desire for interpersonal attachments as a fundamental human motivation. *Psychological Bulletin, 117*(3), 497–529. https://doi.org/10.1037/0033-2909.117.3.497

Boateng, G. O., Neilands, T. B., Frongillo, E. A., Melgar-Quiñonez, H. R., & Young, S. L. (2018). Best practices for developing and validating scales for health, social, and behavioral research: A primer. *Frontiers in Public Health, 6*(149), 1–18. https://doi.org/10.3389/fpubh.2018.00149

Böckenholt, U. (2019). Contextual responses to affirmative and/or reversed-worded items. *Psychometrica, 84*(4), 986–999. https://doi.org/10.1007/s11336-019-09680-7

Bowlby, J. (1973). *Attachment and loss: Vol 2. Separation: Anxiety and anger*. Basic Books.

Brislin, R. W. (1980). Translation and content analysis of oral and written material. In H. C. Triandis & J. W. Berry (Eds.), *Handbook of cross-cultural psychology* (Vol. 1, pp. 389–444). Allyn & Bacon.

Byrne, B. M. (2012). *Structural equation modeling with Mplus: Basic concepts, applications, and programming*. Routledge.

Deci, E. L., & Ryan, R. M. (2000). The "what" and "why" of goal pursuits: Human needs and the self-determination of behavior. *Psychological Inquiry, 11*(4), 227–268. https://doi.org/10.1207/S15327965PLI1104_01

Ezenweke, E. O., & Nwadialor, L. K. (2013). Understanding human relations in African traditional religious context in the face of globalization: Nigerian perspectives. *American International Journal of Contemporary Research, 3*(2), 61–70.

Feeney, B. C., & Collins, N. L. (2015). Thriving through relationships. *Current Opinion in Psychology, 1*, 22–28. https://doi.org/10.1016/j.copsyc.2014.11.001

Frey, L. L., Beesly, D., & Newman, J. L. (2005). The relational health indices: Reanalysis of a measurement of relational quality. *Measurement and Evaluation in Counselling and Development, 38*(3), 153–163. https://doi.org/10.1080/07481756.2005.11909776

Goodboy, A. K., & Bolkan, S. (2011). Attachment and the use of negative relational maintenance behaviors in romantic relationships. *Communication Research Reports, 28*(4), 327–336. https://doi.org/10.1080/08824096.2011.616244

Hofstede, G. (2011). Dimensionalizing cultures: The Hofstede model in context. *Online Readings in Psychology and Culture*. Retrieved from http://scholarworks.gvsu.edu/orpc/

Howard, J. L., Gagné, M., Morin, A. J. S., & Forest, J. (2018). Using bifactor exploratory structural equation modeling to test for a continuum structure of motivation. *Journal of Management, 44*(7), 2638–2664. https://doi.org/10.1177/0149206316645653

Hu, L., & Bentler, P. M. (1999). Cutoff criteria for fit indexes in covariance structure analysis: Conventional criteria versus new alternatives. *Structural Equation Modeling, 6*(1), 1–55. https://doi.org/10.1080/10705519909540118

Jennrich, R. I., & Bentler, P. M. (2011). Exploratory bi-factor analysis. *Psychometrica, 76*, 537–549. https://doi.org/10.1007/S11336-011-9218-4

Jordan, J. V. (1986). *The meaning of mutuality. Work in Progress* (Vol. 23). Stone Center for Developmental Services and Studies.

Jordan, J. V. (1997). The relational model is a source of empowerment for women. In M. R. Walsh (Ed.), *Women, men, and gender: Ongoing debates* (pp. 373–382). Yale.

Jordan, J. V. (2000). The role of empathy in relational-cultural therapy. *Journal of Clinical Psychology, 56*(8), 1005–1016.

Jordan, J. V. (2001). A relational-cultural model: Healing through mutual empathy. *Bulletin of the Menninger Clinic, 65*(1), 92–103. https://doi.org/10.1521/bumc.65.1.92.18707

Jordan, J. V. (2008). Recent developments in relational-cultural theory. *Women and Therapy, 31*, 1–4. https://doi.org/10.1080/02703140802145540

Jordan, J. V. (2010). *Relational-cultural therapy*. American Psychological Association.

Jordan, J. V. (2017). Relational-cultural theory: The power of connection to transform our lives. *Journal of Humanistic Counselling, 56*(3), 228–243. https://doi.org/10.1002/johc.12055

Keyes, C. L. M. (2002). The mental health continuum: From languishing to flourishing in life. *Journal of Health and Social Behavior, 43*(2), 207–222.

Keyes, C. L. M. (2005). Mental illness and/or mental health? Investigating axioms of the complete state model of health. *Journal of Consulting and Clinical Psychology, 73*(3), 3–11.

Keyes, C. L. M. (2007). Promoting and protecting mental health as flourishing: A complementary strategy for improving national mental health. *American Psychologist, 62*(2), 95–108. https://doi.org/10.1037/0003-066X.62.2.95

Kline, R. (2013). Exploratory and confirmatory factor analysis. In Y. Petscher, C. Schatschneider, & D. L. Compton (Eds.), *Applied quantitative analysis in education and the social sciences* (pp. 171–207). Routledge.

LeFebvre, R., & Franke, V. (2013). Culture matters: Individualism vs. collectivism in conflict decision-making. *Societies, 3*(1), 128–146. https://doi.org/10.3390/soc3010128

Lenz, A. S., Balkin, R. S., Soler, I. G., & Martinez, P. (2016). Development and evaluation of a Spanish-language version of the relational health indices. *Psychological Assessment, 28*(5), e62–e69. https://doi.org/10.1037/pas0000170

Liang, B., Tracy, A., Taylor, C. A., Williams, L. M., Jordan, J. V., & Miller, J. B. (2002). The relational health indices: A study of women's relationships. *Psychology of Women Quarterly, 26*(1), 25–35.

Liang, B., Tracy, A., Glenn, C., Burns, S. M., & Ting, D. (2007). The relational health indices: Confirming factor structure for use with men. *The Australian Community Psychologist, 19*, 35–52.

Mbiti, J. (1970). *African religions and philosophies*. Doubleday.

Mbiti, J. S. (1990). *African religions and philosophy*. Heinemann.

McDermott, R. C., Cheng, H.-L., Lopez, F. G., McKelvey, D., & Bateman, S. L. (2017). Dominance orientations and psychological aggression in college student relationships: A test of an attachment theory-guided model. *Psychology of Violence, 7*(4), 508–520. https://doi.org/10.1037/vio0000061

McNeish, D., An, J., & Hancock, G. R. (2018). The thorny relation between measurement quality and fit index cutoffs in latent variable models. *Journal of Personality Assessment, 100*(1), 43–52. https://doi.org/10.1080/00223891.2017.1281286

Merz, E.-M., & Jak, S. (2013). The long reach of childhood. Childhood experiences influence close relationships and loneliness across life. *Advances in Life Course Research, 18*(3), 212–222. https://doi.org/10.1016/j.alcr.2013.05.002

Miller, J. B. (1976). *Toward a new psychology of women*. Beacon Press.

Miller, J. B. (1986). *What do we mean by relationships? Work in Progress, 22*. Wellesley College.

Miller, J. B., & Striver, I. P. (1997). *The healing connection: How women form relationships in therapy and in life*. Beacon Press.

Morin, A. J. S., Arens, A. K., & Marsh, H. W. (2016). A bifactor exploratory structural equation modeling framework for the identification of distinct sources of construct-relevant psychometric multidimensionality. *Structural Equation Modeling: A Multidisciplinary Journal, 23*(1), 116–139. https://doi.org/10.1080/1070551.2014.961800

Morin, A. J. S., Arens, K., Tran, A., & Caci, H. (2016). Exploring sources of construct-relevant multidimensionality in psychiatric measurement: A tutorial and illustration using the composite scale of morningness. *International Journal of Methods in Psychiatric Research, 25*(4), 277–288. https://doi.org/10.1002/mpr.1485

Muthén, L. K., & Muthén, B. O. (1998–2019). *Mplus (Version 8.3) [Computer software]*. Author.

Olafsen, A. H., Niemiec, C. P., Halvari, H., Deci, E. L., & Williams, G. C. (2017). On the dark side of work: A longitudinal analysis using self-determination theory. *European Journal of Work and Organizational Psychology, 26*(2), 275–285. https://doi.org/10.1080/1359432X.2016.1257611

Perreira, T. A., Morin, A. J. S., Hebert, M., Gillet, N., Houle, S. A., & Berta, W. (2018). The short form of the workplace affective commitment multidimensional questionnaire (WACMQ-S): A bifactor ESEM approach among healthcare professionals. *Journal of Vocational Behavior, 106*, 62–83. https://doi.org/10.1016/j.jvb.2017.12.004

Rigby, C. S., & Ryan, R. M. (2018). Self-determination theory in human resource development: New directions and practical considerations. *Advances in Developing Human Resources, 20*(2), 133–147. https://doi.org/10.1177/1523422318756954

Roos, V., Keating, N., & Khal, C. (2019). Loneliness of older black South African women subjected to forcible relocation. *Global Health Action, 12*, 1672329. https://doi.org/10.1080/16549716.2019.1672329

Sánchez-Oliva, D., Morin, A. J. S., Teixeira, P. J., Carracxa, E. V., Palmeira, A. L., & Silva, M. N. (2017). A bifactor exploratory structural equation modeling representation of the structure of the basic psychological needs at work scale. *Journal of Vocational Behavior, 98*, 173–187. https://doi.org/10.1016/j.jvb.2016.12.001

Suárez-Alvarez, J., Pedrosa, I., Lozano, L. M., García-Cueto, E., Cuesta, M., & Muñiz, J. (2018). Using reversed items in Likert scales: A questionable practice. *Psichothema, 30*(2), 149–158. https://doi.org/10.7334/psicothema2018.33

Teo, K., Chow, C. K., Vaz, M., Rangarajan, S., & Yusuf, S. (2009). The prospective urban rural epidemiology (PURE) study: Examining the impact of societal influences on chronic noncommunicable diseases in low-, middle-, and high-income countries. *American Heart Journal, 158*(1), 1–7. https://doi.org/10.1016/j.ahj.2009.04.019

Van de Vijver, F., & Hambleton, R. J. (1996). Translating tests: Some practical guidelines. *European Psychologist, 1*(2), 89–99. https://doi.org/10.1027/1016-9040.1.2.89

Van de Vijver, F. J. R., & Leung, K. (1997). *Methods and data analysis for cross-cultural research*. Sage.

Wilson, A., Wissing, M. P., & Schutte, L. (2019). "We help each other": Relational patterns among older individuals in South African samples. *Applied Research in Quality of Life, 14*(5), 1373–1392. https://doi.org/10.1007/s11482-018-9657-5

Wissing, M. (2008/2012). *The prevalence of levels of psychosocial health: Dynamics and relationships with biomarkers of (ill) health in South African social contexts (FORT3)*. Research project with ethical approval registered at the North-West University.

Wissing, M. P. (2014). Meaning and relational well-being: Reflection on the state of the art and the way forward. *Journal of Psychology in Africa, 24*(1), 115–121. https://doi.org/10.1080/14330237.2014.904100

Wissing, M. P., & Delle Fave, A. (2013). *Meaning and relational well-being: Towards a model*. In Paper presented at the second conference on positive psychology (CPPC) in Brno, Czech Republic.

Wissing, M. P., Schutte, L., & Wilson Fadiji, A. (2019). Cultures of positivity: Interconnectedness as a way of being. In I. Eloff (Ed.), *Handbook of quality of life in African societies*. Springer. https://doi.org/10.1007/978-3-030-15367-0_1

Wissing, M. P., Wilson Fadiji, A., Schutte, L., Chigeza, S., Schutte, W. D., & Temane, Q. M. (2020). Motivations for relationships as sources of meaning: Ghanaian and South African experiences. *Frontiers in Psychology, 11*, 2019. https://doi.org/10.3389/fpsyg.2020.02019

Xia, Y. (2016). *Investigating the chi-square based model-fit indexes for WLSMV and ULSMV estimators (Doctoral dissertation)*. Florida State University.

Xia, Y., & Yang, Y. (2018). The influence of number of categories and threshold values on fit indices in structural equation modeling with ordered categorical data. *Multivariate Behavioral Research, 53*, 731–755. https://doi.org/10.1080/00273171.2018.1480346

Part III
Manifestations and Dynamics of Well-Being in Africa

Chapter 7
Resilience in the Context of Chronic, Complex Stressors: An Emerging Adult's Account

Linda Theron and Michael Ungar

Abstract This chapter presents a single case study that illustrates the complexity of emerging adult resilience in the context of relentless socio-ecological risk. The case, which is instrumental, is drawn from the Resilient Youth in Stressed Environments (RYSE) study, South Africa. It foregrounds the positive adjustment over time of Simphiwe, an isiZulu-speaking young man, to the challenges of unemployment and environmental risk. When asked to explain his resilience (using a variety of qualitative methods), Simphiwe consistently foregrounded the resilience-enabling power of a personal vision for an improved future and associated habits. Of interest is his lived experience of community apathy towards such youth vision, how he navigated this constraint, and the implications of his journey for a deeper understanding of social-ecological resilience. In short, Simphiwe's case calls for a greater emphasis on social and ecological factors if the wellbeing of emerging adults is to be meaningfully championed.

Keywords Case study · Emerging adult · Resilient youth in stressed environments (RYSE) · Resilience · South Africa · Youth unemployment

7.1 Introduction

Emerging adulthood (EA) is a distinctive phase of development that spans the ages of 18 to 29 (Arnett, 2000). Whilst some have disputed its universal applicability (Côté, 2014; Hendry & Kloep, 2010; Syed, 2016), EA is generally characterised by instability that arises from emerging adults' search for identity, lasting romantic ties,

L. Theron (✉)
Department of Educational Psychology, University of Pretoria, Pretoria, South Africa
e-mail: Linda.Theron@up.ac.za

M. Ungar
Resilience Research Centre, Dalhousie University, Halifax, NS, Canada

L. Schutte et al. (eds.), *Embracing Well-Being in Diverse African Contexts: Research Perspectives*, Cross-Cultural Advancements in Positive Psychology 16,
https://doi.org/10.1007/978-3-030-85924-4_7

and gainful employment (Arnett et al., 2014; Wood et al., 2018). This search, and its attendant uncertainties, is believed to be fairly common across social classes and/or ethnicities (Arnett, 2000, 2014, 2016).

Although it can be a period of opportunity, the volatility of this developmental stage is frequently associated with threats to young people's wellbeing, including deterioration in mental health (Arnett et al., 2014; Newcomb-Anjo et al., 2017; Wood et al., 2018). High youth unemployment and/or limited access to social capital are more strongly associated with negative experiences of instability and decreased wellbeing. Given the service industry's monopoly over the world of work and tertiary education requirements for securing or sustaining employment in the service-focused world of work, negative experiences of EA and decreased wellbeing are even more pronounced for 18- to 29-year-olds with limited education (Arnett, 2014; Maree, 2016). In contrast, studies of emerging adult resilience have advanced an understanding that EA can provide significant turning point opportunities for young people challenged by past and/or present disadvantage (Madewell & Ponce-Garcia, 2016).

Thus, in the global context of troubling and apparently intractable levels of youth unemployment (Mayer et al., 2019), it is important to better understand what protects the wellbeing of emerging adults who live in countries with high levels of unemployment and associated disadvantage. Put differently, it is important to understand the resilience of EA challenged by economic and other environmental stressors. It is especially important to include EA from sub-Saharan Africa in this focus, given the exponential growth of sub-Saharan Africa's youth population; the region's apparently relentless socioeconomic challenges and the negative impacts thereof on youth wellbeing; and forecasts that the wellbeing of Africa's youth will have decisive impacts on regional and global economies (O'Malley et al., 2014; Owusu-Sekyere, 2019). Even though some consider South Africa to be socioeconomically better off than most other countries in sub-Saharan Africa, its EA population is believed to be particularly vulnerable to socioeconomic challenges (StatsSA, 2019). Thus, understanding and promoting the resilience of South African EA is a pressing agenda.

7.1.1 Emerging Adult Resilience: A Brief Review of the Relevant Literature

Resilience is the ability of a system (e.g., a human being) to adjust successfully to challenges (e.g., unemployment) that have the potential to disrupt development or functioning (Masten, 2014; Masten & Cicchetti, 2016). Various theoretical approaches have been used to explain this capacity (Windle, 2011). In this chapter, which reports a South African case study of resilience, we follow an ecosystems or social-ecological approach to resilience. As in other parts of the world, a social-ecological approach to resilience is the preferred approach in South African studies of child and youth resilience (Van Breda & Theron, 2018).

A social-ecological approach underscores that positive adjustment to significant challenges is a process that is co-facilitated by individuals and the ecologies in which they find themselves (Rutter, 2012; Ungar, 2011; Wright & Masten, 2015). In contrast to earlier studies of resilience that emphasised individual strengths, social-ecological approaches value both the individual and the ecological (Masten, 2014). In fact, Ungar (2012, p. 15) contended that resilience is "as, *or more*, dependent on the capacity of the individual's physical and social ecology to potentiate positive development under stress than the capacity of individuals to exercise personal agency during their recovery from risk exposure".

Reviews of South African and other sub-Saharan studies of child and adolescent resilience attest to the systemic nature of resilience (Theron & Theron, 2010; Theron, 2020; Van Breda & Theron, 2018). For instance: in addition to personal strengths (such as agency, optimism, or diligence), the resilience of sub-Saharan young people draws on social-ecological supports (especially contextually and culturally relevant ones, such as supportive relationships, access to microloans or other forms of financial support, or spiritual belief systems) that bolster wellbeing (Adegoke & Steyn, 2017; Betancourt et al., 2011; Ebersöhn et al., 2018; Vindevogel et al., 2015). Although frequency counts in the Van Breda and Theron (2018) and Theron (2020) review suggest that relational supports are more prominent than personal resources in accounts of child and adolescent resilience, the numerical differences are slight. This led to Theron (2020) concluding that "relational and personal supports matter more-or-less equally for the resilience of children and adolescents living in sub-Saharan Africa".

Burt and Paysnick's (2012) review of studies of emerging adult resilience reinforces social-ecological understandings of resilience. In other words, their review showed that emerging adult resilience is part personal capacity and part ecological support. As intimated by Ungar (2012), their review considered ecological supports to be particularly influential. Following their summation of key longitudinal studies that followed children exposed to various forms of adversity into adulthood, Burt and Paysnick (2012) concluded that relationships (historical ones as well as new ones formed during the period of EA) were most critical to the resilience of emerging adults. Their conclusion also fit with authoritative resilience scholars' conclusions about the centrality of supportive relationships to human resilience (Luthar, 2006; Masten, 2014). However, Burt and Paysnick's (2012) consideration of specific cross-sectional studies conducted with emerging adults facing varied risks (such as aging out of care or histories of chronic physical or mental illness) also drew attention to the resilience-enabling importance of personal strengths, such as planfulness (i.e., "the ability to plan ahead, delay gratification, and make positive choices" p. 502) and self-efficacious future-orientation (i.e., "a drive for mastery ... resilient emerging adults have experienced difficult times without defining themselves by their adversity" p. 502). Since Burt and Paysnick's (2012) review, only a limited number of studies has specifically accounted for the resilience of emerging adults (Madewell & Ponce-Garcia, 2016). These studies have also reinforced social-ecological understandings of resilience. For instance, emerging adult resilience was associated with optimism and positive future orientation but also with support systems and social interaction (e.g., Harper et al., 2019; Miller & Bowen, 2019).

Interestingly, a 2019 review of the resources associated with lifespan resilience following maltreatment has drawn attention to the developmental variability of what enables resilience (Yoon et al., 2019). Specifically, this synthesis found that for persons transitioning into adulthood (i.e., emerging adults) resilience was more often conceptualised as a personal response or set of personal strengths than an ecologically supported one. Rather than mean that ecological resources were unimportant to the resilience of emerging adults, Yoon et al.'s (2019) conclusion suggests that ecological resources were less pronounced. As argued by Yoon et al. (2019), the emphasis on the personal could mirror the developmental importance in EA of individuation or, to quote Arnett et al. (2014, p. 571), the developmental specificity of "self-focus".

7.2 Purpose of this Chapter

To date, South African resilience studies have under-explored the resilience of emerging adults. A number focused on the resilience of university students (e.g., Theron & Theron, 2013, 2014; Van Breda, 2018; Zulu, 2019). Others included participants who fall into the age range of EA (e.g., Malindi, 2014; Phasha, 2010; Van Breda, 2015; Van Breda & Dickens, 2017). However, none detailed how the reported resilience processes fit with the developmental stage of EA and its emphasis on a search for identity, stable love relationships, and gainful employment. As such it is unclear which of the reported resilience processes, if any, are particularly developmentally appropriate for emerging adults (as per Yoon et al.'s, 2019 conclusion about personal factors for emerging adults).

Moreover, StatsSA (2019) put the unemployment rate of South Africans aged 15 to 24 at 55.2% for the first quarter of 2019 and noted that the "burden of unemployment is concentrated amongst the youth (aged 15–34 years) as they account for 63,4% of the total number of unemployed persons". When emerging adults are neither employed, nor in education or training, their vulnerability is generally heightened and concomitant declines are noted in their wellbeing (Holte et al., 2019). Although there are multiple studies that focus on or include South African youth who are unemployed (e.g., De Witte et al., 2012; Griep et al., 2014; Paver et al., 2019; Van der Vaart et al., 2018), these studies have not focused on this population's resilience.

The above prompted us (i.e., the authors) to reconsider the case studies that were generated by in the Resilient Youth in Stressed Environments (RYSE) study, South Africa, to determine how emerging adults—who are neither employed, nor in education or training—explain their resilience. RYSE is a multi-year (2017–2021), multi-site study of youth resilience in contexts of environmental and economic stress in Canada and South Africa (see www.ryseproject.org). Accordingly, the question that directed this chapter is as follows: How do emerging adults account for their resilience in the face of challenges associated with living in a stressed environment and being neither employed, nor in education or training?

7.3 The Case of Simphiwe

To answer this question, we selected a single case study: Simphiwe,[1] a Zulu young man who is an active RYSE participant. When he first participated in the RYSE study in 2017, Simphiwe was 21 years old. He explained that he and his brother lived with their grandfather and had intermittent contact with their biological parents. Because of financial and other constraints, Simphiwe had lived with his grandparents from when he was in primary school. His grandmother died when he was in high school. At the start of the RYSE study (2017), Simphiwe was unemployed. Although he had completed matric, he had not gained university exemption. In response he diligently tried to improve his marks, but the inaccessibility of quality tuition to support this intention obstructed his attempts. He tried various avenues to gain training or employment (e.g., he applied to the South African military), but these were not successful. Still, he persisted in searching. By late 2019 he had gained employment at the local petrochemical industry and considered this a steppingstone to achieving the future he dreamed of.

Although the RYSE study, South Africa, includes multiple case studies we decided to report only Simphiwe's case. Our decision was informed by Creswell's (2007, p. 74) guidance that a researcher "focuses on an issue or concern, and then selects *one* bounded case to illustrate this issue". It was also informed by Yin's (2014) reference to the value of a critical case. The critical case offers a valuable illustration when it can confirm or challenge theory because it reports "a contemporary phenomenon . . . in depth and within its real-world context" (Yin, 2014, p. 16). Similarly, Eisenhardt and Graebner (2007) advised that one case is ample, so long as it provides critical insights. As detailed below, Simphiwe's case provides grounds for theorising about emerging adult resilience because it is distinctively rich in its explicit reference to pathways of resilience in the face of challenges relating to living in a stressed environment and being neither employed nor in education or training. Further, his case raises compelling questions about the primacy of ecological contributions (as theorised by Burt & Paysnick, 2012; Ungar, 2012) to emerging adult resilience in stressed environments.

[1] His real name, as per his choice for us not to use a pseudonym when referring to him

7.3.1 Methodological Snapshot

As explained elsewhere (Theron & Ungar, 2019), the South African research site is a township that was built for the blue-collar workers of a large petrochemical plant that manufactures petrochemical products from coal. Simphiwe has resided in this township since he was a little boy. Residents of Simphiwe's township are vulnerable to the pollutants of the adjacent petrochemical industry as well as those emitted by nearby coal mines. Like many other South African townships, the township in question is densely populated and characterized by multiple, chronic risks. Amongst others, violence, crime, communicable disease, and structural disadvantage challenge residents' wellbeing. In the 2017–2019 period, the community was repeatedly shut-down by protesting residents who were exasperated by an ongoing lack of service delivery, local government and other corruption, wide-ranging unemployment, and general penury. In one of these shut-downs, protestors torched municipal assets and the local mall. Such rage is not unique to this specific community—across South Africa, oppressed people are increasingly engaging in violent protest in a desperate attempt to draw attention to their ongoing struggle for survival (Canham, 2018).

RYSE-affiliated research in this community was approved by the Faculty of Education Ethics Committee and the Faculty of Health Sciences Research Ethics Committee (ethics number: UP 17/05/01). The informed consent documentation explicated that all participation was voluntary and invited participants to stipulate how they would prefer to be identified in publications of the study's findings (e.g., by their real name or a pseudonym). It also clarified that some research activities could be conducted in a group format, along with the potential limitations to privacy and confidentiality.

As advised for resilience studies (e.g., McCubbin & Moniz, 2015), a community-based advisory panel (CAP) invited voluntary participation from local youth (aged 14–24) who believed they could contribute meaningful information about what enabled and constrained the resilience of local young people and who were comfortable communicating with researchers in English. The first person whom the CAP recruited was Simphiwe. From 2017 to 2019 Simphiwe engaged in seven qualitative research activities (see the timeline in Fig. 7.1), including arts-based activities, the creation of digital stories, individual interviews, and focus group interviews. The arts-based activities involved draw-and-write techniques (see Mitchell et al., 2011) and body-maps (see Ebersöhn et al., 2016). The prompts for the arts-based activities and the digital stories were resilience focused (e.g., draw/map/make a story of what enables you to be resilient [to be OK even when your life is hard]). The same focus informed the questions in the follow-up discussions about the created artefacts and in the interviews (e.g., What are the biggest challenges youth in your community face/you face? What do youth do/do you do to overcome these challenges? What/who makes it possible for young people/you to be OK when their lives are affected in negative ways? How would you explain youth/your resilience? Do you consider yourself resilient—how come?). In summary, although we used different qualitative

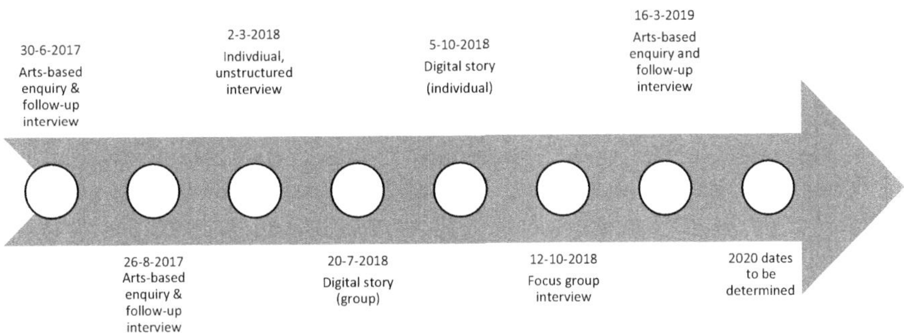

Fig. 7.1 Timeline of Simphiwe's participation in qualitative RYSE research (at time of chapter)

methods to generate data, all of them facilitated rich narrative data that we recorded and transcribed verbatim. Because Simphiwe spoke English to us, translation was not necessary.

For the purposes of this chapter, we reviewed the narrative data relating to how Simphiwe explained his resilience. Our focus was on data that related to the research question guiding this chapter (i.e., we focused on how he accounted for resilience in the face of challenges associated with living in a physically and economically stressed environment and being neither employed nor in education or training). Following Braun and Clarke's (2006) guidelines for inductive, thematic analysis, we coded each transcript for instances where the data explained such risk or resilience. This means we labelled segments of the text with a phrase that summarised what that segment explained about the risks that Simphiwe faced or what enabled resilience to the identified risks. We grouped similar labels into themes and interrogated what these themes revealed about Simphiwe's capacity to adjust successfully to his residence in a stressed environment where unemployment was rampant. We invited an independent researcher to audit the meaning we had made. We asked Simphiwe to do the same. Although they were generally in agreement with our analyses, we used their comments to refine what we report in this chapter.

7.3.2 *Learning About Emerging Adult Resilience from Simphiwe*

In summary, the story of Simphiwe's resilience is rooted in a context that is largely disabling. He responds to this context by foregrounding a vision for an improved future; and, in commitment to this vision, he nurtures resilience-enabling habits, some solo, some cooperative. Each of these aspects is detailed next.

7.3.2.1 "I Suffer a Lot": The Challenge of a Disabling Physical and Social Ecology

Simphiwe's physical ecology was not conducive to health. Like the other participants, Simphiwe referred to the health risks of living in a stressed environment, including water and air pollution and associated respiratory and digestive ailments. In 2017 he said: "*I suffer a lot; especially when I am about to sleep, my nose gives me a lot of problems*". He added that a younger brother had suffered more from exposure to air pollution and believed that this had culminated in his untimely death. In 2019 Simphiwe was still concerned about the pollution that he and his community were exposed to: "*When you inhale it, or it gets in ... it rots inside of your body.*"

Simphiwe described the social ecology as similarly toxic. It was characterised by unemployment and financial stress, neither of which seemed to be easily redressed by tertiary qualifications. For instance, in 2018 Simphiwe reported:

> We do have very educated people, but they are unemployed. For example, there's a guy who is an accountant, but he has no job. He's been looking, he's not just sitting on his bed. And another guy, he's a media specialist. Same. Education is the key to success, yes, but I feel in [name of township] you also need a little bit of luck.

However, the chances for "*a little bit of luck*" seemed to be restricted by community members' tendency to not share information that would heighten individuals' chances of being lucky. Simphiwe explained this tendency as follows:

> Important knowledge is—like, they keep it for themselves, it's secretive ... Because it's sort of a competition to succeed. It's something that people want—to achieve. Just to spite other people or to be seen as better than others. Hence, they don't want to share their recipes or the way they do things ... we end up fighting for the same jobs.

One consequence of such secrecy and competitiveness was Simphiwe's experience that community members were disinclined to encourage one another to succeed. The net result was accepting that motivation needed to be self-generated. He said:

> It's very rare to find someone who will motivate you. You're very lucky if someone motivates you because success has become a competition. So, motivating yourself is your own job; I can easily say to [name of a friend], 'Let's go'in party' but I won't motivate him coz then he might get what I could have.

In addition to Simphiwe's experience that community members were generally not willing to help others succeed or inspire an achievement-oriented way-of-being, he perceived many community members as preoccupied with status symbols or "*fake*" pursuits. For him, their preoccupation with impressing others meant that they could not be trusted to provide meaningful advice or to be true to enabling or altruistic values. In 2018 he described the consequence of this as: "*One of the hardest things for me to cope with in* [name of township] *is the social expectations because they do not resonate with my beliefs and my life interests.*" In 2019 he said: "*It affects me socially ... they drain you.*"

This lack of trust was worsened by the influx of migrant workers and subsequent negative changes to local culture. For instance, Simphiwe recounted:

> This place is crowded by people from different tribes or different places in South Africa. As you know here in South Africa, we have 11 official languages. [In my community] we have almost 10 or 15 people from each tribe or from each culture who speak a different language, who come from a different environment and come and influence this place ... such as the initiation schools. So, some boys will go to initiation school and come back like these monsters, these violent people who mug people, who rob people. So, it affects me in a negative way ... a few weeks back I was at a funeral burying one of the guys—we finished matric together. He was stabbed by his "friends".

In short, for Simphiwe and others this disabling physical and social ecology meant that life was "*hard, really hard*". As explained next, for Simphiwe the solution was "*Thinking about a better tomorrow*". Focusing on the future supported him "*to be OK regardless of the current situation; it helps to think about tomorrow, a better tomorrow; today might be like this but tomorrow might be a totally different story*".

7.3.2.2 "I Can Still Make It": A Vision for the Future

Over time, Simphiwe was committed to a future that transcended his present reality: "*I believe I'm on my journey to success.*" This belief inspired action and hope: "*The thoughts about the future inspire me to grow and to learn, and that there's still room for me and I can still make it.*" His immediate plan for 'making it' largely entailed gaining secure employment:

> I feel that job security is very, very, very vital because it gives you the privilege to budget and to plan for things and to take each thing step by a step. Compare [job security] to someone who just lost their contract—it's back to square one, having to start again, make your way up and fall again. ... I want a better one [a secure job] where I can start with a certain path and continue with it, until it takes me where I want to go

His "*end goal*", however, was "*to be an entrepreneur*"; secure employment was something for the interim: "*I believe I have to go through different things and work towards that* [being an entrepreneur]." Taken together, his immediate and future goals constituted his drive to "*build a runway*". In his words:

> There's something people call a runway. Meaning that some kids have the opportunity to go to school [university]; some have family businesses that from school they join, they start working there; ... stuff like that. As for me when I finished school, I never had such [a runway]. But, I wanna create such.

"*Building a runway*" was partly about enabling himself and partly about enabling present and future family: "*I want to build the runway for my* [future] *kids and better the conditions in my home and for myself*". It also had altruistic intent:

> It hurts me if maybe my locals, people I grew up with, my siblings or my peers don't utilise or are not given the opportunity to actually access opportunities in the petrochemical industry or to ... open up businesses or ... access land ... I wanna create employment for other people

Simphiwe's commitment to 'making it' persisted over time. Over time, he was also unequivocal that becoming successful (i.e., economically independent) was a personal duty (rather than one that would be co-facilitated by his ecology). In 2017 he stated: "*I developed a sense of self-belief . . . I can reach my potential*". In 2018 he stated:

> I feel that my happiness is my responsibility and it's my job to give it to myself. Every time I see young kids grow in front of my eyes, I learn a lesson that life gives each and every one an opportunity to grow and build themselves

His 2019 wording was slightly different, but the gist of personal responsibility for an optimal future was consistent:

> I believe that my future is in my hands and no one is coming to give it to me, I already have it in my hands and it's my responsibility to make my dreams a reality and my imagination, to bring them to life . . . It's very personal. My dream is my biggest thing. If I stop dreaming, I stop living. So, my dreams are my life; my tomorrow is my life; my future, my kids is my life—I don't have any [kids] at the moment but that's who I aspire to be.
>
> So, there's a difference between someone who had a runway and someone who is trying to create one. It's much more demanding if you're trying to create one rather than having one already there. So, that's why I want to equip myself . . .

To 'equip' himself he cultivated the three habits described next.

7.3.2.3 "It's a Habit I Started"

Habit 1: "I Try to Make as Much Time as I Can for my Health"
Simphiwe indicated that physical health was important to his vision and so he took care to nurture his health. He attributed the fact that he was generally healthy, despite daily exposure to pollution, to his exercise routine: "*Exercise decreases my chances of being sick . . . I go to the gym and in my room before I sleep, I do push ups and sit ups and I do some exercises before I go to work sometimes.*" [2019]. Simphiwe's appreciation of exercise seemed to be rooted in childhood experiences of friends who loved to play sport:

> I didn't even have much time for TV, because these friends would come and say, 'Let's go run, let's go run!' And we would run and run and run. These other ones would come, 'Let's go and play soccer outside'. We would go and play soccer, the other day it's cricket. [2018]

The habit was also facilitated by local exercise facilities that were sponsored by the petrochemical industry:

> I wanted to speak about the petrochemical industry: as much as it affects us [negatively] it also affects us in a positive way. It creates jobs, it offers bursaries, it builds recreational centres, it also builds sports facilities . . . [2019]

Habit 2: "I Search for Knowledge"

Simphiwe explained that knowledge was crucial to becoming successful. He reported that he was continuously searching for information or motivation that might be relevant to his future goals. To this end, he used a variety of sources to learn how to navigate his negative social ecology: "*I read books or listen to podcasts or maybe socialise so that I can learn, or login to my social media to see if there's something new I can learn. ... I watch motivational videos and listen to motivation most of the time*" [2019].

He and his friends shared relevant books (mostly ones they downloaded) with one another:

> The things we [friends] talk about ...: 'I read this and this and this in such a book and it got my attention' ... and then I will say, 'Please borrow me that book when you are done with it' ... and we would come and discuss the book and how it made sense to us and how it relates to living. To a living that we all share.

Given his general mistrust of the local community (see Sect. 7.3.2.1), Simphiwe was fastidious about human sources of knowledge. He regarded only his close friends and his grandfather as reliable sources of advice or information:

> I have a very small circle of friends that I can share my ideas with and maybe my problems or ask if they can help and resolve something. Maybe someone will tell me this and not that. I can use what they share to come up with a resolution to the problem ... I cannot trust them [friends] to an extent where I would let them do a decision on my behalf concerning my life, but I trust them enough for the opinions they can give and that they could maybe bring up the solution I am looking for. ...With my grandfather, I actually do what he tells me and sometimes it works well and sometimes, since he is old and it's the modern context now, some things they don't work ... [So] it goes from not only hearing advice but actually listening and taking the advice and looking for ways to understand the advice and how can it apply in the modern day too, into my life at the moment.

Habit 3: "I Choose the Positive"

Simphiwe was unambiguous about the importance of a positive way-of-seeing and -being for becoming successful: "*I choose the positive because I feel that the negative energy will just delay me or maybe derail me from where I want to go, but the positive energy keeps one going...*" For the most part, Simphiwe generated this positive energy on his own: "*I try, by all means, to give myself the solution because sometimes you can rely on people, but they won't be always there, or sometimes they themselves are the cause of the issue*". He used various techniques to maintain or regain a positive outlook. For example:

> ... being alone and spending time with myself and meditating sometimes. Or, thinking through, what is actually the matter and going through it again—it's worth the energy and the time and everything ... I believe as humans we have a limited amount of emotional energy per day and so if I lose all my energy I will be sleeping and I will be depressed and life will be still on that point and the problem will still be hanging there and waiting for me. But, if I can sit and think it through and come up with a solution, I think it can be a better way to attend to the matter. So, I try and cheer myself up that I can solve it ... [laughter] And music ... a chilled music will sometimes bring up my mood; I will rest a bit and listen to

> such music and maybe snooze, sleep a bit, but when I wake up I would have a different view and different amount of energy [2018]

> … I think about my past challenges … things I've overcome in life or things I've been through and I see myself as a bigger person because I went through all these things and they didn't kill me or drag me down. And I tell myself that I'm strong enough to have gone through that and I can still go through other things in life, so it gives me that edge to go forward in a way [2019]

At other times, his friends or family scaffolded a positive focus. For instance, one of Simphiwe's friends (with a similar history of hardship) had succeeded in living out his dream of being a musician and this encouraged Simphiwe to remain positive about his own dreams. Again, because Simphiwe was aware that negative others could detract from his focus, he was circumspect in his choice of friends:

> I have a very strict circle around me, I don't just make friends—I don't just make anyone my friend … As I grew older, I just could see the difference between my habits and the habits other people do ... so I discovered that my friends would play a huge role in the person I have become. So, if I allow just anybody [to be my friend], I won't have direction of where I am going in life

Religion also played a role in Simphiwe's capacity to focus on the positive and to focus on the future. As he explained: "*Religion it's very important, I must say… What you believe in … has a huge role in your lifestyle and it plays a huge role in your lifestyle choices also; the choices in my life as a Christian are different to the choices you make as a traditional person*". He attributed the genesis of his valuing of religion to his social ecology:

> … in most cases it starts from our families and we take religion from our parents. I remember it was hard for me to swear, even now, because of the religion my grandparents taught me. They were Christians. It was hard for me to swear at somebody or anything, but it helped me to respect people, it helped me to interact better with people … I spent a lot of time in church and it was an environment where I would think about the future coz in Christianity they teach about the coming of Jesus or the hope of glory … so it gives you that think-ahead thinking about something ahead of your current situation. [2019]

7.4 Theorising About Emerging Adult Resilience: Three Propositions

Before we detail three insights that are implicit in Simphiwe's account of resilience, it is important to acknowledge some limitations. They are similar to the ones we reported elsewhere about the RYSE study (see Theron & Ungar, 2019). First, Simphiwe's account (as reported in this chapter) reflected multiple engagements with the RYSE team between 2017 and 2019 (see Fig. 7.1). Following from the findings of Theron and Van Rensburg (2018) with similarly disadvantaged South African youth, it is possible that Simphiwe's future accounts might emphasize different aspects of resilience. Put differently, the fact that this chapter draws on data that cohered over time does not necessarily mean that the reported findings are immutable. Also, English was not Simphiwe's mother tongue. Even though he was willing to communicate in English (he was schooled in English) and did so competently, his account might have been even richer had he communicated in his mother tongue (i.e., isiZulu). Despite these limitations, we believe that the detail of Simphiwe's account has important pointers for the conceptualisation and facilitation of emerging adult resilience.

7.4.1 Personal Resources Trump Ecological Ones

Simphiwe's case is heavily skewed toward individual resources of resilience. His account of what it means to adjust well to unemployment and environmental stress underscores his personal capacity to be oriented to a brighter future and to cultivate specific habits that support his use of the present as a pathway toward this envisaged future. In so doing his account echoes Burt and Paysnick's (2012) mention of the personal resources that mattered for emerging adult resilience, namely planfulness and a self-efficacious future-orientation.

On the one hand this emphasis on the individual fits with the tasks of EA (e.g., a search for personal identity and for gainful employment) (Arnett, 2000, 2014; Arnett et al., 2014) and with EA's "self-focus" (Arnett et al., 2014, p. 571). It also fits with Yoon et al.'s (2019) review of publications documenting resilience over the lifespan following maltreatment and their finding that emerging adult resilience was more often conceptualised as a personal response or set of personal strengths than an ecologically supported one. On the other hand, it does not fit with Burt and Paysnick's (2012) finding that relational resources were pivotal to the resilience of emerging adults in the longitudinal studies that they reviewed, or with Ungar's (2012) contention that ecological resources matter as much, if not more, than personal ones for human resilience. It also contradicts Theron's (2020) conclusion that sub-Saharan child and adolescent resilience is informed "more-or-less equally" by relational and personal supports.

To be clear, Simphiwe's account did include some mention of ecological resources. These comprised enabling relationships with his grandfather and a select and restricted group of trusted friends; the local petrochemical industry that provided access to sports and recreational facilities and created some employment opportunity; faith-based beliefs (that were largely passed on by his grandparents); and access to social media and books. These ecological resources have been previously documented in the studies of child and adolescent resilience in South and sub-Saharan Africa (Theron, 2020; Theron & Theron, 2010; Van Breda & Theron, 2018). As in these previous reviews, when Simphiwe referenced ecological resources they were more often relational resources than structural or cultural ones. However, unlike previous studies of South and sub-Saharan African child and adolescent resilience, his account flagged the resilience-enabling importance of being discriminatory in the choice of relational supports. As detailed next, this emphasis provides a clue to a possible reason for personal resources trumping ecological ones.

7.4.2 Ecological Constraints Likely Explain the Emphasis on Personal Strengths

Simphiwe's account of his ecology is generally not a positive one. It foregrounds a community that is contaminated by pollution, distrust, and rivalry. The distrust and rivalry are at odds with traditional African values of interdependence and harmony (often called *ubuntu*) (Motsamai, 2017; Ramphele, 2012). As has been documented by various African writers (see the volume edited by Mhlongo, 2019), it is possible that the state of Simphiwe's social ecology reflects a decline in *ubuntu*-aligned ways-of-being. There are concerns that younger, more affluent Africans have acculturated to traditionally Western or culturally atypical ways-of-being (i.e., individualist rather than interdependent; Ramphele, 2012). Although some would contest a declining allegiance to *ubuntu* values or *ubuntu's* worth to the current day South Africa (Chimakonam, 2016; Van Breda, 2019), others report that ever-worsening economic conditions are constraining Africans' capacity to be charitable and supportive (Mhlongo, 2019). It is therefore possible that distrust and rivalry can be explained by the oppressive resource-constraints that besiege Simphiwe's community, as in other disadvantaged South African communities (Canham, 2018; Mhlongo, 2019). One wonders what his account of resilience might have been, had he been the member of a disadvantaged community that was nevertheless characterised by community connectedness and altruism (such as the one imagined by youth participants in the study by Mosavel et al., 2015). Would he still then have highlighted his personal role, almost to the exclusion of all other resources, in his successful adjustment to ongoing hardship? It is our contention that this would likely *not* have been the case. Arguably, had Simphiwe's community been more resilient he would have had access to ecological resources (such as mentors, entrepreneurial courses, or start-up loans) that could have co-facilitated his vision for the future. Put differently, we assert that a more enabling ecology would have freed Simphiwe from having to rely almost exclusively on his personal capacity to adjust to adversity. In this regard, we found it telling that his vision of the future included the altruistic intention to enable his family (present and future) and peers. In Simphiwe's vision for the future, a benevolent collective obviates the need for almost exclusive self-reliance.

At the time of writing this chapter, Simphiwe had just been promoted. We wondered, though, how he would have construed his resilience had he been less successful. Would he have blamed himself, rather than a lack of ecological support? A danger of resilience accounts that foreground personal vision and personal agency is that the individual can be blamed if outcomes are not positive (Masten, 2014). This is particularly problematic when ecological factors (such as a lack of employment opportunities, social injustice, or marginalisation) limit the potential of personal vision and personal agency to effect meaningful change (Munford & Sanders, 2015). Given this caveat, there is an urgent need to shift the focus away from initiatives that are solely focused on enabling personal agency in the face of adversity to ones that include a focus on enabling ecologies to be resilience promoting.

7.4.3 *Facilitate Ecological Supports to Amplify the Resilience of Emerging Adults in Stressed Environments*

In addition to supporting communities to be resilient, a key pathway to the resilience of emerging adults is equitable access to meaningful employment. In South Africa, multiple role-players are committed to enabling such access (Paver et al., 2019), and government is constantly advertising its commitment to solving the employment crisis (SAnews, 2019). Even so, more needs to be done if the wellbeing of emerging adults, like Simphiwe, is to be safeguarded. In this regard, Simphiwe's account points to the importance of opportunities to maintain physical health and mental wellbeing. Everyday resources such as gymnasiums or libraries (including electronic ones) with a good supply of motivational and educational resources would be valuable, so long as access to them is affordable for those without a source of income. It is worth mentioning that Simphiwe explained that the gym he referred to is sponsored by the local petrochemical industry and free-to-use for local community residents.

Simphiwe's account also alludes to the potential value attached to entrepreneurial skill. Although this value is formally recognised in South Africa's basic education curriculum and elsewhere in sub-Saharan Africa (Ajufo, 2013), accessible opportunities for post-school entrepreneurial training are important too. In addition, emerging adults need financial support for their entrepreneurial plans. In addition to the provision of microloans (albeit of sometimes dubious value; Bateman & Chang, 2012), there is vast potential benefit in teaching adolescents and emerging adults about responsible membership of informal savings groups and their potential to support emerging adults' entrepreneurial plans for income-generation activities. Elsewhere in sub-Saharan Africa, youth savings groups are typically used to initiate youth financial inclusion and economic empowerment. Membership has the added benefit of providing access to social capital and enabling positive behavioural change (Flynn & Sumberg, 2018).

In summary, there is indisputable value to assisting individual emerging adults (e.g., by supporting them to reflexively manage employment instability; Di Fabio et al., 2019) and to celebrating the personal contributions that emerging adults make to their resilience. There is something remarkable in an emerging adult, like Simphiwe, experiencing relentless hardship "without defining themselves by their adversity" (Burt & Paysnick, 2012, p. 502). Even so, our argument is for greater attention to the social-ecological. In contexts, such as Simphiwe's, where community connectedness, resources, and opportunities are constrained it is imperative to also facilitate ecological supports—such as opportunities for recreation or savings groups—to amplify the resilience of emerging adults in stressed environments.

7.5 Conclusion

We used Simphiwe's case to illustrate that the resilience of an emerging adult to unemployment and additional environmental stress is a process that is partly informed by personal resources and partly ecological ones. In Simphiwe's case, the emphasis was on personal resources. Whilst this emphasis fits with EA theory (Arnett, 2000, 2014, 2016; Arnett et al., 2014) and developmentally sensitive accounts of resilience (Yoon et al., 2019), it is at odds with social-ecological theories of resilience (Ungar, 2012), reviews of child and adolescent resilience in South and sub-Saharan Africa (Theron, 2020; Van Breda & Theron, 2018), and a review of emerging adult resilience (Burt & Paysnick, 2012). We make sense of this contradiction by theorising that the ecological constraints that dominate Simphiwe's context probably translated into his need for self-reliance. Although his capacity is admirable, it also signals the need for urgent attention to the ecologies of emerging adults. When these ecologies are resource-constrained and characterised by low human connectedness, a first step is to foster community resilience and to amplify young adult access to structural resources that will promote employment and sustain wellbeing.

References

Adegoke, C. O., & Steyn, M. G. (2017). A photo voice perspective on factors contributing to the resilience of HIV positive Yoruba adolescent girls in Nigeria. *Journal of Adolescence, 56*, 1–10. https://doi.org/10.1016/j.adolescence.2017.01.003

Ajufo, B. I. (2013). Challenges of youth unemployment in Nigeria: Effective career guidance as a panacea. *African Research Review, 7*(1), 307–321. https://doi.org/10.4314/afrrev.v7i1.21

Arnett, J. J. (2000). Emerging adulthood: A theory of development from the late teens through the twenties. *American Psychologist, 55*(5), 469–480. https://doi.org/10.1037/0003-066X.55.5.469

Arnett, J. J. (2014). *Emerging adulthood: The winding road from the late teens through the twenties*. Oxford University Press.

Arnett, J. J. (2016). Does emerging adulthood theory apply across social classes? National data on a persistent question. *Emerging Adulthood, 4*(4), 227–235. https://doi.org/10.1177/2167696815613000

Arnett, J. J., Žukauskienė, R., & Sugimura, K. (2014). The new life stage of emerging adulthood at ages 18–29 years: Implications for mental health. *The Lancet Psychiatry, 1*(7), 569–576. https://doi.org/10.1016/s2215-0366(14)00080-7

Bateman, M., & Chang, H. J. (2012). Microfinance and the illusion of development: From hubris to nemesis in thirty years. *World Economic Review, 1*, 13–36.

Betancourt, T. S., Meyers-Ohki, S., Stulac, S. N., Elizabeth Barrera, A., Mushashi, C., & Beardslee, W. R. (2011). Nothing can defeat combined hands (abashize hamwe ntakibananira): Protective processes and resilience in Rwandan children and families affected by HIV/AIDS. *Social Science & Medicine, 73*(5), 693–701. https://doi.org/10.1016/j.socscimed.2011.06.053

Braun, V., & Clarke, V. (2006). Using thematic analysis in psychology. *Qualitative Research in Psychology, 3*(2), 77–101. https://doi.org/10.1191/1478088706qp063oa

Burt, K. B., & Paysnick, A. A. (2012). Resilience in the transition to adulthood. *Development and Psychopathology, 24*(2), 493–505.

Canham, H. (2018). Theorising community rage for decolonial action. *South Africa Journal of Psychology, 48*(3), 319–330. https://doi.org/10.1177/0081246318787682

Chimakonam, J. O. (2016). The end of Ubuntu or its beginning in Matolino-Kwindingwi-Metz debate: An exercise in conversational philosophy. *South African Journal of Philosophy, 35*(2), 224–234. https://doi.org/10.1080/02580136.2016.1174921

Côté, J. E. (2014). The dangerous myth of emerging adulthood: An evidence-based critique of a flawed developmental theory. *Applied Developmental Science, 18*(4), 177–188.

Creswell, J. W. (2007). *Qualitative inquiry and research design. Choosing among five approaches*. Sage.

De Witte, H., Rothmann, S., & Jackson, L. T. (2012). The psychological consequences of unemployment in South Africa. *South African Journal of Economic and Management Sciences, 15*(3), 235–252. https://doi.org/10.4102/sajems.v15i3.153

Di Fabio, A., Maree, J. G., & Kenny, M. E. (2019). Development of the life project reflexivity scale: A new career intervention inventory. *Journal of Career Assessment, 27*(2), 358–370. https://doi.org/10.1177/1069072718758065

Ebersöhn, L., Ferreira, R., Van der Walt, A., & Moen, M. (2016). Bodymapping to step into your future: Life design in a context of high risk and high diversity. In R. Ferreira (Ed.), *Thinking innovatively about psychological assessment in a context of diversity* (pp. 228–241). Juta.

Ebersöhn, L., Loots, T., Mampane, R., Omidire, F., Malan, V. R. M., Sefotho, M., & Nthontho, M. (2018). An indigenous psychology perspective on psychosocial support in Southern Africa as collective, networking, and pragmatic support. *Journal of Community & Applied Social Psychology, 28*(5), 332–347. https://doi.org/10.1002/casp.2371

Eisenhardt, K. M., & Graebner, M. E. (2007). Theory building from cases: Opportunities and challenges. *Academy of Management Journal, 50*(1), 25–32. https://doi.org/10.5465/amj.2007.24160888

Flynn, J., & Sumberg, J. (2018). Are savings groups a livelihoods game changer for young people in Africa? *Development in Practice, 28*(1), 51–64. https://doi.org/10.1080/09614524.2018.1397102

Griep, Y., Baillien, E., Vleugels, W., Rothmann, S., & De Witte, H. (2014). Do they adapt or react? A comparison of the adaptation model and the stress reaction model among South African unemployed. *Economic and Industrial Democracy, 35*(4), 717–736. https://doi.org/10.1177/0143831x13495719

Harper, G. W., Wagner, R. L., Popoff, E., Reisner, S. L., & Jadwin-Cakmak, L. (2019). Psychological resilience among transfeminine adolescents and emerging adults living with HIV. *AIDS (London, England), 33*(Suppl 1), S53–S62. https://doi.org/10.1097/QAD.0000000000002174

Hendry, L. B., & Kloep, M. (2010). How universal is emerging adulthood? An empirical example. *Journal of Youth Studies, 13*(2), 169–179. https://doi.org/10.1080/13676260903295067

Holte, B. H., Swart, I., & Hiilamo, H. (2019). The NEET concept in comparative youth research: The Nordic countries and South Africa. *Journal of Youth Studies, 22*(2), 256–272. https://doi.org/10.1080/13676261.2018.1496406

Luthar, S. (2006). Resilience in development: A synthesis of research across five decades. In D. Cicchetti & D. Cohen (Eds.), *Developmental psychopathology: Risk, disorder, and adaptation* (Vol. 3, 2nd ed., pp. 739–795). Wiley.

Madewell, A. N., & Ponce-Garcia, E. (2016). Assessing resilience in emerging adulthood: The resilience scale (RS), Connor–Davidson resilience scale (CD-RISC), and scale of protective factors (SPF). *Personality and Individual Differences, 97*, 249–255. https://doi.org/10.1016/j.paid.2016.03.036

Malindi, M. J. (2014). Exploring the roots of resilience among female street-involved children in South Africa. *Journal of Psychology, 5*(1), 35–45. https://doi.org/10.1080/09764224.2014.11885503

Maree, J. G. (2016). Career construction counseling with a mid-career black man. *The Career Development Quarterly, 64*(1), 20–34. https://doi.org/10.1002/cdq.12038

Masten, A. S. (2014). *Ordinary magic: Resilience in development*. Guilford.

Masten, A. S., & Cicchetti, D. (2016). Resilience in development: Progress and transformation. In D. Cicchetti (Ed.), *Developmental psychopathology, Vol. 4: Risk, resilience, and intervention* (3rd ed., pp. 271–333). Wiley. https://doi.org/10.1002/9781119125556.devpsy406

Mayer, T., Moorti, S., & McCallum, J. K. (Eds.). (2019). *The crisis of global youth unemployment*. Routledge.

McCubbin, L. D., & Moniz, J. (2015). Ethical principles in resilience research: Respect, relevance, reciprocity and responsibility. In L. C. Theron, L. Liebenberg, & M. Ungar (Eds.), *Youth resilience and culture: Commonalities and complexities* (pp. 217–229). Springer.

Mhlongo, N. (Ed.). (2019). *Black tax: Burden or ubuntu?* Jonathan Ball.

Miller, B., & Bowen, E. (2019). "I know where the rest of my life is going": Attitudinal and behavioral dimensions of resilience for homeless emerging adults. *Journal of Social Service Research*. https://doi.org/10.1080/01488376.2019.1607647

Mitchell, C., Theron, L. C., Stuart, J., Smith, A., & Campbell, Z. (2011). Drawings as research method. In L. C. Theron, C. Mitchell, A. Smith, & J. Stuart (Eds.), *Picturing research: Drawings as visual methodology* (pp. 19–36). Rotterdam, NL.

Mosavel, M., Ahmed, R., Ports, K. A., & Simon, C. (2015). South African, urban youth narratives: Resilience within community. *International Journal of Adolescence and Youth, 20*(2), 245–255. https://doi.org/10.1080/01488376.2019.1607647

Motsamai, M. (2017). Personhood and rights in an African tradition. *Politikon, 2017*, 1–15. https://doi.org/10.1080/02589346.2017.1339176

Munford, R., & Sanders, J. (2015). Young people's search for agency: Making sense of their experiences and taking control. *Qualitative Social Work, 14*(5), 616–633. https://doi.org/10.1177/1473325014565149

Newcomb-Anjo, S. E., Barker, E. T., & Howard, A. L. (2017). A person-centered analysis of risk factors that compromise wellbeing in emerging adulthood. *Journal of Youth and Adolescence, 46*(4), 867–883. https://doi.org/10.1007/s10964-016-0603-2

O'Malley, J., Wardlaw, T., You, D., Hug, L., & Anthony, D. (2014). Africa's child demographics and the world's future. *The Lancet, 384*(9945), 730–732. https://doi.org/10.1016/S0140-6736(14)61331-3

Owusu-Sekyere, E. (2019). Africa's demographic dividend: Fact or farce? *AfricaGrowth Agenda, 16*(Jan/Mar), 10–12. Retrieved from https://hdl.handle.net/10520/EJC-1477183935

Paver, R., Rothmann, S., Van den Broeck, A., & De Witte, H. (2019). Labour market interventions to assist the unemployed in two townships in South Africa. *SA Journal of Industrial Psychology, 45*, 1–14. https://doi.org/10.4102/sajip.v45i0.1596

Phasha, T. N. (2010). Educational resilience among African survivors of child sexual abuse in South Africa. *Journal of Black Studies, 40*(6), 1234–1253. https://doi.org/10.1177/0021934708327693

Ramphele, M. (2012). *Conversations with my sons and daughters*. Penguin Books.

Rutter, M. (2012). Resilience: Causal pathways and social ecology. In M. Ungar (Ed.), *The social ecology of resilience* (pp. 33–42). Springer.

SAnews. (2019, May 14). *Government focused on tackling unemployment*. South African Government News Agency. Retrieved from https://www.sanews.gov.za/south-africa/government-focused-tackling-unemployment

StatsSA. (2019, May 15). *Youth graduate unemployment rate increases in Q1: 2019*. Retrieved from http://www.statssa.gov.za/?p=12121

Syed, M. (2016). Emerging adulthood: Developmental stage, theory, or nonsense. In J. Arnett (Ed.), *The Oxford handbook of emerging adulthood* (pp. 11–25). Oxford University Press.

Theron, L. C. (2020). Resilience of sub-Saharan children and adolescents: A scoping review. *Transcultural Psychiatry*. https://doi.org/10.1177/1363461520938916

Theron, L. C., & Theron, A. M. C. (2010). A critical review of studies of South African youth resilience, 1990-2008. *South African Journal of Science, 106*(7/8). https://doi.org/10.4102/sajs.v106i7/8.252

Theron, L. C., & Theron, A. M. C. (2013). Positive adjustment to poverty: How family communities encourage resilience in traditional African contexts. *Culture & Psychology, 19*(3), 391–413. https://doi.org/10.1177/1354067x13489318

Theron, L. C., & Theron, A. M. C. (2014). Education services and resilience processes: Resilient black South African students' experiences. *Children and Youth Services Review, 47*(Part 3), 297–306. https://doi.org/10.1016/j.childyouth.2014.10.003

Theron, L. C., & Ungar, M. (2019). Adolescent resilience in the face of relentless adversity: The role of strong, black women. In I. Eloff (Ed.), *Handbook of quality of life in African societies* (pp. 97–111). Springer.

Theron, L. C., & Van Rensburg, A. (2018). Learning from school-attending adolescents living in conditions of structural inequality. *Journal of Adolescence, 67*, 167–178. https://doi.org/10.1016/j.adolescence.2018.06.012

Ungar, M. (2011). The social ecology of resilience: Addressing contextual and cultural ambiguity of a nascent construct. *American Journal of Orthopsychiatry, 81*(1), 1–17. https://doi.org/10.1111/j.1939-0025.2010.01067.x

Ungar, M. (2012). Social ecologies and their contribution to resilience. In M. Ungar (Ed.), *The social ecology of resilience* (pp. 13–32). Springer.

Van Breda, A. D. (2015). Journey towards independent living: A grounded theory investigation of leaving the care of Girls & Boys Town South Africa. *Journal of Youth Studies, 18*(3), 322–337. https://doi.org/10.1080/13676261.2014.963534

Van Breda, A. D. (2018). Resilience of vulnerable students transitioning into a South African university. *Higher Education, 75*(6), 1109–1124. https://doi.org/10.1007/s10734-017-0188-z

Van Breda, A. D. (2019). Developing the notion of Ubuntu as African theory for social work practice. *Social Work, 55*(4), 439–450. https://doi.org/10.15270/55-4-762

Van Breda, A. D., & Dickens, L. F. (2017). The contribution of resilience to one-year independent living outcomes of care-leavers in South Africa. *Children and Youth Services Review, 83*, 264–273. https://doi.org/10.1016/j.childyouth.2017.11.009

Van Breda, A. D., & Theron, L. C. (2018). A critical review of South African child and youth resilience studies, 2009-2017. *Child and Youth Services Review, 91*, 237–247. https://doi.org/10.1016/j.childyouth.2018.06.022

Van der Vaart, L., De Witte, H., Van den Broeck, A., & Rothmann, S. (2018). A psychosocial typology of the unemployed in South Africa. *South Africa Journal of Psychology, 48*(2), 179–192. https://doi.org/10.1177/0081246317721600

Vindevogel, S., Ager, A., Schiltz, J., Broekaert, E., & Derluyn, I. (2015). Toward a culturally sensitive conceptualization of resilience: Participatory research with war-affected communities in northern Uganda. *Transcultural Psychiatry, 52*(3), 396–416. https://doi.org/10.1177/1363461514565852

Windle, G. (2011). What is resilience? A review and concept analysis. *Reviews in Clinical Gerontology, 21*(2), 152–169. https://doi.org/10.1017/s0959259810000420

Wood, D., Crapnell, T., Lau, L., Bennett, A., Lotstein, D., Ferris, M., & Kuo, A. (2018). Emerging adulthood as a critical stage in the life course. In N. Halfon, C. B. Forrest, R. Lerner, & E. M. Faustman (Eds.), *Handbook of life course health development* (pp. 123–143). Springer.

Wright, M. O., & Masten, A. S. (2015). Pathways to resilience in context. In L. C. Theron, L. Liebenberg, & M. Ungar (Eds.), *Resilience and culture: Commonalities and complexities* (pp. 3–22). Springer.

Yin, R. K. (2014). *Case study research: Design and methods* (5th ed.). Sage.

Yoon, S., Howell, K., Dillard, R., McCarthy, K. S., Napier, T. R., & Pei, F. (2019). Resilience following child maltreatment: Definitional considerations and developmental variations. *Trauma, Violence, & Abuse*. https://doi.org/10.1177/1524838019869094

Zulu, N. T. (2019). Resilience in black women who do not have fathers: A qualitative inquiry. *South Africa Journal of Psychology, 49*(2), 219–228. https://doi.org/10.1177/0081246318782187

Chapter 8
Psychological Well-Being Among Young People Living with HIV: Role of Social Support, Self-Esteem and Socio-Demographic Variables

Charles Magoba Muwonge, Annet Kembabazi, Gladys Nakalema, Margaret Ekatushabe, Diana Kwarikunda, Henry Kibedi, and Joseph Ssenyonga

Abstract The focus of the present study was two-fold: (a) to examine the relations between demographic characteristics and the psychological well-being of Young People Living with HIV (YPLWH) and (b) to assess the extent to which self-esteem mediated the relationship between social support and psychological well-being of YPLWH. The sample consisted of 181 YPLWH selected from four Primary Health Care clinics in South-Western Uganda who responded to anonymous self-administered questionnaires. Data were analyzed using t-tests, ANOVA, and path analysis. We noted that females had significantly higher purpose in life scores than males ($p < .05$). General family support exerted direct effects on purpose in life ($\beta = .40, p < .001$) and positive relations ($\beta = .15, p < .001$). The effects of general family support on personal growth were mediated by self-esteem ($\beta = .14$, $p < .001$). Conversely, the total contributions of support from friends on personal growth and positive relations were mostly direct rather than being mediated by self-esteem. The study highlights a need to enhance the social support networks as a way of enhancing self-esteem and ensuring psychological well-being among YPLWH in Uganda.

C. M. Muwonge (✉) · A. Kembabazi · G. Nakalema · M. Ekatushabe · J. Ssenyonga
Department of Educational Foundations and Psychology, Mbarara University of Science and Technology, Mbarara, Uganda

D. Kwarikunda
Department of Educational Foundations and Psychology, Mbarara University of Science and Technology, Mbarara, Uganda

Department of Educational Psychology, University of Potsdam, Potsdam, Germany

H. Kibedi
Department of Psychology, Kyambogo University, Kyambogo, Uganda

L. Schutte et al. (eds.), *Embracing Well-Being in Diverse African Contexts: Research Perspectives*, Cross-Cultural Advancements in Positive Psychology 16,
https://doi.org/10.1007/978-3-030-85924-4_8

Keywords Psychological well-being · Self-esteem · Social support · Socio-demographic variables, young people living with HIV

8.1 Introduction

According to the Joint United Nations Program on HIV/AIDS (UNAIDS, 2019), globally, HIV and AIDS remain a major public health concern, with over 37.9 million people estimated to have been infected with HIV by 2019. In 2019, worldwide, there were 460,000 new HIV infections among young people aged 10–24 years, of which over 170,000 infections were recorded among adolescents aged 10–19 years (United Nations International Children's Emergency Fund, 2020). The UNAIDS (2019) report further indicated that 2.8 million young people living with HIV (YPLWH) reside within sub-Saharan Africa. In Africa, HIV/AIDS accounts for the highest number of deaths among young people aged 10–24 years (Avert, 2020). The projected increase in the young people's population threatens to further escalate the HIV prevalence on the African continent. Low and middle-income countries have the highest number of YPLWH, with over 84% of all YPLWH residing in sub-Saharan Africa (Avert, 2020). According to the Uganda AIDS Commission (UAC), by 2018, approximately 160,000 young people aged 15–24 years were infected with HIV in Uganda (UAC, 2019).

Over an extended period of time, YPLWH experience numerous psychological threats and other forms of challenges to their well-being. These challenges include discrimination, lack of enough social and emotional support, domestic violence, financial constraints, and other challenges related to adherence to antiretroviral therapy (ART) (Ashaba et al., 2018, 2019; Kihumuro et al., 2021; Kimera, Vindevogel, Kintu, et al., 2020). Such challenges emanate from the families, schools, health centers, and communities—where these young people interact with other people daily (Kimera et al., 2019; Osafo et al., 2017). For example, Kimera et al. (2019) indicated that within the East-African region, schools present highly stigmatizing environments for YPLWH due to some insensitive and bullying students and teachers who hold opprobrious views about HIV/AIDS.

Additionally, within their families, YPLWH are taken to low-ranking schools, served meals on separate utensils, and are given little financial and emotional support compared to their counterparts who are HIV negative (Kimera, Vindevogel, Kintu, et al., 2020; Kimera, Vindevogel, Reynaert, et al., 2020). In their study, Kidman and Violari (2018) reported that the perinatal-HIV infected young people experience physical, sexual, and intimate partner-violence as they transition into the dating life. Other challenges include grief and bereavement owing to the death of their caretakers, and the trauma posed by the prospect of their own 'imminent' death (Ashaba et al., 2019). There are concerns about the sexuality of YPLWH and the fear of having to disclose their HIV status to family members or spouses before starting family life (Ssali et al., 2010). Coupled with their emerging psychological and physical development, the above threats could trigger several mental problems, leading to poor psychological well-being and psychosocial adjustment of YPLWH (Ashaba et al., 2018).

Among YPLWH, poor psychological well-being has been associated with poor adherence to ART (Leserman, 2008; Mavhu et al., 2013; Okawa et al., 2018), high risk of mental health problems such as depression and suicidal ideation (Abebe et al., 2019; Ashaba et al., 2018; Lyons, 2010; Okawa et al., 2018) and increase in the likelihood of spreading HIV to other people. Additionally, poor psychological well-being among YPLWH has been linked to poor adherence to doctors' advice and lack of compliance with medical prescriptions and treatments (Okawa et al., 2018).

Young adulthood is a very critical period in human development as it is at this stage when individuals develop social and human capital alongside other resources that can enable them to live an enjoyable adult-life later. Among YPLWH, their well-being is even more threatened as their survival and livelihood are already encumbered by AIDS-related morbidity, mortality and low quality of life since some of them are not able to access good medical and psychological support. In Africa, projections have indicated that the number of YPLWH will rise by 40% between 2015 and 2030 (Govindasamy et al., 2020). Therefore, as Govindasamy et al. (2020, p. 2) assert:

> Models predict that investment in the quality of life among the growing youth population in sub-Saharan Africa, particularly via addressing health needs, could increase labor productivity and resultantly accelerate economic growth. If long-run economic growth is to be achieved, then public health policies need to also promote the well-being among YPLWH, a vulnerable and growing population in this region.

Researchers in sub-Saharan Africa should even be concerned about the well-being of YPLWH as there is compelling evidence that "the stocks and intergenerational transfer of human capital to young people in this region have already been eroded by the HIV/AIDS epidemic" (Govindasamy et al., 2020, p. 12).

Although Sustainable Development Goal 3 roots for the promotion of well-being among individuals of all ages, campaigns for the advancement of mental well-being and high quality of life among YPLWH have not been satisfactory in sub-Saharan Africa (Govindasamy et al., 2020), Uganda inclusive. Therefore, there is need to focus attention on individual considerations that result in better health-status and general well-being of YPLWH, especially in low and middle-income sub-Saharan African countries.

As Walakira et al. (2014) assert, the psychosocial well-being of HIV-infected people is a growing area of concern, and efforts are being made to understand the factors that relate to or promote their welfare. In order to develop interventions that are context-specific and fit for given sub-Saharan populations, there is need to examine how different socio-demographic variables (e.g., gender, religious affiliation, age, etc.) are related to the well-being of YPLWH, especially in developing countries. There is convincing evidence that such socio-demographic variables are highly associated with various aspects of psychological and mental well-being in the general population (e.g., Keyes & Waterman, 2003; Khumalo et al., 2012). Therefore, there is need to further examine variations in the psychological well-being of

YPLWH with respect to their socio-demographic variables, especially in sub-Saharan Africa.

Social support and self-esteem have also been identified to be protective against mental illnesses and psychological distress among People Living with HIV (PLWH) (Lyons, 2010; Mavandadi et al., 2009) including YPLWH (Abebe et al., 2019). For example, people with HIV who report satisfying social relationships exhibit high life satisfaction, are happier, and are less likely to be depressed (e.g., Mavandadi et al., 2009). Among youth, lower social support is highly correlated with more poor mental-health symptoms (Lam et al., 2007). Lee et al. (2007) have indicated that among young people aged 11–18 years, better social support was significantly associated with lower depression and reductions in general misconduct.

Additionally, low self-esteem among people living with HIV is associated with high stigma and discrimination, depression, and other related mental health issues (Kalomo, 2018). Manhas (2014) also indicated that high self-esteem was positively correlated with high quality of life, high psychological health, and higher levels of independence among PLWH.

Given that social support varies across different cultures (Taylor, 2007), and that many studies examining social support have been conducted in the Western countries (which are more individualistic), there is need to further examine the correlates of social support in African settings which value interdependence. Such studies will inform culturally specific interventions to enhance social support and self-esteem among YPLWH in Uganda with a view to improving their overall quality of life and well-being.

Although the relationships between self-esteem and social support have been well studied (e.g., Kong et al., 2013; Lyons, 2010), the structural relationship among these variables is loosely understood especially among YPLWH in sub-Saharan Africa. Therefore, the present cross-sectional study focused on examining the differences in the psychological well-being of YPLWH in Uganda for different socio-demographic groups, and how social support and self-esteem factors relate to psychological well-being in this group.

8.1.1 Relationship Between Socio-Demographic Variables and Psychological Well-Being Among YPLWH

Psychological well-being among people living with HIV has been associated with several socio-demographic variables such as age, gender, socio-economic status, number of people in the family, and characteristics of caregivers among other factors (Asante, 2012; Cederfjäll et al., 2001; Liping et al., 2015; Mavandadi et al., 2009; Vorster et al., 2000). Examining how certain demographic variables are linked to well-being provides an insight into which group is most vulnerable, and hence, helps to design interventions consistent with specific sub-Saharan populations. In the following section, we discuss the relations between socio-demographic variables and psychological well-being among people living with HIV.

Across all age groups of people living with HIV, YPLWH have been, arguably, the most affected group (Avert, 2020). This is partly because they are not only battling challenges associated with their HIV status, but also the emotional, physical, and psychological changes associated with the transitions from childhood and adolescence to adulthood. Although adolescents' awareness of their HIV status has no negative impact on their mental health as compared to those who are unaware of their status (Menon et al., 2007), the disclosure and/or fear of disclosure of the HIV status of YPLWH to schoolmates or other less closely related individuals in the community significantly impacts their psychological health and well-being (Kimera, Vindevogel, Kintu, et al., 2020; Lam et al., 2007). However, disclosure to trusted family and friends who provide emotional support does not threaten the psychological health of YPLWH (Lam et al., 2007).

Some studies have found age to be positively associated with the positive mental health of PLWH. For example, Mavandadi et al. (2009) found that older people (54+ years), especially those who grow up with HIV, have been found to show better psychological well-being and health adjustment compared to the younger ones ($\leq$54 years). Older people receive much support from their colleagues and family members thereby reducing social isolation, leading to better mental health. Liping et al. (2015) evaluated the association between socio-demographic variables and quality of life among people living with HIV in China. In contrast with the results of Mavandadi et al. (2009), Liping et al. (2015) found individuals aged 30 years and below had a higher quality of life compared to those who were older. Other studies have indicated no significant differences in psychological well-being between age groups (e.g., Asante, 2012; Flannelly & Inouye, 2001). For instance, Asante (2012) conducted a study among adults, many of whom had received higher education, and although higher levels of social support were associated with lower levels of depression, there were no significant correlations between age and their general psychological well-being.

Although some studies agree that there are no variations in the well-being and mental health of YPLWH based on their gender (Flannelly & Inouye, 2001; Mellins et al., 2006; Worthington & Krentz, 2005), other researchers seem to disagree. For example, a study among people aged 18–58 years living with HIV in Ghana indicated that females experienced higher levels of depression, anxiety, and stress compared to their male counterparts (Asante, 2012). This agreed with earlier studies conducted among adolescents living with HIV (ALWH, e.g., American ALWH between 1993 and 1995 [Lee et al., 2007]; Malawian ALWH [Kim et al., 2015]; and Spanish ALWH [Ramiro et al., 2013]). Among Kenyan YPLWH, depressive symptoms were higher among males than females—which were attributed to exposure to more negative events in life or conflicts at home. Nevertheless, specific phobias were more prevalent among females (Kamau et al., 2012).

Worthington and Krentz (2005) examined the relationships between education level, socio-economic status, and well-being (indicated by health-related quality of life; HRQL) among HIV-positive adults in Canada. After controlling for clinical characteristics, results indicated that educational levels, employment status, and income significantly predicted HRQL, while other factors like living with a partner and the mode of HIV transmission did not. In China, family annual income was significantly and positively associated with high physical health and mental health scores among adults living with HIV (Xiao et al., 2019). Similarly, Flannelly and Inouye (2001) indicated that among Hawaiian adults aged 25–54 years, socio-economic status combined with other variables such as religious affiliation and faith explained HIV patients' well-being. These studies suggested that high socio-economic status is linked to access to better medical services, better social networks, and better psychosocial support, all of which can lead to improved mental health among people living with HIV.

The psychological well-being of YPLWH can also be influenced by the characteristics of the caregiver. For example, children living with HIV-infected parents or caregivers are at higher risk of psychological stress resulting from uncertainty regarding the health of the caregiver than those living with non-infected ones. Additionally, Lee et al. (2007) have indicated high depression levels among young people whose parents had disclosed their HIV status to them. On the contrary, other studies suggest that the characteristics of the caregiver have no impact on a child's mental health. For example, Mellins et al. (2006) study among an American population indicated that the caregivers' gender, race, and biological relationship had no significant effect on the child's (9–16 years) psychiatric condition. The same study indicated that the caregiver's HIV status had no influence on the child's mental condition. In Uganda, studies have indicated that the mental health of many orphaned YPLWH living with other relatives (e.g., grandparents) or in child-headed homes was poor (Atwine et al., 2005; Sengendo & Nambi, 1997). In a resource-poor Kenya urban community, Kamau et al. (2012) indicated that the characteristics of the primary guardian, parental status (i.e., whether single parent, both parents alive, or orphaned), and ART were not associated with the psychiatric morbidity of a sample of children and ALWH.

In summary, previous studies have indicated variations in the psychological well-being of people living with HIV with respect to their demographic characteristics. Based on the results discussed above, it is evident that the relationship between socio-demographic variables and psychological well-being is context-specific and varies according to the population and circumstances under study. Nevertheless, many studies examining these relationships have been conducted with older people living with HIV/AIDS in Western and Asian countries. In terms of HIV management, Western and Asian societies differ significantly from African societies. For example, leaving aside the cultural differences, there is better access to HIV treatment and psychosocial support for HIV-infected individuals in Western countries compared to their counterparts in sub-Saharan Africa. Consequently, such findings from European, American, and/or Asian contexts cannot necessarily be used to inform practices in Africa. The present study responds to this research gap by exploring whether the psychological well-being of YPLWH differs in accordance with their socio-demographic variables.

8.1.2 *Relationships Between Social Support, Self-Esteem, and Psychological Well-Being Among YPLWH*

In the following sections, we highlight the relationships between social support, self-esteem, and psychological well-being.

8.1.2.1 Associations Between Social Support and Self-Esteem

Social support is defined as "the perception or experience that one is loved and catered for, esteemed and valued, and part of the social network of mutual assistance and obligations" (Kong et al., 2013, p. 152). Perceived social support is significantly associated with high self-esteem (Kong et al., 2013; Lyons, 2010; Sung et al., 2012; Tian et al., 2013). When young people have warm and positive relationships with their colleagues, they experience acceptance, encouragement, and support from interactions in such relationships thereby developing a high positive regard for themselves, high self-confidence, and high self-esteem (Wilson et al., 1990). Among young people aged 10–19 years, high self-esteem has been reported from those who receive a lot of support from fellow peers and their families (Huurre, 2000). When young people have supportive role models (e.g., teachers and parents), they are more likely to have higher self-esteem as such models help in shaping and correcting their attitudes.

8.1.2.2 Relationship Between Self-Esteem and Well-Being

Self-esteem is a component of self-concept that refers to the person's positive or negative orientation towards him/herself. People with high self-esteem are highly optimistic, have high hopes about the future, and exhibit high life satisfaction compared to those with low self-worth. Low self-esteem has been associated with unhealthy and anti-social habits such as drug abuse, rape, and engagement in high-risk behaviors that lead to poor mental health and psychological distress (Chernaskey, 2017).

In the general population, self-esteem has been strongly associated with high levels of psychological well-being. For example, high self-esteem correlates strongly with life satisfaction, positive affect (Diener & Diener, 1995) and predict the cognitive component of subjective well-being among young people aged 10–19 years (Zhang & Leung, 2002). In China, Xi et al. (2017) indicated that self-esteem and self-efficacy predicted subjective well-being among Chinese college students. The above results dovetailed with those of Sung et al. (2012) who found that high self-esteem was associated with lower depression levels among institutionalized adolescents in Korea. Compared to individuals with high self-esteem, those with lower self-esteem lack sufficient coping mechanisms necessary to prevent spiraling downward into depression when faced with traumatic events or challenging situations (Orth et al., 2009).

In summary, individuals with high esteem and self-acceptance develop a positive view about themselves which leads to high optimism and hopes for the future—which consequently boosts their personal growth, psychological adjustment, and well-being compared to those with low self-esteem.

8.1.2.3 Social Support and Well-Being

The positive associations between social support and well-being are widely documented. This is also the case for people living with HIV/AIDS or other life-long illnesses (e.g., Asante, 2012; Funck-Brentano et al., 2005; Lee et al., 2007; Mavandadi et al., 2009; Neff et al., 2003; Symister & Friend, 2003; Walker et al., 2004). For example, Asante's study involving a Ghanaian sample of PLWH aged between 18 and 58 years found that individuals who reported receiving more social support were less depressed and had lower levels of anxiety than those who reported receiving less social support. This is consistent with the studies of Lee et al. (2007) and Tian et al. (2013) that involved ALWH from the USA and China respectively, and Sung et al.'s (2012) study with a South Korean sample of PLWH. High social support has been linked to low CD4 lymphocyte count and reduced HIV progression (Persson et al., 1994), lower depression levels (Mavandadi et al., 2009; Schrimshaw & Siegel, 2003; Vyavaharkar et al., 2009), more positive moods ($r = .374$), less negative moods ($r = -.276$; Fleishman et al., 2000) and higher medication adherence practices—all of which are indicative of the better psychological well-being of PLWH. In Ethiopia, Abebe et al. (2019) found that, in addition to age and poor medication adherence, low and moderate social support were highly associated with depressive symptoms among youth infected with HIV. Social support promotes well-being through influencing behaviors, emotions, and cognitions that promote positive affect (Cohen et al., 2000).

8.1.2.4 Self-Esteem as Mediator Between Social Support and Well-Being

There is evidence to suggest that the effects of social support on psychological well-being are mediated by self-esteem (Symister & Friend, 2003; Sung et al., 2012). Social support leads to high self-esteem which in turn, leads to better psychological well-being (Bosson et al., 2000; Diener & Diener, 1995). It is therefore reasonable to hypothesize that self-esteem mediates the relationship between social support and well-being (see Fig. 8.1).

The mediation effect of self-esteem on the relationship between social support and psychological well-being has been demonstrated in some studies conducted with adolescent and adult populations (e.g., Kong et al., 2013; Sung et al., 2012; Tian et al., 2013; Xi et al., 2017). In China, Sung et al. (2012) investigated the

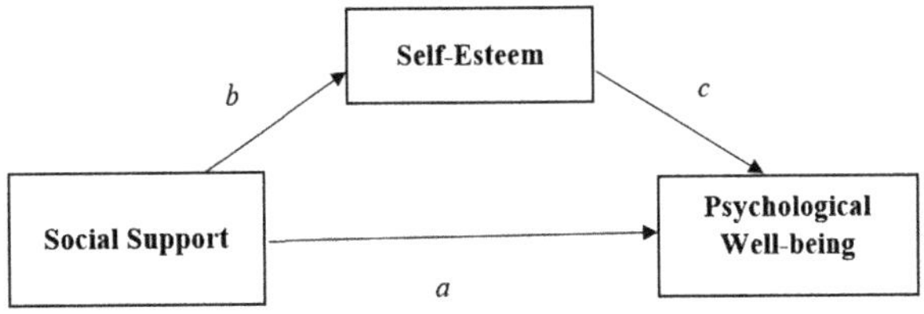

Fig. 8.1 Hypothesized structural relationship between social support, self-esteem, and psychological well-being

relationship between perceived social support, self-esteem, and depression among adolescents from child welfare institutions. A structural equation model indicated that high social support was associated with high self-esteem ($\beta = .47$) and negatively with depression. The same study indicated that self-esteem mediated the relationship between social support and depression. Xi et al. (2017) examined the mediation effects of self-esteem in the relationship between social support and subjective well-being among college students in China. Results indicated that social support positively influenced subjective well-being and that self-efficacy mediated the relationship between social support and well-being. Similarly, Tian et al. (2013) studied the mediation role of self-esteem in the relation between social support and school well-being among middle and early adolescents in China. Among the early adolescents, the relationship between parental support and school well-being was mediated by self-esteem. Additionally, self-esteem mediated the relationship between teacher support and well-being for both early and middle adolescents.

Despite all available evidence, there is a paucity of studies examining the relationship between self-esteem, social support, and well-being of vulnerable groups including PLWH, especially in low and middle-income countries, and particularly in Africa. Therefore, the current study examined the mediation effect of self-esteem on the relationship between social support and well-being among YPLWH in Uganda. This knowledge is important for designing comprehensive interventions that target different aspects of the psychological well-being of YPLWH in the Ugandan context.

8.1.3 The Present Study

In view of the gaps highlighted above, the present study was guided by the following objectives:

(a) To examine whether psychological well-being differs with respect to the demographic characteristics among YPLWH in Uganda.
(b) To assess the extent to which the relationship between social support and psychological well-being is mediated by self-esteem among YPLWH in Uganda.

8.2 Method

8.2.1 Design and Sampling

The study was conducted at four Primary Health Care clinics in South-Western Uganda that provide ART to YPLWH. At the time of the study, there were 400 YPLWH receiving services from these health facilities. In line with the recommendations of Krejcie and Morgan (1970) regarding sample selection, we anticipated including a randomly selected sample of 196 respondents. The study adopted a cross-sectional research design.

8.2.2 Participants

The sample consisted of 181 YPLWH (92% response rate), females (56.9%), aged 12–20 years with a mean age of 16.67 years ($SD = 2.2$). Most of the participants were not in a romantic relationship (102, 56.4%). The sample consisted of Catholics (29.3%), Moslems (24.3%), Anglicans (24.3%), Pentecostals (10.5%), Seventh Day Adventists (5.0%) and other unidentified religions (0.6%). Eleven respondents (6.1%) did not indicate their religion. Most respondents (45.3%) indicated that both biological parents were alive, 32% had one parent who was alive, and 19.9% had lost both parents. Five respondents (2.8%) did not indicate whether their parent (s) were alive or dead. Seventy-one respondents indicated that they lived with both parents compared to 51 and 29 respondents who indicated that they lived with one parent and relatives respectively. Twenty-two respondents indicated they lived with other guardians yet one respondent indicated that he/she lived in a child-care institution. Seven respondents did not indicate whom they lived with at home. Most respondents were taking antiretroviral (ARV) drugs (157, 84.5%) yet 24 respondents (13.3%) indicated that they were not taking ARV drugs. The majority of the participants (42%) were born with HIV, 32.6% acquired HIV through sexual intercourse, and 25.4% acquired HIV through other means such as needle sharing and accidents.

8.2.3 Instruments

A self-report questionnaire consisting of two sections was used to assess the study variables. The first section consisted of items about the YPLWH demographic characteristics such as age, sex, religion, whether one is in a romantic relationship (i.e., relationship status), whether all biological parents were alive, who they live with at home, whether they were taking ARV's or not, and mode of transmission of

HIV. The second section consisted of several subscales that assessed the respondents' psychological well-being, social support, and self-esteem as described below.

8.2.3.1 Psychological Well-Being

Ryff's psychological well-being questionnaire (Ryff, 1989) assessed psychological well-being. This scale comprises six subscales including autonomy, environmental mastery, personal growth, positive relationships, purpose in life, and self-acceptance subscales. Previous studies (e.g., Gao & McLellan, 2018; Springer & Hauser, 2006) have indicated high correlations between subscales of autonomy, environmental mastery, and self-acceptance, indicating a poor discriminant validity of these scales. Consequently, in the present study, only three subscales were adopted as indicators of psychological well-being including the positive relations subscale (4 items), the purpose in life subscale (4 items), and the personal growth subscale (4 items). Sample items from the above subscales included; (a) positive relationships ("I enjoy personal and mutual conversations with family members or friends" and "I know that I can trust my friends, and they know they can trust me"), (b) purpose in life ("I have a sense of direction and purpose in life" and "I enjoy making plans for the future and working to make them a reality"), and (c) personal growth ("For me, life has been a continuous process of learning, changing and growth", and "I think it is important to have new experiences that challenge how I think about myself and the world"). In the present study, Cronbach's alpha values for the positive relations, purpose in life and personal growth subscales were .73, .72 and .81 respectively.

8.2.3.2 Social Support

A 12-item multidimensional scale of perceived social support (Zimet et al., 1988) assessed the YPLWH perceived social support from sources including; (a) family (4 items), (b) friends (4 items), and (c) significant others (4 items).

Initial analysis indicated a very high correlation between the family and significant others' social support subscales ($r = .98$, $p < .01$). In our context, significant others would include the immediate helpers of the young people with whom they share their joys and sorrows, which, in the present study, were the family members of the YPLWH. This could explain the high correlations between these two factors. In fact, previous research indicates that Ugandan adolescents and YPLWH mainly receive social support from their immediate family members (e.g., Damulira et al., 2019; De Nutte et al., 2015; Nabunya et al., 2020; Osafo et al., 2017), hence YPLWH in Uganda consider their family members as also their significant others. Consequently, we merged items from these scales to create a new factor—general family social support (8 items). Sample items from the above subscales included; (a) general family support ("My family really tries to help me" and "I get the emotional help and support I need from my family") and (b) support from friends ("I can talk about my problems with my friends"and "I have friends with whom I can share my joys and sorrows''). In the present study, Cronbach's alpha values for the general family social support and friends' subscales were .94 and .80 respectively.

8.2.3.3 Self-Esteem

Self-esteem was assessed using the unidimensional 10-item Rosenberg self-esteem subscale (Rosenberg, 1985). Sample items from this section included; "I feel that I have a number of good qualities and I am able to do things as well as most other people". The Cronbach's alpha for the self-esteem scale was .80 in the present study.

8.2.4 Procedure

Ethical clearance for the study was sought from the Research Ethics Committee of Mbarara University of Science and Technology, Uganda. Later on, we sought permission from the health clinic's authorities to administer the questionnaires to the YPLWH attending the ART clinic on particular days. The first author explained the aims of the study to the young people before enrolling them in the study. Besides, the potential participants were informed that participation in the study was voluntary and that they were free to withdraw from the study at any time. Additionally, all information that was to be collected was anonymous, confidential, and used for research purposes only. YPLWH were allowed to ask questions on issues where they needed clarifications. Before the participants were enrolled in the study, written assent and parents'/guardians' written consent for participants aged below 18 years, and written consent for participants aged 18–20 years were sought. The participants used approximately 20 min to fill in the questionnaires. The completed questionnaires that were received from the respondents were further checked during submission and participants were encouraged to complete any missing items identified.

8.2.5 Data Analyses

Our analytic strategy followed two main stages including; (a) initial data screening, and (b) analyses related to the study questions—as described below.

Data were screened for (a) multicollinearity, (b) outliers, and (c) missing values—as required before the use of some analyses such as t-tests and structural equation modeling in the subsequent steps. Some subscales' items had missing values of <1%, and hence the full information maximum likelihood method for handling missing values was used, as it is more efficient and less biased compared with other techniques such as list-wise deletion (Geiser, 2013). In line with Kline's (2005) recommendation, all correlations between the variables were below 0.85 (see

Table 8.1 Descriptive statistics and correlations for the Likert-type questionnaires

	M	*SD*	1	2	3	4	5
1. General family support	39.31	10.69					
2. Friends support	19.02	4.41	.57*				
3. Self-esteem	12.37	3.64	.56*	.45*			
4. Positive relations	16.37	4.37	.49*	.51*	.49*		
5. Purpose in life	17.64	3.72	.53*	.29*	.47*	.47*	
6. Personal growth	16.91	4.42	.40*	.42*	.48*	.58*	.52*

*$p < .01$

Table 8.1); hence, there was no significant multicollinearity among the study variables. No outliers were identified in the dataset.

Analysis of Variance (ANOVA) and t-tests were used to examine statistical differences in psychological well-being among YPLWH related to their socio-demographic characteristics. We used a path model (using manifest variables) to examine the mediation effects of self-esteem on the relation between social support and psychological well-being. The use of manifest variables in the structural models is justified when the variables show high levels of reliability indicated by Cronbach's $\alpha > .70$ (Pedhazur, 1982) and when one has many parameters to estimate, as was the case in the present study. We followed the acceptable model fit criteria stated by Hu and Bentler (1999), who proposed Comparative Fit Index (CFI) and Tucker–Lewis index (TLI) values above .90, Standardized Root Mean Square Residual (SRMR) $\leq .08$, and Root Mean-Square Error of Approximation (RMSEA) $\leq .06$ are indicative of adequate fit. Analyses to answer the first research question were conducted in SPSS Version 25 while Mplus 7.4 (Muthén & Muthén, 1998–2015) was used in analysis related to the second research question. The robust maximum likelihood (MLR) estimator was used in model estimations as it is not affected by violations of assumptions of normality (Wang & Wang, 2012).

8.3 Results

8.3.1 Descriptive Statistics

Descriptive statistics of the different Likert-type scales and correlations between scale scores are presented in Table 8.1. Social support variables were positively correlated with self–esteem and psychological well-being.

8.3.2 *Variations in Psychological Well-Being with the Respondents' Demographic Characteristics*

We noted significant differences in purpose in life subscale with respect to gender of YPLWH.

(t (174) $= -2.2$, $p = .03$) with females expressing a higher purpose in life ($M = 18.18$, $SD = 3.33$) compared to males ($M = 16.99$, $SD = 3.92$). There were no significant differences in the psychological well-being of YPLWH with respect to: relationship status, religion, whether parents are alive or not, who they live with at home, whether they are taking ARV's or not, and mode of HIV transmission.

8.3.3 *Mediation Effect of Self-Esteem on the Relationship Between Social Support and Psychological Well-Being*

We examined the mediating effects of self-esteem on the relation between social support and psychological well-being using the two steps below:

8.3.3.1 Analysis of the Direct Effect Model

Prior to the analysis of the indirect model, we first analyzed the direct role of social support on psychological well-being. The effects of gender on purpose for life were controlled for in the analyses. The direct model fitted with the data [CFI = 1.00, TLI = 1.00, RMSEA = .00, SRMR = .00]. General family support had a significant direct effect on personal growth ($\beta = .20$, $p = .03$), positive relations ($\beta = .29$, $p < .001$) and purpose in life ($\beta = .53$, $p < .001$). Support from friends had a direct effect on personal growth ($\beta = .34$, $p < .001$) and positive relations ($\beta = .34$, $p < .001$) but not purpose in life ($\beta = -.03$, $p = .74$).

8.3.3.2 Analysis of Multiple Indirect Effects Model

Based on the direct effect model above, we placed self-esteem in the relation between social support and psychological well-being. The structural equation model was based on the diagrammatic illustration shown in Fig. 8.1. The mediating effect model fitted the data well [CFI = 1.00, TLI = 1.00, RMSEA = .00, SRMR = .01] upon deletion of one non-significant path (from general family support to personal growth). In this model (see Fig. 8.2), both friends support ($\beta = .20$, $p < .001$) and general family support ($\beta = .42$, $p < .001$) significantly contributed to the YPLWH self-esteem. Additionally, self-esteem significantly contributed to YPLWHs' positive relations ($\beta = .25$, $p < .001$), personal growth

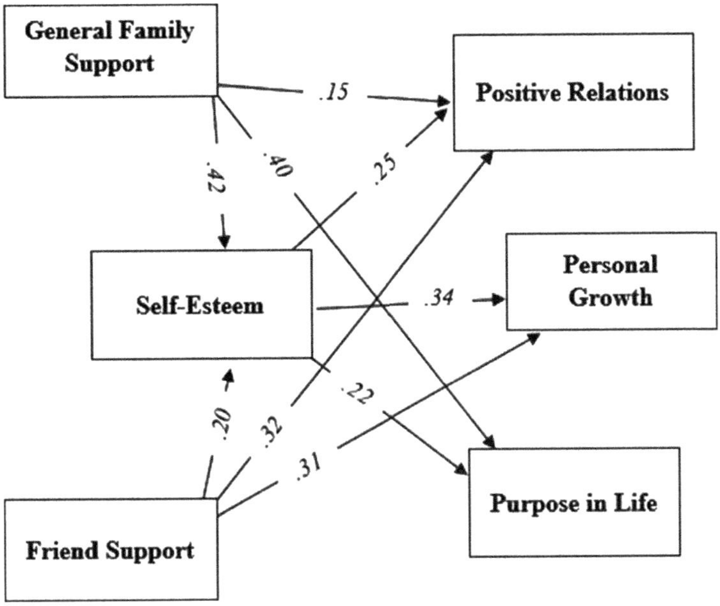

Fig. 8.2 Path model showing the mediation effect of self-esteem on the relation between social support and the indicators of psychological well-being *Note*: Only significant paths have been shown in the model (**$p < .05$)

Table 8.2 Direct and Indirect Effects of Family Support on the Indicators of Psychological Well-being

Path	Direct effect	Indirect effect	Total effect
General family support effect on purpose in life	.40**	.09**	.49**
General family support effect on personal growth	–	.14**	.14**
General family support effect on positive relations	.15**	.11**	.26**
Support from friends' effect on positive relations	.32**	.05	.37**
Support from friends effect on personal growth	.31**	.07**	.38**

**$p < .05$

($\beta = .34, p < .001$), and purpose in life ($\beta = .22, p < .001$). These results indicated that self-esteem mediated the relationship between the social support and psychological well-being of YPLWH.

We then estimated the indirect effects of social support on psychological well-being through self-esteem. As shown in Table 8.2, the total contribution of support from friends on personal growth ($\beta = .38, p < .001$) and positive relations ($\beta = .37$, $p < .001$) was mostly exerted directly ($\beta_{personal\ growth} = .31, p < .001$; $\beta_{positive\ relations} = .32, p < .001$) rather than indirectly ($\beta_{personal\ growth} = .07, p = .03$; $\beta_{positive\ relations} = .05, p = .07$). The total contributions of general family support on personal growth, purpose in life and positive relations were $\beta = .14$, $p < .001$; $\beta = .49$, $p < .001$; $\beta = .26, p < .001$ respectively. The contribution of general family support on purpose in life and positive relations were mostly exerted directly ($\beta_{purpose\ in\ Life} = .40, p < .001$; $\beta_{positive\ relations} = .15, p = .04$) rather than indirectly ($\beta_{purpose\ in\ life} = .09, p = .04$; $\beta_{positive\ relations} = .11, p = .02$) through self-esteem. The effect of general family support on personal growth was entirely indirect ($\beta = .14, p < .001$) through self-esteem. Overall, the variables in the model explained 31.5%, 35.7%, 30.1% and 30.2% of the variance in the respondents' self-esteem, positive relations, purpose in life and personal growth respectively.

8.4 Discussion

The aim of the present study was two-fold: (a) to examine the extent to which socio-demographic variables explain variations in the psychological well-being of YPLWH and (b) to test the mediation effect of self-esteem on the relationship between social support and psychological well-being of YPLWH. Significant differences were noted in the respondents' purpose in life with respect to their sex—with female students exhibiting a more purpose-oriented outlook on life as compared to their male counterparts. Additionally, the contribution of social support on the well-being of YPLWH was exerted both directly and indirectly through self-esteem.

Our finding of the higher levels of purpose in life among females agrees with results elsewhere (García-alandete et al., 2013; Lindfors et al., 2006; Ryff et al., 2003). Our results also dovetail with those of Hendricks-Ferguson (2006) who found that the purpose in life among female young people is higher compared to their male counterparts. A higher purpose in life is particularly important among YPLWH since it has been associated with lower suicidal ideation (Taliaferro et al., 2009), higher self-esteem and life satisfaction (Yakushko, 2005), longevity (Steptoe et al., 2014), and reduced risky behaviors such as drug-abuse (Lamis et al., 2014). Xi et al. (2018) have indicated that the high purpose in life among women compared to men could be explained by the altruistic behaviors and attitudes, and spirituality among women. In the Ugandan context, women and girls are regarded as caregivers in their respective homesteads and communities—which in turn may underpin higher altruistic and empathetic levels thereby enhancing their purpose and meaning in life (Xi et al., 2017).

Additionally, in line with the Sustainable Development Goal 5 ("To achieve gender equality and empower all women and girls"), the Ugandan government has enacted several laws and policies to reduce gender disparities in the different sectors. As such, there have been improvements in societal attitudes towards women and girls, a significant increase in the enrolment of girls in schools at all levels of learning, more representation of women in administrative and legislative positions, and an increase in active participation of women and girls in economic activities such as commercial agriculture and trade (United Nations Development Program, 2017).

Consequently, compared to the previous generations that were traditionally dominated by men, women and girls currently have a greater consciousness of their abilities, competencies, and potentials—which could have led to a higher purpose in life. As García-alandete et al. (2013) assert, "In conditions of cultural and educational equality, certain aspects of women related to their psychological well-being may emerge strongly, surpassing those in men' (p. 23). Therefore, given the women's emancipation programs currently undertaken by the Ugandan government, it may not be surprising that females had higher mean scores on purpose in life compared to the males in the present study.

Contrary to previous findings (e.g., Dalmida et al., 2013; Soulsby & Bennett, 2015), the present study has revealed that YPLWH had non-significant differences on the well-being indicators with respect to other demographic variables. Recently, in Uganda, there has been an increase in the provision of psychosocial support among YPLWH through the establishment of peer-clubs and whose membership does not depend on individuals' demographic variables such as socioeconomic status and level of education among others. Such clubs have significantly improved young people's access to ART services, increased adherence to medication, and increased social networking—all of which have improved the quality of life and well-being of YPLWH in Uganda. For example, in South-Western Uganda where data was collected, *Ariel Adherence Clubs* have been established by the Elizabeth Glaser Pediatric AIDS Foundation, and these have led to increased access and adherence to ART services, increased HIV and other sexually transmitted infections testing services, and increased access to counseling services among members as compared to non-members (Kagoro, 2018; World Health Organization, 2019). Such groups provide a platform to share challenges and collectively find solutions to such problems and, as such, help to cushion YPLWH against challenges such as being lonely, loss of their parents, and having little support in terms of their emotional well-being (Kagoro, 2018).

Additionally, as noted above, there has been an increase in access to ART services among YPLWH in Uganda. This means that nowadays, YPLWH can expect to live longer and enjoy a higher life expectancy just like those individuals who are not infected with HIV and have a high appreciation of what life has to offer (Mutabazi-Mwesigire et al., 2014). Perhaps, this could explain the reasons why there were few significant differences in the well-being of YPLWH with reference to socio-demographic variables.

The mediation effect of self-esteem on the relationship between social support and psychological well-being is well supported in previous studies carried out with the general population (Kong et al., 2013; Sung et al., 2012; Tian et al., 2013; Xi et al., 2017) and among people living with HIV (Lyons, 2010). General family support (but not support from friends) significantly contributed to the respondents' purpose in life. In the Ugandan context, care for young people infected with HIV is borne by their families (Osafo et al., 2017) especially by women such as mothers, sisters, aunts, and grandmothers—thereby making families a major source of emotional, social, and financial support to YPLWH in Uganda (Nabunya et al., 2020). For example, a study conducted to examine the facilitators of school attendance among young people aged 12–19 years living with HIV in Western Uganda, Kimera, Vindevogel, Kintu, et al. (2020) found that for some YPLWH, their sisters and mothers would help to pick ARV's from the hospitals, while they are doing examinations at school. Additionally, high family cohesion and communication are associated with high adherence to HIV medication among YPLWH in Uganda (Nabunya et al., 2020) which in turn leads to a higher purpose in life. Therefore, we advocate for strengthening the capacities of families that care for the YPLWH in Uganda through the provision of education about HIV-related issues, empowering them financially, and encouraging them to form groups for knowledge sharing (Russo, 2014).

Additionally, support from friends and family had a direct influence on self-esteem, which in turn influenced the well-being indicators. When they receive support from friends and family members, YPLWH are convinced that they are valued, catered for, and that other people can offer help in times of need—which enhances their self-worth and esteem (Tian et al., 2013). With high self-esteem, YPLWH can bear with the stigma, discrimination, anxieties, and other mental issues related to HIV thereby leading to better well-being. Therefore, it is important to strengthen social and family networks among YPLWH in Uganda for better psychological well-being (Kagoro, 2018). This could be done by establishing support associations or using social media platforms (such as WhatsApp and Facebook groups) where YPLWH can seek psychosocial guidance and help from others. Self-esteem can also be improved by encouraging YPLWH to exercise frequently, have positive thinking towards oneself, surrounding oneself with supportive friends and persons who trigger positive thinking, use of verbal praises, and use of self-affirmation techniques (Johnson, 2016).

Health workers could also design motivating psychosocial and self-esteem support sessions at hospitals and clinics where YPLWH in Uganda go for treatment. Ashaba et al. (2018) study reported that most YPLWH in Uganda only report to hospitals to collect their medicines and/or for medical check-ups without bothering to attend the organized sessions on psychological support, perhaps due to fear and low self-esteem. This reduces possibilities and opportunities for networking with other YPLWH and/or having in-depth interactions with the health workers. Yet within these designed support sessions, health workers could provide incentives like meal plans, buddies (in the buddy program) that can encourage the YPLWH to look forward to attending these sessions and also provide a platform for further networking.

The following limitations should be taken into consideration when interpreting the above findings. Firstly, self-report questionnaires were used in data collection which are subject to social desirability—a situation where one responds to the items in such a way as to appear good. This could affect the validity of the study findings. Secondly, the study employed a cross-sectional research design; hence causal inferences cannot be drawn from the findings especially those that involve examination of the structural relationships between the study variables. Lastly, the study employed quantitative methods of which the results are limited to the provision of numerical descriptions rather than detailed narratives of respondents' experiences and perceptions; hence future studies could employ a mixed-methods approach.

8.5 Conclusion

As far as we are aware, this study is a first attempt to examine the relations between demographic variables, self-esteem, social support, and the well-being of YPLWH in the Ugandan context, and as such, provides important findings that could potentially contribute to further research and practice among YPLWH in Uganda and on the African continent as a whole. First, significant gender differences in the respondents' purpose in life were noted. Females reported higher levels of purpose in life compared to the males. Hence, more attention and guidance should be directed towards the male gender especially concerning their perceptions about their purpose in life. Second, as predicted, the relationship between perceived social support and the psychological well-being of YPLWH was partially mediated by self-esteem. This suggests the need to consider strengthening and including self-esteem interventions (in addition to providing social support groups) in the care provided to the YPLWH as a means of improving their psychological well-being. There is need to further explore other variables related to the well-being of YPLWH to aid in designing more comprehensive models of their psychological well-being. Additionally, further studies that employ longitudinal and mixed-methods approaches should be undertaken for better insights into the well-being aspects of YPLWH in the Ugandan context. It is important that general well-being is taken as a priority in the health care of YPLWH for better health outcomes, good mental health, high medical adherence, and improving their longevity.

References

Abebe, H., Shumet, S., Nassir, Z., Agidew, M., & Abebaw, D. (2019). Prevalence of depressive symptoms and associated factors among HIV-positive youth attending ART follow-up in Addis Ababa, Ethiopia. *AIDS Research and Treatment, 2019*, 1–7. https://doi.org/10.1155/2019/4610458

Asante, K. O. (2012). Social support and the psychological well-being of people living with HIV/AIDS in Ghana. *African Journal of Psychiatry, 15*(5), 340–345.

Ashaba, S., Cooper-Vince, C., Maling, E. C., Rukundo, S., Akena, G. Z., & D., & Tsai, A. C. (2018). Internalized HIV stigma, bullying, major depressive disorder, and high-risk suicidality among HIV-positive adolescents in rural Uganda. *Global Mental Health, 5*, 1–10.

Ashaba, S., Cooper-Vince, E. C., Vořechovská, D., Rukundo, Z. G., Maling, S., Akena, D., & Tsai, C. A. (2019). Community beliefs, HIV stigma, and depression among adolescents living with HIV in rural Uganda. *African Journal of AIDS Research, 18*, 169–180. https://doi.org/10.2989/16085906.2019.1637912

Atwine, B., Cantor-Graae, E., & Bajunirwe, F. (2005). Psychological distress among AIDS orphans in rural Uganda. *Social Science & Medicine, 61*(3), 555–564.

Avert. (2020). *Young people, HIV and AIDS*. Retrieved from https://www.avert.org/professionals/hiv-social-issues/key-affected-populations/young-people

Bosson, J. K., Swann, W. B., & Pennebaker, J. W. (2000). Stalking the perfect measure of implicit self-esteem: The blind men and the elephant revisited? *Journal of Personality and Social Psychology, 79*(4), 631–643.

Cederfjäll, C., Langius-Eklöf, A., Lidman, K., & Wredling, R. (2001). Gender differences in perceived health-related quality of life among patients with HIV infection. *AIDS Patient Care and STDs, 15*, 31–39. https://doi.org/10.1089/108729101460083

Chernaskey, R. (2017). *How self-esteem affects well-being*. Retrieved from https://www.operationwarm.org/blog/how-self-esteem-affects-well-being/

Cohen, S., Gottlieb, B. H., & Underwood, L. G. (2000). Social relationships and health. In S. Cohen, L. G. Underwood, & B. H. Gottlieb (Eds.), *Social support measurement and intervention: A guide for health and social scientists* (pp. 3–25). Oxford University Press.

Dalmida, S. G., Koenig, H. G., Holstad, M. M., & Wirani, M. M. (2013). The psychological well-being of people living with HIV/AIDS and the role of religious coping and social support. *The International Journal of Psychiatry in Medicine, 46*(1), 57–83.

Damulira, C., Mukasa, M. N., Byansi, W., Nabunya, P., Kivumbi, A., Namatovu, P., Namuwonge, F., Dvalishvili, D., Bahar, O. S., & Ssewamala, F. M. (2019). Examining the relationship of social support and family cohesion on ART adherence among HIV-positive adolescents in southern Uganda: Baseline findings. *Vulnerable Children & Youth Studies, 14*(2), 181–190.

De Nutte, L., Okello, J., & Derluyn, I. (2015). Social relationships and social support among post-war youth in northern Uganda. *International Journal of Psychology, 52*(4), 291–299.

Diener, E., & Diener, M. (1995). Cross-cultural correlates of life-satisfaction and self-esteem. *Journal of Personality and Social Psychology, 68*(4), 653–663.

Flannelly, T., & Inouye, J. (2001). Relationships of religion, health status, and socioeconomic status to the quality of life of individuals who are HIV positive. *Issues in Mental Health Nursing, 22*(3), 253–272.

Fleishman, J. A., Sherbourne, C. D., Crystal, S., Collins, R. L., Marshall, G. N., Kelly, M., Bozzette, S. A., Shapiro, M. F., & Hays, R. D. (2000). Coping, conflictual social interactions, social support, and mood among HIV-infected persons. HCSUS consortium. *American Journal of Community Psychology, 28*(4), 421–453.

Funck-Brentano, I., Dalban, C., Veber, F., Quartier, P., Hefez, S., Costagliola, D., & Blanche, S. (2005). Evaluation of a peer support group therapy for HIV-infected adolescents. *AIDS, 19*(14), 1501–1508.

Gao, J., & McLellan, R. (2018). Using Ryff's scales of psychological well-being in adolescents in mainland China. *BMC Psychology, 6*(17), 1–8.

García-alandete, J., Soucase, L. B., Sellés, N. P., & Martínez, E. R. (2013). Predictive role of meaning in life on psychological well-being and gender-specific differences. *Acta Colombiana de Psicología, 16*(1), 17–24.

Geiser, C. (2013). *Data analysis with Mplus*. The Guilford Press.

Govindasamy, D., Seeley, J., Olaru, I. D., Wiyeh, A., Mathews, C., & Ferrari, C. (2020). Informing the measurement of well-being among young people living with HIV in sub-Saharan Africa for policy evaluations: A mixed-methods systematic review. *Health and Quality of Life Outcomes, 18*, 1–34. https://doi.org/10.1186/s12955-020-01352-w

Hendricks-Ferguson, V. (2006). Relationships of age and gender to hope and spiritual well-being among adolescents with cancer. *Journal of Pediatric Oncology Nursing, 23*(4), 189–199.

Hu, L., & Bentler, P. M. (1999). Cut-off criteria for fit indexes in covariance structure analysis: Conventional criteria versus new alternatives. *Structural Equation Modeling, 6*(1), 1–55.

Huurre, T. (2000). *Psychosocial development and social support among adolescents with visual impairment (doctoral dissertation)*. University of Tampere. Retrieved from https://trepo.tuni.fi/bitstream/handle/10024/67015/951-44-4842-1.pdf?sequence=1&isAllowed=y

Johnson, J. (2016). *What are the techniques to enhance self-esteem?* Retrieved from https://www.psychreg.org/techniques-to-enhance-self-esteem/

Kagoro, B. (2018). *Ariel club restores hope for HIV positive youth in Uganda*. Retrieved from https://www.usaid.gov/uganda/news/ariel-club-restores-hope-hiv-positive-youth-uganda

Kalomo, E. N. (2018). Associations between HIV-related stigma, self-esteem, social support, and depressive symptoms in Namibia. *Aging & Mental Health, 22*(12), 1570–1576.

Kamau, J. W., Kuria, W., Mathai, M., Atwoli, L., & Kangethe, R. (2012). Psychiatric morbidity among HIV-infected children and adolescents in a resource-poor Kenyan urban community. *AIDS Care, 24*(7), 836–842.

Keyes, C. L. M., & Waterman, M. B. (2003). Dimensions of well-being and mental health in adulthood. In M. C. Bornstein, L. Davidson, C. L. M. Keyes, & K. A. Moore (Eds.), *Well-being: Positive development across the life course* (pp. 477–497). Laurence Erlbaum Associates.

Khumalo, I. P., Temane, Q. M., & Wissing, M. P. (2012). Socio-demographic variables, general psychological well-being and the mental health continuum in an African context. *Social Indicators Research, 105*, 419–442. https://doi.org/10.1007/s11205-010-9777-2

Kidman, R., & Violari, A. (2018). Dating violence against HIV-infected youth in South Africa: Associations with sexual risk behavior, medication adherence, and mental health. *Journal of Acquired Immune Deficiency Syndromes, 77*(1), 64–71.

Kihumuro, R. B., Muganzi, D. J., Wandira, E. G., Alinaiswe, R., Nanyunja, J. J., Kugumisiriza, R., Alele, P. E., & Mubangizi, V. (2021). Influence of boarding secondary school environments on HIV positive students in South-Western Uganda. *BMC Public Health, 21*, 1–11. https://doi.org/10.1186/s12889-021-10380-0

Kim, M. H., Mazenga, A. C., Yu, X., Devandra, A., Nguyen, C., Ahmed, S., Kazembe, P. N., & Sharp, C. (2015). Factors associated with depression among adolescents living with HIV in Malawi. *BMC Psychiatry, 15*, 1–12. https://doi.org/10.1186/s12888-015-0649-9

Kimera, E., Vindevogel, S., Rubaihayo, J., Reynaert, D., De Maeyer, J., Engelen, A. M., & Bilsen, J. (2019). Youth living with HIV/AIDS in secondary schools: Perspectives of peer educators and patron teachers in Western Uganda on stressors and supports. *Journal of Social Aspects of HIV/AIDS, 16*, 51–61. https://doi.org/10.1080/17290376.2019.1626760

Kimera, E., Vindevogel, S., Kintu, M. J., Rubaihayo, J., De Maeyer, J., Reynaert, D., Engelen, A.-M., Nuwaha, F., & Bilsen, J. (2020). Experiences and perceptions of youth living with HIV in Western Uganda on school attendance: Barriers and facilitators. *BMC Public Health, 20*, 1–12. https://doi.org/10.1186/s12889-020-8198-7

Kimera, E., Vindevogel, S., Reynaert, D., Justice, K. M., Rubaihayo, J., De Maeyer, J., Engelen, A.-M., Musanje, K., & Bilsen, J. (2020). Experiences and effects of HIV-related stigma among youth living with HIV/AIDS in Western Uganda: A photovoice study. *PLoS One, 15*, 1–21. https://doi.org/10.1371/journal.pone.0232359

Kline, R. B. (2005). *Principles and practice of structural equation modeling*. Guilford.

Kong, F., Zhao, J., & You, X. (2013). Self-esteem as mediator and moderator of the relationship between social support and subjective well-being among Chinese university students. *Social Indicators Research, 112*, 151–161. https://doi.org/10.1007/s11205-012-0044-6

Krejcie, R. V., & Morgan, D. W. (1970). Determining sample size for research activities. *Educational and Psychological Measurement, 30*(3), 607–610.

Lam, P. K., Naar-King, S., & Wright, K. (2007). Social support and disclosure as predictors of mental health in HIV-positive youth. *AIDS Patient Care and STDs, 21*, 20–29. https://doi.org/10.1089/apc.2006.005

Lamis, D. A., West, L. M., Mehta, N., Lisco, C., Tarantino, N., Wilson, C., & Kaslow, N. J. (2014). Existential well-being, drug abuse, and parenting stress in African American women. *International Journal of Mental Health and Addiction, 12*(5), 686–699.

Lee, S. J., Detels, R., Rotheram-Borus, M. J., Duan, N., & Lord, L. (2007). Depression and social support among HIV-affected adolescents. *AIDS Patient Care and STDs, 21*(6), 409–417.

Leserman, J. (2008). Role of depression, stress, and trauma in HIV disease progression. *Psychosomatic Medicine, 70*(5), 539–545.

Lindfors, P., Berntsson, L., & Lundberg, U. (2006). Factor structure of Ryff's psychological well-being scales in Swedish female and male white-collar workers. *Personality and Individual Differences, 40*(6), 1213–1222.

Liping, M., Peng, X., Haijiang, L., Lahong, J., & Fan, L. (2015). Quality of life of people living with HIV/AIDS: A cross-sectional study in Zhejiang Province, China. *PLoS One, 10*(8), 1–14.

Lyons, S. J. (2010). *The role of social support and psychological resources in depression in people living with HIV/AIDS: Examining the mediating role of mastery and self-esteem* (Doctoral thesis). University of Toronto. Retrieved from https://tspace.library.utoronto.ca/bitstream/1807/24230/6/Lyons_Sarah_J_201003_MA_thesis.pdf

Manhas, C. (2014). Self-esteem and quality of life of people living with HIV/AIDS. *Journal of Health Psychology, 19*, 1471–1479. https://doi.org/10.1177/1359105313493812

Mavandadi, S., Zanjani, F., Ten Have, T. R., & Oslin, D. W. (2009). Psychological well-being among individuals aging with HIV: The value of social relationships. *Journal of Acquired Immune Deficiency Syndrome, 51*(1), 91–98.

Mavhu, W., Berwick, J., Chirawu, P., Makamba, M., Copas, A., Dirawo, J., Willis, N., Araya, R., Abas, M. A., Corbett, E. L., Mungofa, S., Laver, S. M., & Cowan, F. M. (2013). Enhancing psychosocial support for HIV positive adolescents in Harare, Zimbabwe. *PLoS One, 8*(7), 1–9.

Mellins, C. A., Brackis-Cott, E., Dolezal, C., & Abrams, E. J. (2006). Psychiatric disorders in youth with perinatally acquired human immunodeficiency virus infection. *Pediatric Infectious Disease Journal, 25*(5), 432–437.

Menon, A., Glazebrook, C., Campain, N., & Ngoma, M. (2007). Mental health and disclosure of HIV status in Zambian adolescents with HIV infection: Implications for peer-support programs. *Journal of Acquired Immune Deficiency Syndrome, 46*(3), 349–354.

Mutabazi-Mwesigire, D., Seeley, J., Martin, F., & Katamba, A. (2014). Perceptions of quality of life among Ugandan patients living with HIV: A qualitative study. *BMC Public Health, 14*, 1–10. https://doi.org/10.1186/1471-2458-14-343

Muthén, L. K., & Muthén, B. O. (1998–2015). *Mplus user's guide (version 7.4)*. Muthén & Muthén.

Nabunya, P., Bahar, O. S., Chen, B., Dvalishvili, D., Damulira, C., & Ssewamala, F. M. (2020). The role of family factors in antiretroviral therapy (ART) adherence self-efficacy among HIV-infected adolescents in southern Uganda. *BMC Public Health, 20*, 1–9. https://doi.org/10.1186/s12889-020-8361-1

Neff, J. A., Amodei, N., Valescu, S., & Pomeroy, E. C. (2003). Psychological adaptation and distress among HIV-positive Latina women: Adaptation to HIV in a Mexican American cultural context. *Social Work in Health Care, 37*(3), 55–74.

Okawa, S., Kabaghe, S. M., Mwiya, M., Kikuchi, K., Jimba, M., Kankasa, C., & Ishikawa, N. (2018). Psychological well-being and adherence to antiretroviral therapy among adolescents living with HIV in Zambia. *AIDS Care: Psychological and Socio-medical Aspects of AIDS/HIV, 30*(5), 634–642.

Orth, U., Robins, R. W., & Meier, L. L. (2009). Disentangling the effects of low self-esteem and stressful events on depression: Findings from three longitudinal studies. *Journal of Personality and Social Psychology, 97*(2), 307–321.

Osafo, J., Knizek, B. L., Mugisha, J., & Kinyanda, E. (2017). The experiences of caregivers of children living with HIV and AIDS in Uganda: A qualitative study. *Globalization and Health, 13*, 1–13. https://doi.org/10.1186/s12992-017-0294-9

Pedhazur, J. (1982). *Multiple regression in behavioral research: Explanation and prediction*. Holt, Rinehart, & Winston.

Persson, L., Gullberg, B., Hanson, B. S., Moestrup, T., & Ostergren, P. O. (1994). HIV infection: Social network, social support, and CD4 lymphocyte values in infected homosexual men in Malmö, Sweden. *Journal of Epidemiology & Community Health, 48*(6), 580–585.

Ramiro, M. T., Teva, I., Bermúdez, M. P., & Buela-Casal, G. (2013). Social support, self-esteem and depression: Relationship with risk for sexually transmitted infections/HIV transmission. *International Journal of Clinical and Health Psychology, 13*(3), 181–188.

Rosenberg, M. (1985). Self-concept and psychological well-being in adolescence. In R. L. Leahy (Ed.), *The development of the self* (pp. 205–246). Academic.

Russo, S. (2014). *Family support groups foster hope in Uganda*. Retrieved from https://www.pedaids.org/2014/12/24/20-family-support-groups-foster-hope-in-uganda/

Ryff, C. D. (1989). Happiness is everything, or is it? Explorations on the meaning of psychological well-being. *Journal of Personality and Social Psychology, 57*(6), 1069–1081.

Ryff, C. D., Keyes, C. L., & Hughes, D. L. (2003). Status inequalities, perceived discrimination, and eudaimonic well-being: Do the challenges of minority life hone purpose and growth? *Journal of Health & Social Behaviour, 44*(3), 275–291.

Schrimshaw, E. W., & Siegel, K. (2003). Perceived barriers to social support from family and friends among older adults with HIV/AIDS. *Journal of Health Psychology, 8*(6), 738–752.

Sengendo, J., & Nambi, J. (1997). The psychological effect of orphanhood: A study of orphans in Rakai district. *Health Transition Review, 7*(Suppl), 105–124.

Soulsby, L. K., & Bennett, K. M. (2015). Marriage and psychological well-being: The role of social support. *Psychology, 6*, 1349–1359. https://doi.org/10.4236/psych.2015.611132

Springer, K. W., & Hauser, R. M. (2006). An assessment of the construct validity of Ryff's scales of psychological well-being: Method, mode, and measurement effects. *Social Science Research, 35*(4), 1080–1102.

Ssali, S. N., Atuyambe, L., Tumwine, C., Segujja, E., Nekesa, N., Nannungi, A., Ryan, G., & Wagner, G. (2010). Reasons for disclosure of HIV status by people living with HIV/AIDS and in HIV care in Uganda: An exploratory study. *AIDS Patient Care and STDs, 24*(10), 675–681.

Steptoe, A., Deaton, A., & Stone, A. A. (2014). Subjective well-being, health, and aging. *Lancet, 385*, 640–648. https://doi.org/10.1016/S0140-6736(13)61489-0

Sung, H. L., Ok, S. K., & Mi, Y. Y. (2012). The impact of social support on self-esteem and depression of adolescents in institutions. *Asia-Pacific Journal of Business Venturing and Entrepreneurship, 7*(2), 207–214.

Symister, S., & Friend, F. (2003). The influence of social support and problematic support on optimism and depression in chronic illness: A prospective study evaluating self-esteem as a mediator. *Health Psychology, 22*(2), 123–129.

Taliaferro, L. A., Rienzo, B. A., Pigg, M. R., Miller, D. M., & Dodd, V. J. (2009). Spiritual well-being and suicidal ideation among college students. *Journal of American College Health, 58*(1), 83–90.

Taylor, S. E. (2007). Social support. In H. S. Friedman & R. C. Silver (Eds.), *Foundations of health psychology* (pp. 145–171). Oxford University Press.

The Joint United Nations Program on HIV/AIDS. (2019). *UNAIDS data 2019*. Retrieved from https://www.unaids.org/sites/default/files/media_asset/2019-UNAIDS-data_en.pdf

Tian, L., Liu, B., Huang, S., & Huebner, E. S. (2013). Perceived social support and school well-being among Chinese early and middle adolescents: The mediational role of self-esteem. *Social Indicators Research, 113*, 991–1008. https://doi.org/10.1007/s11205-012-0123-8

Uganda AIDS Commission (UAC). (2019). *Presidential fast-track initiative on ending HIV and AIDS in Uganda: Fact sheet 2019*. Retrieved from https://uac.go.ug/sites/default/files/2019%20Uganda%20Fact%20Sheet_0.pdf

United Nations Development Programme. (2017). *Annual report, 2017*. Retrieved from https://annualreport.undp.org/2017/

United Nations International Children's Emergency Fund. (2020). *Adolescent HIV prevention*. Retrieved from https://data.unicef.org/topic/hivaids/adolescents-young-people/

Vorster, H. H., Venter, C. S., Kruger, H. S., Kruger, A., Malan, N. T., de Ridder, J. H., Veldman, F. J., Steyn, H. S., Margetts, B. M., & Maclntyre, U. (2000). The impact of urbanization on the physical, physiological and mental health of Africans in the north West province of South Africa: The THUSA study. *South African Journal of Science, 96*, 505–514.

Vyavaharkar, M., Moneyham, L., Corwin, S., Saunders, R., Annang, L., & Tavakoli, A. (2009). Relationships between stigma, social support, and depression in HIV-infected African American women living in the rural southeastern United States. *Journal of Association for Nurses in AIDS Care, 21*(2), 144–152.

Walakira, E. J., Ddumba-Nyanzi, I., & Kaawa-Mafigiri, D. (2014). HIV and AIDS and its impact on child well-being. In A. Ben-Arieh, F. Casas, I. Frønes, & J. E. Korbin (Eds.), *Handbook of child*

well-being: Theories, methods and policies in global perspective (pp. 2355–2377). Springer. https://doi.org/10.1007/978-90-481-9063-8
Walker, J. G., Jackson, H. J., & Littlejohn, G. (2004). Models of adjustment to chronic illness: Using the example of rheumatoid arthritis. *Clinical Psychology Review, 24*(4), 461–488.
Wang, J., & Wang, X. (2012). *Structural equation modeling: Applications using Mplus*. Wiley.
Wilson, P. A., Moore, S. T., Rubin, D. S., & Bartels, P. K. (1990). Informal caregivers of the chronically ill and their social support: A pilot study. *Journal of Gerontological Social Work, 15*, 155–170. https://doi.org/10.1300/J083v15n01_14
World Health Organization. (2019). *Adolescent-friendly health services for adolescents living with HIV: From theory to practice*. Retrieved from https://apps.who.int/iris/bitstream/handle/10665/329993/WHO-CDS-HIV-19.39-eng.pdf?sequence=1&isAllowed=y
Worthington, C., & Krentz, H. B. (2005). Socio-economic factors and health-related quality of life in adults living with HIV. *International Journal of STD & AIDS, 16*(9), 608–614.
Xi, X., Wang, Y., & Jia, B. (2017). The effect of social support on subjective well-being: Mediator roles of self-esteem and self-efficacy. *Advances in Social Science, Education and Humanities Research, 121*, 493–505. https://doi.org/10.2991/ichssr-17.2017.101
Xi, J., Lee, M. T., Carter, J. R., & Delgado, D. (2018). Gender differences in purpose in life: The mediation effect of altruism. *Journal of Humanistic Psychology*. https://doi.org/10.1177/0022167818777658
Xiao, Y., Lin, C., Li, L., & Ji, G. (2019). Individual and family level factors associated with physical and mental health-related quality of life among people living with HIV in rural China. *BMC Public Health, 19*, 1–7. https://doi.org/10.1186/s12889-018-6352-2
Yakushko, O. (2005). Influence of social support, existential well-being, and stress over sexual orientation on self-esteem of gay, lesbian, and bisexual individuals. *International Journal for the Advancement of Counseling, 27*, 131–143. https://doi.org/10.1007/s10447-005-2259-6
Zhang, L., & Leung, J. (2002). Moderating effects of gender and age on the relationship between self-esteem and life satisfaction in mainland Chinese. *International Journal of Psychology, 37*, 83–91. https://doi.org/10.1080/00207560143000252
Zimet, G. D., Dahlem, N. W., Zimet, S. G., & Farley, G. K. (1988). The multidimensional scale of perceived social support. *Journal of Personality Assessment, 52*(1), 30–41.

Chapter 9
Exploring Protective Resources that Facilitate Positive Outcomes among Married Girls in the Northern Region of Ghana

Hajara Baba, Joana Salifu Yendork, and Samuel Atindanbila

Abstract Child marriage has been identified as a violation of human rights and an obstacle to promoting the development goals concerning gender, health and education. All these impacts undermine the development of the girl child. Despite the potential for negative outcomes, the presence of intrinsic and extrinsic resources can buffer the adverse effects (e.g., psychological, physical and economic impact) of early marriage. This study employed a qualitative exploratory, descriptive design to explore and describe protective resources utilised by married girls in the Northern region of Ghana to cope with the challenges in their marriage and to promote positive outcomes. Using semi-structured interviews, data was collected from 21 married girls who were aged between 12 and 19 years. Findings, from a thematic analysis of data, showed that intrinsic resources that promoted positive outcomes included possession of resilience attitudes, the use of help-seeking and active coping, and in some instances avoidance coping for problems they perceived as unsolvable. Extrinsic resources included interpersonal support networks, however, participants reported limited access to community and NGO support, which were also identified as protective resources. Policy makers and clinicians should consider a social justice approach in evaluating and recommending protective resources to girls in early marriages when working to promote their well-being. In so doing, attention should be placed on making external support systems accessible to married girls.

Keywords Child marriage · Married girls · Positive outcomes · Intrinsic and extrinsic resources · Ghana

---

H. Baba · J. S. Yendork (✉) · S. Atindanbila
Department of Psychology, University of Ghana, Accra, Ghana
e-mail: jyendork@ug.edu.gh

L. Schutte et al. (eds.), *Embracing Well-Being in Diverse African Contexts: Research Perspectives*, Cross-Cultural Advancements in Positive Psychology 16,
https://doi.org/10.1007/978-3-030-85924-4_9

9.1 Introduction

Psychological research and practice with adolescents has traditionally focused on risks and pathologies associated with the unpleasant effects of adverse conditions, as this stage is constantly marked by many developmental changes coupled with stress and hardship (Viejo et al., 2018). Alternatively, some researchers have argued that these numerous changes in adolescence represent a form of plasticity, essential in the human development process (Lerner, 1984). This demonstrates an underlying strength which is characterised by the period of adolescence (Lerner, 2009). Therefore, this strength is worth exploring especially within the context of child marriage, which is usually seen as involving several risk factors that can elicit negative health and well-being outcomes (Svanemyr et al., 2015).

As defined by the United Nations Children's Emergency Fund (UNICEF, 2015), child marriage is a girl or boy getting married before the age of 18 years, which is internationally recognised as a violation of human rights. Evidence points to an array of risk factors among married girls (Svanemyr et al., 2015). For instance, young married girls are exposed to sexually transmitted infections (UNICEF, 2013), poor reproductive health outcomes (Godha et al., 2013; Sawant & Venkat, 2013), poor psychological well-being (Ahmed et al., 2013; Duflo, 2011) and inadequate formal education (Klugman et al., 2014; Nguyen & Wodon, 2015) which limits their prospects for employment (Parsons et al., 2015).

Despite the potential for these negative outcomes, research has established an association among the processes of plasticity, adaptive developmental regulation and thriving, suggesting an inherent strength possessed by young people that may be tapped into, to promote thriving throughout the adolescence years (Geldhof et al., 2013). Similarly, studies have shown that many children who experience stress and adversity in life are able to thrive in spite of their severe challenges (Alvord & Grados, 2005; Brooks, 2006; Masten, 2001, 2007). These children have been identified as resilient because they benefit from certain protective resources that enable them to overcome adverse conditions (Zolkoski & Bullock, 2012). These protective resources could be intrinsically found within an individual's personal strengths such as resilience attitudes (Wingo et al., 2010; Youssef et al., 2016); self-efficacy, identified as a useful personal resource in moderating the effects of stress among maltreated children (Day & Kearney, 2016); locus of control (Culpin et al., 2015); and emotional regulation (Schweizer et al., 2016). Furthermore, the individual's sense of belonging to social networks (Bowlby, 1988), as well as having a sense of purpose (Hamby et al., 2018) have been shown to enhance subjective well-being amidst childhood adversity. In the Ghanaian context, Wilson and Somhlaba (2016) found that adolescents in adversity draw a sense of hope from family and religion while realising their set goals. Also a positive self-image emerged as a determinant of positive well-being. Furthermore, the nature of coping strategies adopted by adolescents that could enhance well-being include active coping (Gonzales et al., 2001), help-seeking (Gould et al., 2004), and planning (Aldridge & Roesch, 2008). On the other hand, adolescents' use of self-blame and behavioural disengagement (Horwitz et al., 2011), as well as substance use (Turner et al., 2005) among other avoidance strategies have been found to predict negative outcomes in some instances.

Conversely, extrinsic resources involve strengths that could be tapped into within the environment such as social relationships (Black & Ford-Gilboe, 2004; Walsh, 2003) and external support systems such as social facilities and community support systems (Smokowski et al., 2000). With regard to social support, the family performs a critical role in the household by promoting the psychological well-being of adolescents (Abrinkova et al., 2019; Hoagwood et al., 2010; Wilson & Somhlaba, 2016). Similarly, peers are important sources of support for positive adolescent well-being (Smokowski et al., 2014; Wilson & Somhlaba, 2016). Support from adult figures present in the adolescent's immediate environments (such as home, school, and neighbourhood) may also strengthen the positive impact of social support on their psychological well-being (Capp et al., 2016; Vermuelen & Greeff, 2015).

It has been recognised that some particular groups may be more susceptible to certain risks due to their social identities. Therefore, focusing on the perspectives of young people regarding their own experiences of challenges may increase our understanding of differences in individual resilience (Wright & Masten, 2005). In addition, certain factors such as social changes, the nature of individual's relationship with other people in the society and cultural practices have all been identified as important contextual factors in the analysis of resilience (Bottrell, 2009). With emphasis on context in the development of resilience, social support plays a key role in this regard. For the purpose of this study, married girls' utilisation of protective resources (intrinsic and extrinsic) and coping strategies were explored and described since adaptive regulations increase the potential for healthy and positive outcomes (Geldhof et al., 2013).

In Ghana, 1 in 5 girls married before the age of 18, which translates to 21% of Ghanaian girls being affected (Ghana Statistical Service [GSS], Ghana Health Service [GHS], & The DHS Program [DHS], 2015). Despite the important insights from research (Sarfo et al., 2020) on the scope and range of interventions to address this problem (e.g., enactment of community bylaws, youth and economic empowerment, community education, enforcement of educational policies, role modelling and recruitment, skills development, school reintegration), a great deal of the intervention measures fall short of practicability and are not usually incorporated into larger government or private sector initiatives to promote economic and social change. This has been responsible for the short-term nature of these intervention programmes (Gupta et al., 2008). In order to reduce the incidence of early marriages, a large number of these interventions are tailored towards education to bring about change in societal norms and address poverty and lack of economic opportunities in the local contexts (McCleary-Sills et al., 2015). Apparently, these programmes explicitly emphasise the need for investments in unmarried girls so as to prevent them from going into early marriages (Greene, 2014). However, there is growing evidence that suggest that mitigating the impact of child marriages on victims is equally an important contributing factor to curbing the menace (Edmeades et al., 2016). This makes it compelling to explore the protective resources that are being used by married girls to improve their well-being. Also, it stands to reason that resources that enable children to overcome adverse effects of risks vary by the kind of population studied, the context and outcome (Fergus & Zimmerman, 2005). Hence, introducing protective factors in child marriage contexts may provide effective interventions for change especially among the disadvantaged girls who find themselves in early marriages.

This study adopts a social justice approach to resilience (Hart et al., 2016) by recognising the role of both internal and external resources in the married girls' lives that could play a significant role in mitigating the effects of adversity in their marriages. This is an expansion of the concept of resilience from the micro level of the individual to incorporate meso-level structures (Hart et al., 2016) by exploring the nature of support from the family, local community and external organisations. Hence both intrinsic and extrinsic protective resources were explored and described in the study. The study had two objectives which were to: (1) Explore the intrinsic and extrinsic protective resources used by married girls and (2) Describe how these resources were utilised by married girls to manage challenges and encounter positive outcomes in their marriages.

9.2 Methodology

9.2.1 Research Design

The findings reported in the present paper were part of a broader mixed-method research that was carried out in Northern Ghana. In the broader research, both qualitative and quantitative methods were used to explore the nature of challenges that married girls experienced in their marriages and the kind of protective resources that they used to mitigate the effects of their challenges. The qualitative part, which is reported in the present paper, used a qualitative exploratory, descriptive design. This approach enabled us to explore and describe protective resources utilised by married girls to manage challenges and enhance positive outcomes in their marriages. Data was collected using a semi-structured interview guide.

9.2.2 Research Settings and Socio-Cultural Context

The study was conducted in the Northern region of Ghana, which according to the Ghana Demographic Health Survey in 2014 (GSS, GHS, & DHS, 2015) was shown to have recorded the highest frequency of child marriage practices. This justifies the Northern region as an appropriate context to conduct an exploratory study on child marriage. Data was collected specifically in the Sagnarigu, Tolon and Mion districts. Communities in these districts were chosen because high rates of child marriages have been recorded in there (Naatogmah, 2016).

The Dagomba ethnic group is the dominant ethnic group in the research contexts and the Dagbani language is the widely spoken language in the communities (Ghana Statistical Service, 2010). The Dagomba people practice the patriarchal system where the male is the head and controls the family and inheritance. Due to this male dominance, women are usually marginalized and side-lined when it comes to decision making (Bawah et al., 1999; Takyi & Dodoo, 2005). Moreover, the people of the Dagomba ethnic group observe strict gender role ideologies where the role of women is restricted to the kitchen and childbearing (Bawah et al., 1999). Owing to these strict gender roles, most girls lack access to educational opportunities. Girls who are able to attend school often drop out early to be married off because of poverty (Alhassan, 2013), religious reasons and parents' attempt to prevent girls' involvement in premarital sexual relations (Alhassan, 2013; Awusabo-Asare et al., 2004; Osafo et al., 2014). Early marriages are also encouraged because of cultural norms and the value that is placed on marriage and childbearing by the society (Addai et al., 2015; Alhassan, 2013).

In the research contexts, marriage is considered a prestigious institution and an indicator of social recognition and respect by both men and women. The respect and recognition accorded married individuals result from the high value that the society place on chastity and childbearing. Again, the male dominance enables men to practice polygamy and have as many children as they want, which they use to secure respect and higher social status in the society. On the other hand, women associate themselves with their husbands' identities and bear children to be recognised and respected in the society (Addai et al., 2015; Adinkrah, 2012; Tsekpo et al., 2016).

According to the Dagomba tradition, menarche serves as a yardstick to measure maturity among young girls (Ampofo, 2001) because it is believed that girls can bear children at that stage. Girls are often groomed purposefully for marriage; hence, they are trained from childhood to assume their future roles as housekeepers (Ampofo, 2001). However, boys are allowed to attend school, learn a trade or work (Ampofo, 2001). Islam is the predominant religion in Northern Ghana, which also dominates some aspects of their culture. This dominance is noticeable in their festivals and dress codes (Abdul-Hamid, 2010).

9.2.3 Participants

Twenty-one married girls were purposively sampled and in some cases, snowballing was used due to the restrictedness of the sample. Participants who met the following inclusion criteria were included in the study; (1) if they were female and lived in the research communities, (2) if they married before age 18 years, and (3) if they were willing to participate in the study. Twenty-one participants were considered enough because no new information was being obtained from the participants (Grady, 1998; Saunders et al., 2018). Married girls were entirely made up of school drop-outs within the ages of 12 and 19 years. There were four of them who had no formal education, six dropped out at primary school, eight dropped out at junior high school and three dropped out at senior high school. Participants were mainly Muslim with 16 out of 21 engaged in no economic activity while the rest were engaged in menial jobs.

9.2.4 Procedure

Before data collection, prior visits were carried out by the first author to the communities under study. The aim of this visit was to establish rapport with people of the communities and also to make arrangement for the recruitment of the married girls. Some community stakeholders such as chiefs, head teachers, and assemblymen assisted in the recruitment process. These individuals provided us with information as to where and when it will be easier to meet the girls personally and in some cases they provided gatekeepers who could lead us to some of the girls. The gatekeepers were lay persons who volunteered to assist in the recruitment of participants. Married girls were also identified through some beneficiaries of the NGOs after which the snowball method of participant recruitment was used for further selection. Potential participants were pre-informed about the visit of the researchers. Participants were also approached in person and recruitment was done by word-of-mouth.

Consent was sought verbally from participants and recorded for documentation after the goals of the study, participants' role in the study, and the associated benefits and risks involved were explained to them. Some girls declined to take part in the study because their families were resistant while others were afraid of their husbands seeing them with strangers.

Then, meetings for interviews were scheduled to take place either at school premises, offices of National Health Insurance, or participants' parents' homes. The first author carried out the interviews with married girls in the Dagbani language, their local dialect, which were audio-recorded with tape recorders following participants' consent.

A semi-structured interview guide was used to obtain responses from participants. This allowed them to freely share their experiences with the researchers without distorting the aims of the study. Sample questions included: How do you cope with challenges of being a young wife and mother? How do you utilise the kinds of support available to you? What are the external support systems you are able to access? In order to seek further clarifications on issues discussed by the participants, probes were used. The duration of the individual interviews was between 20 and 30 min.

After the 19th participant, we noticed several similarities in participants' narratives. We went ahead to add two more participants which brought the total number of participants to 21. The additional participants also shared experiences that were similar to those of the 19 previously interviewed participants. This signalled to us that we had attained data saturation hence the need to end data collection (Grady, 1998; Saunders et al., 2018).

9.2.5 Data Analysis

Braun and Clarke's (2006) stages of thematic analyses were followed in analysing data gathered from audio-recorded interviews in the Dagbani language. The stages include familiarisation of researchers with data, generation of codes from data, identification of themes, review of the emerging themes, definition and assignment of names to identified themes, and writing of a report. Thematic analysis was deemed appropriate for this study because of its flexibility and style of presenting experiences, meanings and reality of participants, making room for interpretations to be made in line with both social and psychological perspectives (Braun & Clarke, 2006).

To begin the analysis process, the audio recordings of interviews were listened to several times by the first author to get acquainted with participants' narratives. Being a native of the research context, the first author, conducted a word-to-word translation while transcribing the audio-taped recordings into an English written document. To ensure trustworthiness, a Dagbani language expert based at University of Ghana's Department of Linguistics reviewed the translated transcripts and the audio-taped recordings for accuracy. The goal was to ensure accurate depiction of participants' expressions. Data analysis began with both the first and second authors reading through the translated transcripts several times. This process helped the authors to get a better understanding of participants' narratives and also to generate a strategy for coding. Deductive and inductive coding strategies were used for the coding. For deductive coding, the research objectives guided the process whereas for inductive coding, sub-themes were identified from the data.

The second stage of data analysis was the process of code generation. To achieve this, first author did a line-by-line reading of all the 21 transcripts several times. She then applied the open/in-vivo coding where she identified segment of the transcripts that made meaning after which she labelled them. To manage the data, Microsoft Excel was used. The study objectives (e.g., intrinsic resources utilised by married girls, extrinsic resources utilised by married girls) were used as the heading of each column and participants' pseudonyms were used to label each row.

The third stage of data analysis was the process of reviewing all the codes generated by the first author. Here, all the authors participated in the review process and areas where there was disagreement were revolved. When the authors reached an agreement, codes with similar ideas were grouped and labelled as themes and sub-themes. During this process, it was realised that some codes were not placed under the right headings. These codes were copied from their original cells and they were placed in different cells which fitted the issues they highlighted better. When it was realised that all codes had been placed into broader themes and sub-themes, all the three authors reviewed them again to ensure that all the placements were done correctly. The last stage of data analysis occurred when the themes and sub-themes that were generated in the previous stages were defined and assigned names. The clearly defined themes were then discussed in a report with reference to existing literature.

9.2.5.1 Trustworthiness of Findings

Guba and Lincoln's (1981) procedures for ensuring trustworthiness in qualitative research were followed. Credibility was ensured by taking into consideration the following steps. First, before data collection began, the first author visited the research settings to familiarise herself with the places and also to establish a relationship with potential participants. Second, all the authors engaged in regular debriefing sessions at all stages of the research and data analyses. The debriefing sessions helped the researchers to ensure that any potential researcher biases were checked and corrected. Third, data was recorded carefully by using quality audio tape recorder. This ensured that participants' actual expressions were captured. Fourth, member checks were carried out with some participants who partook in the study. Fifth, the interviews were conducted in the participants' own local language to ensure accuracy in the capturing of experiences shared by the participants. Sixth, Dagbani language expert conducted a review of the translated transcripts to ensure that they accurately captured the participants' experiences.

Transferability was achieved by the provision of sufficient and detailed descriptions of the research contexts and process, as well as the backgrounds of the married girls. This would ensure that readers would understand the research processes well which would enable them to compare the findings of the research with real life situations. Dependability was ensured by the second and third authors reviewing the codes that were initially generated by the first author. Afterwards, all the authors participated in the remaining stages of data analysis. This ensured that the conclusions that were drawn were not based on the researchers' own ideas but were based solely on participants' accounts of their experiences. Additionally, we documented all the processes that were followed during the interviews, data transcription and analysis in order to ensure that the research can be replicated. Confirmability was ensured by the researchers keeping audit trails which encompassed a transparent description of the steps taken throughout the research, the methodology, how data were analysed, and the nature of interpretations made from the data, were documented and reported in this paper.

9.2.6 Ethical Considerations

Ethics clearance was obtained from the University of Ghana's Ethics Committee for Humanities (reference number: ECH 022/17-18). We also sought and obtained permission from the Department of Social Welfare in Accra, Ghana, because the married girls formed part of the people managed by the institution. The goals of the study were carefully explained to participants verbally in their local dialect. This was done to ensure that they understood the study and their role in it and could withdraw if they found it inconvenient. Participants were informed of the prospective benefits that they may get from participating in the study. They were told that they may get relief from some distresses that they may be experiencing in their marriages if they speak with someone concerning such challenges as keeping these distresses could harm their wellbeing. Also, participants were told that if they share their experiences, researchers could understand their situation better and the information that would be generated from their experiences could be helpful in mobilising support for them through the NGOs. Besides the positive benefits, they were told about the potential risks of them participating in the research. They were told that they could breakdown emotionally or they may remember painful events that happened to them in the past that could be distressing for them. Following thorough explanation of the content of the informed consent form, verbal consent, as opposed to written consent, was audio recorded before they were recruited into the study. Verbal assent was taken because of the low literacy levels of participants.

Although some participants were below the legal age of majority (18 years) in Ghana, they were considered adults by virtue of their marital status and their consent was taken without the involvement of their parents or husbands. In the context in which the study was conducted and considering the nature of the population used in this study, the status of participants as married individuals has cultural implications that cannot be ignored. Punch (2002) argues that how a society perceives childhood influences how they treat such individuals. Similarly, Ibrahim (2015) argues that children's maturity, age and capacities differ in different societies. Thus, while the national criterion for adulthood in Ghana is age-based and pegged at 18 years, there are variations across cultures within the country (Ibrahim, 2015). According to Ibrahim (2015), in the Dagomba culture where the study was conducted, childhood and adulthood is not determined by the individual's chronological age but by the assumption of certain responsibilities. Marriage is considered a symbol of maturity and responsibility and confers on teenage boys and girls adulthood status with its associated benefits and recognition as full-fledged adults in comparison to the unmarried peers of the same age or even older. Thus, married adolescent girls are considered responsible and valued members of the community and are given all the benefits and support offered to older members of the community (Ibrahim, 2015). As adults, they are admitted into community/family meetings, they have voting rights at meetings, they can express their views and make financial contributions. Based on this, married girls who gave consent to be part of the study were included in the study. This decision was indicated in the research protocol, which was approved by the ethics committee. In addition to consent from married girls, the researchers also sought consent from parents of some married girls who had just given birth and were temporarily living with their parents. In the Dagomba communities, it is a common practice for women who had just given birth to move in briefly to live with their parents. During this period, they are guided and taught strategies for caring for their new born children (Baba et al., 2020).

The researchers also assured the participants of confidentiality and anonymity by not demanding names and other forms of identity that could later link information to them. Rather, their narratives were identified using pseudonyms. In our quest to ensure confidentiality, we interviewed participants in private settings that were provided by the gatekeepers and, in some cases, the NGOs in order to protect the information obtained from the married girls. Some girls who were approached at home were interviewed in their homes. However, measures were put in place to carry out those interviews in private rooms and spaces provided by the girls themselves. This was to guarantee the safety of participants who participated in the study and to avoid them getting into trouble with their families. To cater for participants who may experience emotional upheavals during the course of interviews, a clinical psychologist was made available and participants were encouraged to use this service. However, no participants requested for this service. A standard monetary compensation of 5 Ghana cedis (equivalent to USD 1 at the time of data gathering) was offered, after the interview, for participants' time.

9.3 Findings

This study explored some intrinsic and extrinsic resources and described how these resources enabled married girls to deal with the challenges they face in their marriages as young wives and young mothers. Intrinsic resources were identified as the coping strategies that they employed in dealing with situations and their individual attitudes. With regard to extrinsic resources, the study explored the nature of social support received, whether or not the participants could utilise community and NGO support and the impact of such support on their well-being. Details of the findings are discussed below.

9.3.1 Intrinsic Resources

In identifying the intrinsic resources, coping strategies used by married girls to deal with their various challenges were identified. The strategies that emerged included active coping, help seeking and avoidance strategies. Additionally, it emerged that some married girls demonstrated resistance towards dominant marriage norms which was identified as a personal strength that enabled them to cope with their adverse marriage experiences.

9.3.1.1 Coping Strategies

Although early parenthood among adolescent girls may increase risk for negative life outcomes, some young girls were able to adapt fairly well and accomplish positive outcomes for themselves and their children through various coping strategies. The themes surrounding coping that were identified were mainly help seeking, active coping and avoidance strategies.

Help-seeking and active coping strategies, which involved determining effective strategies for reducing distress levels, were used to manage problems that the participants encountered in their marriages. Most young mothers raised issues concerning their ability to identify and reach out to significant others in their lives for support. This approach to seeking support is treated as an intrinsic resource in the sense that it involves seeking material assistance from the people available in order to solve a particular problem. They talked about the support they sought from their husbands, in-laws and healthcare providers that helped them to cope with the distress associated with marriage and early motherhood. The nature of support that was sought was in the form of assistance with nursing and caring for their babies or financial aid:

> When the child is sick and his father is around, I give him to his father and he too will hold him for some time, when the child is hungry then I collect him back. He can finish eating and keep quiet then [I] can put him down to sleep. [Hajara; 17 years, 1 year of marriage]

> When the baby is crying, he [husband] can collect him so I can do my work...Yes. He [husband] teaches me [how to nurse the baby]. [Zumera; 17 years, 1 year of marriage]

Another coping strategy that the young mothers employed was seeking help from health professionals. This form of support seeking involved searching for solutions to medical problems and seeking professional advice from healthcare givers. The excerpts below support this point:

> When it [Pain and discomfort in pregnancy] happens, I take it to the hospital because when it was like that for me it was the hospital that I went to. [Zulfawu; 18 years, 1 year of marriage]

> ...he [my son] had problem in the chest...When he was delivered he wasn't crying but just breathing heavily and the nurses tried their best to restore back his breathing again. They then told us that if we go home and the breathing changes again, we should come back tomorrow so they can write a note for us. [Salamat; 13 years, 1 year of marriage]

Active coping was also identified as a form of coping for young mothers. This strategy involved the young mothers actively taking initiatives to deal directly with challenges associated with caring for their children by finding solutions to them. The strategies they employed involved soothing the baby when the baby was in distress or refused to sleep, and getting medicine for the child when he/she was sick. Although these actions on a face value portray a normal response expected in such situations, however, in highly stressful situations like child marriages, it can be very challenging to make appropriate decisions and choices for survival amidst the numerous stressors. Therefore, having that sound judgement to make the appropriate decisions in these circumstances becomes a strength (active coping strategy) in dealing with that situation, unlike others who might resort to doing nothing out of frustration. Also active coping methods included actively following instructions and professional medical advice to ensure their health and that of their babies. This was indicated by the following married girls' excerpts:

> When the child is not sleeping or is disturbed, I just carry him at my back till he sleeps. When he is sick, I would force and buy the drugs for him... [Amina; 18 years, 3 years of marriage]

. . . You know as a pregnant woman, when you go to the hospital, you are told what to eat and what not to eat, so that it can facilitate childbirth. So [I was] able to follow their advice. [Latifa; 16 years, 1 year of marriage]

Also identified was the use of some avoidance strategies to deal with young motherhood challenges that they perceived as uncontrollable. The strategies employed were disengagement and distraction. Disengagement was one avoidance strategy employed by an 18 year old mother who was married for a year. She resorted to giving up or doing nothing at all to deal with the pains she experienced in her pregnancy condition as a way of coping. Another participant also used distraction strategies by spending time with her friends or engaging in some form of entertainment. These strategies served as interim relief from distress that they were unable to deal with. The excerpts presented below show how some young mothers used avoidance strategies to deal with the challenges they experienced during pregnancy:

. . . Eih Madam! I am not able to do anything [during pregnancy]. . . Yes. I wait till it [pain] subsides then I go back to sleep." [Adiza; 18 years, 1 year of marriage]

When I wanted to stop thinking about it [disturbances in pregnancy], I went to sit and chat with my friends or if there is any entertainment, then I go and watch so that I won't think about it. [Salamat; 13 years, 1 year of marriage]

9.3.1.2 Attitudes Towards Dominant Marriage Norms

Married girls demonstrated some strength in their narratives concerning their attitudes towards some dominant marriage norms. Overall, the narratives of the participants showed divergent views reflecting either compliance with dominant marriage norms or resistance to dominant marriage norms. This was an interesting finding because both compliance and resistance towards dominant marriage norms were used differently by these girls to reflect both positive and negative outcomes. Six married girls showed attitudes of compliance towards what was required of them per their cultural norms. This conversely indicated a potential sign of vulnerability among the girls as this compliance could limit their autonomy and agency and could negatively affect their well-being. Early marriage was acceptable for girls who were interested in getting married and glorified in their quest to fulfil parents' wishes and societal expectations. An illustration of this is evident in the excerpt below:

. . .Yes we are supposed to listen to our parents [Even when they are forcing you into an early marriage]. [Rahina; 17 years, 2 years of marriage]

Some girls who held on to these cultural norms also made justifications to register their claims. They accepted the idea of restriction often given to married girls in their new homes as a form of prevention of extra marital affairs, a form of rationalisation to reduce any cognitive distress that might be accompanied by their restriction and lack of agency. This can be observed in the excerpt below:

> ... yes, it's good [A married woman should be restricted]... because some ...can just get married and still be having boyfriends... Even she can just get pregnant and it will ... be for another boy. [Ramatu; 17 years, 1 year of marriage]

On the other hand, four married girls demonstrated resistant attitudes towards cultural norms. Again, resistance here could also serve both positive and negative consequences depending on the manner it is being utilised. For some married girls, resistance towards dominant marriage norms was a strength which enabled them to develop stronger identities of themselves that are devoid of social pressures and expectations. These girls registered their dissatisfaction with social and cultural norms which marginalized females and robbed them of their childhood and sense of autonomy to pursue their own dreams and aspirations. This was highlighted in the excerpts below:

> ... No, I am not in favour of it [the female having no choice]...It is possible that the man they [parents] impose on you does not even love you. There is the likelihood that he will beat you every day, and you will always be quarrelling with him. Every day, even if he has money, he wouldn't give you since he was not in love with you but you were imposed on him. So you will not be happy with him. Every day you will be sad. [Leila; 18 years, 2 years of marriage]

> ... If I had the power I would change the situation [forcing young girls into early marriages]... [Samira; 16 years, 2 years of marriage]

On the other hand an attitude of resistance towards dominant marriage norms in this early marriage context could be a weakness in that, married girls who demonstrated this attitude could be at risk of psychological distress if they uphold an attitude that is contrary to the behaviour they exhibit in order to conform to societal expectations.

9.3.2 *Extrinsic Resources*

With regard to the kind of extrinsic resources available to the married girls, the nature of received social support, access to Non-Governmental Organisations (NGOs) and community support systems were explored and described. Here, the married girls were asked about their access to social support networks, NGO support and the nature of support they get from the community. The participants were asked about NGO support because all the communities involved in the study had NGO operations running in them. Some of these NGOs included Action AID Ghana, Right to Play Ghana and NORSAAC (Northern Sector Action on Awareness Centre) which provided support to victims of child marriage. Hence, we wanted to find out how accessible these organisations were to the participants and whether or not the participants reached out to them for support. The themes generated are discussed as follows:

9.3.2.1 Receipt of Social Support

A central theme that emerged was that marriage was a source of social support and satisfaction of basic needs to the married girls. They reported that their marriage provided them access to support that satisfied their needs. Some girls admitted that their husbands provided them with their needs such as food, clothing and gifts. This helped them to adjust to the assumption of their new roles as wives and enhanced positive experiences:

> To be frank, if I ask him[husband] to buy me something he gets it for me. If he doesn't have money he tells me to exercise patience. Truly, when he gets money he gets me what I asked for. [Rahina; 17 years, 2 years of marriage]

> He [husband] gives me money for upkeep. Sometimes his mother also gives me some [money]. This also makes me happy. Apart from these, my own hard work also makes me happy. [Salima, 17 years, 1 year in marriage]

Besides their husbands, assistance from in-laws in taking care of their children also enhanced positive experiences. For these girls, assistance from their new families helped them to build resilience and experience positive outcomes:

> When it is at night, you or one of the people you are sleeping with [family] will wake up and soothe the baby. His grandmother can wake up and help or his father too can come in and collect him. [Mari; 18 years, 2 years in marriage]

> The dresses he [husband] buys me, and when he helps me with the baby when he is crying and I am busy with house chores. And when we eat together and also play games sometimes. [Ramatu; 17 years, 1 year of marriage]

9.3.2.2 NGO Support

When asked about access to NGO support, most (16) of the girls reported of having no access to external support from organisations although the communities of focus had prevailing NGOs activities for married girls. A few of the girls admitted to being aware of NGOs operating in their communities although they reported that they had not gotten access to them yet. They believed that having access to NGOs depended on luck. The excerpts below accounted for this assertion:

> Yes, we see them coming to help people. They [NGOs] come [to help people] but because it has to do with luck so I haven't been lucky yet. [Habiba; 17 years, 1 year of marriage]

> Yes. They [NGOs] come but for me, I don't know if I am not always lucky or what? Whenever they come and they select people, my name is not always part of them. There was one that I did and they gave me their things and made me do a lot of photo copies and passport pictures, but when they came and selected, I wasn't part. [Rabia; 17 years, 5 years of marriage]

Other married girls reported that they had no idea of any external support such as NGO services that were available to them. By virtue of some married girls often being restricted, they had limited contacts with friends and other individuals who might have provided information on how to effectively access some of these support systems. This led to their inability to access some of the support systems which would have enabled them to deal with the adverse conditions of their early marriages. Below are excerpts that illustrated this point:

> ... I have not seen them but some people talk about them. People say that some NGOs are coming but I don't get to see them and what they do. [Fatima; 18 years, 1 year of marriage]

> ...Madam, I don't know. Maybe they [NGOs] are there but I don't know them. [Adiza; 18 years, 1 year of marriage]

The report of married girls' unawareness of NGO services suggested that these girls might be demonstrating ignorance or lack of adequate information on the kinds of external opportunities available to support them. It was also possible that they were unaware of the procedures involved in accessing support systems of the NGOs.

Inasmuch as most girls reported to have no access to external support such as NGOs, there were three out of 21 girls who reported that they had access to some of the support from NGOs. This finding suggests that there were available external support systems that married girls could benefit from, but the problem was with how well they were able to identify these opportunities and use them to their advantage. Married girls' narratives showed that most of them were not aware of the NGOs because they had no information as to when personnel of the organisations visited their vicinities. Therefore, those who were able to access the NGOs were girls who got out to either work or school. The excerpts below explained this:

> ...We do have [NGOs that come to support the community]...They [NGOs] are many. Because we go to work, they normally come to the workplace. And they don't come every day. Four of them can come within the space of three weeks for a very long time before they come back. But there are times you go home and you are informed that some of them came around and that they do offer help to people. And for about three months, they wouldn't meet you in the house and they would be informed that you've gone. [Leila; 18 years, 2 years of marriage]

> ... No [NGOs do not come]. It was only when we were in school that they came to give us maize. [Memuna; 18 years, 5 years of marriage]

9.3.2.3 Community Support

Concerning married girls' access to community support systems, participants were asked about the availability of community women support groups and community-based intervention programmes. Most of the girls (12) reported that they lacked access to these kinds of support or were unaware of the existence of such support systems. Some of them emphasised that there were entirely no such support systems in their communities. The excerpts below explained this point:

> I don't know if they [community] do that [provide support] and I am not aware of it because they can be doing some things that I am not aware of. [Zulfawu; 18 years, 1 year of marriage]

...No. I have never known such a thing [any source of community support available to the community]. [Memuna; 18 years, 5 years of marriage]

On the other hand, some of the girls reported being aware of community support groups for older women, however, they reported that they had no access to them because of their young ages. From the excerpts below, it appeared that some of the community groups were made up of only older women and were not accessible to young married girls. They reported:

...They [community support groups] are there but ... they are older women [am not a part of it]. [Safia; 18 years, 1 year of marriage]

There are [Community support groups], only I am not part of them. [Rahina; 17 years, 2 years of marriage]

9.4 Discussion

For most women, motherhood is generally not experienced as entirely negative as it can provide an important opportunity for positive behavioural change (Leadbeater & Way, 2001). This suggests that although early parenthood among adolescent girls may increase risk for negative life outcomes, some young women are able to adapt fairly well and accomplish positive outcomes for themselves and their children due to the presence of intrinsic resources such as their coping strategies. Some of the themes that emerged as coping strategies used by the young mothers were mainly help-seeking, active coping and avoidance coping. With regard to help seeking and active coping, married girls sought support from their husbands, in-laws and healthcare providers. This clearly supports the notion that promoting beneficial relationships between adolescents and their environment is necessary for their well-being (Geldhof et al., 2013; Wilson & Somhlaba, 2016).

Seeking social support proved resourceful in promoting access to resources such as food, clothing, shelter, education, medical assistance and economic support (Ungar et al., 2007) which are important for coping. Also, active coping strategies were used by young mothers and could be accounted for by the contribution of gender norms concerning division of labour in the household which limits a woman's roles to reproduction and domestic work, while a man's role is reserved for leadership and provision for the household (Pereznieto & Taylor, 2014; UNFPA, 2012). With this, married girls accepted their irrevocable fate of solely shouldering reproduction responsibilities and therefore resorted to actively dealing with their own challenges and finding solutions to them.

We also found in the girls' narratives that some of them used avoidance coping methods such as distraction and disengagement to manage problems that they perceived were uncontrollable. They resorted to doing nothing about their problems or using other activities such as conversing with friends and other forms of entertainment to keep their minds away from the source of stress. This reflected existing literature that has highlighted that behavioural distraction and disengagement methods are often employed by adolescents and children in dealing with conditions that are unbearable and uncontrollable to manage (Zimmer-Gembeck & Skinner, 2011). In the present study, when married girls felt they could not bear the pain and discomfort associated with pregnancy and childbirth, they tended to disengage or distract themselves from their source of stress. Whereas avoidance can be helpful in the short term, such strategies however, often have negative consequences (Hofmann & Hay, 2018).

Another intrinsic resource which reflected aspects of strength were demonstrated in married girls' attitudes towards negative dominant marriage norms. The findings showed divergent views reflecting compliance with and resistance to those norms. These identified attitudes nonetheless turned out to have both positive and negative outcomes. Bottrell (2007) argued that young people often have to accept or reject some cultural norms and ideals in order to negotiate for the constraints and opportunities for expressing their self-identities. This usually mirrors the collective establishment of social life that continues to offer powerful frameworks, constraining young people's experiences and their life chances (Furlong & Cartmel, 1997). Most of the girls maintained an attitude of compliance towards the cultural norms surrounding marriage in their societies. Here, some girls had accepted their fate and what was required of them per their cultural norms, reflecting a form of compliance in which self-efficacy and competence may be compromised. This may expose them to vulnerabilities and the risks of being bullied and oppressed by negative norms that threaten their independence and personal growth. Again, compliance could be utilised effectively when it serves as a defence mechanism to rationalise and create harmony between the individual's attitudes and their behaviours. This would work well for the married girls in the current research context where they must comply with the norms of society against their personal beliefs or choices.

On the other hand, a few of the married girls demonstrated some amount of resistance to cultural norms that seemed to limit their agency and freedom to pursue their own goals and aspirations. There has been some established evidence of strength among young people. These young people resist prevailing cultural norms in their society and they also try to refute and criticise negative stereotypes despite adversity (Bottrell, 2007). According to Bottrell (2007), in response to marginalization, difficult circumstances and competing demands, young people show resistance in attempt to nullify the negative images people have of them and to create new ones for themselves. In the case of these married girls, some of the negative images included the fact that they are meant for the kitchen, child birth and to submit to their husbands who are perceived to be more intelligent and better at decision making. Therefore, demonstrating resistance towards these negative ideas about themselves could go a long way to enhance well-being by helping them develop more positive self-concepts. This form of resistance served as strength which enabled married girls to cope successfully in their stereotypical and marginalizing social environment. However, merely professing a resistant attitude may sometimes be detrimental when that same attitude is not reflected in one's behaviour. This would likely lead to cognitive dissonance, a form of distress which Festinger and Carlsmith (1959) associates with acting in ways that are contrary to our attitudes. By virtue of this, married girls who act in conformity to these norms while holding strong negative attitudes towards those same norms are more likely to go through this cognitive distress which compromises well-being. Therefore, it is important to express these attitudes in behaviours or practices which can be done by empowering married girls through education (formal or informal) and also providing them with the necessary protective resources to enable them express themselves and limit distress.

The study also explored the kind of extrinsic resources available and how these resources were being utilised by the married girls. Married girls' access to social support networks, NGOs and community support systems were the focus of the study. Some of the girls were able to identify various kinds of social support networks, including support from their husbands, in-laws and siblings that enabled them to cope with the challenges in their marriages. The main forms of social support reported by married girls included financial and emotional support from husbands and in-laws. These kinds of support led to positive experiences in their marriages. This finding support previous research which has shown that girls are usually brought up with the idea that once a girl is married, her husband is supposed to provide for her financially (Ampofo, 2001). When these expectations or goals are met in their marriages, it leads to feelings of satisfaction, fulfilment of needs and happiness which are important for well-being.

Support from NGOs was also explored because the communities of focus were beneficiaries of NGOs. This is because Northern Ghana is said to be a host to over half of Ghana's Non-Governmental Organisations that are committed to helping communities tackle issues of poverty by assisting them to raise economically viable and sustainable projects (Mwakideu, 2016). The community support systems that were explored included married girls' access and participation in women and youth group activities, as well as community welfare initiatives. Excerpts from married girls' accounts revealed that most of them had no access to external support from organisations and community support systems. Some of them reported having heard of them but had not gotten access to their services while others reported having absolutely no knowledge about their existence. Married girls' limited access to these extrinsic resources could be attributed to lack of awareness, limited access to informed choices, restricted mobility and social interactions due to the conditions in their marriages (Santhya & Jejeebhoy, 2003). It has been reported that married girls often suffer social isolation which limits their access to support from family and friends and other sources of external support (UNFPA, 2012; UNICEF, 2013). This limited contact with family and friends make them lose out on some important information that is available to the public which might provide assistance on how to effectively access some of these external support systems.

Inasmuch as most girls reported to have no access to external support such as NGOs and community support systems, there were a few girls who were able to access some of the support from NGOs available to them. This suggested that there were external support systems that married girls could benefit from, but the problem was associated with the girls' lack of awareness of the existence of these opportunities and how best to use them. This reflected resilience attitudes in that, people who have a sense of control and efficacy are those who are able to amass more concrete types of assistance, or at least recognise the availability and access to the kinds of supports options available to them (Green & Rodgers, 2001). The girls who reported having access to these support systems were either engaged in some form of economic activity or social support network that enabled them to explore their environment. This meant that girls who were more exposed to social networks such as family and peers had the chance to develop confidence and self-efficacy that helped them to explore their environment and to identify other external support options.

These findings demonstrate an emphasis on the micro (individual) level approaches to resilience as against the role of meso-level (social structures and systems). However, mechanisms that promote resilience have been proven to reside both internally and externally across the different levels of the systems (Hart et al., 2016). This information is important for determining the kind of resources available and those that are lacking when drawing resilience interventions.

9.5 Implications for Intervention

Given the lack of awareness of the existence of external support networks, interventions should focus on educating married girls on the existence of support systems and how these supports could be accessed. This lack of access to external support networks also demonstrates some inequalities which can be addressed by adopting interventions that target social structures and systemic transformations. Therefore, researchers and practitioners are urged to adopt a holistic approach to resilience by considering a variety of resources both within the individual and those within the society, as well as environmental interactions (Hart et al., 2016).

Married girls may benefit from education on a variety of adaptive coping strategies that could be adopted to manage challenges of early marriage and motherhood. Married girls could also be supported to develop healthy ways of developing resistance and compliance towards stereotypical dominant norms that prevent them from achieving their dreams. This could be achieved through training on skills of assertiveness, decision making, social skills, agency, self-efficacy and self-worth. Empowerment can also be achieved by amending societal systems and structures that breed inequalities and place girls at a disadvantaged position.

9.6 Limitations and Recommendations for Future Studies

The present study used a small sample of girls in some communities in only the Northern region and of the Dagomba ethnicity. It is possible that married girls in other regions and ethnic groups may have different experiences. Future studies should consider including a large and diverse sample that is representative of the married girls in Ghana. Findings from such study may provide data that could inform policy making at the national level. The use of gatekeepers for participant recruitment could have affected the kind of married girls that participated in the present study. It is also possible that only participants with similar characteristics were selected for the study. Hence, future studies should consider selecting participants randomly in order to ascertain a diverse sample and potentially gain varied experiences.

9.7 Conclusions

Although a previous research study on married girls (Baba et al., 2020) has identified adverse conditions association with child marriage, this current study has demonstrated the role of intrinsic and extrinsic resources in dealing with these challenges. We found that married girls were able to cope with their situations by using some help-seeking, active coping and avoidance coping strategies and also possessed some resilience attitudes. Regarding extrinsic resources, support provided by the husbands, in-laws, friends and siblings were relevant due to their association with positive experiences among the married girls. However, the girls were lacking access to extrinsic resources in the community and NGO support. This limited the benefits that the married girls could have gained from external resources which could have reduced the impact of challenges associated with early marriage and motherhood. This finding further stresses the need for interventions designed for married girls to adopt a social justice approach which emphasises a multi-systemic approach to achieving resilience among at-risk populations. This approach is an essential tool in the promotion of well-being and positive outcomes among these married girls.

References

Abdul-Hamid, M. (2010). The influence of Islam on an African people: The case of the Dagomba of the northern Ghana. In *International conference on universalism, relativism & intercultural philosophy* (pp. 3–5). University of Cape Coast.

Abrinkova, L., Orosova, O., Bacikova-Sleskova, M., Stefanakova, M., & Gajdosova, B. (2019). External resources of resilience in association with the alcohol use among early adolescents. *European Journal of Public Health, 29*(4). https://doi.org/10.1093/eurpub/ckz186.167

Addai, I., Opoku-Agyeman, C., & Amanfu, S. K. (2015). Marriage and subjective well-being in Ghana. *African Review of Economics and Finance, 7*(1), 53–79.

Adinkrah, M. (2012). Better dead than dishonoured: Masculinity and male suicidal behaviour in contemporary Ghana. *Social Science & Medicine, 74*(4), 474–481. https://doi.org/10.1016/j.socscimed.2010.10.011

Ahmed, S., Khan, S., Alia, M., & Noushad, S. (2013). Psychological impact evaluation of early marriages. *International Journal of Endorsing Health Science Research, 1*(2), 84–86.

Aldridge, A. A., & Roesch, S. C. (2008). Developing coping typologies of minority adolescents: A latent profile analysis. *Journal of Adolescence, 31*(4), 499–517. https://doi.org/10.1016/j.adolescence.2007.08.005

Alhassan, E. (2013). Early marriage of young females: A panacea to poverty in the northern region of Ghana? *Research on Humanities and Social Sciences, 3*(12), 18–31.

Alvord, M. K., & Grados, J. J. (2005). Enhancing resilience in children: A proactive approach. *Professional Psychology: Research and Practice, 36*(3), 238–245. https://doi.org/10.1037/0735-7028.36.3.238

Ampofo, A. A. (2001). "When men speak women listen": Gender socialisation and young adolescents' attitudes to sexual and reproductive issues. *African Journal of Reproductive Health, 5*(3), 196–212. https://doi.org/10.2307/3583335

Awusabo-Asare, K., Abane, A. M., & Kumi-Kyereme, A. (2004). *Adolescent sexual and reproductive health in Ghana: A synthesis of research evidence*. Alan Guttmacher Institute.

Baba, H., Salifu Yendork, J., & Atindanbila, S. (2020). Exploring married girls' subjective experiences of well-being and challenges. *Journal of Adolescence, 79*, 193–207. https://doi.org/10.1016/j.adolescence.2020.01.009

Bawah, A. A., Akweongo, P., Simmons, R., & Phillips, J. F. (1999). Women's fears and men's anxieties: The impact of family planning on gender relations in northern Ghana. *Studies in Family Planning, 30*(1), 54–66.

Black, C., & Ford-Gilboe, M. (2004). Adolescent mothers: Resilience, family health work and health-promoting practices. *Journal of Advanced Nursing, 48*, 351–360. https://doi.org/10.1111/j.1365-2648.2004.03204.x

Bottrell, D. (2007). Resistance, resilience and social identities: Reframing 'problem youth and the problem of schooling. *Journal of Youth Studies, 10*(5), 597–616. https://doi.org/10.1080/13676260701602662

Bottrell, D. (2009). Understanding 'marginal' perspectives: Towards a social theory of resilience. *Qualitative Social Work, 8*(3), 321–339. https://doi.org/10.1177/1473325009337840

Bowlby, J. (1988). Developmental psychiatry comes of age. *American Journal of Psychiatry, 145*(1), 1–10.

Braun, V., & Clarke, V. (2006). Using thematic analysis in psychology. *Qualitative Research in Psychology, 3*(2), 77–101. https://doi.org/10.1191/1478088706qp063oa

Brooks, J. E. (2006). Strengthening resilience in children and youths: Maximizing opportunities through the schools. *Children & Schools, 28*(2), 69–76. https://doi.org/10.1093/cs/28.2.69

Capp, G., Berkowitz, R., Sullivan, K., Astor, R., De Pedro, K., Gilreath, T., Benbenishty, R., & Rice, E. (2016). Adult relationships in multiple contexts and associations with adolescent mental health. *Research on Social Work Practice, 26*, 622–629. https://doi.org/10.1177/1049731515624967

Culpin, I., Stapinski, L., Miles, O. B., Araya, R., & Joinson, C. (2015). Exposure to socioeconomic adversity in early life and risk of depression at 18 years: The mediating role of locus of control. *Journal of Affective Disorders, 183*, 269–278.

Day, T., & Kearney, C. A. (2016). Resilience variables and posttraumatic symptoms among maltreated youth. *Journal of Aggression, Maltreatment & Trauma, 25*(9), 991–1005.

Duflo, E. (2011). *Women's empowerment and economic development*. National Bureau of Economic Research. Retrieved from https://ideas.repec.org/p/nbr/nberwo/17702.html

Edmeades, J., Lantos, H., & Mekuria, F. (2016). Worth the effort? Combining sexual and reproductive health and economic empowerment programming for married adolescent girls in Amhara, Ethiopia. *Vulnerable Children and Youth Studies, 11*(4), 339–351.

Fergus, S., & Zimmerman, M. A. (2005). Adolescent resilience: A framework for understanding healthy development in the face of risk. *Annual Review of Public Health, 26*, 399–419. https://doi.org/10.1146/annurev.publhealth.26.021304.144357

Festinger, L., & Carlsmith, J. M. (1959). Cognitive consequences of forced compliance. *Journal of Abnormal and Social Psychology, 58*, 203–210.

Furlong, A., & Cartmel, F. (1997). Risk and uncertainty in the youth transition. *Young, 5*(1), 3–20. https://doi.org/10.1177/110330889700500102

Geldhof, G. J., Bowers, E. P., & Lerner, R. M. (2013). Special section introduction: Thriving in context: Findings from the 4-H study of positive youth development. *Journal of Youth and Adolescence, 42*, 1–5. https://doi.org/10.1007/s10964-012-9855-7

Ghana Statistical Service. (2010). *Population and housing census: National analytical report*. Ghana Statistical Service.

Ghana Statistical Service (GSS), Ghana Health Service 9HGS), and The DHS Program. (2015). *Demographic and Health Survey 2014*. Retrieved from https://www2.statsghana.gov.gh/docfiles/publications/2014%20GDHS%20%20Report.pdf

Godha, D., Hotchkiss, D. R., & Gage, A. J. (2013). Association between child marriage and reproductive health outcomes and service utilization: A multi-country study from South Asia. *Journal of Adolescent Health, 52*(5), 552–558.

Gonzales, N. A., Tein, J. Y., Sandler, I. N., & Friedman, R. J. (2001). On the limits of coping: Interaction between stress and coping for inner-city adolescents. *Journal of Adolescent Research, 16*(4), 372–395. https://doi.org/10.1177/0743558401164005

Gould, M. S., Velting, D., Kleinman, M., Lucas, C., Thomas, J. G., & Chung, M. (2004). Teenagers' attitudes about coping strategies and help-seeking behaviour for suicidality. *Journal of the American Academy of Child & Adolescent Psychiatry, 43*(9), 1124–1133. https://doi.org/10.1097/01.chi.0000132811.06547.31

Grady, M. P. (1998). *Qualitative and action research: A practitioner handbook*. Phi Delta Kappa Educational Foundation.

Green, B. L., & Rodgers, A. (2001). Determinants of social support among low-income mothers: A longitudinal analysis. *American Journal of Community Psychology, 29*(3), 419–441.

Greene, M. (2014). *Ending child marriage in a generation: What research is needed?* Ford Foundation/Greene Works.

Guba, E. G., & Lincoln, Y. S. (1981). *Effective evaluation: Improving the usefulness of evaluation results through responsive and naturalistic approaches*. Jossey-Bass.

Gupta, S. D., Mukherjee, S., Pande, R., Singh, S., & Basu, S. (2008). *Knot ready: Lessons from India on delaying marriage for girls*. International Centre for Research on Women (ICRW). Retrieved from https://www.icrw.org/wp-content/uploads/2016/10/Knot-Ready-Lessons-from-India-on-Delaying-Marriage-for-Girls.pdf

Hamby, S., Grych, J., & Banyard, V. L. (2018). Resilience portfolios and poly-strengths:Identifying protective factors associated with thriving after adversity. *Psychology of Violence, 8*(2), 172–183.

Hart, A., Gagnon, E., Eryigit-Madzwamuse, S., Cameron, J., Aranda, K., Rathbone, A., & Heaver, B. (2016). Uniting resilience research and practice with an inequalities approach. *SAGE Open, 6*(4). https://doi.org/10.1177/2158244016682477

Hoagwood, K. E., Cavaleri, M. A., Olin, S. S., Burns, B. J., Slaton, E., Gruttadaro, D., & Hughes, R. (2010). Family support in children's mental health: A review and synthesis. *Clinical Child and Family Psychology Review, 13*(1), 1–45. https://doi.org/10.1007/s10567-009-0060-5

Hofmann, S. G., & Hay, A. C. (2018). Rethinking avoidance: Toward a balanced approach to avoidance in treating anxiety disorders. *Journal of Anxiety Disorders, 55*, 14–21. https://doi.org/10.1016/j.janxdis.2018.03.004

Horwitz, A. G., Hill, R. M., & King, C. A. (2011). Specific coping behaviours in relation to adolescent depression and suicidal ideation. *Journal of Adolescence, 34*(5), 1077–1085. https://doi.org/10.1016/j.adolescence.2010.10.004

Ibrahim, K. D. (2015). *Exploring the cultural conceptualisations and understandings of child fostering and the concept of the child's best interests among the Dagomba of Northern Ghana* (PhD dissertation). The University of Edinburgh. Retrieved from https://era.ed.ac.uk/bitstream/handle/1842/33296/Ibrahim2015.pdf?sequence=1&isAllowed=y

Klugman, J., Hanmer, L., Twigg, S., Hasan, T., McCleary-Sills, J., & Santamaria, J. (2014). *Voice and agency: Empowering women and girls for shared prosperity*. The World Bank.

Leadbeater, B., & Way, N. (2001). *Growing up fast: Transitions to early adulthood of inner city adolescent mothers*. Lawrence Erlbaum Associates.

Lerner, R. M. (1984). *On the nature of human plasticity*. Cambridge University Press.

Lerner, R. M. (2009). The positive youth development perspective: Theoretical and empirical bases of strengths-based approach to adolescent development. In S. J. Lopez & C. R. Snyder (Eds.), *Oxford handbook of positive psychology* (pp. 149–163). Oxford University Press.

Masten, A. S. (2001). Ordinary magic: Resilience processes in development. *American Psychologist, 56*(3), 227–235. https://doi.org/10.1037//0003-066X.56.3.227

Masten, A. S. (2007). Resilience in developing systems: Progress and promise as the fourth wave rises. *Development and Psychopathology, 19*(03), 921–930. https://doi.org/10.1017/S0954579407000442

McCleary-Sills, J., Hanmer, L., Parsons, J., & Klugman, J. (2015). Child marriage: A critical barrier to girls' schooling and gender equality in education. *The Review of Faith and International Affairs, 13*(3), 69–80. https://doi.org/10.1080/15570274.2015.1075755

Mwakideu, C. (2016, November 13). *Northern Ghana 'poor' despite NGOs presence*. Retrieved from https://p.dw.com/p/2SdTP

Naatogmah, A. (2016, December 16). *Child marriage rampant in 5 districts of Northern Region-Songtaba*. Retrieved from http://citifmonline.com/2016/12/16/child-marriage-rampant-in-5-districts-of-northern-region-songtaba/

Nguyen, M. C., & Wodon, Q. (2015). Global and regional trends in child marriage. *The Review of Faith & International Affairs, 13*(3), 6–11.

Osafo, J., Asampong, E., Langmagne, S., & Ahiedeke, C. (2014). Perceptions of parents on how religion influences adolescents' sexual behaviours in two Ghanaian communities: Implications for HIV and AIDS prevention. *Journal of Religion and Health, 53*(4), 959–971.

Parsons, J., Edmeades, J., Kes, A., Petroni, S., Sexton, M., & Wodon, Q. (2015). Economic impacts of child marriage: A review of the literature. *The Review of Faith & International Affairs, 13*(3), 12–22.

Pereznieto, P., & Taylor, G. (2014). A review of approaches and methods to measure economic empowerment of women and girls. *Gender and Development, 22*(2), 233–251. https://doi.org/10.1080/13552074.2014.920976

Punch, S. (2002). Research with children: The same or different from research with adults? *Childhood, 9*(3), 321–341.

Santhya, K. G., & Jejeebhoy, S. J. (2003). Sexual and reproductive health needs of married adolescent girls. *Economic and Political Weekly, 38*, 4370–4377. Retrieved from http://www.jstor.org/stable/4414138

Sarfo, E. A., Salifu Yendork, J., & Naidoo, A. V. (2020). Working with married girls: The experiences of professionals on the causes, impact and interventions of child marriage. *Journal of Human Right and Social Work*. https://doi.org/10.1007/s41134-020-00130-4

Saunders, B., Sim, J., Kingstone, T., Baker, S., Waterfield, J., Bartlam, B., et al. (2018). Saturation in qualitative research: Exploring its conceptualisation and operationlisation. *Qualitative & Quantitative, 52*, 1983–1907. https://doi.org/10.1007/s11135-017-0574-8

Sawant, L. D., & Venkat, S. (2013). Comparative analysis of normal versus foetal growth restriction in pregnancy: The significance of maternal body mass index, nutritional status, anaemia, and ultrasonography screening. *International Journal of Reproductive Medicine*. https://doi.org/10.1155/2013/671954

Schweizer, S., Walsh, N. D., Stretton, J., Dunn, V. J., Goodyer, I. M., & Dalgleish, T. (2016). Enhances emotion regulation capacity and its neural substrates in those exposed to moderate childhood adversity. *Social Cognitive and Affective Neuroscience, 11*(2), 272–281.

Smokowski, P. R., Evans, C. B. R., Cotter, K. L., & Guo, S. (2014). Ecological correlates of depression and self-esteem in rural youth. *Child Psychiatry and Human Development, 45*, 500–518. https://doi.org/10.1007/s10578-013-0420-8

Smokowski, P. R., Reynolds, A. J., & Bezruczko, N. (2000). Resilience and protective factors in adolescence: An autobiographical perspective from disadvantaged youth. *Journal of School Psychology, 37*(4), 425–448. https://doi.org/10.1016/S0022-4405(99)00028-X

Svanemyr, J., Chandra-Mouli, V., Raj, A., Travers, E., & Sundaram, L. (2015). Research priorities on ending child marriage and supporting married girls. *Reproductive Health, 12*(1), 1–4. https://doi.org/10.1186/s12978-015-0060-5

Takyi, B. K., & Dodoo, F. N. A. (2005). Gender, lineage, and fertility related outcomes in Ghana. *Journal of Marriage and Family, 67*, 251–257. https://doi.org/10.1111/j.0022-2445.2005.00019.x

Tsekpo, K., Afram, A., Boateng, E. S., & Sefa-Nyarko, C. (2016). *Child marriage in Ghana's fishing industry: Analysing the experience of children who have witnessed or undergone child marriage*. Challenging Heights.

Turner, A. P., Larimer, M. E., Sarason, I. G., & Trupin, E. W. (2005). Identifying a negative mood subtype in incarcerated adolescents: Relationship to substance use. *Addictive Behaviours, 30*(7), 1442–1448.

Ungar, M., Brown, M., Liebenberg, L., Othman, R., Kwong, W. M., Armstrong, M., & Gilgun, J. (2007). Unique pathways to resilience across cultures. *Adolescence, 42*(166), 287–310. Retrieved from http://go.galegroup.com/ps/anonymous?id

United Nations International Children's Emergency Fund [UNICEF]. (2013). *Ending child marriage: Progress and prospects*. UNICEF.

United Nations International Children's Emergency Fund [UNICEF]. (2015). *Child marriage*. Retrieved from https://www.unicef.org/protection/child-marriage

United Nations Population Fund [UNFPA]. (2012). *Marrying too young: End child marriage*. UNFPA.

Vermuelen, T., & Greeff, A. P. (2015). Family resilience resources in coping with child sexual abuse in South Africa. *Journal of Child Sexual Abuse, 24*(5), 555–571. https://doi.org/10.1080/10538712.2015.1042183

Viejo, C., Gómez-López, M., & Ortega-Ruiz, R. (2018). Adolescents' psychological well-being: A multidimensional measure. *International Journal of Environmental Research and Public Health, 15*(10), 2325. https://doi.org/10.3390/ijerph15102325

Walsh, F. (2003). Family resilience: A framework for clinical practice. *Family Process, 42*, 1–18. https://doi.org/10.1111/j.1545-5300.2003.00001.x

Wilson, A., & Somhlaba, N. Z. (2016). Psychological well-being in a context of adversity: Ghanaian adolescents' experiences of hope and life satisfaction. *Africa Today, 63*(1), 85–103.

Wingo, A. P., Wrenn, G., Pelletier, T., Gutman, A. R., Bradley, B., & Ressler, K. J. (2010). Moderating effects of resilience on depression in individuals with a history of childhood abuse or trauma exposure. *Journal of Affective Disorders, 126*, 411–414. https://doi.org/10.1016/j.jad.2010.04.009

Wright, M. O., & Masten, A. S. (2005). Resilience processes in development. In S. Goldstein & R. B. Brooks (Eds.), *Handbook of resilience in children* (pp. 17–37). Springer.

Youssef, N. A., Belew, D., Hao, G., Wang, X., Treiber, F. A., Stefanek, M., et al. (2016). Racial/ethnic differences in the association of childhood adversities with depression and the role of resilience. *Journal of Affective Disorders, 208*, 577–581. https://doi.org/10.1016/j.jad.2016.10.024

Zimmer-Gembeck, M. J., & Skinner, E. A. (2011). The development of coping across childhood and adolescence: An integrative review and critique of research. *International Journal of Behavioural Development, 35*(1), 1–17. https://doi.org/10.1177/0165025410384923

Zolkoski, S. M., & Bullock, L. M. (2012). Resilience in children and youth: A review. *Children and Youth Services Review, 34*(12), 2295–2303. https://doi.org/10.1016/j.childyouth.2012.08.009

Chapter 10
Factors Contributing to Student Wellbeing: Student Perspectives

Irma Eloff, Sumari O'Neil, and Herbert Kanengoni

Abstract Globally, the wellbeing of students in tertiary environments is increasingly linked to long-term educational outcomes at the systemic level. In South Africa, the tertiary sector has seen wide-ranging changes at universities across the country in recent years. Universities have seen calls for decolonised curricula and increased access to higher education, and a strong emphasis is placed on throughput and graduation rates. Such an amplified emphasis on academic outcomes frequently disregards the holistic nature of university education and the importance of the subjective wellbeing experiences of university students. This chapter investigates the factors that students identified as important to their wellbeing at a large residential university in South Africa. Data was collected by means of an open-ended question asked and answered during face-to-face interviews with 2439 students from nine university faculties on five campuses, and the findings were analysed by means of thematic analysis. Students' responses revolved around two major themes: the learning environment (relating to the physical environment as well as the facilities on and around campus) and support structures (including social support systems and facilities). The learning environment and support structures are interlinked and together ensure the fulfilment of student needs and their wellbeing.

Keywords Student wellbeing · Higher education · Learning environment · Social support

I. Eloff (✉)
Department of Educational Psychology, University of Pretoria, Pretoria, South Africa
e-mail: irma.eloff@up.ac.za

S. O'Neil · H. Kanengoni
Department of Human Resource Management, University of Pretoria, Pretoria, South Africa

L. Schutte et al. (eds.), *Embracing Well-Being in Diverse African Contexts: Research Perspectives*, Cross-Cultural Advancements in Positive Psychology 16,
https://doi.org/10.1007/978-3-030-85924-4_10

10.1 Introduction

Among the more than 19,000 universities (International Association of Universities World Higher Education Database [IAU WHED], 2019) in the world, there is a growing recognition that student wellbeing is an integral experience of students in tertiary environments (Di Placito-De Rango, 2018; Harmening & Jacob, 2015). While the academic development of students lies at the heart of the task of the university (Crawford & Johns, 2018), researchers worldwide acknowledge that students need to be prepared to take ownership of their own psychological wellbeing and act appropriately when their wellbeing is at risk (Haynes et al., 2012).

The focus on wellbeing at universities stems in part from the alarming levels of psychological distress that students experience when entering higher education (Field et al., 2015; Govender et al., 2018). Statistics from the World Health Organization (WHO, 2019) for instance indicate that among 15- to 29-year-olds, suicide is the second-highest leading cause of death. This is specifically prevalent in low- and middle-income countries, with 79% of global suicides occurring in these contexts (WHO, 2019). Psychological distress is higher among university students than among the general population (Stallman, 2010). A global study involving 14,000 students from Australia, Belgium, Germany, Mexico, Northern Ireland, South Africa, Spain, and the United States, found that 35% of students reported symptoms consistent with at least one psychological disorder (Auerbach et al., 2018). In the United Kingdom (UK), 29% of students report clinical levels of distress (Laidlaw et al., 2016). Similarly, in North America at least 30% to 40% of students experience increased psychological distress or mental disorders (Howell, 2009). In South Africa specifically, 12% to 15% of university students experience moderate to severe symptoms of depression and anxiety (Bantjes et al., 2017). Although deteriorating psychological health is prevalent in both developed and developing countries, students at South African universities may experience higher levels of psychological distress due to contextual factors, resulting in lower levels of wellbeing (Shefer et al., 2018; Young & Campbell, 2014). Local environmental factors such as the high unemployment rates, the increasing levels of inequality and diversity may play a role in decreased student wellbeing in South Africa (Kotzé & Kleynhans, 2013; Young & Campbell, 2014).

Wellbeing levels seem to be especially low during the first semester of the first year (Field et al., 2015; Salmela-Aro, 2010). Students face many new challenges such as leaving home for the first time, increased academic pressure, increased opportunities for substance abuse and greater financial responsibility (Bantjes et al., 2019; Bowman, 2010; Leese, 2010; Nel et al., 2009; Richardson et al., 2017; Wilson-Strydom, 2011). Levels of distress increase shortly after students enter university and fluctuate during the years of study as students transition between different degree levels (Marais et al., 2018; Turner & Tobbell, 2018). Cooke et al. (2006) note, however, that although distress may decrease in the years of study, it never returns to pre-university levels.

Even if no mental distress is present, optimising levels of wellbeing in student populations is important for their positive psychological functioning (Huppert, 2009). Wellbeing has been shown to aid students in adjusting to university life and to promote achievement of academic goals (Kotzé & Kleynhans, 2013; Stallman et al., 2018). For instance, Howell (2009) found that wellbeing levels predict cognitive and behavioural processes that reflect self-regulated learning, where self-regulated learning is instrumental in student success in the higher education context. Students with higher levels of wellbeing are also more flexible and efficient in problem solving and more committed to their academic goals (Salami, 2010). Freire et al. (2016) found that wellbeing is an essential resource for adaptive coping in a university environment that enables students to adjust to and handle the demands placed on them in the university context (Bewick et al., 2010).

The current study was focused on exploring and identifying the factors that contribute to student wellbeing in South Africa, yet backgrounded within the global context. Previous research by Carroll et al. (2009) identified factors that relate to students' successful functioning in the Australian higher education environment. The model of enablers and barriers that students experience at university was extended by Bowles and Brindle (2017). According to this model, factors can be grouped in three dimensions: situational factors, institutional factors, and dispositional factors. Situational factors relate to a student's life circumstances. Institutional factors relate to the procedures, policies and structures of the institution, which include and encourage student participation in the learning activities. Examples are staff responsiveness, the academic programme design, the relevance of the programme to the student's aspirations, and student support systems. The dispositional factors in turn relate to the student's individual and collectively held beliefs, values and perceptions, such as motivation, goal orientation, self-efficacy, and overall satisfaction. Table 10.1 illustrates the facilitating factors identified in the extended model by Bowles and Brindle (2017).

It is evident from Table 10.1 that situational factors include financial aid and positive support networks, such as peer and family support and having basic needs (e.g., accommodation) met (Goenner & Snaith, 2003). Although family support is important, having a family may also be a stressor if their family responsibilities place high social, financial and psychological demands on the student (Carroll et al., 2009). The institution can support positive psychological functioning by providing support services such as orientation programmes, counselling services, or academic planning services to students (Sutherland et al., 2007). Having positive relationships with lecturers, as well as having mentors available, also supports wellbeing (Wilcox et al., 2005). The culture of the institution (e.g., being culturally sensitive and inclusive of indigenous content in the courses) may further provide an enabling learning context (Wilson et al., 2011). The dispositional factors include student age, behaviour, achievement, social engagement, personality factors, as well as lifestyle choices and habits. Previous academic achievement and academic self-efficacy plays an equally important role (Raelin et al., 2014).

In a study conducted specifically among South African students, group factors that were found to contribute to successful and unsuccessful transitions to university

Table 10.1 Facilitating factors that affect student success at University (Adapted from Bowles & Brindle, 2017)

Situational factors	
Financial	*Attaining a scholarship*
Interpersonal	*Social support from family and friends*
Personal	*Accommodation*
Dispositional factors	
Demographics	*Age group (i.e. more mature)*
	Marital status (i.e. being unmarried)
Student behaviour	*Self-determination*
	Study skills
	Time management skills
	Intention to gain knowledge and skills
	Self-motivation
Goal achievement	*Attaining academic success*
	Education is seen as valuable
	Academic momentum
	Psychological needs of the student are met
Social engagement	*Sense of belonging*
	Campus involement
Institutional factors	
Characteristics at the institution	*Institutional climate*
	Cultural sensitivity
Staff at the institution	*Positive student teacher relationships*
	Mentors
	Availability of staff
	Timely feedback on assignments
Availability of support services	*Transtitions programmes*
	On campus support
	Academic planning services
	Counselling services
	Peer mentoring and study groups
	Student advisors
	Library services

included academic, social, socio-economic, financial, as well as cultural issues (Kotzé & Kleynhans, 2013). Academic issues included students' academic expectations and academic skills e.g., time management skills, independent learning, academic writing skills (Conley & French, 2013 Stallman et al., 2018), whereas social issues included factors related to social and academic integration, as well as peer, parental and lecturer support. When entering university, students often lack a stable social support system (Awang et al., 2014), and poor social support is linked to non-completion of degrees (Laidlaw et al., 2016). In South Africa, parental support has been shown to play an important role in student success (Kotzé &

Kleynhans, 2013). For instance, first-generation students who often come from impoverished backgrounds may be under pressure to graduate, so as to better not only their own lives, but also the lives of their family members (Young & Campbell, 2014). Financial and socio-economic factors pertain to a student's ability to sustain a living and afford a livelihood while studying, and hence the cost of attending university may well contribute to student stress and lack of wellbeing (Bewick et al., 2010; Govender et al., 2018; Laidlaw et al., 2016). While many students rely on grants and loans, they may still have concerns about paying for textbooks, accommodation and transport, and about settling other costs related to their studies (Kotzé & Kleynhans, 2013). Lastly, cultural factors may involve matters of diversity and inclusion. Considering the history of South Africa, the dynamics of racial, religious, linguistic and other dimensions of inclusion may play a nuanced, but important, role in the wellbeing of students.

On another front, Denovan and Macaskill (2017) argue that some specific changes in the higher education context over the last couple of years have contributed to decreased levels of wellbeing among students. Increasing numbers of students in classes often make it difficult for students to make friends and experience a sense of belonging, while the decreasing staff-to-student ratios have made it less likely that students receive personal support. In addition, decreased funding to institutions often means that they cannot provide the psychological and support services that higher numbers of students need. In South Africa the importance of student wellbeing has become increasingly evident with rising numbers of students entering universities. The statistics on post-school education and training in South Africa (Department of Higher Education and Training [DHET], 2018) indicate that a total of 975,837 students were enrolled at universities by 2016. Regular student protests on campuses across the country and limitations in terms of the available resources to provide psychological support (Badat, 2016; Van Breda, 2018) further emphasise the need to understand student wellbeing. At the same time, students are more independent and mobile in their approaches towards learning, which means that they are often removed from traditional sources of support such as student counsellors and peers.

At the University of Pretoria (UP)—a large, public, urban university in the Gauteng province of South Africa—student wellbeing has always been prioritised and it has received even more attention recently. Student wellbeing initiatives are applied in numerous strategic planning processes, and platforms have been created where students can engage on matters of wellbeing on a regular basis. The multifaceted nature of wellbeing is furthermore accepted and awareness campaigns address issues such as financial wellbeing, spiritual wellbeing, health and nutrition, emotional wellbeing and safety. As part of a comprehensive commitment to student wellbeing, a research project consisting of three phases has been conducted to assess student wellbeing. The current chapter focuses on the first phase, which explored the factors that support student wellbeing at UP. The aim of this study was therefore to explore and describe the factors that support student wellbeing at the University of Pretoria.

10.2 Method

10.2.1 Approach and Design

A qualitative approach enabled us as the researchers to explore, without setting prespecified categories, the factors that students view as supporting their wellbeing. Since the main aim was exploring and describing, a basic interpretive design (Merriam, 2002)—or what Percy et al. (2015) refer to as a generic qualitative design—was chosen. The reason for this was that the study did not fit within the parameters of other qualitative designs commonly used in psychology (i.e., case study design, ethnography, phenomenology, narrative analysis or grounded theory).

Generic qualitative designs are typically used for descriptive and exploratory studies that require the use of qualitative data collected by means of surveys and where the focus of the survey is on real events (Percy et al., 2015). Data for this study was collected by means of a questionnaire that posed a single open-ended question to students. The idea was to get a broad range of opinions from a large number of students representing the different faculties, campuses and year groups (Kahlke, 2014). The focus of our study was on the actual content and not on the internal subjective structures (as is the interest of phenomenology), the in-depth description of the phenomenon (as in case study designs) or the socio-cultural aspects of the phenomenon (as in the case of ethnography).

10.2.2 Data Collection

UP was established in 1908 and has grown to serve approximately 50,000 students on seven campuses. In the current study, students ($n = 2513$) at five campuses of the university (i.e., Hatfield, Groenkloof, Mamelodi, Prinshof and Onderstepoort campuses) answered a single question in a face-to-face interview with a student fieldworker: "What contributes to your wellbeing as a student at the University of Pretoria?" The participants were asked to write their answer as well as other biographical details on an answer form. The biographical details included age, gender, degree studied, citizenship, home language and province of origin. Data was collected in multiple four-hour blocks from Monday to Friday over a 10-day period in May 2018. Fieldworkers were selected students from the helping professions (e.g., psychology and social work). Prior to the data collection the fieldworkers were trained in ethical research conduct, strategies for data collection in the social sciences, wellbeing research in the world and the role of a research fieldworker.

The completed questionnaires were returned in sealed envelopes after each data collection session. A separate group of students in the helping professions who were trained as data capturers captured the data on password-protected MS Excel spreadsheets. After all the written questionnaires had been captured electronically, the full data set was cleaned and checked for accuracy.

10.2.3 Participants

The distribution of the participants was a fair reflection of the student population of UP. Altogether 2439 usable responses were retrieved from the 2513 questionnaires collected. Data was deemed unusable if it was spoilt because it was incomplete or illegible, or if the age of the respondents was below 18.

The participants represented various faculties, namely Humanities, Economics and Management Sciences, Law, Education, Theology, Natural and Agricultural Sciences, Health Sciences, Veterinary Sciences and Engineering. Most of the participants (94.5%) were South African citizens. Of the remainder, 78 (3.2%) were citizens from other Southern African Development Community (SADC) countries and 31 (1.3%) hailed from other African countries. Only 22 (0.9%) were citizens of countries outside the African continent. In terms of the gender distribution, more than half (58.1%) were female and 40.5% were male. The age of the participants varied between 18 and 58, with a mean age of 20.6. The majority of the participants (83.4%) were 22 years old or younger, and most were probably undergraduate students.

Most of the participants (61.7%) resided in the Gauteng province. The remainder were from Limpopo (10.5%), Mpumalanga (8.8%) and KwaZulu-Natal (8.0%). A few participants represented the other five provinces (9.8%), which included the Eastern Cape (3.2%), North West (3.0%), Free State (1.9%), Western Cape (1.4%) and Northern Cape (0.3%). Thirty respondents (1.2%) indicated that they were not from a particular province. These students were international students who probably stayed on one of the university's campuses. The discrepancy between the number of non-South African citizens (78) and international students may be explained by the fact that although some students were living in South Africa, they did not hold local citizenship. These students would have chosen a particular province of residence in the province question on the questionnaire.

The study acknowledges that race is a social construction and recognises the pertinent racial and historical cartography of South Africa. Institutional requirements to conduct the study however necessitated data capturing for various biographic variables, including students who identify themselves as African (47.2%), White (41.2%), Indian (6.6%), Mixed race (3.0%) or other (1.5%). The distribution by home language was across all nine of the official language groups in South Africa, with 41.0% of the participants indicating their home language as an African language. Slightly more than half of the remaining participants indicated that they speak either Afrikaans (27.6%) or English (27.2%) at home. Only 81 (3.3%) of the participants indicated that they speak languages other than those listed on the questionnaire (see Table 10.2).

Table 10.2 Characteristics of the participants ($N = 2439$) (Adapted from Eloff, 2021)

	f	%		*f*	%
Province			***Gender***		
Gauteng	1504	61.7	Female	1416	58.1
Limpopo	255	10.5	Male	987	40.5
Mpumalanga	214	8.8	Other	10	0.4
KwaZulu-Natal	195	8.0	Missing values	26	1.1
Eastern Cape	77	3.2			
North West	74	3.0	***Age***		
Free state	47	1.9	18–22	2021	82.9
Western Cape	34	1.4	23–27	349	14.4
Northern Cape	7	0.3	28–32	35	1.4
[a]International	30	1.2	33–37	13	0.5
Missing values	2	0.1	≥38	4	0.2
			Missing values	17	0.7
Language					
Afrikaans	672	27.6	***Ethnicity***		
English	663	27.2	African	1152	47.2
IsiZulu	210	8.6	White	1005	41.2
Sepedi	201	8.2	Indian	160	6.6
Setswana	154	6.3	Mixed race	74	3.0
Sesotho	85	3.5	Other	37	1.5
Xitsonga	83	3.4	Missing values	11	0.5
Other	81	3.3			
isiXhosa	80	3.3	***Citizenship***		
SiSwati	70	2.9	South African	2305	94.6
isiNdebele	69	2.8	SADC	78	3.2
Tshivenda	49	2.0	Non- SADC	31	1.3
Missing values	22	0.9	Non-African	22	0.9
			Missing values	3	0.1

[a]International students that do not reside in South Africa

10.2.4 Data Analysis

Although the data was collected from a large participant group ($N = 2439$), the answers on most of the questionnaires were limited to a few words (see Illustration 10.1) or a couple of sentences (see Illustration 10.2). In most of the responses, the students did not present one single aspect that contributes to their wellbeing, but mentioned a cluster of factors that together support their wellbeing.

Illustration 1 Verbatim extract from the responses containing limited words

> Family support. Friendships. Food

Illustration 2 Verbatim extract from the responses containing more words

> I'd say mainly be at the right state of mind which comes from being at the right place with God (spiritually). Also ensuring I take part in societies on campus that just contribute to empowering me mentally and etc., an example of this would be The Business Women Association student chapter UP. The support structure we also have as students, such as lecturers, tutors and people we can consult about anything happening within our lives, contribute to our wellbeing.

The data was analysed by means of thematic analysis (Braun & Clarke, 2006; Clarke & Braun, 2014). Although thematic analysis lends itself to more than mere description of data (Clarke & Braun, 2018), the analysis for the current chapter was explorative and descriptive in that it aimed to identify and describe the factors that the participants voiced as important for their wellbeing. Descriptive coding uses an inductive approach and was therefore the appropriate choice (Saldaña, 2016). The code also identifies the topics in the data content.

The initial codes, assigned by the principal investigator, identified during the familiarisation phase were refined and finalised during the two coding cycles that followed. These cycles were completed by the second author using Atlas.ti 8. After the coding process the codes were grouped into themes. Themes where identified according to Boyatzis's (1998) view that themes may be identified on a manifest level—directly from the observable information—and that they can function as a way to categorise the data into groups of repeating ideas.

After several coding cycles themes and subthemes were identified and discussed with the first author. The themes were grouped and synthesised into two overarching or integrative themes: *learning environment* and *support structures*. The overarching themes and their subthemes will be described in the findings section.

The authors employed the 15-point checklist proposed by Braun et al. (2016) to ensure good practice in conducting the thematic analysis and confirm that the analysis process was "rigorous, deliberate and reflexive" (p. 16). Data was checked for accuracy before the coding started. Each data item was subjected to the coding process in each of the coding cycles to ensure inclusive and comprehensive coding. Using Atlas.ti 8 ensured better data management of coded extracts. Through iterative movement between coding and thematising, the codes and themes were checked against each other and against the original dataset until coherent, consistent and distinctive themes emerged.

10.2.5 Ethical Considerations

Ethics approval for the project was obtained from the relevant institutional ethics committee (Ethics Committee of the Faculty of Humanities, Ref GW0180232HS).

Having been thoroughly trained in the ethical requirements related to data collection, the fieldworkers explained the requirements of participation to each of the participants before they were given the questionnaire. The questionnaire did not ask the participants to identify themselves through student numbers or names. However, demographic details, for instance age, field of study and home language were captured. The huge volume of data and the nature of the question made it difficult to link the responses to a specific person. However, the data was not completely anonymous because of the fact that the answers were collected in a face-to-face situation. Keeping the data confidential was therefore a priority to the research team. Each of the data capturers signed a confidentiality agreement. Data was subsequently sent to the data capturers in a password-protected file and they deleted the files from their computers once the data had been sent back to the research team. Participation was completely voluntary since no incentives were attached. Thirty-nine of the students were under 18, and since informed consent was not obtained from their legal guardians, their data was deleted from the dataset before analysis.

10.3 Findings

The findings are presented in terms of the themes that emerged and then discussed by extracting samples from the raw data. The biographical variables of the participants are also included in order to depict the diversity of participants from various subject fields at the university.

10.3.1 Learning Environment

The learning environment mentioned in the student responses relates to the facilities on campus and in the university residences. These include the library and adequate study facilities; the outside spaces; the information technology, accessible Wi-Fi and online learning systems; safety and security on campus; shops and the availability of food facilities; as well as transportation services. These factors causally relate to students' wellbeing. Facilities related to the basic needs of feeling safe and secure as well as having access to food came across strongly in the responses.

For a 19-year-old female Visual Arts student being safe was the first on the list of factors that contribute to her wellbeing: *"First being the safe and tight security system that has been established in the school."* Some students mentioned concerns regarding security at the smaller campuses. For instance, a 20-year-old female BSc Biological Sciences student said: *"The safety of the campus. Being that Mamelodi is situated outside of Hatfield* [the suburb in which the main campus is situated], *is rather secluded, safety of students is important. A positive frame of mind regarding the campus and a feeling of safety contributes greatly to the achievements academically of students."*

The concern for safety was probably strong because of recent and ongoing protests around higher education institutions in South Africa since 2016 (Griffiths, 2019). As a 19-year-old male BSc Physics student noted: *"The University of Pretoria is one of the safest institutions in South Africa due to 24 hours security. I hardly see any strikes from its employees that could put my studies on standby."* After the 2016 protests, security was significantly increased on the campus and this was mentioned by a 22-year-old male Mechanical Engineering student when he said: *"Safety... Security with regards to strikes."*

For other students, the concern of security related more to being on campus at night. A 20-year-old female Theology student said: *"The security on campus. Usually students come to campus at night and the fact that there are security guards at the library and entrance gates makes the campus much safer."* A 19-year-old female Law student appreciated *"...feeling safe when I leave campus late, being walked by the security"*.

Of course one can understand how security relates to student wellbeing and this was highlighted by a 28-year-old male Theology student: *"The fact that the security is tight and I feel safe when I am around campus, makes me concentrate more on my studies, I don't have to worry about safety but I only have to worry about my studies."*

Many students simply noted *"food"* as part of their responses, for example:

> Being around my loved ones, doing well in all my modules and food. (23-year-old female student, no degree stated)

> Fitness, running, food and how I manage my time in varsity. (29-year-old male student, studying Law).

A 19-year-old male Geology student promptly noted *"...[l]ike the food it's one of the only things that keep me going"*. For the most part, the responses related to food were cryptic and did not provide much detail with regard to the food choices or reasons for food being an important factor related to wellbeing. Some respondents did add a hunch that they referred to the food provided by the residence, as a 24-year-old female Law student stated: *"Good food from residence."* A 20-year-old female Occupational Therapy student said: *"The healthy food options that our cafeteria offers"*, noting that both the existence of food facilities on campus and the type of food may play a role in students' wellbeing.

The accessibility of *"[a]ll the shops like bookmark and coffee shops makes my life easier on campus"* said a 23-year-old male BSc Chemistry student. This indicates that facilities other than food shops in and around campus also contributed to student wellbeing. More students however noted food and coffee shops in their responses than they did any other type of shop. Especially coffee shops resonated with the idea of facilities created for socialising with friends. A 20-year-old female BSc Human Physiology student illustrated this in her response: *"I enjoy the coffee shops as well - where you can sit and relax."*

"Balancing university, social life, sport and family. It is important for me to make time for the things that I enjoy" remarked a 20-year-old female Agricultural Science

student. Considering this sentiment, it came as no surprise that recreational facilities were an important factor for students in maintaining their wellbeing. Recreational facilities include sports facilities as well as spaces for relaxation on campus.

Many students indicated that they enjoy the sports facilities. The following excerpts from the data illustrate this point:

> I play soccer on Tuesdays and Thursdays that help me a lot to deal with stress. Playing soccer helps me to train my mind and help me to focus much on school work. (20-year-old male student, no degree stated)

> Rugby for the university (20-year-old male student studying Agricultural Sciences)

> Our faculty has a netball team on which I participate and it relaxes my mind, at the same time it keeps my body fit/healthy (18-year-old female student, studying Agricultural Science)

Together with many other students, a 19-year-old female Accounting student saw exercise as "*a very important factor as it helps me destress when I feel like I am drowning in my studies*". However, numerous students who probably did not participate in organised sports still enjoyed the spaces that allow walks in between classes, as indicated by a 22-year-old male Electronic Engineering student: "*The distance between classes allows for a short exercise walk.*" A 22-year-old female BSc Social Work student also noted that she enjoyed walks during breaks between classes.

Besides exercising, students also mentioned that they need a "*Chill-out zone*" (20-year-old female Education student). This is a "*place you can relax on campus between lectures*" (19-year-old female Geology student). It may involve "*entertainment on campus*" (21-year-old male Meteorology student), but also "*[o]pen space to sit and relax between lectures*" (29-year-old male student, doing a PhD in Chemistry).

Many students noted the serenity of the outside spaces on campus. "*The open grass spaces to hang out and get some fresh air in breaks*", mentioned a 29-year-old female student, doing a PhD in Biochemistry. "*The atmosphere as well as the ability to sit under a tree between classes to destress*", said an 18-year-old Zoology student. An 18-year-old female BSc Biological Sciences student described the outside spaces as "*peaceful*", while her 18-year-old female class mate noted that the "*[sc]enery of the university (Trees, grass, buildings) definitely help to make the environment "pretty" and contributes to good wellbeing*".

A 24-year-old male Financial Sciences student and a 22-year-old female French honours student remarked that the fact that the environment was clean and well taken care of was an important factor in their wellbeing. The condition of the facilities did not apply to the outside spaces only, but to all the facilities. For instance, a 31-year-old female student, doing a PhD in Genetics, explained: "*Equipment that works such as overhead projectors and computers. These devices eases learning but if they don't work it can be greatly frustrating.*"

The condition of the facilities provided by the university was just as important as their cleanliness. A 20-year-old female Biochemistry student promptly noted that a *"clean campus"* contributes to her wellbeing. *"Bathrooms and classrooms that are neat and clean, helps to give a sense of professionalism"* said a 21-year-old Education student. A 22-year-old female Medical student responded *"[a] clean and comfortable space (campus and facilities) that make it easy for me to learn/ study/practice"*, while a 22-year-old male BCom Financial Sciences student stated that *"[c]leanliness, a clean environment promotes a productive day"*.

In terms of learning spaces, students noted that an adequate study environment was important to their wellbeing. This included the library, study facilities, the online learning system and other facilities related to information technology and internet connectivity. *"The library is helpful, one can borrow a book and librarians are helpful"* said a 19-year-old male BCom Accounting Sciences student. The library not only contributed to students' wellbeing by providing resources such as books, it also provided a space for studying. An 18-year-old female Radiology student said: *"I go to the library and study alone quietly."* The library also provided an overall resources centre with facilities to print, connect to the internet or use a computer. A 19-year-old female Medical student referred to the library as a "*place to study and print*", while a 27-year-old male Biological Sciences student remarked: *"The Mamelodi library* (library on the Mamelodi campus) *helps entirely when it comes to my assignments and tasks which overall contribute to my wellbeing."*

Some students were very specific as to which aspects of the learning environment contributed to their wellbeing: *"The learning environment such as lecture halls, the library and the labs are well conducive for teaching and learning"* (26-year-old female Education student). A Mechanical Engineering student thought that "*[t]he learning environment such as lecture halls, the library and the labs are well conducive for teaching and learning. It is great to be a student at UP, I like the way we study, the clickUP* [Blackboard online learning system] *tests lecture slides that are online make every everything ease even when you missed the lecture you still going to find what was done in class, click up tests every week make me know where we are, and make me feel happy about being a student at UP."*

The internet accessibility on campus was mentioned by numerous students: "*The Wi-Fi on campus helps with studies and research*", said a 20-year-old male Business Management student. A student of Food Sciences shared thoughts along similar lines: *"Also the computer facilities that are available on campus for students like me who do not have access to the internet at home, it enables us to be able to access information on the internet"*. Access to the internet as well as computer facilities on campus helps students who do not have these facilities at home. For example, a 21-year-old female Commerce student noted: *"The computer labs and the wifi help me do my school work so I won't have to worry about data and computers I do not have"*. Internet connectivity specifically did not only enable students to connect to the online learning system and access online information, but also to connect with their family and friends:

> Wi-fi which allows me to keep in contact with the university, friends and family. (20-year-old female Education student).

The online learning system (called clickUP at UP) was in itself seen as important to the respondents' wellbeing: *"Blackboard helps to keep me up to date and that I didn't miss any important dates"* (20-year-old female Education student).

The last important facility mentioned by the respondents was transportation to and among campuses:

> A bus (shuttle) service which transports us to and from campus - making travel to university (Mamelodi campus) safer under more controlled circumstances. (18-year-old female BSc student)

> The transportation to Mamelodi is reliable, the drivers are kind. (21-year-old female Physics student)

> In general attending university can be stressful and therefore contributes negatively to my wellbeing. However, some things are a true light at the end of the tunnel. Such as the golf carts that transport us from the entrance to the parking area and back. (22-year-old female Nursing student)

> Being able to get from the Gautrain station to Groenkloof campus each day safely and vice versa. The buses from Hatfield campus even though it would be nice if there were buses directly from the train to main campus. This affects many students." (19-year-old female Education student)

The factors described in this section show the importance of a quality learning environment in influencing students' wellbeing. From our analysis, we included the following facilities under quality learning environment: security; food and shops in and around campus; recreational facilities; the library and other venues where learning activities take place; transportation services; and facilities related to information technology (including laboratories, printing facilities, online learning system and internet connectivity). From the responses it was also clear that the outside spaces on campus contribute to students' wellbeing. The existence of these facilities, their accessibility, as well as their condition have an important effect on the respondents' wellbeing. The quality learning environment therefore relates to the physical infrastructure and facilities offered by the institution.

10.3.2 Support Structures

The single factor that was mentioned most by the respondents was the social support provided by their peers. Or as a 24-year-old male Economics student stated: *"Peer communication. Connections."* Peers include classmates, friends and other university students whom the respondents meet and interact with. According to a 22-year-old female Law student, *"[m]y wellbeing is contributed by my friends at the university. They help with everyday life and support you."*

The notion of interaction and communication with peers as a form of support came out strongly in the responses:

> Eating well, talking to people about my issues and working out. (22-year-old female student, degree not given)

> Interactions with other students outside the classroom. (26-year-old female Veterinary student)

> Happy study environment with a comfortable social interaction between students. (32-year-old male Veterinary Nursing student)

However, for some respondents it was not so much about the interaction with peers as about the company: *"It's not even about talking about your life, just the company makes the ride easier"* (21-year-old female Computer Sciences student). This sense of belonging that peer connection provides was strongly indicated in their responses:

> Student interaction - study groups, similar struggles (you're not alone), figuring out what you've missed in classes, different perspectives to learning. (23-year-old female Law student)

> I also need friends and or a support system to help me through difficult times and make me feel that I belong. (19-year-old female Consumer Sciences student)

Belonging emphasises the importance of friendships and the social support that comes from social and sport clubs, as well as societies at the universities. As a 19-year-old female student (no degree stated) said: *"Inclusiveness, being part of social groups/sports/committees."* A 19-year-old male Business Management student agreed with this and remarked: *"Being part of degree and day house helped me grow into a student that actually enjoys university. Trying to be a part of everything definitely contributes to the wellbeing of a student."*

It is interesting that some respondents noted that the diversity of the student body they interacted with contributed to their wellbeing. For example, a 24-year-old female Education student observed: *"Engaging in different groups around the campus; the diversity of the campus, since we have different backgrounds and how we think are different, we share our ideas, and that helps a lot*". Her sentiment was shared by a 19-year-old female Law student: *"Diversity of many students on campus helps to contribute to my wellbeing."*

From the responses related to social support by peers it was clear that the residences and day houses provided important locations for friendships to be made and interactions to take place. Similar to societies and clubs on campus, residences also provided a sense of belonging and emotional support. For instance, a 21-year-old female BSc Biological Sciences student mentioned: *"Definitely being part of residence culture. Having a support system in residence has really contributed to my wellbeing … Doing residence activities has helped a lot with the balance in my life."* Similarly, an 18-year-old female Law student said: *"Staying in Res* [the residence] *allows me to have many channels that can help with my wellbeing. We have wellbeing sessions every Wednesday and we learn how to deal with stressors of university. There is also student support that also helps me when I am not coping."*

Another important support structure mentioned by the respondents was family:

> Communication with my family back at home. (21-year-old male Medical Sciences student)

> My mom and dad for helping get past the course and other family members also supporting. (19-year-old male Commerce student)

> Having a brother who supports and encourages me is also helpful to me. (22-year-old male Physiology student)

Spirituality and religion constituted another factor that students reported to contribute to their wellbeing. *"Going to church and having a small group that knows what you going through and supports you"*, an 18-year-old female Medical Sciences student declared. Her statement was echoed by a 21-year-old female Medical student: *"My wellbeing comes from things like church activities and groups."*

On the other hand, spirituality and religion to some of the respondents went beyond the social gathering and support provided by a church, and included also being spiritual and finding meaning in a god:

> I am a very spiritual person, meaning that my God is important to me which helps me a lot in whatever situation I encounter. (20-year-old female Education student)

> Happy and knowing that God is protecting and guiding me in all that I do as a student contributes to my wellbeing. (23-year-old female Nursing student)

In terms of support structures provided by the university as an institution, academic support provided by lecturers and tutors, as well as student support services were mentioned. A 19-year-old male Actuarial Sciences student noted: *"The university also has faculty advisors, a health care centre of which is very beneficial to me."* The healthcare centres that he referred to offered support by medical staff as well as psychologists and counsellors. *"Having doctors and nurses around campus for whenever I am not feeling well"*, said a 20-year-old female Human Genetics student. A 26-year-old female Education student remarked that *"[t] here is great student support such as FSA's* (Faculty student advisors) *who assisted me with academic, personal and career goals"*. The student also mentioned specific university-wide initiatives that support student wellbeing: *"FLY@UP workshops and activators also disseminate useful information that helps students such as exam preparations and health and wellness."*

For other students, access to psychological support was important: *"The fact that I can see a psychologist whenever I have stress or I am under pressure with my school work. Ease of access to support from staff regarding academic issues/needs. Support structures in a place for students with any issues or problems"*—as stated by a 20-year-old female Human Genetics student.

The role of supportive lecturers at the university seemed to be integrally linked to the wellbeing of students. Students mentioned various aspects that support their learning, among which they indicated the role of supportive lecturers. For instance, a 20-year-old male Information Sciences student said: *"I will conclude by saying the lecturers for my course also contribute to my wellbeing because they are very supportive to me, in general to all their students and they all want what is best for us; which is to succeed.*"

"*Attitudes and enthusiasm of lecturers*", responded a 20-year-old female Education student, and an 18-year-old male Actuarial Economics student said: "*Most lecturers seem to have sincere concern about me*". According to a 19-year-old female BA student, "*(l)ecturers that are well scheduled; lecturers who are understanding and willing to help*" contribute to her wellbeing.

"*The lecturers are always willing to help when you have specific questions.*" So said a 20-year-old female Industrial Engineering student when she considered the factors supporting her wellbeing at university.

"*Having lecturers who give their best during lessons as we do during exams and the submission of assignments*", commented a 20-year-old female Education student. A 21-year-old male Public Administration student agreed along the same lines: "*My personal wellbeing at UP stems from in terms of academics, being able to attend lectures with component lecturers who teach my modules as well as having free and open use to all the academic tools and support I need.*"

Not only did the lecturer's concern and teaching play a role in the respondents' wellbeing, but also the involvement of tutors who provide academic support.

> We get extra help from the tutors and the lecturers to make sure to go through the work and make sure that we understand it as good as possible. (19-year-old female student, no degree stated)

> The tutors that provide us with extra work to help improve our studies. (18-year-old female Law student)

To summarise, responses related to support structures included the social support provided by peers and family, academic support provided by lecturers and tutors, as well as medical support provided by psychologists, doctors and nurses at the clinics and medical centres on campus.

10.4 Discussion

The findings from this study highlight particular aspects of student wellbeing at a large urban university in South Africa. The intricate links between the *learning environment* and student wellbeing are evident. Students mention the reciprocal effect between their wellbeing and the physical environment repetitively, across campuses and from a wide variety of study fields. They refer to "big picture" aspects such as the aesthetic dimensions of campuses, but they also zoom in on seemingly minute aspects, such as the temperature in lecture halls and the efficiency of teaching technology. In terms of students' perception of the influence of the different aspects that make up a quality learning environment, our findings are similar to those of Muhammad et al. (2014). They described the academic buildings on campuses as a physical resource that may provide in various student needs, including the need for comfort, health and safety; quality facilities; and provision for areas of study, socialisation, relaxation and recreation. Specifically, academic buildings on university campuses need to enhance and foster both knowledge creation and knowledge dissemination.

Muhammad et al. (2014) found that buildings should not only serve as a place of learning, but also have a restorative capacity to help students overcome mental fatigue. Their findings indicate that academic buildings may have positive or negative effects on learning activities. To have a positive impact, buildings should be comfortable, have the correct temperature, lighting, control for noise, comfortable seating and enough space to accommodate the number of students. Spacious and well-equipped classes were also found to be an important factor relating to students' overall satisfaction with the institution in another South African study by Tait and De Jager (2009).

Students' emphasis on the importance of the built and natural environment also supports the dynamic campus learning model of Strange and Banning (2001), which emphasises the interdependence of the physical environment and learning behaviour. According to this model, the physical conditions, design and layout of the campus are a key component in influencing student behaviour. In the current study, great emphasis was placed on the tranquillity of the outside landscape on campus. This was also an aspect mentioned by Muhammad et al. (2014), in that the greenery and landscape of the external environment had a positive psychological effect on their respondents. Abraham et al. (2010) found that the external environment is a health resource that promotes physical, mental and social wellbeing. From our student responses it was clear that the greenery was restorative to the students, in that they could relax and recuperate by "sitting on the grass" and "walking between buildings". The restorative function of landscapes as described by Abraham et al. (2010) can be explained according to four characteristics. Firstly, they allow distance from one's daily life; secondly, they attract attention without being tiring; thirdly, they enable discovery of new things; and lastly, they are in line with the needs of the user. The latter implies that the landscape enables its users to do what they want to do, for example allowing students to get more exercise by walking between classes. The study of Abraham et al. (2010) also explains that the natural environment reduces stress and enables people to express positive feelings. According to Seligman (2011), expressing positive emotions is a key pathway to wellbeing.

Access to facilities such as wi-fi, computers and printers, was also an important aspect noted by the respondents in our study. Similar results were found in the study by Muhammad et al. (2014) who found that access to the internet enhanced both learning and social interaction. In agreement with the current study, Muhammad et al. (2014) also found that computers and office equipment are important for students, but doubted if it is economically feasible to provide such facilities in buildings. The students in the current study noted that these facilities were available in the library, which made the library a "one-stop shop" for completing assignments and university work. This may be especially true for campuses that are remote and situated in rural areas that are further away from shops and facilities.

Students in the current study stressed the importance of adequate study facilities, which according to them required a quiet space on campus. Muhammad et al. (2014) found that study facilities should be optimal for different modes of study. Self-study facilities should be provided for quiet self-study, and other spaces should be available for group discussions. Students in the current study seemed to prefer the facilities available in the library for study purposes on campus. The fact that the library seemed to play an important role in student wellbeing supports the findings of Bowles and Brindle (2017), namely that it is an institutional facilitating factor that can affect student satisfaction and retention.

Accessibility to refreshments was an important contributing factor to student wellbeing, and according to Muhammad et al. (2014), learning is a demanding mental activity for which replenished nourishment is important. In their study, the students demanded that refreshments should be readily available at vending machines. Although the buildings at UP provide vending machines, students did not note them specifically, but rather focused on the restaurants, coffee shops and food stores that are on campus. Interestingly, our study found that access to refreshments did not only serve a recuperative function, but also gave students a chance to interact with one another. It therefore links to what Abraham et al. (2010) referred to as a structure for bonding.

Findings that are more unique in the current study include comments related to transportation services and the safety and security of students. In another South African study by Shefer et al. (2018), safety was a central narrative especially with regard to female students. The need for safety and security can be traced back to students' basic human needs as defined by various theorists such as Maslow (1970) and Murray (1938), who all consider safety as an inherent human need and linked to behaviour. While shelter and safety are *deficiency needs* in Maslow's theory, they should be satisfied before *being needs* such as self-actualisation are attended to. The basic need for safety as conceptualised by Maslow (1970) was later used to conceptualise the dynamic campus learning model of Strange and Banning (2001), in which safety is one of the four major elements on university campuses that have an impact on student learning. Glasser (1999) stressed the importance of individual basic needs in understanding behaviour and specified five basic needs that should be met for psychological and physiological health to be achieved, namely survival, love and belonging, power, freedom, and fun (Burns et al., 2006). Students' safety, as well as their need for food and shelter, is categorised under the physiological need of survival. This implies that wellbeing can only be achieved if the five basic needs are sufficiently met. A study involving first-year Turkish students revealed that survival was the least met need of students, yet the mean scores indicated that it was not a deficiency (Turkdogan & Duru, 2012). The researchers argued that food and shelter needs are met at the minimum level and may be a natural (an inherent) aspect of university life. Although this may explain the responses regarding food in the current study, the major concern for safety is not sufficiently explained by their (Turkdogan & Duru, 2012) argument. It strongly suggests that contextual factors such as the current climate in South African higher education, and possibly high crime levels in the country overall, may be related to the students' concerns. It may also indicate that safety and security is a larger society-wide problem within our study. This view is supported by the study of Gbadamosi and De Jager (2009), who found that students of two South African universities rated security and safety conditions on campus as the most important services the institutions should offer. Their finding can be contrasted to a study conducted in the United States in which safety did not emerge at all as a theme relating to students' experiences of wellbeing on campus (Harmening & Jacob, 2015).

Many of the students in the current study mentioned transportation services between the different campuses and between home and campus as important to their wellbeing. In the study conducted by Gbadamosi and De Jager (2009), transportation was found to be especially important to students living farther away from the university. These students' satisfaction with their transportation was directly correlated to trust in management and how students perceived the university administration. Trust in management also significantly predicted students' satisfaction with the institution where they were studying.

In terms of the *support structures,* our study indicated the importance of social support from family members and peers, as well as academic support from lecturers and tutors. From a Study Demands Resources (SD-R) model (Mokgele & Rothmann, 2014), social support from lecturers as well as peers can also be viewed as study resources. Resources in the case of the SD-R model are those factors that promote student engagement and help them cope with the demands of student life. Social integration and the need for positive relationships are also important factors in various wellbeing theories, including Ryff's (1995) Psychological Wellbeing and Seligman's (2011) PERMA model of wellbeing. Relationships take an eudaimonic perspective on wellbeing (Chang et al., 2015) and are linked to the basic human need of wanting to be part of a social network, as well as being able to make and maintain social relationships (Deci & Ryan, 2008; Glasser, 1999; Maslow, 1970). Social support is significantly positively related to wellbeing of university students (Stallman et al., 2018) and has been identified as offering protection against psychological distress (Väisänen et al., 2017). It is also a situational factor in the model of Bowles and Brindle (2017) that facilitates positive learning behaviour.

For university students, it is especially important to be part of a peer group (Nel et al., 2009). Peers are seen both as friends and as mentors (Harmening & Jacob, 2015). An important site for peer interaction is residences and societies. Especially residences offer vested programmes that focus on student wellbeing through mentorship and support groups. Residences also foster social integration (Nel et al., 2009). The importance of residences in fostering student engagement was highlighted by Harmening and Jacob (2015) and Bowles and Brindle (2017) identified the student residence as a dispositional factor that facilitates positive learning behaviour.

An important theme in our study was that students linked residence life to a sense of belonging and being included. Glasser (2001) defined belonging as a student's need to be with others and be part of a wider network of cooperative relationships. According to Strange and Banning (2001), inclusion is linked to safety, in that students feel safe and free to be themselves within a group. Residence activities, campus activities and society membership, as well as being part of religious activities, all gave students in the current study a sense of belonging. This is in line with the student involvement theory of Astin (1984, p. 518), who describes involvement as the "physical and psychological energy that the student devotes to the academic experience". Involvement directly affects student development, both on an academic level and on a social, emotional and psychological level. Involvement implies not only time in class and time on learning tasks, but also time spent on campus, participation in student organisations, interaction with faculty members and peers. Involvement creates feelings of connectedness and student satisfaction (Krumrei-Mancuso et al., 2013). This view is supported in the model of Bowles and Brindle (2017), in which a sense of belonging is a facilitating dispositional factor for positive learning behaviours. Learning from others' world views has a positive impact on student wellbeing (Harmening & Jacob, 2015). Therefore, it is not surprising that students in the current study also noted that the diversity on campus and in the class enhanced their sense of belonging.

Being part of the residence or campus community also fits in with Maslow's (1970) need for self-actualisation through membership of a community. In Strange and Banning's (2001) model, community would imply being an involved member who engages in meaningful and purposeful activities within the larger campus community. In the current study, students mentioned the sense of community in their residence and student societies, but they mostly valued being part of the larger campus of like-minded individuals, working towards the same goals.

Although positive relationships with peers (friends and classmates) were the most mentioned factor that contributed to students' wellbeing, the important role of academic staff (both lectures and tutors) was also mentioned. According to Bowles and Brindle (2017), positive student-lecturer relationships were found to be a facilitating institutional factor. In a South African study by Tait and De Jager (2009), it was found that approachable and well-informed academic staff was the most important factor relating to academic issues that students selected from a list of eight factors. It was also slightly more important to senior students than to their junior counterparts. The impact of involvement with faculty/lecturers is furthermore related to students' self-efficacy (Harmening & Jacob, 2015). Similar to the current finding about the value of genuine care, Harmening and Jacob (2015, p. 8) noted that the "importance of faculty who seemed to truly care about them, cared about their lives, and encouraged them along their educational pathways" was an important contributing factor to wellbeing. Väisänen et al. (2017) argue that social support from the lecturer includes emotional (i.e., empathy, trust and caring), informational (i.e., useful information to deal with daily and task stressors) and instrumental support (i.e., guidance in terms of task feedback). Nielsen et al. (2017) maintain that lecturer support is important to student wellbeing for two reasons. Firstly, the social support from lecturers provides the social and emotional assistance through comfort, care and encouragement and will therefore assist the students in appraising situations more positively. Secondly, instructor support provides material resources such as practical advice and assistance on how to deal with university demands. Social support from family was also mentioned by the students in our study. It is interesting that Nielsen et al. (2017) found that family support compensates for low instructor support, which shows that both instructor support and family support play an important and interactive role in student wellbeing.

According to Bowles and Brindle (2017), on-campus support structures are an institutional factor that facilitates positive learning behaviour and student retention. Students in the current study found the social, emotional and physical support given by psychologists, student advisors, clinic doctors and nurses to be invaluable to their wellbeing.

10.5 Limitations and Strengths of the Study

Limitations of the study include lack of in-depth questioning and opportunities for follow-up with specific participants. The lack of in-depth questioning is mostly due to the hard-copy questionnaire mode used. Whereas open-ended questionnaires are known not to produce in-depth detailed answers, research suggests that hard-copy versions deliver even shorter answers than their electronic counterparts (Denscombe, 2007). However, owing to the exploratory nature of our research, the research team aimed to reach larger numbers of students for insight, rather than fewer for more in-depth answers. Although open-ended questions in questionnaires allow elaborate and comprehensive answers, they do not leave room for further questioning, unless the details of the participant are captured. Further limitations might include possible language barriers, the fact that data was only collected during the first semester of the academic year, and the fact that fieldworkers were predominantly female.

The large sample size ($n = 2439$) counterbalanced some of the limitations of the study and good geographical coverage was achieved across all university campuses (among undergraduate students). The sample was fairly representative and showed high diversity. The frank and succinct responses, that is, "first thoughts", which were elicited with the direct face-to-face method, also potentially contributed to authentic responses on student wellbeing. Student-to-student interaction for data collection further contributed to a high-quality data set.

10.6 Implications for Theory and Practice

The deliberate connection between physical environments, spaces and aesthetics within learning environments signals the importance of understanding subjective human wellbeing within its environmental situatedness (Evans & McCoy, 1998). For researchers studying student wellbeing, it also supports the trend towards increasing inter-and transdisciplinary research within wellbeing studies. Where and how students learn directly affects their wellbeing. As such, learning environments can enhance or confine student wellbeing and they should be designed and developed accordingly.

Within the overarching theme of support structures, the consistent theme of lecturer support as a key factor in enhancing student wellbeing is pertinent for a variety of reasons. First, while students indicate lecturer support as important to their wellbeing, this aspect is rarely acknowledged as a critical performance area for university lecturers. Rather, the performance of university lecturers is measured in terms of throughput rates, the academic success of students and their own research outputs. Supporting the wellbeing of the students under their tutelage is seldom captured on performance output agreements of academic staff members. Yet, the students in this study consistently emphasise the caring, accessible and supportive nature of their lecturers as critical to their wellbeing. Students in our study also acknowledge the important role of student counsellors and psychologists, but they often do so in conjunction with describing their interactions with their lecturers. This finding—the role of lecturers in the wellbeing of students—therefore has clear implications for the ways in which the work of university lecturers should be articulated, conceptualised and acknowledged. Secondly, the role that well-prepared and supportive lecturers play in respect of student wellbeing speaks to the nature of the teaching and learning dynamics in tertiary lecture halls. While current trends in the use of technology are creating dynamic learning environments that afford creative opportunities to optimise learning, findings from this study indicate that university students are still attaching value to the personal interaction with their lecturers. When distance and online learning modules are considered, creative measures should be taken not to lose the interaction between lecturers and students.

It is important to note that students also allude to the role of *well-prepared* lecturers when they consider factors that support their wellbeing. They mention the enthusiasm of lecturers during lectures, and them "giving their best". Students in the current study highlighted the indirect support to student wellbeing provided by lecturers who are passionate about their own teaching. Students rely on their lecturers for academic support and in some cases this may inadvertently provide emotional support. It is therefore important to invest effort into supporting academics by putting in place mechanisms to encourage, enhance and develop academic staff's teaching, studying and advisory skills. This can be done through staff induction seminars, workshops, peer support and mentoring. In addition, ongoing technical training of both academic and support staff is necessary to ensure quality service to the students.

The subthemes related to *safety and security, infrastructure,* and *residence* elucidate aspects that are not necessarily always consciously connected to student wellbeing. Yet, participants in this study provided ample evidence of these aspects supporting their wellbeing. Therefore, when investment in student wellbeing at universities is considered, decision makers should take a holistic view that correlates student wellbeing comprehensively with a wide variety of systemic factors that support student wellbeing.

Academic and student support services are also frequently related directly to matters of student wellbeing (Basson & Rothmann, 2018; Daniels & Jooste, 2018). Data from this study confirms this position and reiterates the importance of accessible psychological and health support services for students on or near campus, especially in light of the high student numbers in today's universities.

Finally, an analysis of the individual responses of the student participants in this study shows that their 'wellbeing responses' almost always referred to only two or three domains of wellbeing. Even though students provided clusters of responses, it was only in rare instances that students referred to factors from several domains of wellbeing (for instance, relationships *and* positive emotions *and* engagement *and* meaning *and* achievement) when they considered the factors supporting their wellbeing. This phenomenon bodes well for the future design of student wellbeing interventions, because thematic expansion would in all likelihood find fertile ground.

10.7 Conclusion

Wellbeing research has grown exponentially in the last two decades. Student wellbeing research at the tertiary level is, however, still an emerging field, with many aspects of student wellbeing for today's students being under-explored and specifically under-reported. Furthermore, it is becoming increasingly clear that students consider the university experience to extend well beyond the academic task for students. Student experiences are influenced by their satisfaction with academic and social aspects of their learning. However, satisfaction with both academic and social life on campus is also influenced by students' satisfaction with the facilities and learning services. Physical aspects of the learning environment may influence student interaction, participation and inclusiveness, access to quality facilities, as well as comfort.

The current study highlighted the importance of the quality of the learning environment as well as the support of lecturers and peers to improve student wellbeing. The study also revealed aspects in support of student wellbeing that might not be thought to be directly connected to student wellbeing, yet which clearly supported the wellbeing of the students in this study. In the South African context, safety and security in particular seemed to be an important contextual factor related to student wellbeing. Safety, student residences and existing student support mechanisms may be factors that protect and enhance students' wellbeing.

Since university students nowadays function in a digitally driven world, a stronger emphasis needs to be placed on aspects of human connection, engagement and wellbeing during their years of study. Our study points to the fact that higher education institutions bear acute responsibility for helping their students to develop their own wellbeing and for supporting the wellbeing of the learning communities within which they operate.

References

Abraham, A., Sommerhalder, K., & Abel, T. (2010). Landscape and well-being: A scoping study on the health-promoting impact of outdoor environments. *International Journal of Public Health, 55*(1), 59–69. https://doi.org/10.1007/s00038-009-0069-z

Astin, A. W. (1984). Student involvement: A developmental theory for higher education. *Journal of College Student Development, 25*(4), 297–308.

Auerbach, R. P., Mortier, P., Bruffaerts, R., Alonso, J., Benjet, C., Cuijpers, P., Demyttenaere, K., Ebert, D. D., Green, J. G., Hasking, P., Murray, E., Nock, M. K., Pinder-Amaker, S., Sampson, N. A., Stein, D. J., Vilagut, G., Zaslavsky, A. M., & Kess, R. C. (2018). WHO World Mental Health Surveys International College Student Project: Prevalence and distribution of mental disorders. *Journal of Abnormal Psychology, 127*(7), 623–638.

Awang, M., Kutty, F., & Ahmad, A. (2014). Perceived social support and well-being: First-year student experience in university. *International Education Studies, 7*(13), 261–270.

Badat, S. (2016). Deciphering the meanings and explaining the South African Higher Education student protests of 2015–16. *Pax Academica, 1*, 71–106.

Bantjes, J., Lochner, C., Saal, W., Roos, J., Taljaard, L., Page, D., Auerbach, R. P., Mortier, P., Bruffaerts, R., Kessler, R. C., & Stein, D. J. (2019). Prevalence and sociodemographic correlates of common mental disorders among first-year university students in post-apartheid South Africa: Implications for a public mental health approach to student wellness. *BMC Public Health, 19*, 922. https://doi.org/10.1186/s12889-019-7218-y

Bantjes, J., Lochner, C., Stein, D. J., & Taljaard, L. (2017). *Global study aims to unpack mental health issues facing university students*. University of Cape Town. Retrieved from https://www.news.uct.ac.za/article/-2017-05-11-global-study-aims-to-unpack-mental-health-issues-facing-university-students

Basson, M. J., & Rothmann, S. (2018). Antecedents of basic psychological need satisfaction of pharmacy students: The role of peers, family, lecturers and workload. *Research in Social and Administrative Pharmacy, 14*(4), 372–381.

Bewick, B., Koutsopoulou, G., Miles, J., Slaa, E., & Barkham, M. (2010). Changes in undergraduate students' psychological well-being as they progress through university. *Studies in Higher Education, 35*(6), 633–645. https://doi.org/10.1080/03075070903216643

Bowles, T. V., & Brindle, K. A. (2017). Identifying facilitating factors and barriers to improving student retention rates in tertiary teaching courses: A systematic review. *Higher Education Research & Development, 36*(5), 903–919. https://doi.org/10.1080/07294360.2016.1264927

Bowman, N. A. (2010). The development of psychological well-being among first-year college students. *Journal of College Student Development, 51*(2), 180–200. https://doi.org/10.1353/csd.0.0118

Boyatzis, R. E. (1998). *Transforming qualitative information: Thematic analysis and code development*. Sage.

Braun, V., & Clarke, V. (2006). Using thematic analysis in psychology. *Qualitative Research in Psychology, 3*(2), 77–101.

Braun, V., Clarke, V., & Weate, P. (2016). Using thematic analysis in sport and exercise research. In B. Smith & A. C. Sparkes (Eds.), *Routledge handbook of qualitative research in sport and exercise* (pp. 213–227). Routledge.

Burns, M. K., Vance, D., Szadokierski, I., & Stockwell, C. (2006). Student needs survey: A psychometrically sound measure of the five basic needs. *International Journal of Reality Therapy, 25*(2), 4–8.

Carroll, D., Ng, E., & Birch, D. (2009). Retention and progression of postgraduate business students: An Australian perspective. *Open Learning: The Journal of Open, Distance and e-Learning, 24*(3), 197–209. https://doi.org/10.1080/02680510903201599

Chang, J. H., Huang, C. L., & Lin, Y. C. (2015). Mindfulness, basic psychological needs fulfillment, and well-being. *Journal of Happiness Studies, 16*(5), 1149–1162. https://doi.org/10.1007/s10902-014-9551-2

Clarke, V., & Braun, V. (2014). Thematic analysis. In A. C. Michalos (Ed.), *Encyclopedia of quality of life and well-being research* (pp. 6626–6628). Springer.

Clarke, V., & Braun, V. (2018). Using thematic analysis in counselling and psychotherapy research: A critical reflection. *Counselling and Psychotherapy Research, 18*(2), 107–110. https://doi.org/10.1002/capr.12165

Conley, D. T., & French, E. M. (2013). Student ownership of learning as a key component of college readiness. *American Behavioral Scientist, 58*(8), 1018–1034. https://doi.org/10.1177/0002764213515232

Cooke, R., Beswick, B. M., Barkham, M., Bradley, M., & Audin, K. (2006). Measuring, monitoring, and managing the psychological well-being of first year university students. *British Journal of Guidance and Counselling, 34*(4), 505–517. https://doi.org/10.1080/03069880600942624

Crawford, N. L., & Johns, S. (2018). An academic's role? Supporting student wellbeing in pre-university enabling programs. *Journal of University Teaching and Learning Practice, 15*(3), 2.

Daniels, A. D., & Jooste, K. (2018). Support of students by academics in a nursing foundation programme at a university in the Western Cape. *Curationis, 41*(1), 1–7. https://doi.org/10.4102/curationis.v41i1.1927

Deci, E. L., & Ryan, R. M. (2008). Self-determination theory: A macrotheory of human motivation, development, and health. *Canadian Psychology/Psychologie Canadienne, 49*(3), 182–185. https://doi.org/10.1037/a0012801

Denovan, A., & Macaskill, A. (2017). Stress and subjective well-being among first-year UK undergraduate students. *Journal of Happiness Studies, 18*(2), 505–525.

Denscombe, M. (2007). The length of responses to open-ended questions. *Social Science Computer Review, 26*(3), 359–368. https://doi.org/10.1177/0894439307309671

Department of Higher Education and Training (DHET). (2018). *Statistics on post-school education and training in South Africa*. Department of Higher Education and Training.

Di Placito-De Rango, M. L. (2018). Situating the post-secondary instructor in a supportive role for the mental health and well-being of students. *International Journal of Mental Health Addiction, 16*, 284–290. https://doi.org/10.1007/s11469-017-9740-4

Eloff, I. (2021). Student wellbeing and access to technology: new landscapes in student support. In N. Ferreira, I. L. Potgieter, & M. Coetzee (Eds.), *Agile Coping in the digital workplace: Emerging Issues for research and practice* (pp. 299–311). Springer Nature.

Evans, G. W., & McCoy, J. M. (1998). When buildings don't work: The role of architecture in human health. *Journal of Environmental Psychology, 18*(1), 85–94. https://doi.org/10.1006/jevp.1998.0089

Field, R., Duffy, J., & Huggins, A. (2015). Teaching independent learning skills in the first year: A positive psychology strategy for promoting law student well-being. *Journal of Learning Design, 8*(2), 1–7.

Freire, C., Ferradás, M. D. M., Valle, A., Núñez, J. C., & Vallejo, G. (2016). Profiles of psychological well-being and coping strategies among university students. *Frontiers in Psychology, 7*, 1554. https://doi.org/10.3389/fpsyg.2016.01554

Gbadamosi, G., & De Jager, J. (2009). What you see is what you get: Service quality, students' perceptions and satisfaction at South African universities. *South African Journal of Higher Education, 23*(5), 877–893.

Glasser, W. (1999). *Choice theory: A new psychology of personal freedom*. Harper Perennial.

Glasser, W. (2001). *Choice theory in the classroom*. Harper Collins.

Goenner, C. F., & Snaith, S. M. (2003). Predicting graduation rates: An analysis of student and institutional factors at doctoral universities. *Journal of College Student Retention: Research, Theory and Practice, 5*(4), 409–420.

Govender, K., Bhana, A., McMurray, K., Kelly, J., Theron, L., Meyer-Weitz, A., Ward, C. L., & Tomlinson, M. (2018). A systematic review of the South African work on the well-being of young people (2000–2016). *South Africa Journal of Psychology, 49*(1), 52–69. https://doi.org/10.1177/0081246318757932

Griffiths, D. (2019). #FeesMustFall and the decolonised university in South Africa: Tensions and opportunities in a globalising world. *International Journal of Educational Research, 94*, 143–149.

Harmening, D. S., & Jacob, S. A. (2015). Institutional factors that positively impact first-year students' sense of well-being. *Journal of Case Studies in Education, 7*, 1–16.

Haynes, C., Bulosan, M., Citty, J., Grant-Harris, M., Hudson, J., & Koro-Ljungberg, M. (2012). My world is not my doctoral program... or is it? Female students' perceptions of well-being. *International Journal of Doctoral Studies, 7*(1), 1–17.

Howell, A. J. (2009). Flourishing: Achievement-related correlates of students' well-being. *The Journal of Positive Psychology, 4*(1), 1–13. https://doi.org/10.1080/17439760802043459

Huppert, F. A. (2009). Psychological well-being: Evidence regarding its causes and consequences. *Applied Psychology: Health and Well-Being, 1*(2), 137–164. https://doi.org/10.1111/j.1758-0854.2009.01008.x

International Association of Universities World Higher Education Database (IAU WHED). (2019). *The world of higher education at your fingertips*. Retrieved from https://www.whed.net/home.php

Kahlke, R. M. (2014). Generic qualitative approaches: Pitfalls and benefits of methodological mixology. *International Journal of Qualitative Methods, 13*(1), 37–52. https://doi.org/10.1177/160940691401300119

Kotzé, M., & Kleynhans, R. (2013). Psychological well-being and resilience as predictors of first-year students' academic performance. *Journal of Psychology in Africa, 23*(1), 51–59. https://doi.org/10.1080/14330237.2013.10820593

Krumrei-Mancuso, E. J., Newton, F. B., Kim, E., & Wilcox, D. (2013). Psychosocial factors predicting first-year college student success. *Journal of College Student Development, 54*(3), 247–266.

Laidlaw, A., McLellan, J., & Ozakinci, G. (2016). Understanding undergraduate student perceptions of mental health, mental well-being and help-seeking behaviour. *Studies in Higher Education, 41*(12), 2156–2168.

Leese, M. (2010). Bridging the gap: Supporting the student transition into higher education. *Journal of Further and Higher Education, 34*(2), 239–251. https://doi.org/10.1353/csd.2013.0034

Marais, G. A., Shankland, R., Haag, P., Fiault, R., & Juniper, B. (2018). A survey and a positive psychology intervention on French PhD student well-being. *International Journal of Doctoral Studies, 13*, 109–138.

Maslow, A. (1970). *Motivation and personality* (2nd ed.). Harper & Row.

Merriam, S. B. (2002). Basic interpretive qualitative research. In S. B. Merriam (Ed.), *Qualitative research in practice* (pp. 37–39). Jossey-Bass.

Mokgele, K. R., & Rothmann, S. (2014). A structural model of student well-being. *South Africa Journal of Psychology, 44*(4), 514–527.

Muhammad, S., Sapri, M., & Sipan, I. (2014). Academic buildings and their influence on students' wellbeing in higher education institutions. *Social Indicators Research, 115*(3), 1159–1178. https://doi.org/10.1007/s11205-013-0262-6

Murray, H. A. (1938). *Explorations in personality: A clinical and experimental study of fifty men of college age*. Oxford University Press.

Nel, C., Trotskie-de Bruin, C., & Bitzer, E. (2009). Student transition from school to university: Possibility for pre-university intervention. *South African Journal of Higher Education, 23*, 974–991.

Nielsen, I., Newman, A., Smyth, R., Hirst, G., & Heilemann, B. (2017). The influence of instructor support, family support and psychological capital on the well-being of postgraduate students: A moderated mediation model. *Studies in Higher Education, 42*(11), 2099–2115.

Percy, W. H., Kostere, K., & Kostere, S. (2015). Generic qualitative research in psychology. *The Qualitative Report, 20*(2), 76–85. Retrieved from http://nsuworks.nova.edu/tqr/vol20/iss2/7

Raelin, J., Bailey, M., Hamann, J., Pendleton, L., Reisberg, R., & Whitman, D. (2014). The gendered effect of cooperative education, contextual support and self-efficacy on undergraduate retention. *Journal of Engineering Education, 103*, 599–624.

Richardson, T., Elliott, P., Roberts, R., & Jansen, M. (2017). A longitudinal study of financial difficulties and mental health in a national sample of British undergraduate students. *Community Mental Health Journal, 53*(3), 344–352. https://doi.org/10.1007/s10597-016-0052-0

Ryff, C. D. (1995). Psychological well-being in adult life. *Current Directions in Psychological Science, 4*(4), 99–104.

Salami, S. (2010). Emotional intelligence, self-efficacy, psychological well-being and students' attitudes: Implications for quality education. *European Journal of Educational Studies, 2*(3), 247–257.

Saldaña, J. (2016). *The coding manual for qualitative researchers* (3rd ed.). Sage.

Salmela-Aro, K. (2010). Personal goals and well-being: How do young people navigate their lives? *New Directions for Child and Adolescent Development, 130*, 13–26. https://doi.org/10.1002/cd.278

Seligman, M. E. (2011). *Flourish: The new positive psychology and the search for well-being*. Free Press.

Shefer, T., Strebel, A., Ngabaza, S., & Clowes, L. (2018). Student accounts of space and safety at a South African university: Implications for social identities and diversity. *South Africa Journal of Psychology, 48*(1), 61–72. https://doi.org/10.1177/0081246317701887

Stallman, H. M. (2010). Psychological distress in university students: A comparison with general population data. *Australian Psychologist, 45*(4), 249–257.

Stallman, H. M., Ohan, J. L., & Chiera, B. (2018). The role of social support, being present and self-kindness in university student well-being. *British Journal of Guidance and Counselling, 46*(4), 365–374. https://doi.org/10.1111/ap.12271

Strange, C., & Banning, J. (2001). *Educating by design*. Jossey-Bass.

Sutherland, A., Hamilton, M. J., & Goodman, N. (2007). Affirming at-risk minorities for success (ARMS): Retention, graduation and success on the NCLEX-RNO. *Journal of Nursing Education, 46*, 347–353.

Tait, M., & De Jager, J. W. (2009). Image and academic expectations of different levels of university students: A South African case. *South African Journal of Higher Education, 23*(5), 1026–1038.

Turkdogan, T., & Duru, E. (2012). The role of basic needs fulfillment and prediction of subjective well-being among university students. *Educational Sciences: Theory & Practice, 12*(4), 2440–2446.

Turner, L., & Tobbell, J. (2018). Learner identity and transition: An ethnographic exploration of undergraduate trajectories. *Journal of Further and Higher Education, 42*(5), 708–720.

Väisänen, S., Pietarinen, J., Pyhältö, K., Toom, A., & Soini, T. (2017). Social support as a contributor to student teachers' experienced well-being. *Research Papers in Education, 32*(1), 41–55.

Van Breda, A. D. (2018). Resilience of vulnerable students transitioning into a South African university. *Higher Education, 75*(6), 1109–1124.

Wilcox, P., Winn, S., & Fyvie-Gauld, M. (2005). It was nothing to do with the university, it was just the people: The role of social support in the first-year experience of higher education. *Studies in Higher Education, 30*(6), 707–722.

Wilson, D., McKinney, C., & Rapatahanning, M. (2011). Retention of indigenous nursing students in New Zealand: A cross-sectional survey. *Contemporary Nurse, 38*, 59–75.

Wilson-Strydom, M. (2011). University access for social justice: A capabilities perspective. *South African Journal of Education, 31*(3), 407–418.

World Health Organization (WHO). (2019). *Fact sheets: Suicide*. Retrieved from https://www.who.int/news-room/fact-sheets/detail/suicide

Young, C., & Campbell, M. (2014). Student wellbeing at a university in post-apartheid South Africa: A comparison with a British university sample using the GP-CORE measure. *British Journal of Guidance & Counselling, 42*(4), 359–371. https://doi.org/10.1080/03069885.2013.779638

Chapter 11
Nature and Role of Student Hope and Meaning in Goal Setting: Implications for Higher Education in South Africa

Itumeleng P. Khumalo, Werner de Klerk, and Angelina Wilson Fadiji

Abstract This chapter presents an exploration of the nature of student goals and obstacles, and the role played by meaning in life and hope thinking in distinguishing them. Male and female ($n = 101$) students between 18 and 34 years (mean = 22 years) participated in a concurrent equal status, exploratory, mixed-method design study. They were asked about the nature of their goals and anticipated obstacles using open-ended formatted questions, and completed the Dispositional Hope Scale and Meaning in Life Questionnaire. Latent classes of Hope-Meaning were extracted, and compared for the nature of goals and perceived obstacles. Qualitative data were subjected to content analysis. Results show a division of the sample into two Hope-Meaning latent classes: "High hope, high meaning" (92.1%) and "Low hope, search for meaning" (7.9%). The identified and prioritised goals were: tertiary education, employment and career, mobility, secure accommodation, and support for family. Their prioritisation of tertiary education and employment was explained by the need to secure a better material future and support their families. Five obstacles were reported: lack of resources, poor self-regulation, employment problems, fear of failure, and health problems. No goal and obstacle content distinction was made between the two emergent Hope-Meaning latent classes.

I. P. Khumalo (✉)
Department of Psychology, University of the Free State, Bloemfontein, South Africa
e-mail: KhumaloIP@ufs.ac.za

W. de Klerk
Department of Psychology, North-West University, Potchefstroom, South Africa

COMPRES, North-West University, Potchefstroom, South Africa

A. W. Fadiji
Department of Educational Psychology, Faculty of Education, University of Pretoria, Pretoria, South Africa

Africa Unit for Transdisciplinary Health Research, Faculty of Health Sciences, North-West University, Potchefstroom, South Africa

L. Schutte et al. (eds.), *Embracing Well-Being in Diverse African Contexts: Research Perspectives*, Cross-Cultural Advancements in Positive Psychology 16,
https://doi.org/10.1007/978-3-030-85924-4_11

Keywords Hope · Goals · Life satisfaction · Higher education · Meaning · South Africa

11.1 Introduction

The question of "what kinds of goals and values are most likely to promote a person's growth and happiness?" remains relevant to contemporary social scientists (Sheldon et al., 2019, p. 191). The pursuit of goals by students forms part of the developmental process, often accompanied by the simultaneous experience of life as meaningful while also searching for meaning in life (Steger et al., 2008). One of the main existential concerns of young people is to understand themselves and seek purposeful lives. Thus, goal thinking is ubiquitous among the youth (Lopez et al., 2009). Meaningful goals and engagement in meaning-making activities is associated with greater self-concordance (Ho et al., 2010). It makes sense that young people would constantly engage in searching for meaning (Steger et al., 2008).

The desirability of a goal is considered to be high when the goal is aligned with personal needs for autonomy, competence and social integration, higher order goals of identity, and the expected value of achieving the goal (Ryan, 2012). If people feel that these goals cannot be achieved, it is important to know what could be the possible obstacles. Among a large variety of possible obstacles which may act to prevent students from achieving their goals are poverty and the related socioeconomic circumstances, such as generational low levels of literacy (see Møller & Radloff, 2013). Many poor students expect to find upward mobility and break out of the cycle of poverty (Howard, 2001), yet there is a South African reality, including the high unemployment rate, among other hindrances, that stunts this trajectory (Badat & Sayed, 2014).

11.1.1 The Student Context in South Africa

Students in South Africa face the reality of having to set, pursue and achieve their goals in a socioeconomic and political context of hardship, inequality and uncertainty (Badat & Sayed, 2014). With only approximately 17% of South Africans completing Grade 12 at school and accessing higher education (Ramrathan & Pillay, 2015), post-school education remains a limited luxury. Furthermore, most such students are first-generation university entrants, with about 70% having parents who never graduated from a university and 45% having had no family member who graduated from higher education (Universities South Africa, 2017). Ramrathan and Pillay (2015) report an estimated graduation rate of 15%. A 2017 survey by Universities South Africa (Universities South Africa, 2017) found that many South African students are responsible for caring for others. It is not uncommon for students to report suffering from stress due to problems unrelated to the academic project, for example financial problems and the death of family members (Pillay & Ngcobo, 2010). In addition, a lack of digital technology knowledge and support is a major problem for students in South Africa (Khoza & Manik, 2015).

In 2015 and 2016, a period overlapping with the time during which the data for this study were collected, South African universities were experiencing a series of student protest movements. These protests began at the University of Cape Town (UCT) with the Rhodes Must Fall (RMF) call and migrated to finally culminate in a national movement calling for a reduction in university fees among other demands (i.e., #FeesMustFall), with a nodal point at the University of the Witwatersrand (WITS) (Jansen, 2017). The #FeesMustFall movement was born out of a concern that fees for higher education in South Africa are too high and unaffordable for many students who want to study and who are deserving of doing so (Jansen, 2017). It presented the view that education must be freely accessible to all students and that government must subsidise higher education institutions. These calls were made against the backdrop of many South African students' reality which is characterised by poverty and social welfare system support (Pillay & Ngcobo, 2010), among other structural violence ills.

11.1.2 Goals

Not only are goals the units of motivation, but they are at the centre of human functioning, contributing to long-term levels of well-being (Emmons, 2003b; Talevich et al., 2017). Goals represent anything an individual aspires to experience, create, get, do, or become (Lopez et al., 2009). Thus, goals of any nature, mundane or significant, brief or long-term, big or small, abstract or concrete, propel people into action and serve as anchor points for purposive behaviour (Feldman & Snyder, 2005; Snyder, 2002, 2004). In line with Bishop and Willis's (2014) assertion that hope is socially produced, the contribution made by the current study contextualises the measured levels of hope agency within the choices of student goals, as they express their aspirations and potential obstacles. Group membership (Raco, 2009), gender (Anderson et al., 2005; Patterson & Forbes, 2012), and socioeconomic status (Senior & Chenhall, 2012; Threadgold, 2011) serve as determinants of hope. Therefore, young people's hope is integrally connected to the societal and global state of affairs (Eckersley et al., 2008).

As much as hope is an important component of human life (Bishop & Willis, 2014), its importance in the lives of South African students has not been empirically tested. Guse and Vermaak (2011, p. 527) observed that "there is limited knowledge about the prevalence and dynamics of hope among South African youth". Many studies concerned with youth have focused on their fears, worries and anxieties (Bishop & Willis, 2014), instead of positive functioning. Yet, hope (Snyder, 2002), meaning (Steger, 2012) and goals (Emmons, 2003a; Hope et al., 2016; Zhang & Zhang, 2017) are central to all people across the lifespan and multiple life domains, and especially among young people. It is through hope that people often pull through obstacles in life (Lopez et al., 2003). Feldman and Dreher (2012) argue that such obstacles may be associated with lower levels of hope, while higher levels of hope have been associated with individuals' ability to cope constructively with problem-solving (Snyder et al., 1991).

11.1.3 Hope and Meaning

Hope is seen as more than a happy feeling about the future; it is a source of motivational drive to thrive, applicable in all life domains (i.e., work, education, health and personal meaning). According to Snyder et al. (1999), pathways thinking, considered the first of the three concepts, begins in early childhood when children start to add pieces together until they are able to understand that there is causation, or that one thing leads to another. The second concept of Snyder's hope model is agency, which begins at the age of a year when a sense of identity develops (Snyder et al., 1991). At this point, children begin to be aware that they have the capabilities to make things happen. Goals form the third component of this model. Individuals combine pathways and agency thinking in order to pursue their goals. Snyder et al. (1991) found that students who scored higher on the hope measure were more successful in achieving their goals than those with low scores. Students who are hopeful thinkers have greater potential to achieve more academically (Snyder et al., 2000).

When Bishop and Willis (2014) asked young people why hope was important in their lives, they learnt that hope was a source of goals and happiness, it enabled the pursuit of goals, was thought to remain when all else was lost, and that "a life without hope is no life at all". Hope is considered an important determinant of positive development (e.g., Snyder et al., 2003; Valle et al., 2006). According to Nalkur (2009) and Seginer (2008), being hopeful is perceived to be the most significant part of future planning and the development of young adults' identity, and it has also been correlated with students' academic achievement (Ciarrochi et al., 2007; Gilman et al., 2006).

While meaning in life allows people to explore and experience their purpose, significance and belonging (Lambert et al., 2013), hope connects them cognitively and emotionally to their future (Park et al., 2004; Snyder, 2002, 2004). Hope and meaning are therefore forces of direction and motivation (Bryant & Ellard, 2015; Siwek et al., 2017). Meaningful living contributes to positive life experience and embodies the pursuit of personally significant goals (Emmons, 2003a). Among South Africans, Wissing et al. (2019) found that along the mental health continuum, meaning was a sought-after quality with different underlying motives and was prominently tied to relationships, religion and work.

11.1.4 Aim and Objectives of the Study

The purpose of this study was to explore and understand the nature and role of meaning and hope in South African students' goal setting. This purpose was achieved by fulfilling three objectives. The first objective was to establish the latent class membership of students according to the extent to which they experienced their lives as characterised by hope and meaning. In the second objective, the study explored the content of the goals the students set and the kinds of obstacles they perceived to be in their way of achieving their goals. The third objective was concerned with how meaning and hope class membership distinguished the nature of goals and obstacles. A similar approach was followed by Wissing et al. (2019) in their pursuit of exploring and comparing the construals of meaning, goals and relatedness between flourishing and languishing respondents in South Africa. This chapter serves as an extension of previous research (e.g., Wilson et al., 2019) in a number of ways. It deliberately takes the contextualised realities of the students' lives into account. Self-generated goals, the motives behind them, as well as the encountered obstacles, provide the contextual texture of the students' lives. While other studies have been nomothetic by either taking a qualitative or a quantitative methodological route, this one took a mixed-methods approach (Leech & Onwuegbuzie, 2009). The person-centred approach of latent class analysis is also important because, unlike the popular variable-oriented approaches often used, it explores the naturally occurring profiles of people (Rosato & Baer, 2012). It allows for the investigation of how multiple variables are configured within individuals and therefore observes patterns that differentiate groups on the basis of their responses (Dezutter et al., 2014).

11.2 Method

11.2.1 Design

In the study reported here, the researchers collected, analysed and interpreted qualitative and quantitative data in the same group of students, therefore complying with the fully mixed, concurrent, equal status exploratory design (Leech & Onwuegbuzie, 2009). Using an inductive approach, the qualitative responses were subjected to conventional content analysis for text categories and contextual understanding (Hsieh & Shannon, 2005). This approach has been previously used by Wissing et al. (2019).

11.2.2 Participants and Setting

A convenience sample of students who were enrolled for various courses at a university of technology in South Africa participated. The sample of 155 students was made up of 101 female and 54 male students, ranging in age between 18 and 34, with an average age of 23 years (*SD* = 3.55). They were mostly single people who had never been married, with this group making up 50.3% of the sample, the rest were in a relationship (37.4%), married (5.8%) or living together (4.5%), and one person was divorced.

11.2.3 Measuring Instruments

In addition to providing socio-demographic information, participants responded to the Dispositional Hope Scale (DHS; Snyder et al., 1991), and Meaning in Life Questionnaire (MLQ; Steger et al., 2006). The quantitative data provided responses to the following variables: meaning (presence and search), hope (agency and pathways thinking), life satisfaction, age, gender, perception of future expectation, and relationship/marital status. The one-item inquiry of future expectation is an operationalisation of optimism as a generalised expectancy of a positive future (Bruininks & Malle, 2005; Scheier & Carver, 1985). The participants also responded to open-ended questions, which inquired about the goals they wished to achieve in the next 12 months and the obstacles they perceived or experienced as hindering their goal attainment. The three open-ended questions to which they were asked to respond to were: 1. *Please list and describe three (3) goals that you would like to achieve in your life in the next 12 months*; 2. *Now choose the one most important goal and explain why it is important*; and 3. *Please list and describe three (3) obstacles that you think could stand in your way of achieving the goals you want for yourself and your life.*

11.2.3.1 Dispositional Hope Scale (DHS; Snyder et al., 1991)

The DHS is a two-factor, 12-item scale measuring hope as agency-thinking (4 items) and pathways-thinking (4 items). The four additional items are distractor items. The instrument uses an eight-point Likert-type scale. The DHS has been found to be reliable, with Snyder et al. (1991) reporting Cronbach's alphas of between .74 and .84 among students and patients. In the same studies, the Agency subscale attained a Cronbach's alpha coefficient ranging between .71 and .76, and the Pathways subscale between .63 and .80 (Snyder et al., 1991). In the present study, agency-thinking attained an omega reliability index of .74, while pathways-thinking scored .70. To demonstrate construct validity, the two-factor structure (Agency and

Pathways) solution presented excellent goodness-of-fit indexes: χ^2 (19) = 35.57, p = .0119, CFI = .947, TLI = .923, RMSEA = 0.075 [90%CI: .035; .113].

11.2.3.2 Meaning in Life Questionnaire (MLQ; Steger et al., 2006)

The MLQ is a 10-item measure designed to measure presence of meaning (MLQ-P; 5 items) and search for meaning (MLQ-S; 5 items). The two-factor structure of the scale has been reproduced in multiple other studies all over the world including in South Africa (e.g., Temane et al., 2014). All items were scored on a seven-point scale. In the original study, Steger et al. (2006) found reliability indices of .81 for MLQ–P and .84 for MLQ–S at Time 1, and .86 for MLQ-P and .92 for MLQ-S at Time 2. In South Africa, Temane et al. (2014) found Cronbach's alpha values of .85 for MLQ-P and .84 for MLQ-S. Most empirical investigations have found the two subscales to be moderately negatively correlated. The omega reliability indices in the current study were .86 for MLQ-P, and .88 for MLQ-S. In this study, the first-order two-factor structure (presence of meaning and search for meaning) solution presented good fit after error covariance between MLQ-8 "*I am seeking a purpose or mission for my life*" and MLQ-10 "*I am searching for meaning in my life*" was effected. The improved model demonstrated the goodness-of-fit indexes: χ^2 (33) = 75.354, $p < .000$, CFI = .945, TLI = .924, RMSEA = .092 [90% *CI*: .064; .119].

11.2.4 Procedure and Ethical Aspects

This study was approved by the North-West University Research Ethics Review Board and awarded the number: NWU-HS-2014-0012. The first author approached the lecturers for assistance with recruitment and data collection. All details pertaining to the study were shared with the participants and only students who had given written informed consent took part in the study. Students were advised to complete the questionnaires at a time convenient for them and to return them within a maximum of a week. Anonymity was assured by assigning numbers to participants' responses, and their own names were not used.

11.2.5 Data Analysis

Quantitative and qualitative data were analysed in a way that allowed for integration in keeping with the concurrent mixed-method design (Leech & Onwuegbuzie, 2009).

11.2.5.1 Quantitative

Latent class analysis (LCA) in Mplus 8.1 (Muthén & Muthén, 1998–2017) was used to identify classes of hope-meaning combination. The factor scores of the subscales (Hope-Agency and Hope-Pathways, and Meaning- Presence and Meaning-Search) were used. In a progressive sequence, three models (one, two and three-class latent models) were tested. Assessment for choosing the best model was based on fit indices: LRχ^2 (likelihood ratio chi square), BIC (Bayesian information criterion), SSABIC (sample size adjusted BIC), AIC (Akike information criterion), LMR-LRT (Lo-Mendall-Rubin adjusted likelihood ratio test), and entropy, as well as class membership size and theoretical interpretation. For good fit, BIC, SSABIC and AIC were expected to be lower, and LRχ^2 lower and not significant, but the LMR-LRT had to be statistically significant (Nylund et al., 2007), and a higher entropy value (ranging between 0 and 1) would be an indication of good fit. In order to consider the possible impact of unequal group sizes, robust indicators of group differences were used. The class mean scores were compared using 1000 sample bootstrapped t-test computation (see Field, 2018).

11.2.5.2 Qualitative

Qualitative data in the form of participants' responses to open-ended questions about their goals and obstacles were obtained. Their content entailed goals; prioritised goals and reasons for prioritising them; and experienced/ perceived obstacles. After familiarising ourselves with the whole dataset, we inductively analysed, coded and arranged the responses into categories with frequencies. This procedure makes for conventional qualitative content analysis (see Hsieh & Shannon, 2005). Examples of previous studies applying content analysis include those of Eloff et al. (2008) and Wissing et al. (2019). Before the resultant categories were given names/labels, meaningful clusters were formed by an aggregate process of sorting and categorising the codes that had been derived from carefully reading and rereading the text. The rigour, credibility and validity (Crowe et al., 2015; Nieuwenhuis, 2016; Onwuegbuzie & Leech, 2007) of the analysis was enhanced through the process of coding, re-coding as well as co-coding by all researchers. As seen in the subsequent Results section, the following identification system is used to link the qualitative content data with the participant being quoted: participant (with participant abbreviated as "P") number; age; gender.

11.3 Results

11.3.1 *Optimism*

The participants were asked how they viewed the future. Eighty-five percent ($n = 133$) expected that life would get better, while only two viewed it as getting worse; the rest (10.3%) thought things would remain the same.

11.3.2 *Latent Class Membership and Characteristics*

11.3.2.1 Model Fitting and Class Assignments

Although the three-class solution, as seen in Table 11.1, was the one that fitted best, the two-class solution was chosen for application on the basis of sample size percentages and theoretical interpretation. The latent class profile plot, as displayed in Fig. 11.1, shows the two emergent classes: 1. High Hope, High Meaning (92.1%); and 2. Low Hope, Searching for Meaning (7.9%). Table 11.2 shows the class membership likelihood by percentage.

11.3.2.2 Mean Score Differences

As seen in Table 11.3, the two groups differ significantly on their mean scores for Hope Pathways, Hope Agency, and Presence of Meaning, but not for Searching for Meaning, which remains high in both groups. With regard to Hope Agency, the participants in Class 1 reported higher scores ($M = 25.98$, $SD = 3.13$) than those in Class 2 ($M = 13.70$, $SD = 5.68$). The mean difference = 12.28, $BC_a95\%CI$ [8.49, 15.66], was significant, $t(139) = 11.15$, $p < .000$, $d = 2.68$. Regarding Hope Pathways, the participants in Class 1 reported higher scores for Hope Pathways ($M = 26.71$, $SD = 3.66$) than those in Class 2 ($M = 17.17$, $SD = 5.54$). The mean difference = 9.53, $BC_a95\%CI$ [6.05, 12.57], was significant, $t(147) = 8.27$, $p < .000$, $d = 2.03$. With regard to Meaning-Search, the participants in Class 1 reported lower Searching for Meaning ($M = 24.37$, $SD = 8.03$) than those in Class 2 ($M = 26.70$, $SD = 7.41$). However, the mean difference of −2.33, $BC_a95\%$ CI [−6.63, 2.30], was not significant, $t(142) = -0.89$, $p = .374$, $d = 0.302$. For Meaning-Presence, the participants in Class 1 reported higher Presence of Meaning ($M = 27.42$, $SD = 5.46$) than those in Class 2 ($M = 18.00$, $SD = 7.19$). The mean difference = 9.42, BCa95%CI [4.97, 13.41], was significant, $t(145) = 5.57$, $p < .000$, $d = 1.48$.

Table 11.1 Latent class solution model fit indices

Model	Log likelihood	AIC	BIC	SSA BIC	Entropy	L-M-R adjusted LRT		Percentage of sample		
						Estimate	*p*-value	Class 1	Class 2	Class 3
1 class	−880.903	1777.805	1802.101	1776.780				100%		
2 classes	−801.789	1629.577	1669.058	1627.911	0.966	152.00	.2717	92.1%	7.9%	
3 classes	−713.892	1463.784	1518.449	1461.477	0.906	169.079	.0234	2.6%	44.8%	52.6%

Note. AIC = Akaike information criterion; BIC = Bayesian information criterion; SSA BIC = sample size adjusted Bayesian information criterion; p = probability estimate; L-M-R adjusted LRT = Lo-Mendell-Rubin adjusted likelihood ratio test

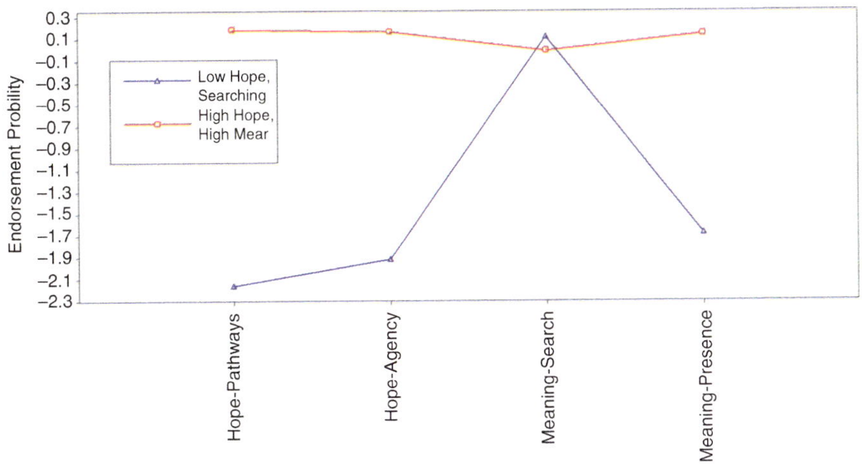

Fig. 11.1 Plot of latent class solution of student hope/meaning

Table 11.2 Most likely class membership (row) by Latent Class (column) by Percentage (%)

	Class 1 (%)	Class 2 (%)
Class 1	.995	.005
Class 2	.046	.954

11.3.3 Goal and Obstacle Content

11.3.3.1 Goals

Self-generated goals mentioned by the particiapnts are dysplayed in Table 11.4. Through an inductive data analysis process using content analysis (Hsieh & Shannon, 2005), five categories were found in the data: tertiary education, employment and career, transport and mobility, own accommodation, and support family.

11.3.3.1.1 Tertiary Education

This category was mentioned 150 times; as goal 1 (93 times), goal 2 (33 times) and goal 3 (24 times). It had no distinguishable subcategories. Participants mostly expressed the goal of getting an education with a sense of agency and the promise it holds for them. They often used the phrase "*pass in record time*". As Participant 126 (24, F) illustrates: "*I want to get myself a degree in order to get myself a job*".

Table 11.3 Descriptive statistics: mean values (using factor scores) of the latent variables per class

Variable	*N*	Mean	*SD*	Min	Max	BC_a 95% CI		Kurtosis	(SE)	Skewness	(SE)
						Lower	Upper				
Latent class 1: High hope, high meaning											
Hope-pathways	137	26.70	3.36	17	32	26.09	27.22	−0.26	0.41	−0.66	0.21
Hope-agency	131	25.98	3.13	17	32	25.47	26.49	−0.14	0.42	−0.40	0.21
Meaning-search	134	24.37	8.03	5	35	22.99	25.64	0.01	0.42	−0.85	0.21
Meaning-presence	135	27.41	5.46	9	35	26.43	28.44	−0.38	0.41	−0.52	0.21
Latent class 2: Low hope, searching for meaning											
Hope-pathways	12	17.17	5.54	8	25	14.16	20.71	−1.20	1.23	−0.20	0.64
Hope-agency	10	13.70	5.68	4	22	10.32	17.22	−0.62	1.33	−0.23	0.69
Meaning-search	10	26.70	7.41	9	35	2.44	10.33	3.40	1.33	−1.68	0.69
Meaning-presence	12	18.00	7.19	8	33	14.11	22.47	0.23	1.23	0.67	0.64

Note. *N* = sample size; *SD* = standard deviation; min = minimum; max = maximum; BC_a = Bias-corrected and accelerated bootstrap interval; SE = standard error

Table 11.4 Frequency of goal categories in the whole sample and by latent class

	Total sample				Class 1				Class 2			
Theme	Goal 1	Goal 2	Goal 3	Total	Goal 1	Goal 2	Goal 3	Total	Goal 1	Goal 2	Goal 3	Total
1. Get tertiary education	93	33	24	150	85	29	22	136	8	4	2	14
2. Employment and career	46	73	34	153	43	69	30	142	3	4	4	11
3. Transport/mobility	2	22	22	46	2	19	21	42	0	3	1	4
4. Own accommodation	0	8	10	18	0	8	10	18	0	0	0	0
5. Support for family	1	1	11	13	1	1	10	12	0	0	1	1

11.3.3.1.2 Employment and Career

This category was mentioned a total of 153 times; as goal 1 (46 times), goal 2 (73 times) and goal 3 (34 times). Three subcategories could be distinguished. The subcategories and their exemplar verbatim phrases are shown here: (1) Becoming employed: "*This is very essential because it will enable me to be able to take care of myself, buy a vehicle and a place*" (P 87, 21, M); (2) Business aspirations: "*Opening a recruitment company. I would like to see myself as a CEO of my own recruitment company in years to come*" (P 10, 23, F), and "*Start a business, I would love to start an events coordination company alongside a clothing business whereby I sell clothes (more like trendy)*" (P 144, 23, F); (3) Career-related growth: "*Get the internship that will help me grow*" (P 38, 21, F); "*Promotion at work and excel in executing my duties*" (P 24, 33, F). This subcategory illustrates the need for personal growth albeit in work domains.

11.3.3.1.3 Transport/Mobility

This, the third category, was mentioned 46 times. In discussing their goals of transport and mobility, participants indicated that getting a driver's licence and buying their own car were necessary. These are indicated by concrete and straightforward statements such as "*get a driver's licence*" (P 90, 20, F; Participant 128, 33, M), and "*[to] buy a car*" (P 20, 25, F; P 63, 24, M; P 70, 31, F; P 85, 21, M; P 88, 21, M; P 89, 22, F). Having a car is associated with easy mobility and fewer hassles: "*Get myself a licence so that one day when I get a car I won't struggle*" (P 4, 23, M).

11.3.3.1.4 Own Accommodation

This category was observed 18 times; as goal 2 (8 times) and goal 3 (10 times). This is exemplified by statements such as: "*To be able to find my own place rather than staying with my parents*" (P 139, 24, F), and "*I want to buy my own house*" (P 132, 22, F).

11.3.3.1.5 Support for Family

This, the last category, was mentioned 13 times; once as goal 1, once as goal 2, and 11 times as goal 3. The need to provide support for the family was divided into financial and housing support. For financial support "*we need to take care of our family*" (P 4, 23, F). Regarding providing housing support, participants indicated the need to work towards this goal: "*Saving account – I want to have an account where I can save up money in order to get a proper house for my parents*" (P 102, 21, F), and "*build my mom a house and take care of my siblings*" (P 135, 22, F) (Table 11.4).

11.3.3.2 Prioritised Goals and Reasons

It was not surprising that the goals prioritised by this group of students were education (68 times) and employment (65 times). The reasons for prioritising these goals are highlighted together the goals in Table 11.5.

11.3.3.2.1 Education

The reasons for prioritising education were underscored by the perceived benefits which include the promise of employment and a pathway to success. The students who prioritised education for the reason that it promised employment said: "*It will open doors for me in getting and applying for jobs in higher level departments*" (P 10, 23, F) and "*the reason this goal is important to me is because if I will be job hunting I will be able to get the job quick because I will be having the needed qualification*" (P 95, 18, M). Education was also prioritised as a way of becoming successful; this view was expressed as follows: "*I really believe that my diploma is my key to happiness, after I obtain my diploma, I really think all my financial problems will be history then I will be able to provide a better life for myself and my whole family, at last everything will be cool and my level of thinking gonna be more relaxed while am happy, successful and enjoying my personal goals and enjoying my life as a whole*" (P 103, 22, M) and "*This is very important because acquiring my BTech I'll be the first person in my family and relatives to have such a recognised qualification from a recognised university of technology. Obtaining this qualification will enable me to be a suitable qualified candidate in the contest for a position within HRM/HRD. It is also important for me to complete my qualification I'll be one of the few educated people in my community*" (P 156, 22, M). The expectation was that as long as a person has an adequate education, there would be limitless opportunities for advancement.

11.3.3.2.2 Employment

This was prioritised for the following reasons: (1) Securing a better future (32 times), (2) Having a better financial position (17 times), (3) Supporting families (13 times), (4) Getting work experience (12 times). The motives for finding employment for the purposes of securing a better future is illustrated by phrases such as: "*Finding a job would be an achievement, considering the current unemployment rate in South Africa*" (P 89, 22, F); "*Because it will help me and pave a way for all the things I want in my life and live an independent life*" (P 134, 25, F); "*So that I can be able to have enough money to have my own business and be able to sustain my family*" (P 160, 22, F). Others wanted to find employment so as to achieve a better financial position: "*Because I need an income to take care of my life without my parents' assistance*" (P 85, 21, M); "*This will basically maintain my want and needs*

Table 11.5 Frequency of prioritised goals and reasons for the whole group and by latent class

Reason for prioritising the goal	Class 1			Class 2			Total sample		
	Reason 1	Reason 2	Total	Reason 1	Reason 2	Total	Reason 1	Reason 2	Total
	The priority goal is Education								
1. Becoming employment	19	0	19	3	0	3	21	0	21
2. Better future	35	1	36	2	0	2	37	1	38
3. Be successful	10	6	16	0	0	0	10	6	16
	The priority goal is employment								
4. Better future	28	0	28	4	0	4	32	0	32
5. Support family	8	3	11	1	1	2	9	4	13
6. Get work experience	10	2	12	0	0	0	10	2	12
7. Better financial position	14	3	17	0	0	0	14	3	17

and basically my daily living" (P 147, 21, F). Linked to securing a better future, employment was also to ensure that families could be supported: "*I come from a very unstable family that is having many dependents with less income in the family so they sacrificed and sent me to varsity so that I can try to change the family situation which is going to take time. When I get a job I will make a huge difference in my family*" (P 142, 23, M). The desire for work experience also motivated some to seek employment: "*This is important to me since I am a graduate with no work experience. I want to achieve this goal because it is the first step for me to start pursing my career*" (P 84, 23, F); "*... give me the platform to practise and grow myself in my chosen field*" (P 128, 33, M) (Table 11.5).

11.3.3.3 Obstacles

As shown in Table 11.6, many obstacles mentioned as possibly obstructing the attainment of goals rest at the personal (internal) and socio-environmental (external) levels. Five categories of obstacles were found in the data.

11.3.3.3.1 Lack of Support/Resources (External)

This category was mentioned 116 times, as obstacle 1 (51 times), obstacle 2 (32 times) and obstacle 3 (33 times). The participants experienced the lack of support as manifested on the financial, family and social levels. Financial support as an illustration of a lack of support or resources was expressed as: "*Financial problems. If I don't get a bursary these will cause problems for me to be able to continue with my studies*" (P 64, 33, F); "*Finance. Without money nothing will happen no matter how good are plans*" (P 72, 20, F). The lack of financial support was critical because it determined whether the student would be able to achieve the goals of education and employment. Regarding poor family support, participants mentioned: "*Lack of support from my family*" (P 29, 22, F); and "*... it's not easy to study whilst you have challenges at home like personal problem*" (P 27, 22, F).

11.3.3.3.2 Poor Self-Regulation (Internal)

The second category to emerge was poor self-regulation (internal), which appeared 103 times. It was mentioned as obstacle one 35 times, as obstacle two 37 times, and obstacle three 31 times. Poor internal self-regulation was linked to the lack of motivation, poor time management skills, and the experience of low self-esteem. To illustrate the lack of motivation student indicated that: "*Laziness, If am lazy I cannot learn hard so my knowledge and skills will not be enhanced*" (P 84, 23, F); and "*Determination, I really have to work hard in order to achieve my dream, I believe that a dream without action is meaningless*" (P 103, 22, M). Participants

Table 11.6 Frequency of obstacle categories in the whole sample and by latent class

	Total sample				Class 1				Class 2			
Theme	Obstacle 1	Obstacle 2	Obstacle 3	Total	Obstacle 1	Obstacle 2	Obstacle 3	Total	Obstacle 1	Obstacle 2	Obstacle 3	Total
1. Lack of support/ resources	51	32	33	116	47	29	29	105	4	3	4	11
2. Poor self-regulation	35	37	31	103	31	33	28	92	4	4	3	11
3. Employment problems	29	31	15	75	27	30	15	72	2	1	0	3
4. Fear of failure	14	13	12	39	14	13	12	39	0	0	0	0
5. Health problems	9	10	5	24	8	10	5	23	1	0	0	1

recognised that although they required external support, there was the need for agency expressed by being motivated to exert the necessary effort for success. On poor time management, a student noted that: "*Failing to plan how I wonna do my things, planning it's imperative to me, if there is no plan I can lose focus easy*" (P 29, 22, F); and "*Time management. I need to manage my time in order to achieve my goals*" (P 67, 21, F). The finding on low self-esteem as an illustration of poor self-regulation showed that participants were aware of the need to evaluating their capabilities positively in order to motivate them to exert the necessary efforts to succeed. A participant noted that: "*Thinking negatively. Always thinking negative stuff about myself will actually not boost my confidence. So I don't think something better will come out of the things I will be doing*" (P 67, 21, F); and "*Lack of self-esteem not believing in myself*" (P 113, 20, F).

11.3.3.3.3 Employment Problems (External)

This third category was mentioned 75 times; 29 times as obstacle 1, 31 times as obstacle 2, and 15 times as obstacle 3. The lack of opportunities, lack of work experience and high unemployment were presented as external career or work-related challenges to student achieving their goals. Lack of opportunities as an illustration of employment problems is evident in this excerpt: "*Not enough job opportunities so one could be absorbed in labour marker due to the economy not performing well*" (P 137, 23, M); "*Lack of career development opportunities in the organisations that I would like to be employed at*" (P 148, 23, M). Participants also felt that the lack of work experience would negatively affect their ability to achieve their goal of getting a good job: "*Not having the necessary skills and experience to get the job I want*" (P 134, 25, F) and "*Lack of experience finding a job won't be easy because I don't have much experience, especially a well-paying job*" (P 87, 21, M). Students noted that the general high unemployment in the country put them in a precarious position: "... *the high rate of unemployment in South Africa*" (P 148, 23, M); "*The country which we are in doesn't have that much opportunities one can apply over two years without getting one single job*" (P 158, 22, F). Finding a job is also prioritised against the backdrop of high levels of unemployment in South Africa, as seen in the case of Participant 89, 22, F.

11.3.3.3.4 Fear of Failure (Internal)

This was the fourth category, appearing 39 times, as obstacle 1 (14 times), obstacle 2 (13 times), and obstacle 3 (12 times). "*Failure. If I fail I won't get my qualification*" (P 72, 20, F); "*The fear of failure or disappointing people around you*" (P 119, 26, M). Participant 111 (20, F), who is concerned that their parents might not continue to afford and pay for their fees is also worried that their mother might become sick and be lost to them. For some of the participants, time management problems occur in the context of having to meet the demands of multiple life domains (e.g., P 113, 20, F). Fear of failure, as illustrated by for example, P 119 (26, M) is not only a problem on the part of the individual, but is also especially a function of not disappointing others who are close to the individual such as family. Participant 142, 23, M is an illustration of how the social difficulties can be incapacitating.

11.3.3.3.5 Health Problems

In fifth place was *health problems, which include fear of and anticipation of death* which were mentioned 24 times; as obstacle 1 (9 times), obstacle 2 (10 times), and obstacle 3 (5 times), and had no subcategories. The category of health problems as an obstacle was expressed by respondents saying: "*Death: you can die before achieving the goals that you want for your life*" (P 26, 24, M); and "*Sick: It might be a challenge, I need to stay healthy so that I can think healthy*" (P 27, 24, F) (Table 11.6).

11.4 Discussion

This chapter explored the different specific configurations of meaning and hope dimensions within students who have contextually bound goals and obstacles. We used a concurrent mixed-method approach to explore the nature of student goals, and the role played by meaning in life and hopeful thinking in distinguishing these goals. Qualitative data were subjected to content analysis to aid the understanding of goal content, goal prioritisation, motives for the goals, and perceived and/or experienced obstacles to goal attainment. Latent class analysis was used for analysing the quantitative data to attain Hope-Meaning latent classes. Methodological, analysis and interpretation integration (Leech & Onwuegbuzie, 2009) were achieved by investigating the way in which the Hope-Meaning latent classes distinguish the goal-setting and obstacles.

11.4.1 The Context of the Perception that Things Are Getting Better

The optimistic view that things are going to get better provides the context within which the findings are understood. The majority of the participants (85%) expected that life would get better, with only two people expecting things to get worse, and the rest (10.3%) thinking that things would remain the same. This provides the context within which the rest of the findings are to be interpreted. At face value, this sense of heightened optimism can be attributed to youth, however this may be anchored in the socio-political state of the South African nation. In a survey by Møller and Radloff (2013), it was the Black South Africans in particular who were most optimistic about the future. The view, compared to reality, would of course render the situation an irony. The high promise of the freedom of education and prosperity, expressed by politicians as "a better life for all" (see Møller, 2013), continues to dominate social discourse even against evidence of contradicting reality. As Badat and Sayed (2014, p. 127) so poignantly put it, "the doors of learning remain shut to the majority of South Africans". A compounding factor which challenges and threatens to thwart the young people's great optimism is the high unemployment rate. Møller and Radloff (2013) refer to the co-occurrence of high unemployment together with high hopes for finding paid work to support households as the "employment paradox".

11.4.2 Hope and Meaning Latent Classes

The emergent two latent classes based on responses to the measures of Hope and Meaning were (a) High Hope, High Meaning (92.1%); and (b) Low Hope, Searching for Meaning (7.9%). This finding is unsurprising as previous studies have pointed to high levels of hope being accompanied by meaning in life (Guse & Shaw, 2018; Yalçın & Malkoç, 2015). Perceiving goals as achievable (high hope) is not only instrumental for facilitating well-being but also meaning in life. This reality is especially true when individuals perceive their goals to be aligned with personal values and self-identity (Yalçın & Malkoç, 2015). Vidwans and Raghvendra (2016) argue that the experience of hope and meaning in life coexists because the eudaimonic experience of meaning is linked to pathway thinking (sense of direction) and a determination of sense of purpose.

It is likely that the emergent classes were due to the tendency of South African students to be hopeful despite the challenges they encounter. Hope pathways for them would represent the pursuit of goals while making sense of their challenging situations. Thus, hopeful thinking would allow them to forge pathways while providing the sense of agency that is necessary for goal fulfilment and purposeful living (see Snyder, 2002). Not only is this trend observed in the quantitative data which show high levels of hope (Agency and Pathways); it is also seen in the qualitative accounts of the future. The dominance of high hope and meaning could be explained by the stage of life in which they found themselves. As young people, students have the opportunity to enact new pathways targeted at achieving specific goals (see Freund et al., 2012). The fact that the two classes reported high levels of searching for meaning is indicative of the expected existential quest of youth; they were more likely to be engaged in meaning searching (Orang et al., 2018).

11.4.3 Goals Set by Students

The participants exhibited pragmatic pathways thinking as opposed to more abstract wishful thinking. Given that the study sample comprised university students, it was unsurprising that education was prioritised as the most important goal. The perceived linear pathway from education to a better and more successful life remains the dominant belief among these students, rendering education an undisputed panacea. There is a perception that educational attainment will result in the achievement of all other intended life goals. Educational aspirations are deemed important because of the context of poverty (Wilson & Somhlaba, 2017). Employment was also prioritised for reasons closely related to educational aspirations. Common to both aspirations is the need to escape the poverty trap.

The intergenerational entrenchment of poverty affecting the psychological well-being of young adults is a reality for the majority of the Black population in South Africa (Savahl et al., 2013). It would seem that greater priority was placed on education and employment because of the associated perceived benefits, one of which could be to provide the means to support the family. Given that these students were from low socioeconomic backgrounds, it was not surprising to find that they had already assumed the responsibility of providing for their family's needs. This is not uncommon in most African families, as the younger generation are expected to give back. Building a house for one's parents is an essential aspiration for the upwardly mobile young entrants to the job market in Black communities in South Africa. Accommodation is an often unfulfilled basic need for the majority of the South African population, as indicated by the vast number of informal settlements across the country. It is also an essential need for the first generation graduates who will likely become intra-country migrant workers away from their families of origin.

University students therefore tend to be more desperate for the upward social mobility provided by being employed. Unfortunately, "South Africans set great store by the instrumental value of an education that will lead to a job" (Møller & Radloff, 2013, p. 60). As often happens, and as was found by Møller and Radloff (2013), older people's pension money is often used to subsidise the education needs of younger ones. Møller and Radloff (2013) question the wisdom of this behaviour, and ask "whether this investment is a wise one for poor households" (p. 660). Against the backdrop of an economy which fails to absorb school leavers and graduates, they may have a valid point. What we observe here is that the preoccupation with finding a job was not only for material need satisfaction but also for the preservation of social ties. This goal is relational in nature as it was a pathway to being able to take care of the student's family.

11.4.4 Obstacles Perceived and Experienced by the Students

The most frequently mentioned and dominant obstacle perceived and experienced by the participants was lack of support in the form of socio-emotional and financial resources. It would be expected that these two needs would top the list among individuals embedded in a collectivistic African cultural orientation and for whom every day is a struggle for survival. The inability of family members to provide the needed support for education made it difficult for the students to focus on achieving their education pursuits. In fact, the expectations of the families of origin regarding the students seemed very high. Lack of support for educational aspirations can manifest in a lack of know-how and material resources (Wilson & Somhlaba, 2017).

11.4.5 Comparison of Hope-Meaning Latent Classes in Qualitative Accounts

Hope-Meaning latent classes showed no noticeable differences in the qualitative nature of goals, motives and obstacles. This means that the goals set, the reasons for deeming their choice important, as well as the perceived obstacles, were ubiquitous across the two groups of High Hope High Meaning, and Low Hope High Search for Meaning. The strength of the ecological factors driving the aspirations for improved quality of life appears to have been the greater determinant for reported goals, motives and obstacles. These two groups are comparable to the flourishing and the languishing groups of Wissing et al. (2019). While we examined differences between Hope-Meaning latent classes, Wissing et al. (2019) investigated the possible similarities and differences between flourishing and languishing groups for construals of meaning, goals and relatedness. Although they found the groups mostly similar in terms of the content of meaning, goals and relatedness, the participants' motives (underlying reasons) differed. At the top of their list of goals were relationships, finances, life goals, and health. The similarity in context of content of goals for both groups in Wissing et al. (2019) dovetails with our findings on the congruence of goals and obstacles in both latent classes.

11.5 Conclusion

Our findings reveal that a high percentage of the current sample are experiencing high hope and high meaning in life. Despite the challenges and obstacles highlighted, it would seem that clear pathway thinking and individual agency are more apparent. A reflection on the South African educational landscape shows gross socioeconomic challenges. In the face of these challenges, it would seem that our sample tend to be trapped in the circumstances of their present lives, and unable to express the goals and hope which transcend them. However meaningful the goals set by the students seem to be, we observe that they lack a level of abstraction; they tend to be concrete, instrumental and pragmatic and, like the disadvantaged youth interviewed by Bryant and Ellard (2015) in Australia, the students in the present study seem to find difficulty with articulating a future beyond their present circumstances. Interventions to improve the quality of life and well-being of students at South African universities need to be able foster a sense of coherence of the student's life experience while improving the amount of education-related support. Given that our qualitative findings pointed to more external than internal challenges, education-related support should not focus on academic skills alone, but also on social and material support to the extent possible. The preoccupation with need satisfaction, as evidenced in the goals of the students, reflects the dominant discourse on material deprivation. Although the current sample was not large, our findings reiterate the need for more social interventions in order to facilitate the transition of students from the institutions of higher learning setting to the world of work.

As the use of a mixed-method design did not allow for adequate in-depth exploration of the goals and obstacles, further research could focus on this. This important topic would also benefit from a nationwide longitudinal survey of institutions of higher learning, as opposed to the cross-sectional design used in this study, in order to inform policymakers on the need for further reforms in this setting. Therefore, as the report by the Universities South Africa, (2017) suggests, it is time for South African universities and the public to focus on meeting students where they are, and making optimal use of their existing attributes, aspirations and skills, rather than trying to force them into a traditional and possibly redundant university mould.

References

Anderson, M., Bechhofer, F., McCrone, D., Jamieson, L., Li, Y., & Stewart, R. (2005). Timespans and plans among young adults. *Sociology, 39*(1), 139–155.

Badat, S., & Sayed, Y. (2014). Post-1994 South African education: The challenge of social justice. *Annals of the American Academy of Political and Social Science, 652*(1), 127–148. Retrieved from https://ezproxy.ufs.ac.za:8253/10.1177/0002716213511188

Bishop, E. C., & Willis, K. (2014). 'Without hope everything would be doom and gloom': Young people talk about the importance of hope in their lives. *Journal of Youth Studies, 17*(6), 778–793.

Bruininks, P., & Malle, B. F. (2005). Distinguishing hope from optimism and related affective states. *Motivation and Emotion, 29*, 324–352.

Bryant, J., & Ellard, J. (2015). Hope as a form of agency in the future thinking of disenfranchised young people. *Journal of Youth Studies, 18*(4), 485–499.

Ciarrochi, J., Heaven, P. C. L., & Davies, F. (2007). The impact of hope, self-esteem, and attributional style on adolescents' school grades and emotional well-being: A longitudinal study. *Journal of Research in Personality, 41*, 1161–1178.

Crowe, M., Inder, M., & Porter, R. (2015). Conducting qualitative research in mental health: Thematic and content analyses. *Australian & New Zealand Journal of Psychiatry, 49*(7), 616–623.

Dezutter, J., Waterman, A. S., Schwartz, S. J., Luyckx, K., Beyers, W., Meca, A., Kim, S. Y., Whitbourne, S. K., Zamboanga, B. L., Lee, R. M., Hardy, S. A., Forthun, L. F., Ritchie, R. A., Weisskirch, R. S., Brown, E. J., & Caraway, S. J. (2014). Meaning in life in emerging adulthood: A person-oriented approach. *Journal of Personality, 82*(1), 57–68.

Eckersley, R., Cahill, H., Wierenga, A., Wyn, J., Waugh, M., Woodman, D., Waters-Lynch, J., McCalman, J., & Gidley, J. (2008, April). *Generations in dialogue about the future: The hopes and fears of young Australians*. Ethos. Social Education Victoria. Retrieved from https://search.informit.org/doi/10.3316/aeipt.170370

Eloff, I., Achoui, M., Chireshe, R., Mutepfa, M., & Ofovwe, C. (2008). Views from Africa on positive psychology. *Journal of Psychology in Africa, 18*(1), 189–194.

Emmons, R. A. (2003a). *The psychology of ultimate concerns*. The Guilford Press.

Emmons, R. A. (2003b). Personal goals, life meaning, and virtue: Wellsprings of a positive life. In C. L. M. Keyes (Ed.), *Flourishing: The positive person and the good life* (pp. 105–128). American Psychological Association.

Feldman, D. B., & Dreher, D. E. (2012). Can hope be changed in 90 minutes? Testing the efficacy of a single-session goal-pursuit intervention for college students. *Journal of Happiness Studies, 13*, 745–759.

Feldman, D. B., & Snyder, C. R. (2005). Hope and the meaningful life: Theoretical and empirical associations between goal-directed thinking and life meaning. *Journal of Social and Clinical Psychology, 24*(3), 401–421.

Field, A. (2018). *Discovering statistics sing IBM SPSS statistics* (5th ed.). Sage.

Freund, A. M., Hennecke, M., & Mustafic, M. (2012). On gains and losses, meaning and ends: Goal orientation and goal focus across adulthood. In R. M. Ryan (Ed.), *The Oxford handbook of human motivation* (pp. 280–300). Oxford University Press.

Gilman, R., Dooley, J., & Florell, D. (2006). Relative levels of hope and their relationship with academic and psychological indicators among adolescents. *Journal of Social & Clinical Psychology, 25*(2), 166–178.

Guse, T., & Shaw, M. (2018). Hope, meaning in life and well-being among a group of young adults. In A. Krafft, P. Perrig-Chiello, & A. Walker (Eds.), *Hope for a good life: Social indicators research series, 72*. Springer.

Guse, T., & Vermaak, Y. (2011). Hope, psychosocial well-being and socioeconomic status among a group of South African adolescents. *Journal of Psychology in Africa, 21*(4), 527–533.

Ho, M. Y., Cheung, F. M., & Cheung, S. F. (2010). The role of meaning in life and optimism in promoting well-being. *Personality and Individual Differences, 48*, 658–663.

Hope, N. H., Milyavskaya, M., Holding, A. C., & Koestner, R. (2016). The humble path to progress: Goal-specific aspirational content predicts goal progress and goal vitality. *Personality and Individual Differences, 90*, 99–107.

Howard, A. (2001). *Students from poverty: Helping them make it through college*. Retrieved from http://www.colby.edu/education/courses/ed215/Howard.pdf

Hsieh, H.-F., & Shannon, S. E. (2005). Three approaches to qualitative content analysis. *Qualitative Health Research, 15*(9), 1277–1288.

Jansen, J. (2017). *As by fire: The end of the South African university*. Tafelberg.

Khoza, S. B., & Manik, S. (2015). The recognition of "digital technology refugees" amongst postgraduate students in a higher education institution. *Alternation Special Edition, 17*, 190–208.

Lambert, N. M., Stillman, T. F., Hicks, J. A., Kamble, S., Baumeister, R. F., & Finchman, F. D. (2013). To belong is to matter: Sense of belonging enhances meaning in life. *Personality and Social Psychology Bulletin, 39*(11), 1418–1427.

Leech, N. L., & Onwuegbuzie, A. J. (2009). A typology of mixed methods research designs. *Quality & Quantity: International Journal of Methodology, 43*(2), 265–275.

Lopez, S. J., Rose, S., Robinson, C., Marques, S. C., & Pais-Ribeiro, J. (2009). Measuring and promoting hope in schoolchildren. In R. Gilman, E. S. Huebner, M. J. Furlong, R. Gilman, E. S. Huebner, & M. J. Furlong (Eds.), *Handbook of positive psychology in schools* (pp. 37–50). Routledge/Taylor & Francis Group.

Lopez, S. J., Snyder, C. R., & Pedrotti, J. T. (2003). Hope: Many definitions, many measures. In S. J. Lopez & C. R. Snyder (Eds.), *Positive psychological assessment: A handbook of models and measures* (pp. 91–108). American Psychological Association.

Møller, V. (2013). South African quality of life trends over three decades, 1980–2010. *Social Indicators Research, 113*, 915–940.

Møller, V., & Radloff, S. (2013). Perceptions of fortune and misfortune in older South African households: Social assistance and the "good life". *Social Indicators Research, 111*, 633–664. https://doi.org/10.1007/s11205-012-0026-8

Muthén, L. K., & Muthén, B. O. (1998–2017). *Mplus statistical analysis with latent variables: Users' guide* (8th ed.). Muthén & Muthén.

Nalkur, P. (2009). Adolescent's hopefulness in Tanzania: Street youth, former street youth and school youth. *Journal of Adolescent Research, 24*(6), 668–690.

Nieuwenhuis, J. (2016). Analysing qualitative data. In K. Maree (Ed.), *First steps in research* (2nd ed., pp. 104–130). Van Schaik.

Nylund, K. L., Asparouhov, T., & Muthen, B. O. (2007). Deciding on the number of classes in latent class analysis and growth mixture modelling: A Monte Carlo simulation study. *Structural Equation Modeling, 14*(4), 535–569.

Onwuegbuzie, A. J., & Leech, N. L. (2007). Validity and qualitative research: An oxymoron. *Quality and Quantity, 41*, 233–249.

Orang, S., Razini, H. H., Ramshini, M., & Orang, T. (2018). Investigating the meaning of life psychological well-being, in youth, adults and elderly. *Iranian Journal of Ageing, 13*(2), 182–197.

Park, N., Peterson, C., & Seligman, M. E. P. (2004). Strengths of character and well-being. *Journal of Social and Clinical Psychology, 23*, 603–619.

Patterson, L., & Forbes, K. (2012). Doing gender in the imagined futures of young New Zealanders. *Nordic Journal of Youth Research, 20*(2), 119–136.

Pillay, A. L., & Ngcobo, H. S. B. (2010). Sources of stress and support among rural based first year university students: An exploratory study. *South Africa Journal of Psychology, 40*(3), 234–240.

Raco, M. (2009). From expectations to aspirations: State modernisation, urban policy, and the existential politics of welfare in the UK. *Political Geography, 28*(7), 436–444.

Ramrathan, L., & Pillay, D. (2015). Re-imagining and expanding the discourse of student access, throughput and dropout within the South African higher education context. *Alternation Special Edition, 17*, 6–27.

Rosato, N. S., & Baer, J. C. (2012). Latent class analysis: A method for capturing heterogeneity. *Social Work Research*, 61–69. https://doi.org/10.1093/swr/svs006

Ryan, R. M. (2012). Motivation and the organization of human behaviour: Three reasons for the re-emergence of a field. In R. M. Ryan (Ed.), *The Oxford handbook of human motivation* (pp. 3–10). Oxford University Press.

Savahl, S., Isaacs, S., Adams, S., Carels, C. Z., & September, R. (2013). An exploration into the impact of exposure to community violence and hope on children's perceptions of well-being: A South African perspective. *Child Indicators Research, 6*(3), 579–592.

Scheier, M. F., & Carver, C. S. (1985). Optimism, coping, and health: Assessment and implications of generalized outcome expectancies. *Health Psychology, 4*(3), 219–247.

Seginer, R. (2008). Future orientation in times of threat and challenge: How resilient adolescents construct their future. *International Journal of Behavioral Development, 32*, 272–282.

Senior, K. A., & Chenhall, R. D. (2012). Boyfriends, babies and basketball: Present lives and future aspirations of young women in a remote Australian aboriginal community. *Journal of Youth Studies, 15*(3), 369–388.

Sheldon, K. M., Corcoran, M., & Prentice, M. (2019). Pursuing eudaimonic functioning versus pursuing hedonic well-being: The first goal succeeds in its aim, whereas the second does not. *Journal of Happiness Studies, 20*, 919–933.

Siwek, Z., Oleszkowicz, A., & Slowinska, A. (2017). Values realised in personal striving and motivation, and meaning in life in Polish university students. *Journal of Happiness Studies, 18*, 549–573.

Snyder, C. R. (2002). Hopeful theory: Rainbows in the mind. *Psychological Inquiry, 13*(4), 249–275.
Snyder, C. R. (2004). Hope and the other strengths: Lessons from animal farm. *Journal of Social and Clinical Psychology, 5*, 624–627.
Snyder, C. R., Cheavens, J., & Michael, S. T. (1999). Hoping. In C. R. Snyder (Ed.), *Coping: The psychology of what works* (pp. 205–231). Oxford University Press.
Snyder, C. R., Feldman, D. B., Taylor, J. D., Schroeder, L. L., & Adams, V. H., III. (2000). The roles of hopeful thinking in preventing problems and enhancing strengths. *Applied and Preventative Psychology, 9*, 249–270.
Snyder, C. R., Harris, C., Anderson, J. R., Holleran, S. A., Irving, L. M., Sigmon, S. T., Lauren, Y., June, G., Charyle, L., & Harney, P. (1991). The will and the ways: Development and validation of an individual-differences measure of hope. *Journal of Personality and Social Psychology, 60*(90), 570–585.
Snyder, C. R., Lopez, S. J., Shorey, H. S., Rand, K. L., & Feldman, D. B. (2003). Hope theory, measurements, and applications to school psychology. *School Psychology Quarterly, 18*, 122–139.
Steger, M. F. (2012). Experiencing meaning in life: Optimal functioning at the nexus of well-being, psychopathology, and spirituality. In P. T. Wong (Ed.), *The human quest for meaning* (2nd ed., pp. 165–184). Routledge.
Steger, M. F., Frazier, P., Oishi, S., & Kaler, M. (2006). The meaning in life questionnaire: Assessing the presence of and search for meaning in life. *Journal of Counseling Psychology, 53*(1), 80–93.
Steger, M. F., Kashdan, T. B., Sullivan, B. A., & Lorentz, D. (2008). Understanding the search for meaning in life: Personality, cognitive style, and dynamic between seeking and experiencing meaning. *Journal of Personality, 76*(2), 199–227.
Talevich, J. R., Read, S. J., Walsh, D. A., Iyer, R., & Chopra, G. (2017). Toward a comprehensive taxonomy of human motives. *PLoS One, 12*(2), e0172279. https://doi.org/10.1371/journal.pone.0172279
Temane, L., Khumalo, I. P., & Wissing, M. P. (2014). Validation of the meaning in life questionnaire in an African context. *Journal of Psychology in Africa, 24*(1), 81–95.
Threadgold, S. (2011). Should I pitch my tent in the middle ground? On 'middling tendency' Beck and inequality in youth sociology. *Journal of Youth Studies, 14*(4), 381–393.
Universities South Africa. (2017). *Understanding students: A key to systemic success*. Retrieved September 22, 2019, from http://www.usaf.ac.za/wp-content/uploads/2018/04/Understanding-students_WEB.pdf
Valle, M. F., Huebner, E. S., & Suldo, S. M. (2006). An analysis of hope as a psychological strength. *Journal of School Psychology, 44*(5), 393–406.
Vidwans, S. S., & Raghvendra, P. (2016). A study of meaningful work, hope and meaning in life in young professional artists. *Indian Journal of Positive Psychology, 7*(4), 469.
Wilson, A., & Somhlaba, N. Z. (2017). Ghanaian school-going adolescents' self-perceived barriers of access to quality education: A qualitative study. *Development Southern Africa, 34*(5), 652–665.
Wilson, A., Wissing, M. P., Schutte, L., & Kruger, I. M. (2019). Understanding goal motivations in deprived contexts: Perspectives of adults in two rural South African communities. *Applied Research in Quality of Life, 14*(1), 113–129.
Wissing, M. P., Schutte, L., Liversage, C., Entwisle, B., Gericke, M., & Keyes, C. (2019). Important goals, meanings, and relationships in flourishing and languishing states: Towards patterns of well-being. *Applied Research in Quality of Life*. https://doi.org/10.1007/s11482-019-09771-8
Yalçın, İ., & Malkoç, A. (2015). The relationship between meaning in life and subjective well-being: Forgiveness and Hope as Mediators. *Journal of Happiness Studies, 16*, 915–929. https://doi.org/10.1007/s10902-014-9540-5
Zhang, K. C., & Zhang, A. (2017). Dare to dream: Personal values, life goals, and international students in New Zealand. *Journal of Religion and Health, 56*, 1503–1514.

Chapter 12
Virtues and Character Strengths, Subjective Well-Being and Academic Achievement: An Exploratory Study with Angolan University Students

Rutnilson da Silva, Ana Maria Rocha, and Dilson Francisco

Abstract This study aimed to understand the existing relationships between virtues, character strengths, subjective well-being and academic achievement in Angolan university students. Two hundred and eighteen students from the Catholic University of Angola participated in this research. Virtues and character strengths were assessed with the VIA survey 24; subjective well-being with the Mental Health Continuum—Short Form—for youth, and academic achievement with cumulative grade-point average and the number of previous school retentions. Regarding virtues and character strengths, transcendence, hope and love had the higher values, and temperance, self-regulation and creativity the lower ones. Our participants had higher levels of psychological well-being, and lower levels of social well-being. The correlations between virtues and character strengths, well-being and academic achievement showed that the overall well-being score is positive and significantly correlated with all virtues and the majority of character strengths. On the other hand, psychological well-being was more strongly related to virtues and character strengths. Finally, the correlations with academic achievement were scarce, in which only love of learning, temperance, appreciation of beauty and excellence and forgiveness seem to have correlations with the first variable. There is a further need to understand how these variables interact with academic achievement.

Keywords Virtues · Character strengths · Subjective well-being · Academic achievement · Angola

R. da Silva · A. M. Rocha (✉) · D. Francisco
Universidade Católica de Angola, Luanda, Angola
e-mail: ana.rocha@ucan.edu

L. Schutte et al. (eds.), *Embracing Well-Being in Diverse African Contexts: Research Perspectives*, Cross-Cultural Advancements in Positive Psychology 16,
https://doi.org/10.1007/978-3-030-85924-4_12

12.1 Introduction

More than 2500 years after Plato claimed that education should help students find pleasure in their learning, it seems this pleasure has seldom been integrated into educational goals. Today, education is still attached to the main focus on academic problem-solving. In education that seeks excellence, in education for all students, its focus should change from products (school results in themselves are valuable) to processes (results are a consequence of the pursuit of excellence). Achieving excellence will require acknowledgment that the cognitive domain must be considered along with the socio-emotional one, focusing on developing the new three "r's" of education: reasoning, resilience, and responsibility (Sternberg, 2008).

In this vein, the Organization for Economic Cooperation and Development ([OECD], 2017) considers that academic achievement and subjective well-being are both needed for high-performing education systems, mentioning that successful students perform well academically, and are satisfied at school as well. On one hand, higher education provides youth with the chance to develop knowledge and perspective, personal identity and personal growth (Giovazolias et al., 2008); on the other hand, it can generate several challenges that may be a source of stress for students, such as coping with academic work, anxiety when being separated from their family, financial worries, as well as developing new social and romantic relationships.

Traditionally, Psychology has focused on the dark side of the human functioning (e.g., psychological problems, psychopathology, weaknesses and deficits) until the emergence of Humanistic Psychology, which started to acknowledge human potential for self-actualization. In 2000, Seligman and Csikszentmihalyi coined the term Positive Psychology, in their editorial in the millennium issue of the American Psychologist, turning to focus on positive behavior, human strengths, virtues and "what makes life worth living" (p. 13), focusing on the conditions and processes that may contribute to the optimal functioning of human beings and organizations (Gable & Haidt, 2005).

12.1.1 Subjective Well-Being

Subjective well-being (SWB) has been frequently studied in Positive Psychology, framed by two major theoretical approaches: hedonic and eudaimonic (Ryan & Deci, 2001). Stemming from the Greek philosopher Aristippus of Cyrene's hedonic perspective, which asserts that to be happy, people need to increase pleasurable situations, Diener's (Diener, 2012; Diener et al., 1999) definition of SWB differentiates between a cognitive and an affective component of SWB; the first is related to individuals' cognitive evaluations of their lives as a whole (i.e., global life satisfaction) and in specific life domains (e.g., job and marital satisfaction); and the second is related to the affective components such as individuals' reports of pleasant emotions (e.g., joy, enthusiasm) and negative emotions (e.g., sadness, depressed mood).

The eudaimonic perspective stems from Aristotle's philosophy, who said that the ultimate purpose of human existence was happiness, which was reached through the activity of expressing virtue and attaining "*daimon*" or the perfect self (not pleasure), or in other words, achieving one's highest needs: self-realization (Ryan & Deci, 2001). Csikszentmihalyi's (2008) flow conceptualization, Seligman's (2011) PERMA[1] model and Keyes's (2002) continuum of mental health are included in this eudaimonic perspective. Generally, these authors' perspective focuses on self-realization and considers well-being as a degree to which an individual is fully functioning. Seligman (2011) proposed the PERMA model, published in his book *Flourish*, in which the term *flourishing* is central to SWB. For an individual to flourish, they must experience more positive emotions, engage in meaningful activities, have positive relationships and achieve meaning in their lives, and reach a stage of accomplishment.

In this research, we followed the eudaimonic perspective, with the underlying assumption that when students recognize and use their positive strengths, are more able to experience more positive emotions, find meaning in life and their activities, and relate to others in meaningful ways, this ultimately leads to greater achievement in life.

More specifically, we focused on Keyes's (2002) approach, which was the first to use the term *flourishing* as part of SWB. For Keyes (2010), mental health is conceived on a continuum from *languishing* (as the state of mental health in which the individual considers they are not feeling emotionally well and its not functioning at their optimal level), to *flourishing* (the state in which individuals are directed to self-actualization and are free of psychopathology, having high degrees of emotional, psychological and social well-being). Keyes's definition of SWB is in line with the World Health Organization's (WHO, 1948) definition of health as "a state of complete physical, mental and social well-being and not merely the absence of disease or infirmity" and positive mental health as "a state of well-being in which the individual realizes his or her own abilities, can cope with the normal stresses of life, can work productively and fruitfully, and is able to make a contribution to his or her community" (WHO, 2001).

According to previous studies, in general, higher levels of SWB are associated with a lower risk of several psycho-social problems, such as depression and maladaptive relationships with others (e.g., Furr & Funder, 1998; Lewinsohn et al., 1991; Park, 2004). Among youth, SWB is associated with better physical and healthy behaviors (Frisch, 2000); fewer discipline problems at school (McKnight et al., 2002), and lower risk behaviors, such as alcohol, tobacco and marijuana use (Zullig et al., 2001).

[1] PERMA is the acronym for positive emotion, engagement, meaning, positive relationships, and accomplishment.

12.1.2 Character Strengths and Virtues

Within the eudaimonic background, Peterson and Seligman (2004) presented the Values-In-Action (VIA) strengths classification system, in opposition to the Diagnostic and Statistical Manual of Mental Disorders (DSM), which contends that character strengths are the core characteristics or traits that facilitate individuals to be virtuous. The authors suggest that these strengths are universal, internally valuable and morally oriented, can be developed, and when used, lead to increased happiness. They are used as ways to reach virtues (Park et al., 2004).

Peterson and Seligman (2004) proposed 24 character strengths, being grouped in 6 universal virtues: wisdom, courage, humanity, justice, temperance, and transcendence. See Table 12.1 for further details about these virtues and character strengths.

According to Peterson and Seligman (2004), the five dominant strengths are to be considered as an individual's signature strengths, the strengths one identifies with. They are central to identity and make an individual feel content, energetic and authentic when using them. Seligman and Csikszentmihalyi (2000) underlined that when individuals use their character strengths, they experience a sense of fulfillment and more satisfaction with life. Seligman (2002) argued that the greatest successes and satisfaction in life emanate from enhancing and using one's character strengths rather than focusing on one's weaknesses. Later on, Seligman (2011), contended that the frequent use of these strengths is associated with flourishing, i.e., generating more positive emotions, engagement in meaningful activities, having positive relationships, achieving meaning in life, and reaching self-realization.

12.1.3 Academic Achievement

Academic achievement is a performance outcome of instruction (Steinmayr et al., 2018) and is central in mastering developmental tasks during school years and young adulthood. Steinmayr et al. (2014) underline the importance of academic achievement as a basis for a nation's wealth. Higher academic achievement is associated with higher self-concept (Guay et al., 2003), higher self-efficacy (Zajacova et al., 2005), higher social competence (Izard et al., 2001; Ragozzino et al., 2003; Mostow et al., 2002), as well as positive health behavior and health (Eide et al., 2010; SigfúSDóttir et al., 2007). This variable can be measured with a wide range of indicators (Steinmayr et al., 2014). In this study, we considered the student's cumulative grade-point average (GPA), which is viewed as the most important indicator of college student performance (Astin, 1993; Pascarella & Terenzini, 1991), as well as previous academic retentions (Almeida & Lemos, 2005).

In a cross-national study, Schaufeli, Martinez, et al. (2002) and Schaufeli, Salanova, et al. (2002) found that Higher Education students' engagement was positively correlated with academic achievement. Longitudinal studies have also shown that engaged students in secondary school were more likely to obtain better

Table 12.1 Peterson and Seligman's (2004) classification of virtues and character strengths

Virtue and character strength	Definition
Wisdom and knowledge	**Cognitive strengths that foster acquisition and use of knowledge**
Creativity	Thinking in a different and productive way in order to do things
Curiosity	Manifesting interest in all experience
Open-mindedness	Analyzing things through and examining them from all sides
Love of learning	Being interested about mastering new skills and bodies of knowledge
Perspective	Being able to provide wise advice to others
Courage	**Emotional strengths that require the exercise the will to accomplish goals when facing internal or external opposition**
Authenticity	Speaking the truth and presenting oneself genuinely
Bravery	Not shrinking in face of threat, challenge, difficulty or pain
Persistence	Finishing what one starts
Zest	Approaching life with excitement and energy
Humanity	**Interpersonal skills that involve "tending and befriending" others**
Kindness	Doing favours and good deeds for others
Love	Valuing close relationships with others
Social intelligence	Being aware of the needs and feelings of oneself and others
Justice	**Civic strengths that underlie healthy community life**
Fairness	Treating all people the same according to fairness and justice
Leadership	Supervising group activities
Teamwork	Working cooperatively as a member of a group or a team
Temperance	**Strengths that protect oneself form excess**
Forgiveness	Forgiving those who have done something wrong
Modesty	Letting one's accomplishments speak for themselves
Prudence	Being careful about one's choices
Self-regulation	Regulating what one feels and does
Transcendence	**Strengths that forge connections to the larger universe and provide meaning**
Appreciation of beauty and excellence	Noticing and appreciating beauty, excellence and/or skilled performance in different domains of life
Gratitude	Being aware of and thankful for the good things that happen to oneself
Hope	Expecting the best and working to achieve it
Humour	Enjoying to laugh and to make others laugh
Spirituality	Having coherent beliefs about the higher purpose and meaning of life

academic outcomes in the long term, such as finishing university degrees (Tuominen-Soini & Salmela-Aro, 2014).

12.1.4 Character Strengths, Subjective Well-Being, and Academic Achievement

Several studies have been carried out around the world regarding the contributions of character strengths to college students' adaptive functioning, such as SWB and academic achievement.

Regarding **academic achievement**, several studies reported a positive correlation with character strengths (Choudhury & Borooah, 2017; Jackson et al., 2014; Kern & Bowling III, 2015; Lounsbury et al., 2009). In the last mentioned study, the strengths showing a greater correlation with academic achievement were persistence, judgment, self-regulation, love for learning, and prudence, with correlations ranging from $r = .25$ to $r = .31$.

Several studies have found correlations between **academic achievement and SWB** (Bücker et al., 2018; Crede et al., 2015; Kirkcaldy et al., 2004; Steinmayr et al., 2014; Suldo et al., 2008). Lounsbury et al. (2009) found that persistence ($r = .31$), judgment ($r = .27$), love for learning ($r = .26$) and self-regulation ($r = .26$) had stronger positive correlations with GPA. On the other hand, Jackson et al. (2014), using structural equation modeling, found that psychological strengths (self-efficacy, gratitude and hope) were significant predictors of SWB (self-esteem and satisfaction with life), with hope and gratitude having the highest coefficients. Kirkcaldy et al. (2004), using data from 30 countries, found that the countries with high performance in the PISA survey (academic achievement in scientific, mathematical and reading literacy) had higher average SWB scores, especially with reading achievement ($r = .63$).

Similarly, positive correlations between **character strengths and SWB** have been found both in cross-sectional (Botha & Mostert, 2014; Douglass & Duffy, 2015; Harzer & Ruch, 2013; Huber et al., 2017; Linley et al., 2010; Littman-Ovadia et al., 2017; Park et al., 2004; Proctor et al., 2011) and longitudinal studies (Wood et al., 2011).

Considering the specific character strengths, zest ($r = .48$), love ($r = .45$), hope ($r = .43$), self-regulation ($r = .41$) and curiosity ($r = .41$) had the highest correlations with SWB (Lounsbury et al., 2009).

12.1.5 The Current Study

This study aims to examine how character strengths are related to two key outcome variables (academic achievement and SWB) in Angolan university students.

The domains under study have been studied in depth worldwide, but hardly at all in Africa, the exceptions being South Africa (Botha & Booysen, 2014; Ebrahim et al., 2013; Møller, 2013) and Ghana (Addai et al., 2014; Pokimica et al., 2012). To our knowledge, no Angolan study has been published in this field.

Lomas (2015) proposes the development of Positive Cross-cultural Psychology to determine the existence of commonalities between people across cultures and the differences between people of different cultures in search of specific contents and processes by which positive processes occur. For instance, Becker and Marecek (2008) underline that the American culture is more individualistic regarding the goals of self-realization. It may be possible that collectivist societies such as Angola (Hofstede Insights, n.d.) have a more societal and family orientation towards SWB.

A great number of African countries, among them Angola, have significant development challenges (Kamoche et al., 2004). Angola was a Portuguese colony for almost 500 years. It became independent in 1975 and faced a civil war lasting more than 30 years. Looking at the current scenario of Angola: it has had impressive economic growth rates in the last 16 years: its average gross GDP growth is 6.5%, ranging from 14.9% (in 2005) to −3.6% % (in 2016), according to the 2006 Angola Economic Report (Universidade Católica de Angola/Centro de Estudos e Investigação Científica, UCAN/CEIC, 2017). It is the second largest oil producer in Africa and the 13th largest in the world. It has the second most polarized economy (around oil) in the world (UCAN/CEIC, 2015), which makes it especially fragile at times of crisis in the sector. Its Human Development Index in 2016 was 0.533 (considered low and occupying the 150th position of 188 countries evaluated by the United Nations, UN). Besides, Angola's Corruption Perceptions Index (Transparency International, 2016, quoted by UCAN/CEIC, 2017) is among the highest in the world, reaching 18 points (corresponding to the 16th position of 176 countries). According to Helmke and Levitsky's (2004, cit. by Cunha et al., 2016), classification, "Angola can be considered more as an 'informally dominated market economy' in which organizational decisions are more influenced by informal institutions, defined as 'socially shared rules', usually unwritten, that are created, communicated, and enforced outside of officially sanctioned channels" (p. 5).

Angola has a very young population with around 65% of people aged below 24 years old. The unemployment rate among young people aged between 20 and 24 years old is high (34.2% for men; 36.7% for women) (Instituto Nacional de Estatística, 2016). The increase in schooling up to Higher Education can generate an increase in the employability of these young people, so it is relevant to study the factors that affect academic performance and school dropout. Additionally, understanding the mechanisms underlying the emergence and maintenance of virtues and character strengths can be relevant in developing a more transparent, democratic and just society, in order to promote higher levels of human development.

12.2 Method

This study followed a quantitative, descriptive-correlational and transversal design. We implemented self-report questionnaires that allow the quantification of variables, in order to describe the existing relations between the variables under study (Vilelas, 2009).

12.2.1 Sample

Using a non-probabilistic and convenience sampling procedure (selecting the students that were available and interested in participating in this study), 218 Angolan university students from the Catholic University of Angola participated in this study, of which 50.90% (n = 111) were female, 48.60% (n = 106) were male; one participant did not indicate gender. The mean age was 22.46 years (SD = 4.61), with a minimum of 18 and a maximum of 52 years.

Regarding students' B.A. course, the majority were studying Accounting (n = 49; 22.50%), Law (n = 34; 15.60%) and Work and Organizational Psychology (n = 34; 15.60%), as shown in Table 12.2.

Considering year of study, 73 (33.50%) were in the third year, 62 (28.40%) were in the fourth year, 51 (23.40%) in the first year, and 32 (14.70%) were in the second year.

12.2.2 Instruments

12.2.2.1 Academic Achievement

To characterize academic achievement, the participants were asked to self-report cumulative grade-point average (GPA) as well as previous academic retentions.

Table 12.2 Student's B.A. Course

B.A. Course	Frequency	Percentage
Accounting	49	22.50%
Law	34	15.60%
Work and Organizational Psychology	34	15.60%
Oil Engineering	24	11.00%
Telecommunications Engineering	22	10.10%
Clinical Psychology	12	5.50%
Business and Administration	12	5.50%
Informatics Engineering	9	4.10%
Nutrition	8	3.70%
Languages and Administration	6	2.80%
Public Health	5	2.30%
Economics	2	0.90%
Missing	1	0.50%
Total	**218**	**100.00%**

12.2.2.2 Subjective Well-Being

Participants responded to the Portuguese version of Mental Health Continuum—Short Form—for youth (MHC-SF; Keyes, 2009), which has been translated and validated by a research team from the University of Lisbon (Matos et al., 2010), who authorized us to use it in Angola. This instrument assesses mental health states, which are estimated from the perceived level of well-being. MHC-SF is a short version of another Questionnaire from the same author previously used with adults.

A Likert scale was used (1—never; 2—from 2 to 3 times a week; 3 - from 3 to 4 times a week; 4—almost every day and 5—everyday). It has 14 items distributed in 3 dimensions: emotional well-being (3 items) which "consists of symptoms that reflect 'emotional vitality' (positive emotions assessed by the degree of happiness, interest and satisfaction in life" (Matos et al., 2010, p. 132); social well-being (5 items) related to the fact that "the mentally healthy person, on a social level, perceives society as meaningful to him/herself, considers that it allows his/her personal development, perceives him/herself as accepted, integrated and understands that he/she contributes to the evolution of that same society" (Matos et al., 2010, p. 133); and psychological well-being (6 items) which is related to "(...) a continuous process of personal development, has goals, perception of meaning and direction in life, has intimate and warm relationships, deals with the surrounding context in order to satisfy needs and has a significant degree of self-determination" (Matos et al., 2010, p. 133).

In this study, the questionnaire subscales have adequate internal consistency indices: general subjective well-being $\alpha = .83$; emotional well-being $\alpha = .74$; social well-being $\alpha = .54$ and psychological well-being $\alpha = .77$. Keyes's (2009) original study with an American sample had values of .84 (emotional), .80 (social) and .78 (psychological). In Setswana-speaking South Africans, Keyes et al. (2008) had the following alphas: .74 (general scale); .67 (emotional); .59 (social) and .67 (psychological). Generally, reliability coefficients are considered acceptable when above .70 (Nunnally, 1978), which means the alphas of emotional and psychological well-being are adequate. Accordingly, the social well-being scale has low internal consistency reliability. Considering an early version of Nunnally's work (1967), in exploratory research (which is the case here) values between .50 and .60 are considered acceptable. On the other hand, "*self-judgments are more situation specific than judgments by others, which tend to be more trait-like*" (Ford, 1982, p. 330). As Anastasi and Urbina mentioned (2000), the instrument's goal itself should be considered for the purpose of item analysis, not taking into account only the statistical information.

12.2.2.3 Virtues and Character Strengths

Character strengths were assessed with the VIA Survey-24, based on the Peterson and Seligman (2004) theoretical model and is a very brief version of the original VIA

Survey (with 240 items). This survey assesses the 24 character strengths which are grouped in 6 virtues, as described in Table 12.1. The VIA Institute on Character provided authorization to translate the scale into Portuguese and use it in Angola. We followed international guidelines in the matter of translating psychological assessment instruments (International Test Commission, 2001). We used two independent Angolan bilingual researchers: firstly, the English version was translated into Portuguese by the first author; secondly, the Portuguese version was back-translated into English by the second author, and, finally, the two versions were compared and discussed until consensus was reached. A Likert type scale was used: 1—totally disagree; 2—strongly disagree; 3—disagree; 4—neutral; 5—agree; 6—strongly agree, and 7—totally agree.

The questionnaire subscales yielded the following internal consistency reliability indices: Wisdom and Knowledge $\alpha = .64$; Courage $\alpha = .54$; Humanity $\alpha = .57$; Justice $\alpha = .37$; Temperance $\alpha = .61$ and Transcendence $\alpha = .64$. According to Nunnally's (1967) guidelines, all the values indicate acceptable internal consistency reliability for an exploratory research, except for the Justice subscale. McGrath (2019) reported Cronbach's alpha values only for character strengths ranging from .71 (modesty) to .84 (leadership, social intelligence and zest). In a South African Sample using the 240-item questionnaire version (Khumalo, 2005), alphas ranged from .56 (self-regulation) to .83 (fairness and leadership). We didn't find any published data related to VIA-24 Survey in any other African country, therefore comparisons between our results and existing studies such as McGrath (2019) and Khumalo (2005) should be made with caution.

12.2.3 Procedure

At the beginning, an authorization from the Catholic University of Angola was given for data collection among its students. Then, having the translated versions of the mentioned instruments, a pilot study was undertaken with 49 undergraduate students of Psychology who were asked to provide adjustments to the Portuguese used in the questionnaires. The final versions of the questionnaires were delivered in group sessions by two senior undergraduate Psychology students, who explained the study purposes, the ethical principles used regarding confidentiality and about the possibility of withdrawing from the study.All data were analyzed using SPSS 24.0.

12.3 Results: Analysis and Discussion

12.3.1 Descriptive Results

12.3.1.1 Academic Achievement

Considering the Cumulative GPA, generally, the participants reported an average value of 12.48 ($SD = 1.45$) on a 0–20 scale. The courses where the cumulative GPA was highest were Nutrition ($M = 13.13$; $SD = 1.65$) and Telecommunications Engineering ($M = 12.73$; $SD = 0.98$). On the other hand, the lowest cumulative GPA was found in Oil Engineering ($M = 11.92$; $SD = 1.07$), Economics ($M = 12.00$), and Informatics Engineering ($M = 12.00$; $SD = 0.71$). For further information, see Table 12.3.

Regarding previous academic retentions, 76 participants (34.9%) have reported that they already had previous academic retentions, while as long as 133 students (61.0%) did not. Nine students (4.1%) didn't answer this question.

Table 12.4 reflects the frequencies of the number of previous academic retentions, in which 52 students (23.90%) had one previous retention and 19 (8.70%) had two.

12.3.1.2 Subjective Well-Being

Table 12.5 provides the descriptive results of MHC-SF. The sample obtained a mean of 3.37 ($SD = 0.65$) in a scale of 1–5, which may be considered an average value. The highest results are present in the psychological well-being domain ($M = 3.77$; $SD = 0.82$) and the lowest in social well-being ($M = 2.73$; $SD = 0.79$).

Comparing these results to other studies, it is interesting to note that they are more similar to a Setswana-speaking South African sample (Keyes et al., 2008), than to a

Table 12.3 Cumulative GPA in the different B.A. Courses

B.A. Course	Mean	*SD*	Min.	Max.
Public Health	n.a.	n.a.	n.a.	n.a.
Nutrition	13.13	1.65	11.50	15.00
Telecommunications Engineering	12.73	0.98	11.50	14.50
Languages and Administration	12.67	1.61	11.50	14.50
Clinical Psychology	12.63	1.36	11.00	14.00
Work and Organizational Psychology	12.61	1.76	10.00	16.00
Accounting	12.56	1.67	10.00	19.00
Business and Administration	12.32	1.08	11.00	14.50
Law	12.23	1.46	9.70	15.00
Informatics Engineering	12.00	0.71	11.50	12.50
Economics	12.00	–	12.00	12.00
Oil Engineering	11.92	1.07	10.50	13.85
General	**12.48**	**1.45**	**9.7**	**19.00**

Table 12.4 Table of frequencies of the number of previous academic retentions

Number of previous academic retentions	Frequency	Percentage
0 previous retention	133	65.80%
1 previous retention	52	23.90%
2 previous retentions	19	8.70%
3 previous retentions	3	1.40%
4 previous retentions	0	0.00%
5 previous retentions	1	0.50%
Missing	10	5.00%
Total	218	100%

Portuguese sample (Cadime et al., 2016). In both Angolan and Setswana-speaking South African samples, the higher results were on psychological well-being and the lowest were in social well-being. On the other hand, in the Portuguese sample the results were in the opposite direction.

These results may be related to a lower perception of control regarding the social environment. We must remember that Angola has a low level of human development and a high level of corruption, as mentioned earlier, which may contribute to a lower belief that people can improve their social conditions. Even so, youth seem to keep on showing psychological resilience.

12.3.1.3 Virtues and Character Strengths

Generally, the sample obtained a mean score of 5.31 ($SD = 0.66$), which may be considered medium-high since the scale ranges from 1–7 points, and were similar in all the 6 virtues. The highest values were in transcendence ($M = 5.51$; $SD = 1.02$) and the lowest in temperance ($M = 5.08$; $SD = 1.02$). Regarding character strengths, the highest results were in hope ($M = 5.79$; $SD = 1.28$) and love ($M = 5.68$; $SD = 1.13$). The lowest results were in self-regulation ($M = 4.73$; $SD = 1.56$) and creativity ($M = 4.88$; $SD = 1.27$).

Comparing these results with others from the USA (Lounsbury et al., 2009), Brazil (Oliveira et al., 2016) and South Africa (Khumalo, 2005), the highest results were in the following strengths: love and kindness; hope and gratitude; spirituality and hope, respectively. The lowest results were in modesty, self-regulation and prudence; prudence and modesty; love of learning and self-regulation. Therefore, generally, Angolan results seem more similar to those of Brazil and South Africa.

The higher results in Angola in the transcendence virtue may be due to higher levels of perception of control, as mentioned above. This, in turn, may lead to people having higher spiritual beliefs and religious practices that cultivate strengths such as love and hope.

According to the 2014 Angolan Population Census, 87.7% of people say they practice a religion (the most frequent were catholic - 41% and protestant—38%) (Instituto Nacional de Estatística, 2016).

Table 12.5 Descriptive statistics of MHC-SF and VIA Survey-24

Dimensions	Mean	*SD*	Min.	Max.
Emotional well-being	3.60	0.92	1000	5.00
Social well-being	2.73	0.79	0.60	4.60
Psychological well-being	3.77	0.82	0.00	5.00
General well-being	**3.37**	**0.65**	**1.22**	**4.81**
Wisdom and knowledge	**5.26**	**0.79**	**2.40**	**7.00**
Creativity	4.88	1.27	1.00	7.00
Curiosity	5.48	1.10	2.00	7.00
Open-mindedness	5.22	1.34	1.00	7.00
Love of learning	5.33	1.17	1.00	7.00
Perspective	5.47	1.19	2.00	7.00
Courage	**5.24**	**0.89**	**2.50**	**7.00**
Authenticity	5.32	1.33	2.00	7.00
Bravery	5.32	1.28	1.00	7.00
Persistence	5.54	1.32	1.00	7.00
Zest	4.94	1.35	1.00	7.00
Humanity	**5.46**	**0.95**	**2.33**	**7.00**
Kindness	5.64	1.38	1.00	7.00
Love	5.68	1.13	1.00	7.00
Social intelligence	5.18	1.20	1.00	7.00
Justice	**5.30**	**0.88**	**2.67**	**7.00**
Fairness	5.43	1.28	1.00	7.00
Leadership	5.46	1.30	1.00	7.00
Teamwork	5.07	1.31	1.00	7.00
Temperance	**5.08**	**1.02**	**1.00**	**7.00**
Forgiveness	5.05	1.69	1.00	7.00
Modesty	5.44	1.23	1.00	7.00
Prudence	5.25	1.39	1.00	7.00
Self-regulation	4.73	1.56	1.00	7.00
Transcendence	**5.51**	**1.02**	**0.00**	**7.00**
Appreciation of beauty and excellence	5.30	1.31	1.00	7.00
Gratitude	5.64	1.29	1.00	7.00
Hope	5.79	1.28	1.00	7.00
Humour	5.56	1.44	1.00	7.00
Spirituality	5.65	1.34	1.00	7.00
Overall character strengths	**5.31**	**0.66**	**2.85**	**6.89**

In a Mozambican study, Galinha et al. (2016) found that people tend to compensate for extreme material poverty with level of satisfaction with life in social (relationships with family and friends) and spiritual domains, which is consistent with a study from Ghana (Pokimica et al., 2012). Indeed, the social support people living in poverty receive from religious organizations may be one of the most important for facing life challenges. Cumulatively, hope as a future expectation may be considered as a mechanism to cope with material hardship. In this line, Møller et al. (2008) consider that future expectations are relevant for people's perceptions of SWB in poverty contexts, where hoping for a better future brings happiness to the present.

Regarding the lower results (temperance, self-regulation, and creativity), these may be due to a high level of indulgence and low level of long-term orientation in Angola (Hofstede, n.d.), which may be associated with a low level of self-determination due to the low level of human development, high level of corruption, and a cumulative effect of more than 30 years of war and almost 500 years of colonization, creating a kind of socially learned helplessness, in which people tend to live 1 day at a time. Finally, it is known that the lower the self-determination, the lower the creativity (Hetland et al., 2011; Ryan & Deci, 2001).

12.3.2 Relation Between Variables

The correlations between virtues and character strengths, well-being and academic achievement appear in Table 12.6, showing that the **overall well-being** score is positive and significantly correlated with all virtues and character strengths, except with persistence, love, leadership, modesty and humor. All the correlation coefficients are low to moderate; the highest correlations with virtues are: wisdom and knowledge ($r = .339$; $p < .01$) and courage ($r = .337$; $p < .01$); and with character strengths are with hope ($r = .295$; $p < .01$), zest and perspective (both with $r = .293$; $p < .01$).

Regarding the three dimensions of well-being, **psychological well-being** has the greatest correlations: all the 6 virtues and 16 (out of 24) character strengths have positive and significant correlations, which are highest with wisdom and knowledge ($r = .349$; $p < .01$) and courage ($r = .326$; $p < .01$), for virtues; and bravery ($r = .304$; $p < .01$) and curiosity ($r = .262$; $p < .01$) for character strengths. **Emotional well-being** had highest positive and significant correlations with wisdom and knowledge ($r = .222$; $p < .01$) and courage ($r = .216$; $p < .01$), for virtues; and with zest ($r = .234$; p < .01) and hope ($r = .228$; p < .01). **Social well-being** followed a similar pattern, having higher positive and significant correlations with wisdom and knowledge ($r = .220$; p < .01) and courage ($r = .248$; p < .01), for virtues; and with appreciation of beauty and excellence ($r = .231$; p < .01) and zest ($r = .234$; p < .01).

Our results regarding the relationship between virtues/character strengths and SWB are relatively similar to previous studies (Botha & Mostert, 2014; Douglass & Duffy, 2015; Harzer & Ruch, 2013; Huber et al., 2017; Linley et al., 2010; Littman-Ovadia et al., 2017; Park et al., 2004; Proctor et al., 2011; Wood et al., 2011). Our highest correlation coefficients (hope, zest, and perspective) are somewhat similar to the studies by Lounsbury et al. (2009) and Jackson et al. (2014), in which zest and hope are two of the highest correlations with SWB. Hope is related to transcendence and reflects the importance religion may have on its promotion, as mentioned earlier

Table 12.6 Pearson correlations between virtues and character strengths, well-being and academic achievement

Virtues and character strengths	Overall well-being	Emotional well-being	Social well-being	Psychological well-being	Cumulative GPA	Number previous school retentions
Overall character strengths	.347**	.224**	.266**	.323**	−.017	−.211
Wisdom and knowledge	.339**	.222**	.220**	.349**	.104	−.073
Creativity	.245**	.218**	.126	.221**	−.028	.012
Curiosity	.279**	.178**	.213**	.262**	.031	−.046
Open-mindedness	.164*	.096	.075	.212**	.047	−.015
Love of learning	.165*	.06	.160*	.174*	.178*	−.1
Perspective	.293**	.173*	.226**	.291**	.119	−.189
Courage	.337**	.216**	.248**	.326**	.07	−.05
Authenticity	.266**	.158*	.226**	.242**	.061	.167
Bravery	.269**	.168*	.156*	.304**	−.032	−.094
Persistence	.094	.066	.036	.119	.101	−.167
Zest	.293**	.234**	.230**	.218**	.07	.051
Humanity	.214**	.091	.175**	.241**	−.124	−.12
Kindness	.221**	.119	.182**	.221**	−.063	−.152
Love	.036	−.035	.045	.084	−.104	−.196
Social intelligence	.215**	.131	.123	.249**	−.036	−.024
Justice	.169*	.123	.108	.161*	−.067	−.18
Fairness	.137*	.137*	.073	.106	.013	−.096
Leadership	.025	.03	.049	.046	−.166+	−.208
Teamwork	.204**	.147*	.112	.215**	.006	−.078
Temperance	.212**	.168*	.189**	.137*	027	−.233*
Forgiveness	.140*	.108	.193**	.031	.09	−.300**
Modesty	.09	.101	.072	.034	−.053	−.099
Prudence	.178**	.099	.111	.208**	.053	−.168
Self-regulation	.190**	.173*	.124	.142*	−.017	−.111
Transcendence	.235**	.152*	.201**	.199**	−.058	−.193
Appreciation of beauty and excellence	.224**	.136*	.231**	.162*	−.051	−.264*
Gratitude	.193**	.147*	.108	.190**	−.144	−.015
Hope	.295**	.228**	.203**	.256**	−.058	−.078
Humour	.115	.086	.103	.079	.066	−.194
Spirituality	.108	.066	.101	.087	.063	−.188

Note: $n = 218$. * $p < .05$ level; ** $p < .01$

(and as Galinha et al. (2016) and Pokimica et al. (2012) found in Mozambique and Ghana). As for perspective, which is partly related to the role the individual plays in social interactions as a source of support, once again, this shows the importance of social relations for SWB, as Galinha et al. (2016) found in Mozambique. Finally, we note the higher number and higher coefficients of correlations between virtues/character strengths and psychological well-being, which may be due to this dimension being somewhat related to self-determination and resilience, revealing the importance of this variable to SWB and a way to cope with life's difficulties.

Considering **academic achievement**, cumulative GPA only had a positive and significant correlation with the love of learning ($r = .178$; $p < .05$). It had a negative, marginally significant correlation with leadership ($r = -.166$; $p = .052$).

Finally, regarding the number of previous school retentions, it had negative and significant correlations with the virtues of temperance ($r = -.233$; $p < .05$), forgiveness ($r = -.300$; $p < .01$) and appreciation of beauty and excellence ($r = -.264$; $p < .05$).

Unlike previous studies, our results regarding the relationships between virtues/character strengths and academic achievement are quite modest, showing us that only the love of learning, temperance, appreciation of beauty and excellence and forgiveness seem to be related. These modest correlations between virtues/character strengths and academic achievement may be due, first of all, to the modest internal consistency of VIA survey subscales.

Love of learning, temperance, and appreciation of beauty and excellence seem to make an obvious contribution to academic achievement because they set a mindset and behaviors that are more appropriate for success, related to assumptions of self-determination theory (Ryan & Deci, 2001), which defends that the needs of autonomy, competence and relatedness increase intrinsic motivation, social development and well-being.

According to the broaden-and-build theory of positive emotions (Fredrickson, 1998, 2001), as academic achievement contributes to fulfilling the need for competence, it enhances self-determination. In addition, higher levels of SWB and specifically positive emotions may increase one's openness to experience, memory and attention processes that raise academic achievement. Cumulatively, positive emotions are associated with the adoption of approach and mastery goals (instead of avoidance goals), which is associated with academic success (Anderman & Wolters, 2006). In the same line, academic intrinsic motivation and the sense of future orientation could be raised as a result of higher levels of psychological well-being, which are present in our sample.

Finally, the correlations between well-being and academic achievement are presented in Table 12.7, showing the only significant correlation to be between the number of previous school retentions and social well-being ($r = -.232$; $p < .05$), which makes sense as students begin to believe that their lack of academic success may undermine their social success.

Table 12.7 Pearson correlations between well-being and academic achievement

Well-being	Cumulative GPA	Number previous school retentions
Overall well-being	.043	−.036
Emotional well-being	.06	.139
Social well-being	.049	−.232*
Psychological well-being	−.011	−.024

Note: $n = 218$. * $p < .05$ level

12.4 Conclusions

Positive Psychology is a burgeoning field of research worldwide, but some places are still little studied, especially Africa. This study sought to contribute to improving this panorama by examining how character strengths were related to academic achievement and SWB in Angolan university students.

Using Keyes's (2009) model of SWB, our participants had higher levels of psychological well-being, and lower levels of social well-being, similarly to samples in other African studies, enhancing the role psychological resilience may have in this context.

Regarding virtues and character strengths, transcendence, hope and love had the highest values, and temperance, self-regulation and creativity the lowest. These results are similar to others found in less developed countries in which spiritual/religious beliefs and social relationships have a more important role.

The correlations between virtues and character strengths, well-being and academic achievement showed the overall well-being score to be positive and significantly correlated with all virtues and character strengths, except for persistence, love, leadership, modesty, and humor, being highest with hope, zest and perspective. Psychological well-being is the type of well-being that is more related to virtues and character strengths.

Finally, the correlations with academic achievement were scarce, with only love of learning correlating positively with cumulative GPA. On the other hand, temperance, appreciation of beauty and excellence and forgiveness had negative correlations with the number of previous school retentions. These results show, to some extent, the role of the development of self-determination through fulfilling competence needs, the effect of positive emotions on cognitive processes and the use of mastery goals. These results may be modest due to cumulative GPA being collected by self-reporting, which may not be so reliable, and because the instruments used to assess SWB and virtues/character strengths have not been validated for the Angolan population.

Generally, our results shed light on the importance of developing resilience and self-determination through fulfilling autonomy, competence and relatedness needs, which may increase the various dimensions of SWB. Naturally, some contextual factors not controllable by the individual *per se* need to be considered, such as the quality of education provided in schools, the degree of employability, the level of corruption that may hinder university students' personal and professional development and may affect their perception of social well-being and degree of self-determination.

Considering our results and regarding practical implications for practitioner psychologists, we underline the importance of:

(a) Implementing Positive Psychology promotion programs in order to develop character strengths and subjective well-being, which can contribute to developing higher academic achievement, higher employability and, indirectly, to a higher level of citizenship, agency, resilience and democratic behaviors that can improve the human development levels of Angola. The contributions of Ubuntu philosophy may be useful to frame positive psychology interventions in Angola, considering the cultural proximity.
(b) Implementing psycho-pedagogical support with a focus on study methods and habits that can enhance academic achievement and commitment;
(c) Implementing career counseling for secondary school students so that the choice of an area of study in higher education is in accordance with students' profile. In Angolan schools, career counseling is still very rare, which may impact negatively on students' academic and intrinsic academic motivation, and subjective well-being, which may be a product of arbitrary choices made by students;
(d) Implementing positive career counseling for university students to facilitate the transition to the work context, focusing on the use of character strengths.

12.5 Limitations and Future Studies

The first limitation of this study is related to the fact that the instruments to assess SWB and virtues/character strengths have not been validated for the Angolan population, which may affect the results. Internal consistency values are quite modest to low for the VIA-Survey, for all its subscales and unacceptable for Justice. Therefore, future research should make deeper psychometric studies (convergent, divergent, content and ecological validity) to ensure its qualities. An alternative could be to use the 72 or 120-item VIA-Survey version, considering that an increased number of items per scale increases the likelihood of having better psychometric properties.

Secondly, the use of self-reporting in these variables and in assessing academic achievement has validity limitations that should be addressed by using multi-source and multi-method instruments. Thirdly, the use of a convenience sample is a limitation in terms of the representativeness of these results, which should be analyzed with due care.

It would be useful to study the impact of cognitive and cultural variables in understanding the mechanisms by which the relation between SWB, virtues/character strengths and academic achievement is formed. Finally, it would be constructive to study the role of religion in these relationships and how students cope with the challenges they face during their studies.

References

Addai, I., Opoku-Agyeman, C., & Amanfu, S. K. (2014). Exploring predictors of subjective well-being in Ghana: A micro-level study. *Journal of Happiness Studies, 15*(4), 869–890.

Almeida, L. S., & Lemos, G. C. (2005). Aptidões cognitivas e rendimento académico: A validade preditiva dos testes de inteligência [Cognitive apptitudes and academic achievement: Predictive validity of intelligence tests]. *Psicologia, Educação e Cultura* [Psychology, Education and Culture], *2*(IX), 277–289.

Anastasi, A., & Urbina, S. (2000). *Testagem psicológica [Psychological testing]* (7th ed.). Artes Médicas.

Anderman, E. M., & Wolters, C. A. (2006). Goals, values, and affect: Influences on student motivation. In P. Alexander & P. Winne (Eds.), *Handbook of educational psychology* (pp. 369–389). Lawrence Erlbaum Associates.

Astin, A. W. (1993). *What matters most in college? Four critical years revisited.* San Francisco: Jossey-Bass.

Becker, D., & Marecek, J. (2008). Dreaming the American dream: Individualism and positive psychology. *Social and Personality Psychology Compass, 2*(5), 1767–1780.

Botha, F., & Booysen, F. (2014). Family functioning and life satisfaction and happiness in South African households. *Social Indicators Research, 119*(1), 163–182.

Botha, C., & Mostert, K. (2014). A structural model of job resources, organisational and individual strengths use and work engagement. *SA Journal of Industrial Psychology, 40*, a1135. https://doi.org/10.4102/sajip.v40i1.1135

Bücker, S., Nuraydin, S., Simonsmeier, B. A., Schneider, M., & Luhmann, M. (2018). Subjective well-being and academic achiement: A meta-analysis. *Journal of Research in Personality, 74*, 83–94.

Cadime, I., Pinto, A. M., Lima, S., Rego, S., Pereira, J., & Ribeiro, I. (2016). Well-being and academic achievement in secondary school pupils: The unique effects of burnout and engagement. *Journal of Adolescence, 53*, 169–179.

Choudhury, S. A., & Borooah, I. P. (2017). Character strengths and academic achievements of undergraduate college students of Guwahati, Assam. *Space and Culture, India, 5*(1), 49–64.

Crede, J., Wirthwein, L., McElvany, N., & Steinmayr, R. (2015). Adolescents' academic achievement and life satisfaction: The role of parents' education. *Frontiers in Psychology, 6*, 1–8.

Csikszentmihalyi, M. (2008). *Flow: The psychology of optimal experience.* Harper Perennial Modern Classics.

Cunha, M. P., Fortes, A., Gomes, E., Rego, A., & Rodrigues, F. (2016). Ambidextrous leadership, paradox and contingency: Evidence from Angola. *The International Journal of Human Resource Management, 2016*, 1–26. https://doi.org/10.1080/09585192.2016.1201125

Diener, E. (2012). New findings and future directions for subjective well-being research. *American Psychologist, 67*, 590–597. https://doi.org/10.1037/a0029541

Diener, E., Suh, E. M., Lucas, R. R., & Smith, H. L. (1999). Subjective Well-being: Three decades of progress. *Psychological Bulletin, 125*, 276–302. https://doi.org/10.1037/0033-2909.125.2.276

Douglass, R. P., & Duffy, R. D. (2015). Strengths use and life satisfaction: A moderated mediation approach. *Journal of Happiness Studies, 16*, 619–632.

Ebrahim, A., Botha, F., & Snowball, J. D. (2013). Determinants of life satisfaction among race groups in South Africa. *Development Southern Africa, 30*(2), 168–185.

Eide, E. R., Showalter, M. H., & Goldhaber, D. D. (2010). The relation between children's health and academic achievement. *Children and Youth Services Review, 32*(2), 231–238.

Ford, M. (1982). Social cognition and social competence in adolescence. *Developmental Psychology, 18*(3), 323–340.

Fredrickson, B. L. (1998). What good are positive emotions? *Review of General Psychology, 2*, 300–319.

Fredrickson, B. L. (2001). The role of positive emotions in positive psychology: The broaden-and-build theory of positive emotions. *American Psychologist, 56*, 218–226.

Frisch, M. B. (2000). Improving mental and physical health care through quality of life therapy and assessment. In *Advances in quality of life theory and research* (pp. 207–241). Springer.

Furr, R. M., & Funder, D. C. (1998). A multimodal analysis of personal negativity. *Journal of Personality and Social Psychology, 74*(6), 1580–1591.

Gable, S. J., & Haidt, J. (2005). What (and why) is positive psychology? *Review of General Psychology, 9*, 103–110.

Galinha, I. C., Garcia-Martín, M. A., Gomes, C., & Oishi, S. (2016). Criteria for happiness among people living in extreme poverty in Maputo, Mozambique. *International Perspectives in Psychology: Research, Practice, Consultation, 5*(6), 67–90.

Giovazolias, T., Karademas, E., & Kalantzi-Azizi, A. (Eds.). (2008). *Crossing internal and external borders: Practices for an effective psychological counselling in the European higher education*. Ellinika Grammata.

Guay, F., Marsh, H. W., & Boivin, M. (2003). Academic self-concept and academic achievement: Developmental perspectives on their causal ordering. *Journal of Educational Psychology, 95*(1), 124–136.

Harzer, C., & Ruch, W. (2013). The application of signature character strengths and positive experiences at work. *Journal of Happiness Studies, 14*, 965–983.

Hetland, H. H., Andreassen, C. S., Pallesen, S., & Notelaers, S. (2011). Leadership and fulfillment of the three basic psychological needs at work. *Career Development International, 16*(5), 507–523.

Hofstede Insights. (n.d.). *Compare countries: Angola.* Retrieved August 8, 2020 from https://www.hofstede-insights.com/product/compare-countries/

Huber, A., Webb, D., & Höfer, S. (2017). The German version of the Strengths Uuse Scale: The relation of using individual strengths and Well-being. *Frontiers in Psychology, 8*, 1–11. https://doi.org/10.3389/fpsyg.2017.00637

Instituto Nacional de Estatística (INE). (2016). *Resultados definitivos do recenceamento geral da população e da habitação de Angola 2014 [Final results of general population and habitation census of Angola 2014.]*. INE.

International Test Commission. (2001). International guidelines for test use. *International Journal of Testing, 1*(2), 93–114.

Izard, C., Fine, S., Schultz, D., Mostow, A., Ackerman, B., & Youngstrom, E. (2001). Emotion knowledge as a predictor of social behavior and academic competence in children at risk. *Psychological Science, 12*, 18–23.

Jackson, L. T. B., Van de Vijver, F. J. R., & Fouché, R. (2014). Psychological strengths and subjective well-being in South African white students. *Journal of Psychology in Africa, 24*(4), 299–307.

Kamoche, K., Debrah, Y., Horwitz, F. M., & Muuka, G. (Eds.). (2004). *Managing human resources in Africa*. Routledge, U.K.

Kern, M., & Bowling, D. S., III. (2015). Character strengths and academic performance in law students. *Journal of Research in Personality, 55*, 25–29.

Keyes, C. L. M. (2002). The mental health continuum: From languishing to flourishing in life. *Journal of Health and Social Behavior, 43*(2), 207–222.

Keyes, C. L. M. (2009). The nature and importance of positive mental health in America's adolescents. In R. Gilman, E. S. Huerbner, & M. J. Furlong (Eds.), *Handbook of positive psychology in schools* (pp. 9–23). Routledge.

Keyes, C. L. M. (2010). Change in level of positive mental health as a predictor of future risk of mental illness. *American Journal of Public Health, 100*(12), 2366–2371.

Keyes, C. L. M., Wissing, M., Potgieter, J. P., Temane, M., Kruger, A., & van Rooy, S. (2008). Evaluation of the Mental Health Continuum Short Form (MHC-SF) in Setswana speaking South Africans. *Clinical Psychology and Psychotherapy, 15*, 181–192.

Khumalo, I. P. (2005). *Exploring the validity of the VIA inventory of strengths in an African context.* (Unpublished Master dissertation). North-West University, Potchefstroom campus, South Africa.

Kirkcaldy, B., Furnham, A., & Siefen, G. (2004). The relationship between health efficacy, educational attainment, and Well-being among 30 nations. *European Psychologist, 9*(2), 107–119.

Lewinsohn, P., Redner, J., & Seeley, J. (1991). The relationship between life satisfaction and psychosocial variables: New perspectives. In F. Strack, M. Argyle, & N. Schwartz (Eds.), *Subjective well-being: An interdisciplinary perspective* (pp. 141–169). Plenum Press.

Linley, P. A., Nielsen, K. M., Wood, A. M., Gillett, R., & Biswas-Diener, R. (2010). Using signature strengths in pursuit of goals: Effects on goal progress, need satisfaction, and well-being, and implications for coaching psychologists: Towards positive education a mindful school model. *International Coaching Psychology Review, 5*, 6–15.

Littman-Ovadia, H., Lavy, S., & Boiman-Meshita, M. (2017). When theory and research collide: Examining correlates of signature strengths use at work. *Journal of Happiness Studies, 18*, 527–548.

Lomas, T. (2015). Positive cross-cultural psychology: Exploring similarity and difference in constructions and experiences of wellbeing. *International Journal of Wellbeing, 5*(4), 60–77.

Lounsbury, J. W., Fisher, L. A., Levy, J. J., & Welsh, D. P. (2009). An investigation of character strengths in relation to the academic success of college students. *Individual Differences Research, 7*(1), 52–69.

Matos, A. P., André, R. S., Cherpe, S., Rodrigues, D., Figueira, C., & Pinto, A. M. (2010). Estudo Psicométrico preliminar da Mental Health Continuum – Short Form – For youthnuma amostra de adolescentes portugueses [Preliminary psychometric study of the Mental Health Continuum – Short Form – For youth, in a sample of Portuguese adolescentes]. *Psychologica, 53*, 131–156.

McGrath, R. E. (2019). *Technical report: The VIA assessment suite for adults: Development and initial evaluation* (rev. ed.). VIA Institute on Character.

McKnight, C. G., Huebner, E. S., & Suldo, S. (2002). Relationships among stressful life events, temperament, problem behavior, and global life satisfaction in adolescents. *Psychology in the Schools, 39*(6), 677–687.

Møller, V. (2013). South African quality of life trends over three decades 1980–2010. *Social Indicators Research, 113*(3), 915–940.

Møller, V., Theuns, P., Erstad, I., & Bernheim, J. (2008). The best and worst times of life: Narratives and assessments of subjective well-being by Anamnestic Comparative Self Assessment (ACSA) in the Eastern Cape, South Africa. *Social Indicators Research, 89*, 1–22.

Mostow, A. J., Izard, C. E., Fine, S., & Trentacosta, C. J. (2002). Modeling emotional, cognitive, and behavioral predictors of peer acceptance. *Child Developmental, 73*, 1775–1787.

Nunnally, J. C. (1967). *Psychometric theory*. McGraw-Hill.

Nunnally, J. C. (1978). *Psychometric theory*. McGraw-Hill.

Oliveira, C., Nunes, M. F., Legal, E. J., & Noronha, A. P. (2016). Bem-Estar Subjetivo: estudo de correlação com as Forças de Caráter [Subjective well-being: Correlational study with character strengths]. *Avaliação Psicológica, 15*(2), 177–185.

Organisation for Economic Cooperation Development [OECD]. (2017). *PISA 2015 Results (Volume III): Students' Well-Being*. OECD Publishing.

Park, N. (2004). The role of subjective Well-being in positive youth development. *The Annals of the American Academy of Political and Social Science, 591*(1), 25–39.

Park, N., Peterson, C., & Seligman, M. E. P. (2004). Strengths of character and well-being. *Journal of Social and Clinical Psychology, 23*, 603–619.

Pascarella, E. T., & Terenzini, P. T. (1991). *How college affects students: Findings and insights from twenty years of research*. Jossey-Bass.

Peterson, C., & Seligman, M. E. P. (2004). *Character strengths and virtues: A handbook and classification*. American Psychological Association.

Pokimica, J., Addai, I., & Takyi, B. K. (2012). Religion and subjective well-being in Ghana. *Social Indicators Research, 106*(1), 61–79.

Proctor, C., Maltby, J., & Linley, P. A. (2011). Strengths use as a predictor of well-being and health-related quality of life. *Journal of Happiness Studies, 12*, 153–169.

Ragozzino, K., Resnik, H., Utne-O'Brien, M., & Weissberg, R. P. (2003). Promoting academic achievement through social and emotional learning. *Educational Horizons, 81*, 169–171.

Ryan, R. M., & Deci, E. L. (2001). On happiness and human potentials: A review of research on hedonic and eudaimonic well-being. *Annual Review of Psychology, 52*, 141–166. https://doi.org/10.1146/annurev.psych.52.1.141

Schaufeli, W., Martinez, I. M., Marques Pinto, A., Salanova, M., & Bakker, A. B. (2002). Burnout and engagement in university students: A cross-national study. *Journal of Cross-Cultural Psychology, 33*(5), 464–481.

Schaufeli, W., Salanova, M., González-Romá, V., & Bakker, A. B. (2002). The measurement of engagement and burnout: A two sample confirmatory factor analytic approach. *Journal of Happiness Studies, 3*, 71–92.

Seligman, M. E. P. (2002). *Authentic happiness: Using the new positive psychology to realise your potential for lasting fulfillment*. Atria Paperback.

Seligman, M. E. P. (2011). *Flourish: A visionary new understanding of happiness and Well-being*. Free Press.

Seligman, M. E. P., & Csikszentmihalyi, M. (2000). Positive psychology: An introduction. *American Psychologist, 55*(1), 5–14.

SigfúSDóttir, I. D., Kristjánsson, A. L., & Allegrante, J. P. (2007). Health behaviour and academic achievement in Icelandic school children. *Health Education Research, 22*(1), 70–80.

Steinmayr, R., Heyder, A., Naumburg, C., Michels, J., & Wirthwein, L. (2018). School-related and individual predictors of subjective well-being and academic achievement. *Frontiers in Psychology, 9*, 1–16. https://doi.org/10.3389/fpsyg.2018.0263

Steinmayr, R., Meißner, A., Weidinger, A. F., & andWirthwein., L. (2014). Academic achievement. In L. H. Meyer (Ed.), *Oxford bibliographies online: Education*. Oxford University Press.

Sternberg, R. J. (2008). Excellence for all. *Educational Leadership, 66*(2), 14–19.

Suldo, S. M., Shaffer, E. J., & Riley, K. N. (2008). A social-cognitive-behavioral model of academic predictors of adolescents' life satisfaction. *School Psychology Quarterly, 23*(1), 56–69.

Tuominen-Soini, H., & Salmela-Aro, K. (2014). Schoolwork engagement and burnout among Finnish high school students and young adults: Profiles, progressions, and educational outcomes. *Developmental Psychology, 50*(3), 649–662.

Universidade Católica de Angola/Centro de Estudos e Investigação Científica. (2015). *Relatório Económico de Angola de 2014 [2014 Economic Report of Angola]*. Catholic University Press.

Universidade Católica de Angola/Centro de Estudos e Investigação Científica. (2017). *Relatório Económico de Angola de 2016 [2016 Economic Report of Angola]*. Catholic University Press.

Vilelas, J. (2009). *Investigação: o processo de construção do conhecimento [Research: The process of knowledge construction]*. Edições Silabo.

Wood, A. M., Linley, P. A., Maltby, J., Kashdan, T. B., & Hurling, R. (2011). Using personal and psychological strengths leads to increases in well-being over time: A longitudinal study and the development of the Strengths Use Questionnaire. *Personality and Individual Differences, 50*, 15–19.

World Health Organisation. (1948). *Preamble to the constitution of the World Health Organization*. World Health Organisation.

World Health Organisation. (2001). *The world health report: Mental health: New understanding, new hope*. World Health Organisation.

Zajacova, A., Lynch, S. M., & Espenshade, T. J. (2005). Self-efficacy, stress, and academic success in college. *Research in Higher Education, 46*(6), 677–706.

Zullig, K. J., Valois, R. F., Huebner, E. S., Oeltmann, J. E., & Drane, J. W. (2001). Relationship between perceived life satisfaction and adolescents' substance abuse. *Journal of Adolescent Health, 29*(4), 279–288.

Chapter 13
Adult Attachment and Well-Being in the Medical Education Context: Attachment Style Is Associated with Psychological Well-Being Through Self-Efficacy

Ephraim Chima Maduakor, JohnBosco Chika Chukwuorji, Peace N. Amanambu, and Chuka Mike Ifeagwazi

Abstract Extensive literature has shown the importance of attachment security in psychological well-being (PWB) of several populations, but the impacts of attachment on PWB in African populations have received less attention, and there is no previous research which have considered the adult attachment and PWB in the context of medical education. The present study investigated the relationships between adult attachment and PWB, and further examined whether self-efficacy mediates such relationships in a sub-Saharan African sample of medical students. Participants were 438 medical students from a university in south east Nigeria (62.3% women, aged 18–30 years, $M_{age} = 20.99$ years, $SD = 2.54$). They completed the 18-item version of Ryff's Scales of Psychological Well-Being, Revised Adult Attachment Scale, and Generalised Self-Efficacy Scale. Data were analysed using Hayes PROCESS macro for SPSS. We found that self-efficacy (negatively associated with attachment avoidance) mediated the link between attachment avoidance and PWB, indicating that lower attachment avoidance is associated with PWB via self-efficacy. Self-efficacy was positively associated with PWB. Attachment anxiety was associated with PWB only directly, but not through self-efficacy. Security in relationships and self-efficacy beliefs may be important targets for interventions to improve well-being in the medical education context.

E. C. Maduakor · P. N. Amanambu · C. M. Ifeagwazi
Department of Psychology, University of Nigeria, Nsukka, Enugu State, Nigeria

J. C. Chukwuorji (✉)
Department of Psychology, University of Nigeria, Nsukka, Enugu State, Nigeria

Department of Psychology, College of Sciences and the Health Professions, Cleveland State University, Cleveland, OH, USA

Promotion of Health and Innovation Lab (PHI), Network for Wellbeing, Nsukka, Enugu State, Nigeria
e-mail: johnbosco.chukwuorji@unn.edu.ng

L. Schutte et al. (eds.), *Embracing Well-Being in Diverse African Contexts: Research Perspectives*, Cross-Cultural Advancements in Positive Psychology 16,
https://doi.org/10.1007/978-3-030-85924-4_13

Keywords Adult attachment · Africa · Mediation · Medical education · Self-efficacy · Psychological well-being

13.1 Introduction

The medical profession is one of the most prestigious and highly lucrative occupations all over the world. Therefore, medical education is usually given priority in most parts of the world. The past three decades have witnessed speedy increase in the number of medical schools in Sub-Saharan Africa (see Monekosso, 2014). Some transformations are witnessed in terms of broadening the subject areas, recruitment and retention of well-qualified faculty, employment of state-of-the-art teaching tools, development of regional training centers and upgrade of technology to support distance learning and resource sharing among institutions (Kristiansen, 2012). In most of the higher institutions in Africa, the field of medicine is also gaining increasing interests and admits students more than any other discipline in most of the higher institutions. These medical students are an important segment of the African population because of their evident passion, dedication, and creativity as change agents in bringing attention to health inequities and social injustices (Chapman et al., 2016). They are key leaders in addressing challenges of all ages and population groups (Chapman & Animasahun, 2017). Thus, even with the enormous challenges, significant opportunities abound for increasing capacity in African medical education (Broadhead & Muula, 2002; Chen et al., 2012; International Association of Medical Science Educators, 2017). Essentially, if the gradual rapid growth, interests, innovations, and trends in medical education is to lead to better care and improved health outcomes for the people of Africa, it is necessary to give attention to the well-being of trainees.

The rigorous nature of academic workload characteristic of medical education worldwide has long been known as a major stressor of medical students (Sani et al., 2012), hence the students are not immune to the significant psychological distress for medical practitioners in training, and trainees' well-being have been noted to be poorer in comparison with their peers in other disciplines (Costa et al., 2012; Oku et al., 2015). Wolf and Kissling (1984) reported that an average medical student must cope with the intense pressure of mastering large amounts of information within a relatively short time, foreboding examinations, limited time for leisure and self, in addition to coping with personal issues of daily living and relationships. Therefore, promoting and nurturing psychological wellbeing during medical school is fundamental to promoting professionalism academic achievement, professionalism, and future options (Aktekin et al., 2001; Dahlin et al., 2005; Dyrbye et al., 2005; Kale et al., 2018; Nivert & Jehan, 2010).

Psychological well-being (PWB) in this study is the development of individual potential or self-actualization and engagement in meaningful activities (Ryff, 1989, 2014; Ryff & Singer, 2008). It refers to the qualities associated with eudaimonia such as the pursuit of excellence, self-realization, and feelings of engagement in personally expressive and meaningful activities (Schutte et al., 2013). This conceptualization of components of well-being comprises six components—autonomy, environmental mastery, personal growth, positive relationships, purpose in life, and self-acceptance; and the sensitivity of this approach has been tested when clinical changes as assessed in intervention contexts (Ryff, 2014). Several studies also report a high degree of association between different PWB dimensions (Abbott et al., 2006; Burns & Machin, 2009). Optimal levels of PWB will enable medical students to enjoy their daily life, form positive relationships with their professors and fellow students, as well as family and friends, and to be resilient in adjustments to the challenges of their long professional training. More importantly, substantial literature has shown that higher levels of well-being result to improved health and reduced mortality (Chida & Steptoe, 2008; Pressman & Cohen, 2005; Ryff, 2014), and there is longitudinal evidence that high scores on Ryff's description of PWB was associated with better physical health, fewer increase in chronic conditions and health symptoms, and fewer increments in functional health limitations (Ryff et al., 2015). Apart from health, success in the society is predicted by PWB (see Lyubomirsky et al., 2005 for a review). There is lack of research on the role of attachment and self-efficacy in well-being, particularly in the case of students in medical training. What are the contributions of attachment styles and self-efficacy in well-being among medical students? Does self-efficacy mediate the link between attachment styles and well-being? The present study therefore examines how adult attachment and self-efficacy contribute to PWB. This study further examines whether self-efficacy mediates the link between attachment styles and PWB in a sub-Saharan African sample of medical students. Neither the direct effects of self-efficacy on PWB nor its mediation effect on PWB has been established in an African sample. Demonstrating the explanatory role of self-efficacy contributes to a better understanding of the attachment-well-being relationship in adulthood.

13.1.1 Adult Attachment Typologies

Medical students are mostly emerging adults, or person undergoing through a life stage marked by change and exploration (Arnett, 2000), which is a veritable time to examine attachment. Research on adult attachment has been guided by generalized attachment style (Homan, 2018) which refers to a set of emotions, behaviors, and expectations people have for how others will respond in relationships (Fraley & Shaver, 2000). In the attachment theory, the attachment style is proposed to originate from earliest interactions patterns between infants and their primary caregiver (Bowlby, 1973, 1980). Bowlby contended that children form emotional attachments with their caregiver, which they internalize and utilise as models for future relationships (Bowlby, 1973, 1980). The nature of this early life relationship with one's primary caregiver creates an internal working model of the self and of other persons for an individual thereby allowing individuals to sustain a bond across time (Ainsworth, 1989). These relational patterns remain stable throughout the lifespan and influences one's expectations pertaining to both interpersonal and non-interpersonal aspects of later life through the internal working model (Hazan & Shaver, 1987). The internal working model is the positivity or negativity of the 'cognitive lens' (mental representation) used in interpreting relational life. The model influences personality development, psychological functioning, coping with stress, mental health and affect regulation in later life relational contexts (Mikulincer & Shaver, 2012; Schiffrin, 2013). Thus, individuals behave, think and engage in adult relationships in a manner that is in harmony with their attachment style because different patterns of cognition, affect, and behaviour develop in response to caregivers' availability, sensitivity and responsiveness to the desire of infants for closeness.

Attachment security and insecurity are the two polarities of human attachment, but specific notable dimensions exist. For example, attachment styles have been categorized into four styles—secure, pre-occupied, dismissive-avoidant, and fearful-avoidant patterns of attachment (Bartholomew & Horowitz, 1991). In each of the attachment styles, the critical element is the polarity of a person's model of self or other. As observed by Bartholomew and Horowitz (1991), those with secure attachment styles (low levels of both attachment-related anxiety and avoidance) have positive models (views) of the self and others which enables them to develop healthy relationships with others. Pre-occupied attachment style is characterized by a negative model of self, which gives rise to excessive concern with gaining approval and acceptance from significant others. Fearful avoidant attachment (high levels of both anxiety and avoidance) is marked by relational anxiety because the individuals have negative views of the self and a negative model of others. Thus, they seek validation from the other party in interpersonal relationships (Bartholomew & Horowitz, 1991). Dismissive avoidant attachment style is marked by low levels of attachment related anxiety and high levels of avoidance.

Some other researchers described two attachment dimensions, namely anxious and avoidant (Brennan et al., 1998; Fraley & Waller, 1998). In more recent understanding, scores on Bartholomew and Horowitz's (1991) four attachment prototypes are transformed into scales for two dimensions, namely anxiety and avoidance (e.g., Rapoza et al., 2016). Under the avoidance and anxiety dimensions, there is still the attachment security and insecurity as manifested in either low ends (security) or high ends (insecurity) of each dimension. Akin to dismissive-avoidant, persons having attachment avoidance downplay the importance of relationships, maintain emotional distance in relationships, and fail to draw close to other people in times of distress, while those with attachment anxiety worry excessively about relationships. Aspects of attachment dependency is also described in the literature as ambivalent attachment style—clinging behaviour (pre-occupied) and excessive worry about abandonment (Simpson et al., 1996). Another typology of adult attachment is the close (comfortable with closeness), dependent (feelings of availability of others when needed) and anxious (worry about being rejected or unloved) attachment styles (Collins & Read, 1990). Regardless of the description of each style, the attachment typologies are associated with self-reported "memories of relationships with parents in theoretically predictable ways" (Collins, 1996, p. 811).

13.1.2 Adult Attachment and PWB

Attachment security and insecurity differentially influence PWB because individuals with the various attachment styles have different perspectives of life and the interactions with their psychosocial environment are guided by these views of life (Çıkrıkçı & Gençdoğan, 2020). Specifically, studies among youth have shown that attachment security is linked to higher levels of psychological well-being such as middle school students in the USA (Jiang et al., 2013), and British first year undergraduate students (Carr et al., 2013). The findings on positive associations of attachment security and well-being have even been extended to older adults in primary care (Kirchmann et al., 2013). Other studies have also reported the positive role of secure attachment in life satisfaction among survivors of childhood sexual abuse (Barnum, 2016), and American college students (Wright & Perrone-McGovern, 2010). Among university students in Mozambique, attachment security did not predict PWB measured by combined scale items taping general and domain-specific life satisfaction as well as positive affect (Galinha et al., 2013).

Attachment anxiety have been reported to be associated with lower scores on indices of PWB among undergraduate students in USA (Schiffrin, 2013), Canadian college students (Milyavskaya & Lydon, 2013), elderly persons in the USA (Homan, 2018), and Chinese old adults (Li & Fung, 2014), as well as life satisfaction of Turkish students (Temiz & Comert, 2018). Nonetheless, attachment anxiety was positively related to PWB among UK young adults (Worsley et al., 2018) and Iranian youth (Masomeh & Farideh, 2014). Greater attachment avoidance was related to lower PWB among students in Canada (Milyavskaya & Lydon, 2013), elderly in the USA (Homan, 2018), and Chinese older adults (Li & Fung, 2014); and to life satisfaction among Turkish students (Temiz & Comert, 2018). Attachment avoidance was positively related to PWB among UK young adults (Worsley et al., 2018). One study that had adopted the typology of close, dependent, and anxious attachment styles reported that dependent attachment styles predicted increased life satisfaction, but neither close nor anxious attachment styles predicted lower life satisfaction (Ingram et al., 2017).

Clearly, there is mixed findings concerning the relationship between attachment styles and PWB. Much of the available studies in general have also been conducted outside the African cultural contexts, except Galinha et al. (2013). Generally, attachment research in African context is also scarce in the literature except a few (Ifeagwazi & Chukwuorji, 2011; Ingram et al., 2017). Adult attachment deserves to be given attention by researchers in order to determine its value to well-being research in the African setting. No study has exclusively focused on medical students. Given that these early attachment pattern shapes a person's ability to withstand challenging situations in adulthood (Hazan & Shaver, 1987; Rapoza et al., 2016), questioning attachments role in PWB of medical students is pertinent. In other words, the peculiar nature of their training makes it important to determine how the attachment-wellbeing connection applies in the medical education context.

13.1.3 *Self-Efficacy in the Context of Attachment Styles and Well-Being*

Self-efficacy refers to a person's belief regarding his/her ability to perform certain activities required to attain specific ends (Bandura, 1997). Bandura later described it as the agentic perspective in positive psychology (Bandura, 2008). It is a general perception of one's competence and capcity to fulfill goals in life (Schwarzer & Jerusalem, 1995; Zimmerman, 2000), which was conceptualized by Bandura (1986) as the central construct in his social cognitive theory. Based on the social cognitive perspective, in as much as individuals believe that they can achieve desired outcomes with the help of their own behaviours, the beliefs serve to enact the behaviours in the given situation. In other words, the self-system permits a person to direct and make various adjustments to their own thoughts, emotions and behaviour (Bandura, 1986). Empirical support exists for the role of self-efficacy in PWB among resident doctors in the USA (Milam et al., 2019), Italian youths (De Caroli & Sagone, 2014), Chilean adolescents (Céspedes et al., 2021), Iranian nurses (Dadipoor et al., 2021) as well as undergraduate students in Malaysia (Sabouripour & Roslan, 2015), Spain (Cabanach et al., 2012), India (Siddiqui, 2015) and Turkey (Ersöz, 2017). We could not find a previous research on self-efficacy in relation to PWB among medical students in the African environment.

Theoretically, attachment security is predicted to be related to positive beliefs about the self and confidence in social situations (Collins & Read, 1990). Studies have shown the relevance of attachment styles to self-efficacy beliefs and social attributions (Kogut, 2016; Leenders et al., 2019; Mikulincer & Florian, 1995); with evidence of association between attachment and self-efficacy among youths in Iran (Faraghi & Abedini, 2015; Tavakoli et al., 2014), Turkey (Erzena & Odaci, 2015), Israel (Kogut, 2016), and the USA (Wei et al., 2005). The cognitively developed internal working models espoused in attachment theory explains how the self, including one's self-efficacy, are influenced by various patterns of attachment relationships (Hazan & Shaver, 1987). Theoretically, an infant's 'successes' and 'failures' when finding the closeness of his/her caregiver by prompting distress may parallel what Bandura described as personal performance achievements, and these experiences are essential in forming one's self-efficacy (Kogut, 2016). In other words, a belief in one's ability to achieve desired outcomes is assumed to be contingent on level of attachment security. By its functional property (Bandura, 2012), this belief in one's ability to achieve desired goals would in turn predict PWB such that individuals who can establish secure attachment bonds based on trust and communication, express their feelings and desires with more clarity and are more likely to believe in their ability to take the right actions to achieve desired goals. Thus, they are capable of coping with life's challenges. Positive interactions with childhood attachment figures lead to a positive sense of self, which enhances personal knowledge and skills, and makes the individual able to adjust flexibly to new situations (Mikulincer & Shaver, 2010). Attachment insecurity may engender PWB by lowering a person's efficacy beliefs. The foregoing theoretical postulation and empirical support for the link between attachment styles and self-efficacy in relation to PWB informs the direction of investigation of a mediation pathway in the current study.

Some empirical studies have found evidence of mediation effect for self-efficacy in attachment-wellbeing relationships. Wei et al. (2005) reported that self-efficacy had a mediation effect on relationships of anxious attachment with loneliness and depression. In a sample of American college students (mostly female Caucasians), Wright and Perrone-McGovern (2010) found that self-efficacy mediated between secure attachment and life satisfaction, suggesting that adult attachment is an important source of information about efficacy beliefs and operates as a fundamental component in the way college students perceive their efficacy which influences life satisfaction. The effect of anxious attachment on perceived stress factors and stress symptoms was mediated by self-concept among Turkish undergraduate students (Bayrak et al., 2018). Such mediation effect has also been reported in relation to life satisfaction (Jiang et al., 2013; Lucktong et al., 2018). Among Spanish adults, secure attachment mediated the positive relationship of secure attachment style to PWB, as well as the inverse association of avoidant and anxious attachment to PWB (Marrero-Quevedo et al., 2019).

The present study follows the recent trend of understanding attachment style, by adopting a positive psychology approach to attachment styles in relation to well-being. Self-efficacy was linked to wellbeing in some previous research, and some findings have reported supported self-efficacy as a potential mediator of the attachment styles-wellbeing connection. This study seeks to test whether self-efficacy mediates this link in a sub-Saharan African medical student sample. The interpersonal relationship histories of persons with less attachment avoidance and attachment anxiety are assumed to be mostly positive, the experiences may reinforce their personal efficacy beliefs in attaining certain outcomes (Mikulincer & Doron, 2016). On the other hand, high attachment avoidance and attachment anxiety may weaken one's self-efficacy expectations, due to past experiences of poor relational outcomes and helplessness (Mikulincer & Doron, 2016). Therefore, we expect in the present study that students who are high on attachment avoidance (insecure attachment) are more likely to report less self-efficacy and thereby have diminished PWB. Further, our hypothesis is that medical students with high attachment anxiety (insecure attachment) are more likely to report lower self-efficacy and hence report poor PWB. It is also hypothesized that self-efficacy will be associated with increased PWB. The conceptual illustration of the mediational pathway is shown in Fig. 13.1. The worldview arising from early attachment experiences and efficacy beliefs may have important implications for positive health.

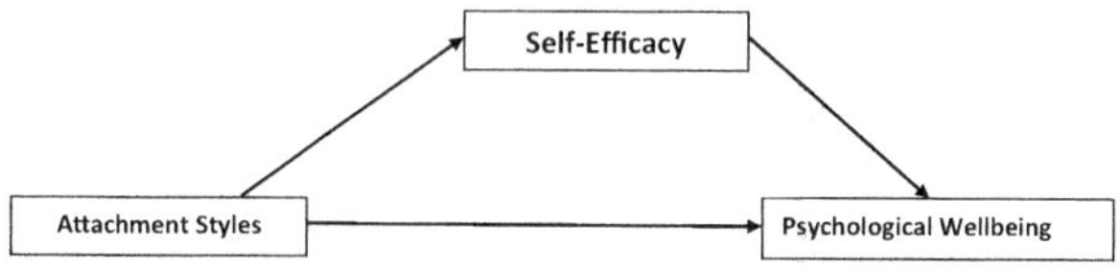

Fig. 13.1 Conceptual model of mediator effects of self-efficacy on adult attachment and PWB relationship

13.2 Method

13.2.1 Participants and Procedure

The sample for this study consisted of 438 medical students from a university in south east Nigeria. They were drawn using purposive sampling, given that the study targeted medical students. The medical students were approached at the end of classes in their classrooms to participate in a study about well-being in medical education. Participants were informed that their responses to the questionnaire will be anonymous as they are not required to write their name or any personally identifying information on any part of the survey. For confidentiality, their responses will also be strictly used for research purposes. The students who were not willing to take part in the study were free to either leave the classrooms or stay quietly without obstructing the exercise. Informed consent was obtained from the students who were willing to take part in the study. They were told that they could withdraw from completing the survey at any time without any consequences to them. The completion of the survey lasted for 15 min on average. There was no reward for participation in the study. Data were collected in April 2018. Ethical approval for the study was obtained from the research review committee of the Department of Psychology in University of Nigeria, Nsukka (D.PSY.UNN/REC/2018-1-IRB000013).

13.2.2 Measures

We obtained the data for this study with a questionnaire form comprising Revised Adult Attachment Scale, RAAS (Collins, 1996), Generalised Self-Efficacy Scale (Schwarzer & Jerusalem, 1995), and the Psychological Wellbeing Scale (PWBS) (Ryff, 1989). A section of the questionnaire also contained relevant demographic information.

13.2.2.1 Revised Adult Attachment Scale (RAAS)

The 18-item RAAS (Collins, 1996) was adopted to measure attachment styles. Originally, it comprised three subscales, each having six items: close, depend, and anxiety. However, Collins (1996) suggested an option for a researcher to measure attachment based on two dimensions: avoidance and anxiety; as informed by the recent understanding on attachment styles, and this pattern is popular in PWB research and other assessment measures of adult attachment (see Barnum, 2016; Fraley et al., 2000; Homan, 2018; Schiffrin, 2013; Temiz & Comert, 2018; Wright & Perrone-McGovern, 2010). Essentially, the two continuous dimensions of attachment—avoidance and anxiety, are believed to reflect a more parsimonious and accurate measurement of the construct as secure attachment is indicated by low scores on both dimensions (Kogut, 2016; Homan, 2018). In RAAS attachment avoidance has 12 items (e.g., "I am not sure that I can always depend on people to be there when I need them"; "I am somewhat uncomfortable being close to others") whereas the attachment anxiety dimension has six items (e.g., "I want to get close to people, but I worry about being hurt"; "I often worry that other people won't want to stay with me"). Each item is rated on a 5-point Likert scale ranging from 1 (*not at all characteristic of me*) to 5 (*very characteristic*). Thus, scores on the attachment avoidance dimension ranged from 12–60, while scores on the attachment anxiety dimension ranges from 6 to 30. The reliability of scores, based on Cronbach's alpha (α), have been reported as .74 (avoidance) and .78 (anxiety) which was found to be stable over a four-month period (Ahmad & Hassan, 2014). Evidence of the utility of the 18-item RAAS exists in Nigeria (e.g., Ottu, 2017). In the present study, the Cronbach's alpha values of the scales were .78 (avoidance) and .72 (anxiety). Higher scores on each of the dimensions show that the individual manifests attachment insecurity, whereas lower scores is evidence of secure attachment.

13.2.2.2 Generalised Self-Efficacy Scale

Self-efficacy was assessed using the 10-item Generalised Self-Efficacy Scale (Schwarzer & Jerusalem, 1995). The scale is designed to assess a person's optimistic self-beliefs to cope with a variety of difficult demands in life. Items on the scale are scored using response options that range from 1 (*not at all true*), to 4 (*exactly true*). Sample items are as follows: "I can always manage to solve difficult problems if I try hard enough"; "It is easy for me to stick to my aims and accomplish my goals"; "I can remain calm when facing difficulties because I can rely on my coping abilities"; etc. Cronbach's alphas between .82 and .93; and evidence of its validity was demonstrated by positive correlations to emotion, optimism, work satisfaction, as well as negative correlations to stress, health complaints, burnout, anxiety and depression (Schwarzer & Jerusalem, 1995). The total score is calculated by summing all the 10 items, and a higher score indicating more self-efficacy. Ecvidence exists to show that the GSE is appropriate for assessment of self-efficacy in the African context (see Gboyega & Popoola, 2010; Okediji et al., 2008; Redelinghuys, 2010; Roos et al., 2013). In the current study, we obtained an α of .81.

13.2.2.3 Psychological Wellbeing Scale (PWBS)

Ryff's (1989) 18-item Psychological Wellbeing Scale (PWBS) was the measure of PWB in the present study. The instruments consist six dimensions: autonomy, environmental mastery, personal growth, positive relationship with others, purpose in life and self-acceptance. Participants responded on a seven-point Likert scale that ranged from 1 (*strongly disagree*) to 7 (*strongly agree*). Sample items in the scale are: "Some people wander aimlessly through life, but I am not one of them"; "I like most parts of my personality"; "When I look at the story of my life, I am pleased with how things have turned out", etc. Negatively worded items are reverse scored, such that higher scores indicate higher psychological well-being. Ryff (1989) reported internal consistency reliability coefficients (α) for the PWBS which ranges from .86 to .93. The scale has been consistently shown to have a one-factor structure among Nigerian students with an acceptable reliability score of .81 (Fagbenro & Olasupo, 2019). For the present study, the α was .83.

13.2.2.4 Socio-Demographic Questionnaire

This was used to obtain relevant demographic information which are as follows: age, gender, educational level and previous degree.

13.2.3 Data Analysis

Pearson's correlation was used to test for the relationship among the variables and Hayes (2018) Process macro was used to test the hypotheses with the aid SPSS (version 23). The macro was used to generate the path coefficients of the regression model and bias-corrected bootstrapped confidence intervals (*CI*s) for total and specific indirect relationships of the attachment styles on PWB via self-efficacy. Bootstrapping in the PROCESS macro narrows the *CI*s by taking all possible random combinations of a study's sample and then estimating a mean. This procedure is widely adopted by researchers for testing the significance of indirect effects due to its several advantages over the traditional approaches in meditation analyses, especially to balance avoidance Type I error and Type II error (e.g., Chukwuorji et al., 2020; Homan, 2018). Path estimates in our study were based on 1000 bootstrapping resamples and are reported with 95% bias-corrected *CI*s. Hence the completely standardised indirect effects of attachment styles on PWB are checked to determine whether zero is straddled in-between the two values. The mediation effect is considered statistically significant when the *CI*s do not include zero (see Hayes, 2018).

13.3 Results

The sample consisted of more women ($n = 273$, 62.3%) than men ($n = 165$, 37.7%). They were aged 18–30 years ($M = 20.99$, $SD = 2.54$). Majority of the participants have had no previous higher education/degree ($n = 424$, 96.8%). The composition of the sample with regards to their ethnic group were as follows: Igbo ($n = 404$, 92.2%), Yoruba ($n = 8$, 1.8%) and other ethnic groups ($n = 26$, 5.9%). By marital status, 99.5% ($n = 436$) had never been married.

Table 13.1 showed that older age was associated with greater number of years in medical school, and having a previous degree in another field of study, but either age nor level of students in medical school correlated significantly with PWB. More female students reported lower number of years in medical school. Students who were in advanced years of medical school had previous degree in another field of study, and they reported lower attachment anxiety Attachment avoidance style was not significantly related to attachment anxiety, but attachment avoidance had a negative relationship with self-efficacy. Attachment anxiety was not significantly associated with self-efficacy. Self-efficacy was positively associated with PWB.

Table 13.2 showed that attachment avoidance was not significantly associated with PWB. Self-efficacy was positively associated with PWB, and the *B* showed that each unit increase in self-efficacy was associated with .60 increase in PWB. The *F* statistics associated with the model was significant, $F(2, 435) = 22.95$, $R^2 = .09$, $p < .001$. The confidence intervals of the completely standardised indirect effect of attachment avoidance on PWB did not include zero ($B = .04$; $95\% CI = .01, .08$), which indicated that self-efficacy mediated the relationship between attachment avoidance and PWB.

Attachment anxiety was positively associated with PWB, and the *B* showed that each unit increase in attachment anxiety was associated with .27 increase in PWB. The *F* statistics associated with the model was significant, $F(2, 435) = 26.37$, $R^2 = .11, p = .004$. The confidence intervals of the completely standardised indirect effect of attachment anxiety on PWB was not significant ($B = -.01$; $95\% CI = -.04$, .02), which indicated that self-efficacy was not a mediator between attachment anxiety and PWB.

13.4 Discussion

This study examined the interrelationships among attachment styles (avoidance and anxiety), self-efficacy, and PWB in Nigerian medical students. Self-efficacy was also considered as a cognitive–behavioural mediator between the attachment styles and

Table 13.1 Descriptive statistics and correlations of demographic variables, attachment styles, emotion regulation self-efficacy, and PWB

Variables		Mean	*SD*	1	2	3	4	5	6	7
1	Age	20.9	2.54	–						
2	Gender	–	–	−.23***	–					
3	Level	–	–	.61***	−.29***	–				
4	Previous degree	–	–	−.32**	−.03	−.22**	–			
5	Avoidance	37.37	5.11	−.03	.07	−.06	.02	–		
6	Anxiety	16.72	5.52	−.07	.03	−.12**	.07	−.08	–	
7	Self-efficacy	30.13	5.64	.05	−.03	.03	−.04	−.15**	−.03	–
8	PWB	75.53	11.41	.06	.02	−.02	−.06	−.11*	.13**	.30***

Note. $^{***}p < .001$; $^{**}p < .01$; $^{*}p < .05$; Gender (coded 0 = males, 1 = females), Previous degree (0 = Yes, 1 = No)

Table 13.2 Hayes PROCESS macro results for mediating role of self-efficacy in relationship between attachment styles and PWB

Predictors	*B*	*SE*	β	*t*	*p*-level	95%*CI*
(a) Avoidance, self-efficacy and PWB						
Avoidance	−.15	.10	−.07	−1.49	−.36	−.05, .36
Self-efficacy	.59	.09	.29	6.32	.000	.41, .77
(b) Anxiety, self-efficacy and PWB						
Anxiety	.27	.09	.13	2.91	.004	.09, .46
Self-efficacy	.62	.09	.30	6.72	.000	.44, .80

PWB. We found that self-efficacy mediated the relationship between attachment avoidance and PWB, but the link between attachment anxiety and PWB was not mediated by self-efficacy. In other words, the students overall psychological well-being was indirectly associated with their levels of attachment avoidance through their levels of efficacy beliefs. This finding is in partial support for our mediation hypotheses, and it is important in the light of previous findings that self-efficacy may serve as a mediator of the relationship between attachment security and subjective well-being of youths (e.g., Marrero-Quevedo et al., 2019; Wright & Perrone-McGovern, 2010). The study where self-efficacy mediated between attachment anxiety and psychological outcomes had loneliness and depression as the criterion variable (Wei et al., 2005).

The individual whose self-related thinking and beliefs are founded on attachment figure's qualities such as being compassionate, sensitive and empathic can apply these same qualities when facing life's challenges (Mikulincer & Shaver, 2004). Empirical research suggests that activation of a person's attachment security can lead to increased positive views of self (Pepping et al., 2015). Findings further suggest how prevention and intervention programs may be helpful in addressing students' PWB, by providing self-efficacy enhancement training programs and opportunities for students and organizing activities that will build essential general life skills. To develop self-efficacy, stakeholders in the community and higher institutions should realize the importance of this social cognitive strength and implement effective strategies to help students acquire this ability to believe in themselves. It would also be valuable to involve families in prevention/intervention programs by educating them on how to enhance efficacy beliefs through attachment relationship and direct modeling.

We also found that attachment avoidance was not significantly associated with PWB. This finding is contrary to our earlier hypothesis. Bartholomew (1990) had distinguished between the fearful avoidants and the dismissing avoidants. Fearful avoidants have a negative model of self and other and so they do not close to others because they worry about being hurt and rejected. On the contrary, dismissing avoidants are characterised by a positive model of self and a negative model of the other and so they desire to be independent and self-sufficient. Since the operationalization of avoidance in the present study did not separate dismissive avoidants and fearful avoidants, it is possible that the combination did not clearly reveal the nuances of avoidant attachment style in terms of whether the participants were most likely to be either fearful or dismissing. Although the general approach in the attachment literature is to look at general avoidance, some recent literature has also reported positive influence or null effect of avoidance on positive health outcomes (e.g., Kogut, 2016). Thus, it may be important for researchers to adopt Bartholomew's (1990) advice for researchers to divide attachment avoidance.

Findings showed that attachment anxiety was associated with increased PWB. We had expected that attachment anxiety would be associated with low PWB. Previous research in large sample of Spanish adults (mean age = 37.2 years) had found an inverse relationship between attachment anxiety and PWB (Marrero-Quevedo et al., 2019), while other studies on student populations reported that attachment anxiety was associated with increased PWB (Masomeh & Farideh, 2014; Worsley et al., 2018). We reason that adults with attachment anxiety have a strong desire for close relationships, but their uncertainty concerning whether they can depend on others and their worry about being rejected and abandoned may sometimes be unhelpful. However, it is possible that even with their concern about being accepted or rejected, they may be open to social relationships in some situations. Additionally, their concern may even motivate them to be their best in any relationship so that they can keep going strong and make effort to adapt to their environment in meaningful ways.

Our finding showed that self-efficacy was associated with increased PWB. This is in support of the study's expectation. If the present result is to be considered in view of previous research findings indicating that self-efficacy helps students to effectively manage the transitions of young adulthood, as well as cope with challenges of education and life (e.g., Cabanach et al., 2012; Ersöz, 2017; Sabouripour & Roslan, 2015; Siddiqui, 2015), it is reasonable to conclude that interventions to enhance self-efficacy can enable successful negotiation of the challenges of medical education. Individuals have increased PWB when they perceive themselves as having the requisite capabilities for successful performance and when they have positive expectation regarding the achievement of relevant goals or valued outcomes (Lent et al., 2005). Self-efficacy is malleable, and self-efficacy improvement interventions have been implemented in several populations including in the medical context (e.g., Long & Stevens, 2004; Moshki et al., 2017; Risucci et al., 2009). Strategies such as positive stress management, coping interventions, and peer mentoring may be particularly helpful in improving perceived and actual capabilities. Medical students may benefit from having peers who show positive qualities in school and by the example of these peers, other students may be helped to believe that the tasks are achievable. Programs that help students to set realistic goals and efficiently focus on the plans would also be necessary. Little improvements in the performance of medical students should also get positive feedback in order to push them to do more.

Although this study has added to knowledge in understanding the pathways to PWB, by indicating a mechanism (self-efficacy) to account for the link between adult attachment and PWB of medical students, it has some obvious weaknesses. Firstly, the sample was from one Nigerian university which does not truly represent the enormous diversity of medical students in African universities. There is need for caution in generalizing the findings of this study. Secondly, although guided by theory and informed by strands of empirical literature, we tested a model that posited that attachment styles was associated with psychological well-being via self-efficacy, our study was cross-sectional in nature, which precludes us from making clear causal inferences. Thirdly, we used self-report measures to collect the data for the study and this mono-method approach affects the extent of confidence in the measurements of key variables. Fourthly, we did not consider the umbrella model of higher order general well-being which embraces both hedonic and eudaimonic conceptualisations and operationalisations of well-being (see Delle Fave et al., 2011, 2013; Joshanloo, 2012; Khumalo et al., 2014; Wissing & Temane, 2008). However, previous studies that have examined the mediation hypotheses have considered mostly the hedonic perspective (life satisfaction), and this study is worthwhile because of its consideration of eudaimonic features. Longitudinal studies, experience sampling techniques, and daily diary studies with larger and more diverse sample of medical students will be helpful in further clarifying the findings of the present study because the defensive strategies of avoidant people may imply that their self-efficacy may be less genuine (Kogut, 2016).

Future research also needs to measure hedonic and eudaimonic well-being in the same sample and assess objective and subjective well-being. Adult attachment could be specified to mother (or mother figure), father (or father figure), and peers, in future research (see Inventory of Parent and Peer Attachment, IPPA; Armsden & Greenberg, 1987). Through these advanced level research methodology, one can more effectively establish whether attachment avoidance and even anxiety are adaptive. Moderated mediation approaches will also determine under what conditions the direct and indirect effects of adult attachment on well-being may be found.

The current study has contributed to the increasing body of scientific investigations into the multifaceted associations between adult attachment and well-being. Our findings demonstrate that attachment avoidance is linked with PWB through self-efficacy; and attachment anxiety is associated with increased PWB but not through self-efficacy. Self-efficacy was associated with increased PWB. The results elucidate one social cognitive pathway (self-efficacy) that may serve as a key mechanism that explains the linkage between attachment avoidance and PWB of youths. Taken together, the findings suggest important psychosocial implications of effective programming at individual, family and societal levels. Our results provide support for continued efforts to promote positive beliefs and trust in one's coping ability. It will be helpful for families and other organizations to realize their crucial roles in making students acquire this strength for positive development and mental well-being.

Conflict of Interest All authors declare that they have no conflict of interests.

References

Abbott, R. A., Ploubidis, G. B., Huppert, F. A., Kuh, D., Wadsworth, M. E., & Croudace, T. J. (2006). Psychometric evaluation and predictive validity of Ryff's psychological well-being items in a UK birth cohort sample of women. *Health and Quality of Life Outcomes, 4*, 76–92. https://doi.org/10.1186/1477-7525-4-76

Ahmad, R., & Hassan, S. A. (2014). Reliability analysis of the revised adult attachment scale (RAAS) instrument in the Malaysian context. *Elixir Social Sciences, 77*, 29098–29100.

Ainsworth, M. D. S. (1989). Attachments beyond infancy. *American Psychologist, 44*, 709–716.

Aktekin, M., Karaman, T., Senol, Y., Erdem, S., Erengin, H., & Akaydin, M. (2001). Anxiety, depression and stressful life events among medical students: A prospective study in Antalya, Turkey. *Medical Education, 3*(5), 12–17.

Armsden, G. C., & Greenberg, M. T. (1987). The inventory of parent and peer attachment: Individual differences and their relationship to psychological well-being in adolescence. *Journal of Youth and Adolescence, 16*(5), 427–454. https://doi.org/10.1007/BF02202939

Arnett, J. J. (2000). Emerging adulthood: A theory of development from the late teens through the twenties. *American Psychologist, 55*, 469–480.

Bandura, A. (1986). *Social foundations of thought and action: A social cognitive theory*. Prentice Hall.

Bandura, A. (1997). *Self-efficacy: The exercise of control*. Freeman.

Bandura, A. (2008). An agentic perspective on positive psychology. In S. J. Lopez (Ed.), *Positive psychology: Exploring the best in people* (pp. 167–196). Praeger.

Bandura, A. (2012). On the functional properties of perceived self-efficacy revisited. *Journal of Management, 38*, 745–752.

Barnum, E. L. (2016). *Attachment, self-esteem and subjective well-being among survivors of childhood sexual trauma* (doctoral dissertation). Ball State University.

Bartholomew, K. (1990). Avoidance of intimacy: An attachment perspective. *Journal of Social and Personal Relationships, 7*(2), 147–178. https://doi.org/10.1177/0265407590072001

Bartholomew, K., & Horowitz, L. (1991). Attachment styles among young adults: A test of a four-category model. *Journal of Personality and Social Psychology, 61*, 226–244.

Bayrak, R., Güler, M., & Şahin, N. H. (2018). The mediating role of self-concept and coping strategies on the relationship between attachment styles and perceived stress. *Europe's Journal of Psychology, 14*(4), 897–913. https://doi.org/10.5964/ejop.v14i4.1508

Bowlby, J. (1973). *Attachment and loss: Vol 2. Separation: Anxiety and anger*. Basic Books.

Bowlby, J. (1980). *Attachment and loss: Vol. 3. Loss, sadness and depression*. Basic Books.

Brennan, K. A., Clark, C. L., & Shaver, P. R. (1998). Self-report measurement of adult attachment: An integrative overview. In J. A. Simpson & W. S. Rholes (Eds.), *Attachment theory and close relationships* (pp. 46–76). Guilford.

Broadhead, R. L., & Muula, A. S. (2002). Creating a medical school for Malawi: Problems and achievements. *British Medical Journal, 325*, 384. https://doi.org/10.1136/bmj.325.7360.384

Burns, R. A., & Machin, M. A. (2009). Investigating the structural validity of Ryff's psychological well-being scales across two samples. *Social Indicators Research, 93*, 359–375.

Cabanach, R. G., Valle, A., Rodríguez, C. F., & del Mar Ferradás, M. (2012). The relations between perceived self-efficacy and psychological well-being in university students. *Revista Mexicana de Psicología, 29*(1), 40–48.

Carr, S., Colthurst, K., Coyle, M., & Elliott, D. (2013). Attachment dimensions as predictors of mental health and psychosocial well-being in the transition to university. *European Journal of Psychology of Education, 28*(2), 157–172. https://doi.org/10.1007/s10212-012-0106-9

Céspedes, C., Rubio, A., Viñas, F., Cerrato, S. M., Lara-Órdenes, E., & Ríos, J. (2021). Relationship between self-concept, self-efficacy, and subjective well-being of native and migrant adolescents. *Frontiers in Psychology, 11*, 620782. https://doi.org/10.3389/fpsyg.2020.620782

Chapman, H. J., & Animasahun, V. J. (2017). More on medical education in Africa. *Academic Medicine, 92*(5), 571–572. https://doi.org/10.1097/ACM.0000000000001634

Chapman, H. J., Animasahun, V. J., Tade, A. E., & Naveed, A. (2016). Addressing the role of medical students using community mobilization and social media in the Ebola response. *Perspectives in Medical Education, 5*, 186190.

Chen, C., Buch, E., Wassermann, T., Frehywot, S., Mullan, F., Omaswa, F., Greysen, S. R., Kolars, J. C., Dovlo, D., El Gali Abu Bakr, D. E., Haileamlak, A., Koumare, A. K., & Olapade-Olaopa, E. O. (2012). A survey of Sub-Saharan African medical schools. *Human Resources for Health, 10*(4), 1–23. https://doi.org/10.1186/1478-4491-10-4

Chida, Y., & Steptoe, A. (2008). Positive psychological well-being and mortality: A quantitative review of prospective observational studies. *Psychosomatic Medicine, 70*, 741–756. https://doi.org/10.1097/psy.0b013e31818105ba

Chukwuorji, J. C., Uzuegbu, C. N., Chukwu, C. V., Ifeagwazi, C. M., & Ugwu, C. (2020). Social support serves emotion regulation function in death anxiety among people living with HIV/AIDS. *South African Journal of Psychology, 50*(3), 395–410. https://doi.org/10.1177/0081246319894700

Çıkrıkçı, Ö., & Gençdoğan, B. (2020). Clarifying the associations among belongingness, setting life goals, need satisfaction and positive orientations: The model testing in accordance with the attachment styles. *Current Psychology*. https://doi.org/10.1007/s12144-019-00587

Collins, N. L. (1996). Working models of attachment: Implications for explanation, emotion, and behavior. *Journal of Personality and Social Psychology, 71*(4), 810–832.

Collins, N. L., & Read, S. J. (1990). Adult attachment, working models, and relationship quality in dating couples. *Journal of Personality and Social Psychology, 58*(4), 644–663. https://doi.org/10.1037/0022-3514.58.4.644

Costa, E. F., Santos, S. A., Santos, A. T., Melo, E. V., & Andrade, T. M. (2012). Burnout syndrome and associated factors among medical students: A cross-sectional study. *Clinics (São Paulo, Brazil), 67*(6), 573–580.

Dadipoor, S., Alavi, A., Ghaffari, M., & Ali Safari-Moradabadi, G. (2021). Association between self-efficacy and general health: A cross-sectional study of the nursing population. *BMC Nursing, 20*(49), 1–6. https://doi.org/10.1186/s12912-021-00568-5

Dahlin, M., Joneborg, N., & Runeson, B. (2005). Stress and depression among medical students: A cross-sectional study. *Medical Education, 39*, 594–604.

De Caroli, M. E., & Sagone, E. (2014). Generalized self-efficacy and well-being in adolescents with high vs. low scholastic self-efficacy. *Procedia - Social and Behavioral Sciences, 141*(25), 867–874.

Delle Fave, A., Brdar, I., Freire, T., Vella-Brodrick, D., & Wissing, M. P. (2011). The eudaimonic and hedonic components of happiness: Quantitative and qualitative findings. *Social Indicators Research, 100*(2), 185–207. https://doi.org/10.1007/s11205-010-9632-5

Delle Fave, A., Brdar, I., Vella-Brodrick, D., & Wissing, M. P. (2013). Religion, spirituality, and well-being across nations: The eudaimonic and hedonic happiness investigation. In H. H. Knoop & A. Delle Fave (Eds.), *Well-being and cultures: Perspectives from positive psychology* (pp. 117–134). Springer.

Dyrbye, L., Thomas, M., & Shanafelt, T. (2005). Medical students' distress: Causes, consequences, and proposed solutions. *Mayo Clinic Proceedings, 80*(12), 1613–1622.

Ersöz, G. (2017). The role of university students' general self-efficacy, depression and psychological well-being in predicting their exercise behavior. *Journal of Education and Training Studies, 5*(3), 110–117. https://doi.org/10.11114/jets.v5i3.2209

Erzena, E., & Odaci, H. (2015). The effect of the attachment styles and self-efficacy of adolescents preparing for university entrance tests in Turkey on predicting test anxiety. *Educational Psychology: An International Journal of Experimental Educational Psychology*. https://doi.org/10.1080/01443410.2014.923555

Fagbenro, D. A., & Olasupo, M. O. (2019). Psychosocial antecedents of psychological wellbeing of local government employees. *Open Journal for Psychological Research, 3*(2), 55–68.

Faraghi, M., & Abedini, M. (2015). The relationship between attachment style with self-efficacy and academic performance of secondary school students in Bandar Abbas. *European Online Journal of Natural and Social Sciences, 4*(1), 716–719.

Fraley, R. C., & Shaver, P. R. (2000). Adult romantic attachment: Theoretical developments, emerging controversies, and unanswered questions. *Review of General Psychology, 4*, 132–154. https://doi.org/10.1037//1089-2680.4.2.132

Fraley, R. C., & Waller, N. G. (1998). Adult attachment patterns: A test of the typological model. In J. A. Simpson & W. S. Rholes (Eds.), *Attachment theory and close relationships* (pp. 77–114). Guilford.

Fraley, R. C., Waller, N. G., & Brennan, K. A. (2000). An item response theory analysis of self-report measures of adult attachment. *Journal of Personality and Social Psychology, 78*, 350–365.

Galinha, I. C., Oishi, S., Pereira, C. R., Wirtz, D., & Esteves, F. (2013). Adult attachment, love styles, relationship experiences and subjective well-being: Cross-cultural and gender comparison between Americans, Portuguese, and Mozambicans. *Social Indicators Research, 119*, 823–852. https://doi.org/10.1007/s11205-013-0512-7

Gboyega, A., & Popoola, S. O. (2010). Demographic variables and self-efficacy as factors influencing career commitment of librarians in federal university libraries in Nigeria. *Library Philosophy and Practice (e-journal)*, 329. Retrieved January 23, 2020, from https://digitalcommons.unl.edu/cgi/viewcontent.cgi?article=1338&context=libphilprac

Hayes, A. F. (2018). *Introduction to mediation, moderation, and conditional process analysis: A regression-based approach*. Guilford Press.

Hazan, C., & Shaver, P. R. (1987). Romantic love conceptualized as an attachment process. *Journal of Personality and Social Psychology, 52*(3), 511–524.

Homan, K. J. (2018). Secure attachment and eudaimonic well-being in late adulthood: The mediating role of self-compassion. *Aging & Mental Health, 22*(3), 363–370.

Ifeagwazi, C. M., & Chukwuorji, J. C. (2011). Mediating effect of self-efficacy on attachment styles and intimacy among students. *International Journal of Communication, 13*, 122–133.

Ingram, A. M., Cox, B. S., Smith, D. M., & Parmelee, P. A. (2017). Attachment style, pain, and psychological well-being in older adults with knee osteoarthritis. *Innovation in Aging, 1*(S1), 128–129.

International Association of Medical Science Educators. (2017, September 28). *Challenges and opportunities for medical education in Sub-Saharan Africa*. Retrieved February 03, 2020 from https://cme.dmu.edu/content/challenges-and-opportunities-medical-education-sub-saharan-africa

Jiang, X., Huebner, E. S., & Hills, K. J. (2013). Parent attachment and early adolescents' life satisfaction: The mediating effect of hope. *Psychology in the Schools, 50*(4), 340–352. https://doi.org/10.1002/pits.21680

Joshanloo, M. (2012). Investigation of the contribution of spirituality and religiousness to hedonic and eudaimonic well-being in Iranian young adults. *Journal of Happiness Studies, 12*, 910–930.

Kale, A., Galadima, B. K., & Egwu, G. (2018). Psychological wellbeing of undergraduate students and its correlation with socio-demographic variables: A study of University of Maiduguri, Borno state, Nigeria. *Scholars Journal of Arts, Humanities and Social Sciences, 6*(2), 383–391. https://doi.org/10.21276/sjahss.2018.6.2.15

Khumalo, I. P., Wissing, M. P., & Schutte, L. (2014). Presence of meaning and search for meaning as mediators between spirituality and psychological well-being in a South African sample. *Journal of Psychology in Africa, 24*(1), 61–72.

Kirchmann, H., Nolte, T., Runkewitz, K., Bayerle, L., Becker, S., Blasczyk, V., Lindloh, J., & Strauss, B. (2013). Associations between adult attachment characteristics, medical burden, and life satisfaction among older primary care patients. *Psychology and Aging, 28*(4), 1108–1114. https://doi.org/10.1037/a0034750

Kogut, E. (2016). Adult attachment styles, self-efficacy, and causal attributional style for achievement-related failures. *Learning and Individual Differences, 50*, 64–72.

Kristiansen, C. (2012). Africa transforms its medical education with medical education partnership initiative (MEPI). *Global Health Matters, 11*(5), 1–2.

Leenders, M. V. E., Buunk, A. P., & Henkens, K. (2019). Attachment avoidance and attachment anxiety as individual characteristics affecting job search behavior. *Journal of Career Development, 46*(5), 487–501.

Lent, R. W., Singley, D., Sheu, H. B., Gainor, K. A., Brenner, B. R., Treistman, D., & Ades, L. (2005). Social cognitive predictors of domain and life satisfaction: Exploring the theoretical precursors of subjective well-being. *Journal of Counseling Psychology, 52*, 429–442.

Li, T., & Fung, H. H. (2014). How avoidant attachment influences subjective well-being: An investigation about the age and gender differences. *Aging & Mental Health, 18*, 4–10.

Long, J. A. D., & Stevens, K. R. (2004). Using technology to promote self-efficacy for healthy eating in adolescents. *Journal of Nursing Scholarship, 36*, 134–139. https://doi.org/10.1111/j.1547-5069.2004.04026.x

Lucktong, A., Salisbury, T. T., & Chamratrithirong, A. (2018). The impact of parental, peer and school attachment on the psychological well-being of early adolescents in Thailand. *International Journal of Adolescence and Youth, 23*(2), 235–249. https://doi.org/10.1080/02673843.2017.1330698

Lyubomirsky, S., King, L., & Diener, E. (2005). The benefits of frequent positive affect: Does happiness lead to success? *Psychological Bulletin, 131*, 803–855.

Marrero-Quevedo, R. J., Blanco-Hernandez, P. J., & Hernandez-Cabrera, J. A. (2019). Adult attachment and psychological well-being: The mediating role of personality. *Journal of Adult Development, 26*(1), 41–56. https://doi.org/10.1007/s10804-018-9297-x

Masomeh, A. Q., & Farideh, F. D. (2014). The relationship between life satisfaction and attachment styles with psychological well-being of children covered by Behzistey in Tehran. *Indian Journal of Fundamental and Applied Life Sciences, 4*(S4), 3336–3344.

Mikulincer, M., & Doron, G. (2016). Adult attachment and self-related processes. In M. Kyrios, R. Moulding, G. Doron, S. S. Bhar, M. Nedeljkovic, & M. Mikulincer (Eds.), *The self in understanding and treating psychological disorders* (pp. 19–28). Cambridge University Press.

Mikulincer, M., & Florian, V. (1995). Appraisal and coping with a real-life stressful situation: The contribution of attachment styles. *Personality and Social Psychology Bulletin, 21*, 406–414.

Mikulincer, M., & Shaver, P. R. (2004). Security-based self-representations in adulthood: Contents and processes. In W. S. Rholes & J. A. Simpson (Eds.), *Adult attachment: Theory, research, and clinical implications* (pp. 159–195). Guilford Publications.

Mikulincer, M., & Shaver, P. R. (2010). *Attachment in adulthood: Structure, dynamics, and change*. Guildford Press.

Mikulincer, M., & Shaver, P. R. (2012). An attachment perspective on psychopathology. *World Psychiatry, 11*, 11–15.

Milam, L. A., Cohen, G. L., Mueller, C., & Salles, A. (2019). The relationship between self-efficacy and well-being among surgical residents. *Journal of Surgical Education, 76*(2), 321–328. https://doi.org/10.1016/j.jsurg.2018.07.028

Milyavskaya, M., & Lydon, J. E. (2013). Strong but insecure: Examining the prevalence and correlates of insecure attachment bonds with attachment figures. *Journal of Social and Personal Relationships, 30*, 529–544.

Monekosso, G. L. (2014). A brief history of medical education in sub-Saharan Africa. *Academic Medicine, 89*(8), S11–S15. https://doi.org/10.1097/ACM.0000000000000355

Moshki, M., Mohammadzadeh, F., & Dehnoalian, A. (2017). The effectiveness of a group-based educational program on the self-efficacy and self-acceptance of menopausal women: A randomized controlled trial. *Journal of Women and Aging, 30*(4), 310–325. https://doi.org/10.1080/08952841.2017.1366753

Nivert, Z., & Jehan, M. I. (2010). Psychiatric morbidity among third year medical students at an Islamic university, Cairo, Egypt. *The Egyptian Journal of Community Medicine, 28*(1), 54–68.

Okediji, A. A., Offiong, U., Umoh, O. O., Sanni, K. B., Ezeh, L. N., & Afolabi, O. A. (2008). The influence of dwelling place and self-efficacy on career decision -making. *Global Journal of Humanities, 7*(1&2), 19–25.

Oku, A., Oku, O., Owoaje, E., & Monjok, E. (2015). An assessment of mental health status of undergraduate medical trainees in the University of Calabar, Nigeria: A cross-sectional study. *Open Access Macedonian Journal of Medical Sciences, 3*(2), 356–362.

Ottu, I. A. F. (2017). Marital closeness: Psychological differences among Ibibio and Yorubas of Nigeria. *IAFOR Journal of Psychology & the Behavioral Sciences, 3*(2), 53–76. https://doi.org/10.22492/ijpbs.3.2.05

Pepping, C. A., Davis, P. J., O'Donovan, A., & Pal, J. (2015). Individual differences in self-compassion: The role of attachment and experiences of parenting in childhood. *Self and Identity, 14*, 104–117. https://doi.org/10.1080/15298868.2014.955050

Pressman, S. D., & Cohen, S. (2005). Does positive affect influence health? *Psychological Bulletin, 131*, 925–971. https://doi.org/10.1037/0033-2909.131.6.925

Rapoza, K. A., Vassell, K., Wilson, D. T., Robertson, T. W., Manzella, D. J., Ortiz-Garcia, A. L., & Jimenez-Lazar, L. A. (2016). Attachment as a moderating factor between social support, physical health, and psychological symptoms. *SAGE Open, 2016*, 1–13. https://doi.org/10.1177/2158244016682818

Redelinghuys, J. (2010). *General self-efficacy as a moderator between stress and positive mental health in an African context* (masters dissertation). Neorth-West University.

Risucci, D., Wolfe, K. C., & Kaul, A. (2009). Promoting self-efficacy in minimally invasive surgery training. *Journal of the Society for Laparaendoscopic Surgeries, 13*, 4–8.

Roos, S. M., Potgieter, J. C., & Temane, M. Q. (2013). Self-efficacy, collective efficacy and the psychological well-being of groups in transition. *Journal of Psychology in Africa, 23*(4), 561–567.

Ryff, C. D. (1989). Happiness is everything, or is it? Explorations on the meaning of psychological well-being. *Journal of Personality and Social Psychology, 57*, 1069–1081. https://doi.org/10.1037//0022-3514.57.6.1069

Ryff, C. D. (2014). Psychological well-being revisited: Advances in science and practice. *Psychotherapy and Psychosomatics, 83*, 10–28.

Ryff, C. D., Radler, B. T., & Friedman, E. M. (2015). Persistent psychological well-being predicts improved self-rated health over 9–10 years: Longitudinal evidence from MIDUS. *Health Psychology Open, 2015*, 1–11. https://doi.org/10.1177/20551029156011582

Ryff, C. D., & Singer, B. H. (2008). Know thyself and become what you are: A eudaimonic approach to PWB. *Journal of Happiness Studies, 9*, 13–39. https://doi.org/10.1007/s10902-006-9019

Sabouripour, F., & Roslan, S. (2015, July). Self-efficacy, psychological well-being and resilience among international students. In *Paper presented at the 7th international conference on education and new learning technologies*, Barcelonam, Spain.

Sani, M., Mahfouz, M., Bani, I., Alsomily, A., Alagi, D., & Alsomily, N. (2012). Prevalence of stress among medical students in Jizan University, Kingdom of Saudi Arabia. *Gulf Medical Journal, 1*, 19–25.

Schiffrin, H. (2013). Positive psychology and attachment: Positive affect as a mediator of developmental outcomes. *Journal of Child and Family Studies, 23*(6), 1062–1072. https://doi.org/10.1007/s10826-013-9763-9

Schutte, L., Wissing, M. P., & Khumalo, I. P. (2013). Further validation of the questionnaire for eudaimonic well-being (QEWB). *Psychology of Well-Being: Theory, Research and Practice, 3*(3), 3. https://doi.org/10.1186/2211-1522-3-3

Schwarzer, R., & Jerusalem, M. (1995). Generalized self-efficacy scale. In M. Johnston, J. Weinman, & S. C. Wright (Eds.), *Measures in health psychology: A user's portfolio. Causal and control beliefs* (pp. 35–37). Windsor, UK.

Siddiqui, S. H. (2015). Impact of self-efficacy on psychological well-being among undergraduate students. *The International Journal of Indian Psychology, 2*(3), 5–16.

Simpson, J. A., Rholes, W. S., & Phillips, D. (1996). Conflict in close relationships: An attachment perspective. *Journal of Personality and Social Psychology, 71*, 899–914.

Tavakoli, N., Jomehri, F., & Farrokhi, N. (2014). The relationship between attachment styles and social self-efficacy with internet addiction in Iranian students. *Bulletin of Environment, Pharmacology and Life Sciences, 3*(Spl issue II), 302–307.

Temiz, Z. T., & Comert, I. T. (2018). The relationship between life satisfaction, attachment styles, and psychological resilience in university students. *Dusunen Adam The Journal of Psychiatry and Neurological Sciences, 31*, 274–283. https://doi.org/10.5350/DAJPN2018310305

Wei, M., Russell, D. W., & Zakalik, R. A. (2005). Adult attachment, social self-efficacy, self-disclosure, loneliness, and subsequent depression for freshman college students: A longitudinal study. *Journal of Counseling Psychology, 52*, 602–614.

Wissing, M. P., & Temane, Q. M. (2008). The structure of psychological well-being in cultural context: Towards a hierarchical model of psychological health. *Journal of Psychology in Africa, 18*(1), 45–56.

Wolf, T., & Kissling, G. (1984). Changes in life-style characteristics, health and mood of freshman medical students. *Journal of Medical Education, 59*, 806–814.

Worsley, J. D., Mansfield, R., & Corcoran, C. (2018). Attachment anxiety and problematic social media use: The mediating role of well-being. *Cyberpsychology, Behavior and Social Networking, 21*(9), 563–568. https://doi.org/10.1089/cyber.2017.0555

Wright, S. L., & Perrone-McGovern, K. M. (2010). An examination of the role of attachment and efficacy in life satisfaction. *The Counseling Psychologist, 38*(6), 796–823. https://doi.org/10.1177/0011000009359204

Zimmerman, B. J. (2000). Self-efficacy: An essential motive to learn. *Contemporary Educational Psychology, 25*, 82–91. https://doi.org/10.1037/a0022511

Chapter 14
Exploration of Harmony as a Quality of Happiness: Findings from South Africa and Ghana

Lusilda Schutte, Marié P. Wissing, Angelina Wilson Fadiji, Sonia Mbowa, Placidia M. Shoko, and Willem D. Schutte

Abstract Harmony is recognized as fundamental to being and functioning well in philosophical traditions and empirical research globally and in Africa. The aim of this study was to explore and describe harmony as a quality of happiness in South Africa (N = 585) and Ghana (N = 420). Using a qualitative descriptive research design, participants' responses to an open-ended question from the Eudaimonic-Hedonic Happiness Investigation (EHHI, Delle Fave et al., Soc Indic Res 100:185–207, 2011) on what happiness meant to them were coded according to the formalized EHHI coding manual. Responses that were assigned any of the following codes were considered: codes from the "harmony/balance" category in the "psychological definitions" life domain; and codes from any other life domain containing the words "harmony", "balance", or "peace". This resulted in 222 verbatim responses from South Africa and 80 from Ghana that were analyzed using content analysis to get a sense of the experiential texture of harmony as a quality of happiness. Findings showed that happiness was often expressed as harmony and balance within and between intrapersonal, interpersonal, transcendental, and universal levels of functioning, with wholeness, interconnectedness, and synergy implied. These findings, resonating with philosophical reflections on harmony from Africa and elsewhere, suggest that harmony as a quality of happiness is essentially holistic

L. Schutte (✉) · M. P. Wissing · S. Mbowa · P. M. Shoko
Africa Unit for Transdisciplinary Health Research, Faculty of Health Sciences, North-West University, Potchefstroom, South Africa
e-mail: Lusilda.Schutte@nwu.ac.za

A. W. Fadiji
Africa Unit for Transdisciplinary Health Research, Faculty of Health Sciences, North-West University, Potchefstroom, South Africa

Department of Educational Psychology, Faculty of Education, University of Pretoria, Pretoria, South Africa

W. D. Schutte
Centre for Business Mathematics and Informatics (BMI), Faculty of Natural Sciences, North-West University, Potchefstroom, South Africa

L. Schutte et al. (eds.), *Embracing Well-Being in Diverse African Contexts: Research Perspectives*, Cross-Cultural Advancements in Positive Psychology 16,
https://doi.org/10.1007/978-3-030-85924-4_14

and contextually embedded and that context-sensitive interdisciplinary approaches to theory building and intervention development pertaining to harmony are needed locally and globally.

Keywords Harmony · Balance · Peace · Happiness · Interconnectedness · South Africa · Ghana

14.1 Introduction

The scientific study of happiness has evolved considerably over the past decades, however, the concept is seemingly still elusive (Oishi et al., 2013), also in Africa. Contributing to the lack of clarity are the cultural differences in how lay people understand happiness, its predictors, and its relations to their daily life experiences and societal changes (Uchida & Ogihara, 2012). Several researchers have empirically explored this still open question across cultural contexts (see Delle Fave et al., 2011, 2016; Pflug, 2009). In this regard, in the Eudaimonic and Hedonic Happiness Investigation (EHHI) across 12 countries from mainly Western, but also some Asian and African contexts, Delle Fave et al. (2016) showed that inner harmony (referring to aspects such as inner peace, inner balance, contentment, and psychophysical well-being) predominated participants' psychological definitions of happiness. This points to the need for a deeper exploration of inner harmony as an important element of happiness in diverse samples, including different African contexts. In addition, relational and spiritual harmony and the interconnectedness of all things play a vital role in notions of the self, well-being and the good life in African people (Metz, 2017; Mkhize, 2020; Nwoye, 2006, 2013, 2015; Wissing et al., 2019, 2020). In view of these gaps, this study attempts to unearth the content of definitions of happiness reflecting inner and contextual harmony to get a sense of harmony as a quality of happiness in South African and Ghanaian samples to shed light on harmony as a universally valued quality of happiness and, at the same time, speak to unique socio-cultural, philosophical and mundane lived experiences of African people.

14.1.1 Some Philosophical and Theoretical Notions of Harmony as an Aspect of Being and Functioning Well

Harmony is fundamental to many philosophical traditions across the world. For example, *He* (harmony, harmonization) is a core concept in ancient Eastern philosophy (Li, 2008) and, as Li (2006) states, "probably the most cherished ideal in Chinese culture" (p. 583). In the Confucian tradition, harmony assumes that different aspects of life co-exist, and implies a certain positive relationship among them. For example, a sensible person is considered to be one who respects diverse viewpoints and can work with different people in a harmonious way, rather than one who seeks sameness (Li, 2006). Harmony is considered to be realized at multiple levels, ranging from internal harmony within a person, harmony with the family and between friends, harmony in the state and the international world, harmony between human society and the natural world, and harmony in the universe (Li, 2006, 2008). While the Confucian tradition does not preclude intrapersonal harmony, that recognizes multidimensionality within a person and refers to internal integration and harmonization of one's mental, moral, and physical dimensions, the emphasis is on interpersonal harmony, harmony with the natural world, and ultimately harmony in the universe (Li, 2006, 2008).

In Western philosophy, harmony has been discussed by Greek philosophers centuries ago (Delle Fave, 2014). For example, Epicure related harmony to *ataraxia*, which refers to being free from worries and anxieties. Harmony also featured in Pythagoras's philosophy of numbers and in Plato's views on a just man, whose reason, spirit and appetites are balanced. The Stoics referred to harmony in their ideal of levelness of judgement and detachment (Delle Fave, 2014).

In African philosophy, a human being's ultimate purpose in life is to reach an actualization of the self as a relational being, which can be done mainly/only by appreciating harmonious relationships (Metz, 2017). This is evident in Desmond Tutu's (1999) account of traditional African values as captured in the concept of *Ubuntu* or *Botho*: "We say, 'a person is a person through other people.' It is not 'I think therefore I am.' It says rather: 'I am human because I belong.' I participate, I share ... Harmony, friendliness, community are great goods. Social harmony is for us the summum bonum—the greatest good" (p. 33). Traditional African thought is built on a number of ontological assumptions, and Mkhize (2008) argues that harmony can be considered to be the principle that ties all the assumptions together. For example, traditional African thought assumes the hierarchy of beings, with God at the apex, then the ancestors (living-dead) serving as God's intermediaries, and then human beings and the rest of the world. Only those who lived morally proceed to ancestorhood, and ancestors act as the wardens of morality (Mkhize, 2008). Morality emerges when there is balance and harmony between people and their milieu, and when there is disequilibrium in relationships, restoration is needed (Mkhize, 2008). Relatedly, traditional African thought is based on the principle of cosmic unity, which assumes a fundamental interconnectedness between God, ancestors, human beings, the natural world, and inanimate objects. To retain harmony and social equilibrium, an ethic is valued that prizes social responsibilities towards other people, the community, and the cosmos (Mkhize, 2008).

An African theory on harmony, the Harmony Restoration Theory, has been developed by Igbokwe and colleagues (Igbokwe et al., 2015; Igbokwe & Ndom, 2008) and defines harmony as "being at peace with one's cosmos (world)" (Igbokwe & Ndom, 2008, p. 61). This theory postulates that, for an individual to have inner peace and inner balance, there must be a peaceful coexistence between the individual and the components of his/her cosmos. Such balance involves peace within the individual (endocosmos), peace between the individual and significant others (mesocosmos) and lastly peace between the individual and a higher power, religion, or ancestral spirits (exocosmos) (Igbokwe & Ndom, 2008). In this theory, an imbalance in one of the cosmoses disrupts the individual's harmony and is the cause of all unwellness, be it physical or psychological (Igbokwe et al., 2015).

Harmony has been appreciated as fundamental to being and functioning well in traditional philosophies across cultural settings. The concept of harmony has been particularly prominent in traditional African thought. Empirical research that aims to get a sense of how the philosophically valued construct of harmony on intrapersonal and contextual levels is expressed as a quality of happiness in African samples will provide insight into the manifestations and qualities of harmony in the everyday lives of African people.

14.1.2 Some Empirical Findings on Harmony as an Aspect of Being and Functioning Well

Empirically, studies across various cultural contexts found that harmony on intrapersonal and contextual levels are key to well-being and functioning well. In several studies that explored happiness/well-being/the good life using bottom-up qualitative methods, harmony and peace emerged as themes from participants' responses. For example, apart from the findings in Delle Fave et al. (2016) cited above, Dela Coleta and Dela Coleta (2006, as cited in Garcia et al., 2015) found that Brazilian students reported harmony/peace as one of the most important facets of a good life. Uchida and Kitayama (2009) found that both American and Japanese students associated happiness with social harmony, but that this was emphasized much more by Japanese participants compared to the American sample. In a study where personal blogs of 12 million people were analyzed, Mogilner et al. (2011) found that, as people get older, they associate happiness more with peacefulness. Pflug (2009) found that German students described happiness as freedom, autonomy, and hedonic pleasure, while black South African students emphasized contentment, social harmony, and tight family relationships in their descriptions of happiness. Osei-Tutu et al. (2020) in examining cultural models of well-being among religious custodians in four Ghanaian languages, discovered that peace of mind was one of the key aspects used to define being well. In all four languages explored (which are spoken in different regions of Ghana), peace or being without worries was a consistent manifestation of well-being. In addition, the content of participants' definitions often referred to low-arousal positive affective states related to contentment, calmness, serenity, and relief that one has met social expectations. In a related study, psychophysical well-being emerged strongly in the findings of Wilson Fadiji et al. (2019) on how Ghanaian adults define well-being. Specifically, emphasis was placed on the absence of ill-being and having a sound mind.

Harmony as a facet of being and functioning well has also been explored in the literature using rating scales or other empirical approaches. For example, on the intrapersonal level, Lee et al. (2013) developed the Peace of Mind Scale to measure affective well-being as valued in Chinese culture, where they defined peace of mind as an internal state of peacefulness and harmony. They found that a sample of Taiwanese students scored higher on peace of mind than a sample of American students. Kjell et al. (2016) developed the Harmony in Life Scale, that measures overall harmony as a cognitive component of subjective well-being, as a complement to the commonly used Satisfaction with Life Scale of Diener et al. (1985). They found that the Harmony in Life Scale explained more unique variance in most of the other well-being-related rating scales included in the study compared to the Satisfaction with Life Scale. Nima, Cloninger, Lucchese, et al. (2020) and Nima, Cloninger, Persson, et al. (2020) argued that the Harmony in Life Scale goes beyond capturing a cognitive component of subjective well-being, and that it actually captures the social/behavioral component thereof, since it focuses on the balance between the individual and the world he or she lives in. Kjell et al. (2019, 2021) developed semantic measures to evaluate a person's level of harmony in life, and found that scores on the semantic measures predicted cooperation as a behavioral outcome, while scores on the Harmony in Life Scale and the Satisfaction with Life Scale, as well as semantic measures of satisfaction with life, did not.

In terms of contextual harmony, Kwan et al. (1997) developed the Interpersonal Relationship Harmony Inventory to measure relationship harmony in an individual's most important close dyadic relationships. They found that relationship harmony, in addition to self-esteem, predicted life satisfaction among students from Hong Kong and America. The Family Harmony Scale (Kavikondala et al., 2016) assesses family harmony, a construct that is postulated to be an important predictor of psychopathology in Chinese culture. In a Hong Kong sample, Kavikondala et al. (2016) found that family harmony had a negative correlation with depressive symptoms after controlling for individual risk factors and general family functioning. Chen et al. (2016) developed the Group Harmony Scale for a workplace setting based on literature on traditional Chinese philosophy and social science research pertaining to the topic of social harmony. They found that group harmony promoted innovative performance by enhancing knowledge sharing among members of the group in a Chinese sample of top management business leaders.

Looking at well-being across intrapersonal and contextual levels of functioning, Igbokwe et al. (2015) operationalized the Harmony Restoration Theory developed in Africa that considers harmony across cosmoses (endocosmos, mesocosmos, and exocosmos) in the Harmony-Disharmony Scale. They found confirmation for the model in a Nigerian sample and suggested that psychopathology in African people arises from disharmony in one or more of the levels, and that psychotherapy should focus on harmony restoration. Hitokoto and Uchida (2015) developed the Interdependent Happiness Scale to measure happiness as experienced by people who have interdependent self-construals (as is typical in East Asian cultures), with a focus on the relational nature of human beings, interdependence, harmony, risk aversion, quiescence, and ordinariness. This scale operationalizes happiness at the level where the intrapersonal and interpersonal/contextual overlap. They found that the subjective well-being of Japanese students was more likely to be explained by interdependent happiness compared to American students. Furthermore, interdependent happiness explained the subjective well-being of working adults in America, Germany, Japan, and Korea, as well as Japanese adults and elders from collectivistic regions of Japan (Hitokoto & Uchida, 2015).

Across cultural contexts, intrapersonal and contextual harmony emerged as core facets of being and functioning well, and attempts have been made to measure and empirically explore harmony on different levels of functioning. However, a deeper and nuanced sense of how people express harmony as a quality of happiness in verbatim responses, especially in the African context, is lacking. This study will address this gap by considering data from South African and Ghanaian samples.

14.1.3 The Present Study

Harmony is a core value in traditional philosophies across the world, including traditional African philosophy. Empirically, inner and contextual harmony have emerged as key facets of well-being and happiness across cultures, also in African samples. What is not known, however, is what the experiential texture of harmony as a quality of happiness is as found in the verbatim definitions of happiness by participants from African settings. The aim of the present study is therefore to explore and describe inner and contextual harmony as a quality of happiness in South African and Ghanaian samples.

14.2 Method

14.2.1 Research Design

This study implemented a qualitative descriptive design (Sandelowski, 2000, 2010) to explore and describe harmony as a quality of happiness. Data gathering for this study partly overlapped with that of the multicountry international Eudaimonic-Hedonic Happiness Investigation (EHHI, Delle Fave et al., 2011, 2016), but focused specifically on oversampled data from two African countries who are currently part of the EHHI project namely South Africa and Ghana. Both these countries gathered data on larger samples than what were required for the EHHI project to allow for additional analyses. The EHHI project included amongst others data collection on a number of open-ended questions including one on happiness. For the purpose of the current study, a selection of responses (see below) to the open-ended question on happiness as formulated and scored in the EHHI study, is relevant, as well as the information of a socio-demographic questionnaire which is used for participant description.

14.2.2 Participants

Participants in the present study had to be 18 years or older and have at least secondary school education. The inclusion criteria were relevant to increase the comparability across the samples, and to heighten the possibility that participants would be able to reflect on the questions posed and provide informative responses, particularly to an open-ended question, which was deemed important for interpretation purposes. In South Africa, adults adhering to the inclusion criteria were recruited by means of snowball sampling through trained research assistants in various provinces of South Africa which enhances variation and diversity in the sample ($N = 585$). In Ghana, participants were recruited by trained research assistants who visited different institutions, such as churches, workplaces, and higher education institutions, to gather data after permission was obtained by the relevant authorities ($N = 420$). See Table 14.1 for a description of the participants per sample.

14.2.3 Data Gathering Instruments

14.2.3.1 Socio-Demographic Questionnaire

A socio-demographic questionnaire was administered in the EHHI project that gathered data on gender, age, standard of living, education level, employment status, marital status, and whether the participant practices religion. This information was used in the present study to describe the participants involved (see Table 14.1).

14.2.3.2 Semi Structured, Open-Ended Question on Happiness

For the purpose of this paper, an open-ended question on happiness from the Eudaimonic-Hedonic Happiness Investigation (EHHI) (Delle Fave et al., 2011) was relevant. The question was phrased as follows: "What is happiness for you? Take your time and provide your definition."

14.2.4 Ethical Considerations and Procedure

In the international EHHI study, each country had to obtain ethical approval for the local study from an authorized ethics committee in the country. In South Africa, data gathering formed part of the FORT3 research program ("The prevalence of levels of psychosocial health: dynamics and relationships with biomarkers of (ill) health in South African social contexts", Wissing, 2008/2012) which obtained ethics approval from the Health Research Ethics Committee of the North-West University,

Table 14.1 Demographic profile of participants

	South Africa ($N = 585$) n (%)	Ghana ($N = 420$) n (%)
Gender		
Female	362 (61.88%)	178 (42.38%)
Male	222 (37.95%)	231 (55.00%)
Missing	1 (0.17%)	11 (2.62%)
Age		
Range, *M* (*SD*)	18–84, 42.15 (11.51)	30–62, 41.37 (9.42)
Level of education		
Secondary	220 (37.61%)	207 (49.29%)
Tertiary	176 (30.09%)	169 (40.24%)
Postgraduate	185 (31.62%)	29 (6.90%)
Missing	4 (0.68%)	15 (3.57%)
Standard of living		
Below average	32 (5.47%)	36 (8.57%)
Average	385 (65.81%)	255 (60.71%)
Above average	147 (25.13%)	45 (10.71%)
Missing	21 (3.59%)	84 (20.00%)
Marital status		
Single	145 (24.79%)	162 (38.57%)
Married	367 (62.74%)	180 (42.86%)
Cohabitating	19 (3.25%)	19 (4.52%)
Separated/divorced	34 (5.81%)	19 (4.52%)
Widowed	11 (1.88%)	23 (5.48%)
Missing	9 (1.54%)	17 (4.05%)
Practicing religion		
No	43 (7.35%)	11 (2.62%)
Occasionally	153 (26.15%)	96 (22.86%)
Regularly	378 (64.62%)	296 (70.48%)
Missing	11 (1.88%)	17 (4.05%)

South Africa, with approval number NWU 00002-07-A2. The University of Ghana Ethics Committee for Human Research approved the Ghanaian study (approval number: ECH 086 16-17). Participants gave written informed consent prior to participating in the study. Participation was voluntary and participants could withdraw at any time during data gathering. To ensure anonymity, the signed informed consent forms were separated from the corresponding answer sheets upon submission of the completed questionnaires. All South African and some Ghanaian participants received the questionnaires to complete at their own time and then submitted it to the field workers. For some other Ghanaian participants, questionnaires were administered in interview format by trained field workers in an attempt to improve the quality of the data.

Since both South Africa and Ghana are multilingual countries where English is the main language for communication between people who speak different languages, questionnaires were administered in English. The researchers deemed it reasonable to expect that participants would be able to complete the questionnaires in English, because the inclusion criteria specified that participants had to have at least Grade 12 education, and English is taught in the education systems of both countries.

After data collection for the EHHI study and for the current oversampled data sets, all responses to the open-ended questions (including that on happiness) were coded and categorized by trained coders in line with the EHHI coding manual. The development of the manualized EHHI coding system by Delle Fave and colleagues was initially based on the responses of participants from eight countries, and later refined and expanded based on data from more countries across six continents (Delle Fave et al., 2011, 2016). Codes for verbatim responses were categorized into meaningful subcategories and categories, which were, in turn, clustered into life domains. The life domains in the EHHI coding system include work, family, standard of living, interpersonal relationships, health, psychological definitions, leisure/free time, spirituality/religion, community/society issues, education, and life in general. We used this coded data to select harmony-related categories and codes for detailed analysis of verbatim responses.

14.2.5 Data Analysis

In this study we explored the content of verbatim responses clustered in harmony-related categories and codes as determined by the EHHI scoring manual. Categories and codes in the manualized EHHI coding system that pertained to harmony were identified and all verbatim excerpts that were assigned these codes were extracted. In total, 222 verbatim responses from South Africa were extracted based on the criteria and 80 verbatim responses from Ghana. These excerpts were then explored in depth to get a sense of harmony as a quality of happiness in these African samples. We will now describe exactly which codes were identified as referring to harmony. First, the EHHI coding system contains a category labelled “harmony/balance” as part of the psychological definitions life domain. We considered all codes within this category in an attempt to get insight into inner harmony as a quality of happiness in our samples. Next, for contextual harmony, we selected all codes in all other life domains that contained the words “harmony”, “balance”, or “peace” in the code descriptions. We selected these terms because “harmony” and “balance” both featured in the category label for inner harmony, and we wanted to do a parallel investigation for contextual harmony. We added the term “peace” because we considered peace to be closely overlapping with harmony, especially on a contextual level. The terms “balance” and “peace” were also some of the most common words mentioned when people had to list ten words that they associate with the word “harmony” in a study by Kjell et al. (2016).

The excerpts (i.e., the literal verbatim expressions of the participants) that were extracted were then scrutinized. This was done by means of a content analysis

(Krippendorff, 2018) of the extracted excerpts, taking a phenomenological and hermeneutic stance towards a deeper and richer understanding of harmony as a quality of happiness. Specifically, data were (re)coded, then (re)clustered into categories which, in turn, were (re)categorized into themes (Krippendorff, 2018). This step in the data analysis process was performed by the first author, and audited by the second and third authors. Discussions were held to clarify and resolve differences. We used an interpretive and naturalistic approach to highlight the quality or texture of harmony experiences described in the content of participants' definitions of what happiness is for them as expressed in their own words.

14.2.6 Trustworthiness

Various elements were built into the different phases of the research to strive towards trustworthiness (Elo et al., 2014; Nowell et al., 2017). Lincoln and Guba (1985) presented four criteria for trustworthiness, namely credibility, transferability, dependability, and confirmability. Credibility holds when there is concordance between what participants reported and how it is presented in the research (Nowell et al., 2017). In the current study, credibility was promoted by setting inclusion criteria that enhanced the probability that participants would be able to reflect on the question asked (Kyngäs et al., 2020); by prolonged engagement with the data, where the authors who conducted the analyses read the excerpts numerous times over the course of an extended period of time (Nowell et al., 2017); by analyst triangulation where several authors checked the findings against the original data (Patton, 1999); and by describing the research process and findings in a transparent manner (Kyngäs et al., 2020). Transferability refers to the extent to which the findings can be transferred to other contexts and fields (Kyngäs et al., 2020). In this study, setting clear inclusion criteria and describing the samples at hand will inform those who seek to apply the findings to their contexts how transferable the findings are (Kyngäs et al., 2020; Nowell et al., 2017). Dependability refers to the quality and coherence of the research process from data collection to data analysis to drawing conclusions and how stable the data is over time (Kyngäs et al., 2020). Dependability was enhanced in this study by the independent data analysis and auditing of the data analysis process and findings by different authors and regular dialogue between the authors about the data and the findings (Kyngäs et al., 2020). Dependability was also promoted by thick description of examples in context and highlighting the complex linking of ideas which were all intended to get a sense of the quality of experiences. Confirmability is achieved when it is clear that the research findings were derived from the data (Nowell et al., 2017). In this study, confirmability was promoted by intentional reflexivity on the side of the researchers, where they aimed to be aware of their own perspectives and positions and how this may influence the results and conclusions drawn, and engaged in repeated dialogues to ensure that personal biases or perceptions did not skew conclusions drawn (Barry et al., 1999; Malterud, 2001).

14.3 Results and Discussion

Three themes emerged and the results will be presented accordingly. The first and second themes echoed the data selection procedures and represented happiness as inner and contextual harmony, respectively. The third theme represented happiness as holistic and dynamic experiences of harmony, balance, and peace. Categories within themes will be presented when the themes are presented. Excerpts to illustrate harmony as a quality of happiness as emerging from the data will be presented, and some information on the participant whose excerpt is cited will be provided in brackets, namely: country (SA denotes South Africa, GH denotes Ghana), gender (F denotes female, M denotes male), age in years, and highest level of education (S denotes secondary education, T denotes tertiary education, P denotes postgraduate education). We corrected small language and grammar errors in the excerpts to ease readability, but ensured that the meaning of the responses did not change.

14.3.1 Happiness as Inner Harmony

The first theme represented responses where participants referred exclusively to inner harmony. Six categories were identified, namely inner peace and contentment, inner harmony despite adversity, inner harmony linked to gratitude and appreciation, self-worth, low-arousal positive emotions and absence of negative emotions, and balance and integration of inner experiences.

14.3.1.1 Inner Peace and Contentment

Many participants referred to inner peace and contentment in their accounts of what happiness is to them. This is evident in responses such as "*Happiness is being fulfilled and content*" (SA, F, 40, P); "*Being content & at peace*" (SA, gender not specified, 31, T); "*Happiness is the inner peace you feel as a person*" (GH, F, 52, S); and "*Happiness for me means being at peace with myself*" (GH, F, 30, T). In the Ghanaian sample, many participants referred to happiness as "peace of mind", as illustrated in the following responses: "*Happiness is peace of mind*" (GH, F, 34, T; GH, M, 44, S; GH, M, 30, T; GH, F, 30, S) and "*Happiness is a peaceful state of mind*" (GH, F, 36, T). "*Happiness is a state of peace of mind*" (GH, 31, F, S; GH, age not provided, M, S).

The prominence of inner harmony in participants' responses is interesting, since one might have expected that inner harmony would not be emphasized to such an extent in African cultures. For example, according to Metz (2017), African ethics typically focuses on relationality between persons, with self-regard and a concept such as intrapersonal harmony not being culturally relevant. However, our findings do concur with Osei-Tutu et al. (2020), who found that "peace of mind" and low-arousal positive affect occurred as a major theme when asking Ghanaian religious leaders (who were considered to be cultural experts) from the three prominent religious groups in Ghana to describe concepts related to well-being implicit in the terminology of four Ghanaian languages. Osei-Tutu et al. (2020) suggested that the peace of mind facet of well-being in Ghanaian culture is related to the contentment, calmness and relief that comes from meeting social expectations embedded in interdependence rather than a self-focused independent experience of peace of mind. The emphasis on the self in definitions of happiness was also seen in the work of Agbo and Ome (2017), where it was argued that a predominant individualistic tendency among the Igbos of Nigeria might explain their findings. Agbo and Ome (2017) also suggested that the inclusion of postgraduate students in their study sample, who tend to adopt more Western dispositions, could have explained their findings. Our findings in this study may support the observation of Wissing et al. (2020) that there may be a dynamic and dialectic pattern of African individualism-collectivism emerging where interdependent and independent value systems flow together.

14.3.1.2 Inner Harmony Despite Adversity

A very prominent element that featured in numerous participants' responses is the notion that happiness is contentment and inner peace despite circumstances and hardship. For example: "*True happiness is being content & at peace from within—no matter what my circumstances*" (SA, F, 41, S); "*Happiness to me is about feeling content and at peace with my life, even if outer circumstances are not ideal*" (SA, M, 38, P); "*A feeling of contentment. A place where I feel at ease despite chaos around me*" (SA, F, 36, P); "*Happiness is peace of mind in the bowl of challenges*" (GH, F, 31, T); and "*Happiness is a state of being relaxed with a peaceful mind no matter the circumstances surrounding one's life*" (GH, M, 48, T). Some participants explicitly described that inner peace despite adversity is the result of a choice or mindset: "*Happiness is a state of mind and a physical mental feeling of contentment, satisfaction and peacefulness. I find happiness is sometimes only achievable as a mental mindset. You have to decide to be happy, and work at it, despite hardships, failure, physical pain, setbacks and achievements. It is training your body and mind to deal with day to day realities in a way that allows you to feel happy most of the time. This is not easy, it takes a lot of work and self-checking but it is achievable. It does become a habit eventually and it does alter the outcome of situations . . . I am a cancer survivor . . .*" (SA, F, 42, P); "*Being at peace with who I am and feeling good about the reality I find myself in. An emotional equilibrium—feeling content despite everything not necessarily being 100% perfect.*" (SA, F, 35, P); and "*Happiness is being content and accepting oneself and one's surroundings. Happiness is a mental outlook on a person's life/well-being*" (SA, F, 24, T).

The emphasis on contentment despite life not being ideal differs significantly from subjective well-being literature where satisfaction with circumstances is often stressed. For example, in the very commonly used Satisfaction with Life Scale

(Diener et al., 1985) three of the five items refer to satisfaction with life circumstances, namely "In most ways my life is close to my ideal" (item 1), "The conditions of my life are excellent" (item 2), and "So far I have gotten the important things I want in life" (item 4). Our findings may be related to context, with South Africa and Ghana not being as affluent as, for example, the United States of America, where the Satisfaction with Life Scale was developed. This finding highlights the contextual embeddedness of experiences. Experiencing happiness as contentment despite bad circumstances may reflect a life attitude (worldview) in which opposites can co-exist as described in philosophical perspectives on harmony. The co-existence or complexity of positive and negative feelings/experiences can be linked to well-being according to Hershfield et al. (2013), and was specifically noted in an African context by Wissing (2016). Our findings can also be interpreted as an expression of resilience in less-than-optimal contexts, where people are able to find happiness even if life is not what they would have wanted it to be. This being said, while it is admirable that people display resilience in the ability to find happiness despite hardship, a subjective evaluation of life conditions should not be disregarded in quality of life research—we should never become complacent about the deprivation and adversity that many people face in daily life. In line with this thought, Hart et al. (2016) indicated that resilience should include "overcoming adversity", while also potentially changing, or even dramatically transforming, the adversity.

14.3.1.3 Inner Harmony Linked to Gratitude and Appreciation

Happiness as contentment and inner peace was often linked to gratitude and appreciation in participants' responses. For example: "*Happiness to me is being content with where you are in life and with what you have. Happiness is appreciating the small & big things in life. Being grateful that you are alive, that you are loved. Happiness to me is an intangible thing and a mindset decision. Its choosing to be happy regardless of everything and/or challenge you may face.*" (SA, F, 27, T); "*To be content with who you are and what you have at the moment. To be thankful in all circumstances*" (SA, F, 30, T); and "*Happiness is contentment with oneself as well as gratitude for all that we have*" (SA, F, 23, T).

The association between gratitude and harmony as a quality of happiness and well-being speaks to the findings of a recent meta-analysis (Portocarrero et al., 2020) which found that dispositional gratitude is moderately to strongly correlated with mental health, considering both positive and negative mental health. Also, using the experience sampling method, Jans-Beken et al. (2019) found that state gratitude, state cheerfulness (as representative of high-arousal positive affect), and state satisfaction (as representative of low-arousal positive affect) reciprocally predicted one another from moment to moment in daily experience. In their study, higher levels of state gratitude predict higher levels of high- and low-arousal positive affect, and vice versa. In South Africa, Guse et al. (2019) found that gratitude was positively associated with satisfaction with life and positive affect and negatively associated with negative affect among South African adolescents. More research on how, why and when gratitude, which is classified as low-arousal positive affect by some (Cavanaugh et al., 2016) and as an empathetic or other-directed positive emotion by others (Tugade et al., 2014), associates with facets such as contentment and inner peace in African settings will be useful.

14.3.1.4 Self-worth

For many participants, happiness was related to having peace with who they are, being worthy, and/or living according to their value system. For example: "*Happiness is feeling good about myself, knowing I am a worthy person. This is created by acting in accordance with my values, doing things for and nurturing others. Keeping fit and healthy, etc.*" (SA, F, 43, P); "*Being honestly content with who you are, what you have and what you give to the people around you*" (SA, F, 32, S); "*If you can live being true to yourself, meaning you can accept who you are, where you are coming from and where you are going to. You accept your strengths and weaknesses.*" (SA, F, 37, T); and "*To be content with who and what I am and where I am going with my life, as well as what I have and what I do*" (SA, M, 60, P).

Living a life and setting goals that are aligned with one's stable values, motives and beliefs, and the benefits thereof for well-being, are emphasized in the self-concordance model (Sheldon, 2014; Sheldon et al., 2004). The findings also resonate with Dzokoto et al. (2018) who found that Ghanaian conceptions of well-being include moral living. This aligns with an African worldview, which emphasizes that being worthy in one's community is essential to being human—being human per definition requires one to be ethical and to practice the values of *Ubuntu* such as justice and caring (Mkhize, 2020). Following on individualist notions of happiness that is expressed as being at peace with oneself, Agbo and Ome (2017) found a relationship between identity need and happiness among Nigerians.

14.3.1.5 Low-Arousal Positive Emotions and Absence of Negative Emotions

Many participants emphasized the presence of low-arousal positive emotions and the absence of stress and other negative emotions in their descriptions of what happiness is to them. For example, "*A state of ultimate peace and relaxation*" (SA, F, 30, P); "*When I feel love and loved. When I feel needed and when I give. When I feel peace and calm.*" (SA, F, 50, S); "*Happiness is the moment where by my soul is very peacefully and not troubled. My life is full of good times and laughter. In other ways good times are more than bad.*" (SA, M, 30, T); "*Is to be free, feel free and relaxed. Have the joy inside and outside that is spiritually, physically and emotionally.*" (SA, M, 51, P); "*Happiness is a free state of mind without worries*" (GH, M, 54, T); and "*It is when one has no problem and is sound in mind, soul and body. It is usually not only about money but personal gains*" (GH, M, 31, T). One participant described the deep-felt experience of this overarching sense of calmness and serenity as "*A feeling I get when embracing my 6 senses, where everything appears to be in a state of ease, calm and tranquility.*" (SA, M, 38, T).

The findings resonate with Pflug (2009) who found that a black South African student sample often described happiness as calm and balanced mental states such as peace of mind and calmness, while a German student sample provided more goal-orientated and hedonic descriptions of happiness. It also concurs with Osei-Tutu et al. (2020) who found that well-being is often understood in terms of low-arousal positive affect in Ghana. Emotional and psychological stability as definitions of well-being in Wilson Fadiji et al. (2019) resonates with our findings on "soundness of mind" as well as the work of Agbo and Ome (2017).

14.3.1.6 Balance and Integration of Inner Experiences

While happiness as low-arousal positive affect is associated with low levels of activation, some participants mentioned "contentment" or "peace" and "energy" together. For example, "*Happiness is a feeling of peace, lightness, harmony, contented energy and enjoyment of the moment*" (SA, F, 41, P) and "*Happiness is being integrated—at peace, energized and able to communicate that energy to others*" (SA, F, 46, P). These excerpts highlight that inner harmony has an integrated and dynamic quality, where contentment and inner peace may provide a basepoint of groundedness and integration, from which focused energy can flow.

The integrated and dynamic quality of harmony was further expressed in participants' responses where happiness was described as an integrated intrapersonal experience highlighting cognitive, affective, physical and/or inner spiritual ("soul") elements being in harmony or in balance. For example: "*Happiness is when my mind, body and spirit (soul) are at a place of peace and joy despite my environment*" (SA, M, 26, S); "*State of contentment—mental, physical, emotional*" (SA, F, 32, P); "*It is when body and soul are in harmony*" (SA, F, 43, S); "*State of mind. When your mind, body and soul is in equal equilibrium and your attitude towards life is positive.*" (SA, M, 30, P). This resonates with the notion of the integrated self of Kuhl et al. (2015) where the fully functioning person is considered to be one whose cognitive, emotional, and behavioral functioning are mutually coordinated and functioning in unity. More so, it supports the work of Igbokwe et al. (2015) on the notions of balance. This suggests that harmony is a holistic intrapersonal experience, where the different facets of intrapersonal functioning are in balance.

14.3.2 Happiness as Contextual Harmony

In the second theme, participants referred exclusively to contextual harmony in their responses. Two categories emerged, namely horizontal and vertical harmony.

14.3.2.1 Horizontal Harmony

Apart from happiness being described as inner harmony and peace, happiness was also expressed as contextual harmony by many participants. For example, happiness was often described as peace and harmony in the house and family. This is illustrated in the following excerpts: "*Happiness for me is living peacefully with my family and understanding each other*" (SA, F, 45, S); "*Happiness is when my family is at peace and all our needs are met*" (GH, F, 45, T); *Happiness is where there is peace and harmony in the house and when everyone is satisfied with what he or she is given and everyone reached their aspiration in life*" (GH, F, 39, T); "*When peace reigns in the house*" (GH, M, 54, P).

Some participants included a wider network of interpersonal relations when describing happiness as contextual harmony, such as those with whom he/she has close relationships, neighbors, friends and the community: "*Happiness for me is peace and contentment in my heart for those I love and care deeply for*" (SA, M, 50, P); "*Happiness for me is being in touch and in good relations with my kids and extended family members and living in harmony with my neighbors. Having money to do what I want.*" (SA, M, 41, S); and "*Happiness is being in harmony with family, friends, work and community*" (SA, F, 50, S).

For others, happiness was to live in harmony with others or one's surroundings more generally: "*Happiness is my most comfortable state where I am at peace with everyone around me and nothing is frustrating me*" (SA, F, 20, T); "*Happiness comes when you are at peace with people around, when your place of achieving something succeeds*" (GH, M, 34, T); "*It is a state of mind when one or two people live or find peace*" (GH, M, 30, S); "*Happiness is living in harmony with everyone without troubles*" (GH, F, 41, S); "*Harmony in social and environmental spheres (including home & children)*" (SA, F, 41, T); "*It is about being free and joyful in a peaceful surrounding and being with the people I love*" (SA, F, 54, S); "*Peace—no conflict. Family—being together. Laughing—laugh a lot.*" (SA, F, 46, S); "*I would say a combination of three things. 1st- spending time with God, 2nd spending time with my family and close friends and 3rd spending quality time by myself to recharge batteries. Being at peace with world brings me immense peace which leads to inner happiness.*" (SA, F, 37, S).

The importance of relationships with others for happiness and well-being is widely recognized (e.g., Demir & Sümer, 2018; Donaldson & Donaldson, 2017; Keyes, 1998; Keyes et al., 2008; Ryff, 2014; Ryff & Singer, 1998, 2000; Seligman, 2011). The findings concur with those of Pflug (2009) where black South African students emphasized close social relationships, and particularly family relationships, in their definitions of happiness, with an emphasis on a stable social environment and regard to others. The prominence of other people in participants' responses resonates with the African worldview emphasizing interdependence between the individual and the community, which is reflected in the notion of *Ubuntu* ("a human is human through other humans", e.g., Nwoye, 2015, p. 109). The results also resonate with values held in Eastern cultures, where interpersonal harmony and adjustment are emphasized (Chen et al., 2016). People reach a sense of well-being through mutual sympathy and harmonious living with others.

14.3.2.2 Vertical Harmony

Other participants described happiness as being in peace and harmony with God and others: "*Happiness is having the peace of God that passes all understanding*" (GH, F, 40, S); "*Happiness is to be in harmony with God and my fellow man. To be content and satisfied with all that I have received from God. To be able to love, work, play and serve. To know that God loves me unconditionally.*" (SA, F, 48, P); "*Peace and Christianity. When our country can be like that then we all would be equal in God and humanity.*" (SA, M, 56, S); "*To be at peace with my Savior, my family, friends and all of mankind*" (SA, F, 54, T); and "*To be at peace with God and others around you. To be loved and have loved ones who accept your love.*" (SA, M, 43, P).

The mentioning of God and spirituality in African participants' responses come as no surprise. For example, Mkhize (2020) identifies "Spirit-ness" as a key tenet of the Afrocentric paradigm in psychology: "Being human is being Spirit; this is more than spirituality . . . Spirit exists before and beyond material existence" (p. 5). Nobles (2013) presents the African meaning of being human as "a divine spirit housed in a physical container having a human experience" (p. 296). Nwoye (2013, 2015) highlights the role of spirituality in Africa peoples. God is assumed to be closely involved in human beings' lives with things only happening upon His approval, which encourage people to submit to God's will when they face problems that they cannot handle or change.

14.3.3 Happiness as Holistic and Dynamic Experiences of Harmony, Balance and Peace

One of the most outstanding trends in the data was that happiness was commonly presented as holistic and dynamic experiences of harmony, balance and peace, resulting in the third theme. No subthemes were distinguished for this theme. Very often, inner and contextual harmony were mentioned simultaneously by participants when expressing what happiness is to them. The following excerpts are examples: "*Happiness to me is being at peace with myself, the people I live with and my extended family.*" (SA, M, 37, S); "*Being content with my life, my family, and my work, but the most important part to be happy with myself.*" (SA, F, 47, T); "*Happiness for me is living in peace with my husband and kids and my in-laws, being in peace with myself emotionally and spiritually.*" (SA, F, 46, S); "*Happiness is achieved when you are at peace with mum, God and yourself. It is a feeling of fulfilment.*" (GH, M, 31, T); "*Happiness is when you got peace with yourself and your surroundings*" (GH, M, 55, S); "*Happiness is a state of being at peace mentally and socially*" (GH, M, 60, S); "*When everything around me is okay and everyone and everything is at peace, that's when I am happy*" (GH, M, 42, T); "*Happiness is a state, notwithstanding negative influences, where a person is at peace with self, one's neighbor and one's place in the universe.*" (SA, M, 63, T); "*Accepting and appreciating yourself—strong as well as weak points. Being in harmony with yourself as well as with nature.*" (SA, F, 53, T). One participant beautifully described this sense of interconnectedness as being "in sync": "*Feeling content with myself and what I have achieved. Feeling in sync with significant others. Being relaxed and confident.*" (SA, M, 51, P). Another participant connected this holistic harmonized experience to beauty: "*Happiness for me, is inner peace and to be able to see all the beauty around me, in nature but as well in other humans and to know that God can be seen everywhere. To love and to be loved for whom I am.*" (SA, F, 43, T).

Other participants described happiness as inner peace, but specifically ascribed this inner peace to relationships with others or God. For example: "*Happiness is the experience (cognitively and emotionally) of peace (not the absence of worry but the presence of Christ), joy, and love. It can include but is not limited to—being with others who make you feel this way and doing things that make you feel this way.*" (SA, F, 33, T); "*Happiness is an inner peace which you experience when all your love-ones are around you. Happiness is to feel good about yourself, to experience health, to feel loved + appreciated.*" (SA, F, 56, T); "*Happiness is being content with who and what you are in life. Also having peace of mind and know who you are and also knowing where you are going in life. God provides that kind of peace.*" (SA, F, 30, T); "*Contentment, joyful, peace, fulfilment but all of this are provided by our Lord and Savior.*" (SA, F, 34, T); "*To have peace within yourself. To accept things the way they are and leaving the rest up to the Lord and to trust Him.*" (SA, 2, 38, P).

Several participants expressed happiness as having balance between different domains of life that they find important: "*Happiness for me is to have a life-work-play balance. To be at your optimal potential in various departments in your life. To be healthy, to have a good relationship with my God, to be happy in my marriage, to be closer to family, to have friends, to be good in the workplace/academics and to spend time with my pet. To be mindful of the moments—All these conclude my definition of happiness.*" (SA, F, 24, P); "*Happiness is a state where I am in balance with people and things around me. Circumstances are under control, most people are at peace with me and I with them and I am attaining my life goals and am on track to continue in this state as far as I can reasonably see into the future.*" (SA, M, 51, T); "*Finding happiness first starts with yourself and inside yourself. If you are an unhappy person, another person cannot make you happy. NB: Believe in Jesus Christ—He gives happiness! Happiness is not only an emotion, but when there is a good healthy balance between the psychological and spiritual, and the physical.*" (SA, F, 43, S); "*It is a state of mind usually experienced when my life is in balance. When I am content with my relationships, physical and mental well-being and feel that I can handle the good and the bad that life may offer. It is influenced by the way I choose to respond to life.*" (SA, F, 34, T).

The findings resonate with a growing body of literature which suggests that happiness is a matter of connectedness (Delle Fave et al., 2016). For example, the Meaning and Relational Well-being model of interconnectedness (Wissing, 2016; Wissing et al., 2019) visually presents the integration of meaning and relatedness in a double spiral helix widening upwards to represent progressively more complex relational systems from the intrapersonal, to the interpersonal, to the social, and then the spiritual/transcendental levels which provide meaning in, to and of life, with all of this being situated in a specific time and place. This dovetails with a strong relational ontology, which assumes the interconnectedness of everything (Slife & Richardson, 2008). Including harmony with nature as part of one's definition of happiness, also concords with relational and holistic conceptions of well-being that emphasizes the interrelatedness between sustainability and well-being (Harrell, 2015; Helne & Hirvilammi, 2015; Kjell, 2011).

The findings clearly reflect some of the main tenets of the Afrocentric paradigm identified by Mkhize (2020). For example, wholeness and balance that speaks to the unity of mind, body and Spirit is core in this paradigm. Also, connectedness and inter-connections is recognized as a constant motif in the Afrocentric paradigm. It speaks to Nobles (2015) who stated that an "African Grand Narrative would privilege the sense of personhood, synergy, interconnectedness, circularity, wholism, and collectivism" (p. 404). It also resonates with Nwoye (2006, 2013, 2015) who explains that, in African thought, the human being is considered to be a complicated organism which is at the same time physical and spiritual in nature, and that there is a dialectical diffusion of the individual and the community in which neither is predominant. Reality is considered to exist of two major levels, namely the visible or material and the invisible or spiritual realms, where the mundane continuously and dynamically interacts with the extra-ordinary. Harmony and ordered development of human beings result when the two levels of reality are in perfect combination (Nwoye, 2006, 2013).

The co-occurrence of inner and contextual harmony in many participants' responses speaks to a trend noticed by Wissing et al. (2020) who found that intrapersonal motives for relationships as common sources of meaning were found in African samples, but at the same time the intrapersonal motives were embedded in contextual relatedness. This could suggest a dialectic pattern of independent-interdependent self-construal in Africa that goes beyond the individualism-collectivism dichotomy to an integrated form of self-construal where the individual is seen as contextually embedded. This also resonates with findings from Ghana presented by Dzokoto et al. (2019) and Osei-Tutu et al. (2020). This concurs with Singelis (1994) who suggested that independent and interdependent self-construals co-exist.

14.3.4 Limitations

While this manuscript contributes to the literature, it is not without limitations. First, participants completed the questionnaire in English and not in their mother tongue. Since languages are specific cultural products (Dzokoto et al., 2018; Osei-Tutu et al., 2020), completion of the questionnaires in English could have led to the incorporation of Western conceptions of happiness in responses, and prevented participants from expressing African conceptions of happiness optimally. Future research should involve similar studies in indigenous African languages. Second, the study only included participants with at least Grade 12 level of education. This requirement excluded large groups of people in the South African and Ghanaian population, and future studies on the topic that are more inclusive are important. Third, race or ethnicity was not measured, and therefore it is not clear what percentage of participants were of African heritage. Especially for the South African sample, it is known that the sample was multiracial and multicultural. Fourth, the responses to the happiness question were short written accounts, rather than rich data obtained from in-depth interviews. Further investigation of the topic by means of in-depth data gathering procedures such as in-depth interviews or focus groups may be informative. Fifth, a restricted set of codes from the EHHI coding system were identified as representative of inner and contextual harmony according to the criteria used for the purpose of this study. It is possible that there were codes and accompanying excerpts that would have been relevant to the topic under study, but were excluded due to the selection procedure used for codes. Sixth, different coders coded the South African and Ghanaian data, and different procedures were used in the two countries to gather data, which limit the comparability of the findings between the two countries. Since the purpose of this study was not to compare the two contexts but rather to get a sense of harmony as a quality of happiness across the samples, this limitation is not fundamentally problematic in this study, but nonetheless deserves mentioning.

14.3.5 Conclusion

In this study, harmony emerged as a quality of happiness in African samples on intrapersonal level, in close interpersonal relationships (for example with family and neighbors), in wider interpersonal relationships (community, society, others in general), in transcendental relationships, and with nature. Importantly, happiness was often expressed as harmony and balance within and between these levels of functioning, with wholeness, interconnectedness, and synergy implied. If interconnectedness represents a prerequisite for happiness and well-being and harmony represents the quality of this interconnectedness, harmony as a lived experience and harmonization as a continuously evolving process are important topics for future research. Pursuit of harmony within and between individuals; within and between groups, communities and societies; between individuals, societies and the transcendental; and between individuals, societies and nature, may contribute not only to healthier and happier individuals, but also to healthier communities, societies, and ecosystems. This suggests that harmony cannot be investigated by a single discipline, but needs to be investigated, understood and promoted from a holistic, and probably interdisciplinary perspective. Also, existing rating scales of harmony and related constructs (see Introduction) do not capture the nuances and extent of the construct as it emerged in this study, which points to a gap to be addressed in future studies.

As per the contributions of the study, we reflect on the paucity of well-being literature among African samples on harmony as a quality of happiness. Apart from the few studies which we have cited, most studies on harmony are theoretical and philosophical in nature. We argue that our study holds potential for theory-building on well-being beyond Western and Eastern cultures. It also provides evidence for interventions aiming to enhance happiness. The use of a multicultural sample across two countries and a wide ranging age group, shows the utility of understanding harmony as a quality of happiness for promotion of psychological well-being. This study points to the need for designing epistemologically and ontologically relevant instruments to measure harmony in African cultures as known scales (Chen et al., 2016; Kavikondala et al., 2016; Kjell et al., 2016; Lee et al., 2013) have been developed and validated mainly in the West and East.

Finally, our findings not only highlight harmony as quality of happiness on inner and contextual levels, but also suggest on a methodological level that the EHHI coding system may be further developed to take into account the categories that we extracted from detailed analysis of verbatim expressions of people from Africa. In particular, the emerged third theme "Happiness as Holistic and Dynamic Experiences of Harmony, Balance and Peace" suggests the inclusion of a harmony-related category in the EHHI coding system to reflect the linkedness and integration of experiences across events and domains of life in general.

Acknowledgements We thank Antonella Delle Fave for her leadership in the EHHI-project, Grace Sogbey for supervising data gathering in Ghana, the team of data capturers, and Leana Meiring and Susan Coetzee for assisting with coding the data. The research was financially supported in part by the National Research Foundation of South Africa (grant numbers: 91557, 106050, 121948). The grantholders acknowledge that opinions, findings and conclusions or recommendations expressed are that of the authors, and that the NRF accepts no liability whatsoever in this regard.

References

Agbo, A. A., & Ome, B. (2017). Happiness: Meaning and determinants among young adults of the Igbos of eastern Nigeria. *Journal of Happiness Studies, 18*(1), 151–175. https://doi.org/10.1007/s10902-016-9722-4

Barry, C. A., Britten, N., Barber, N., Bradley, C., & Stevenson, F. (1999). Using reflexivity to optimize teamwork in qualitative research. *Qualitative Health Research, 9*(1), 26–44.

Cavanaugh, L. A., MacInnis, D. J., & Weiss, A. M. (2016). Perceptual dimensions differentiate emotions. *Cognition and Emotion, 30*(8), 1430–1445. https://doi.org/10.1080/02699931.2015.1070119

Chen, C. C., Ünal, A. F., Leung, K., & Xin, K. R. (2016). Group harmony in the workplace: Conception, measurement, and validation. *Asia Pacific Journal of Management, 33*(4), 903–934. https://doi.org/10.1007/s10490-016-9457-0

Dela Coleta, J. A., & Dela Coleta, M. F. (2006). Felicidade, bem-estar subjetivo e comportamento acadêmico de estudantes universitários [Happiness, subjective well-being and the academic behavior of university students]. *Psicologia em estudo, 11*(3), 533–539. https://doi.org/10.1590/S1413-73722006000300009

Delle Fave, A. (2014). Harmony. In A. C. Michalos (Ed.), *Encyclopedia of quality of life and well-being research* (pp. 2695–2697). Springer.

Delle Fave, A., Brdar, I., Freire, T., Vella-Brodrick, D., & Wissing, M. P. (2011). The eudaimonic and hedonic components of happiness: Qualitative and quantitative findings. *Social Indicators Research, 100*(2), 185–207. https://doi.org/10.1007/s11205-010-9632-5

Delle Fave, A., Brdar, I., Wissing, M. P., Araujo, U., Castro Solano, A., Freire, T., Nakamura, J., Singh, K., & Nafstad, H. E. (2016). Lay definitions of happiness across nations: The primacy of inner harmony and relational connectedness. *Frontiers in Psychology, 7*, 30. https://doi.org/10.3389/fpsyg.2016.00030

Demir, M., & Sümer, N. (2018). *Close relationships and happiness across cultures*. Springer.

Diener, E., Emmons, R. A., Larsen, R. J., & Griffin, S. (1985). The Satisfaction with Life Scale. *Journal of Personality Assessment, 49*(1), 71–75.

Donaldson, S., & Donaldson, S. I. (2017). Other people matter: The power of positive relationships. In M. A. Warren & S. I. Donaldson (Eds.), *Toward a positive psychology of relationships: New directions in theory and research* (pp. 1–8). ABC-CLIO.

Dzokoto, V. A., Osei-Tutu, A., Kyei, J. J., Twum-Asante, M., Attah, D. A., & Ahorsu, D. K. (2018). Emotion norms, display rules, and regulation in the Akan society of Ghana: An exploration using proverbs. *Frontiers in Psychology, 9*(1916), 1–14. https://doi.org/10.3389/fpsyg.2018.01916

Dzokoto, V. A., Osei-Tutu, A., Scollon, C. N., Wallace, D., & Peters-Chitwood, L. (2019). Meaning and perceptions of the good life in Ghana. *Psychological Studies, 64*(1), 11–20. https://doi.org/10.1007/s12646-018-0475-5

Elo, S., Kääriäinen, M., Kanste, O., Pölkki, T., Utriainen, K., & Kyngäs, H. (2014). Qualitative content analysis: A focus on trustworthiness. *SAGE Open, 4*(1), 1–10. https://doi.org/10.1177/2158244014522633

Garcia, A., Pereira, F. N., & de Macedo, M. D. C. (2015). Friendship and happiness in Latin America: A review. In M. Demir (Ed.), *Friendship and happiness* (pp. 225–234). Springer.

Guse, T., Vescovelli, F., & Croxford, S.-A. (2019). Subjective well-being and gratitude among South African adolescents: Exploring gender and cultural differences. *Youth & Society, 51*(5), 591–615. https://doi.org/10.1177/0044118X17697237

Harrell, S. P. (2015). Culture, wellness, and world "PEaCE": An introduction to person-environment-and-culture-emergence theory. *Community Psychology in Global Perspective, 1*(1), 16–49. https://doi.org/10.1285/i24212113v1i1p16

Hart, A., Gagnon, E., Eryigit-Madzwamuse, S., Cameron, J., Aranda, K., Rathbone, A., & Heaver, B. (2016). Uniting resilience research and practice with an inequalities approach. *SAGE Open, 6*(4), 1–13. https://doi.org/10.1177/2158244016682477

Helne, T., & Hirvilammi, T. (2015). Wellbeing and sustainability: A relational approach. *Sustainable Development, 23*(3), 167–175. https://doi.org/10.1002/sd.1581

Hershfield, H., Scheibe, S., Sims, T., & Carstensen, L. (2013). When bad can be good: Mixed emotions benefit physical health outcomes across the life span. *Social Psychological and Personality Science, 4*(1), 54–61. https://doi.org/10.1177/1948550612444616

Hitokoto, H., & Uchida, Y. (2015). Interdependent happiness: Theoretical importance and measurement validity. *Journal of Happiness Studies, 16*(1), 211–239. https://doi.org/10.1007/s10902-014-9505-8

Igbokwe, D., Elegbeleye, A., & Agoha, B. (2015). Harmony-disharmony Scale: Development and initial factorial validation. *Covenant International Journal of Psychology, 1*(1), 1–17.

Igbokwe, D., & Ndom, R. (2008). Harmony-disharmony therapy: A treatment method of African origin. *Nigeria Journal of Clinical Psychology, 6*(1 & 2), 61–77.

Jans-Beken, L., Jacobs, N., Janssens, M., Peeters, S., Reijnders, J., Lechner, L., & Lataster, J. (2019). Reciprocal relationships between state gratitude and high-and low-arousal positive affects in daily life: A time-lagged ecological assessment study. *The Journal of Positive Psychology, 14*(4), 512–527. https://doi.org/10.1080/17439760.2018.1497684

Kavikondala, S., Stewart, S. M., Ni, M. Y., Chan, B. H., Lee, P. H., Li, K.-K., McDowell, I., Johnston, J. M., Chan, S. S., Lam, T. H., Lam, W. W. T., Fielding, R., & Leung, G. M. (2016). Structure and validity of Family Harmony Scale: An instrument for measuring harmony. *Psychological Assessment, 28*(3), 307–318. https://doi.org/10.1037/pas0000131

Keyes, C. L. M. (1998). Social well-being. *Social Psychology Quarterly, 61*(2), 121–140.

Keyes, C. L. M., Wissing, M. P., Potgieter, J. P., Temane, Q. M., Kruger, A., & Van Rooy, S. (2008). Evaluation of the Mental Health Continuum–Short Form (MHC–SF) in Setswana-speaking South Africans. *Clinical Psychology & Psychotherapy, 15*(3), 181–192. https://doi.org/10.1002/cpp.572

Kjell, O. N. (2011). Sustainable well-being: A potential synergy between sustainability and well-being research. *Review of General Psychology, 15*(3), 255–266. https://doi.org/10.1037/a0024603

Kjell, O. N., Daukantaité, D., Hefferon, K., & Sikström, S. (2016). The Harmony in Life Scale complements the Satisfaction with Life Scale: Expanding the conceptualization and measurement of the cognitive component of subjective well-being. *Social Indicators Research, 126*, 893–919. https://doi.org/10.1007/s11205-015-0903-z

Kjell, O. N., Daukantaitė, D., & Sikström, S. (2021). Computational language assessments of harmony in life - not satisfaction with life or rating scales - correlate with cooperative behaviours. *Frontiers in Psychology*. https://doi.org/10.3389/fpsyg.2021.601679

Kjell, O. N., Kjell, K., Garcia, D., & Sikström, S. (2019). Semantic measures: Using natural language processing to measure, differentiate, and describe psychological constructs. *Psychological Methods, 24*(1), 92–115. https://doi.org/10.1037/met0000191

Krippendorff, K. (2018). *Content analysis: An introduction to its methodology* (4th ed.). Sage.

Kuhl, J., Quirin, M., & Koole, S. L. (2015). Being someone: The integrated self as a neuropsychological system. *Social and Personality Psychology Compass, 9*(3), 115–132. https://doi.org/10.1111/spc3.12162

Kwan, V. S., Bond, M. H., & Singelis, T. M. (1997). Pancultural explanations for life satisfaction: Adding relationship harmony to self-esteem. *Journal of Personality and Social Psychology, 73*(5), 1038–1051.

Kyngäs, H., Kääriäinen, M., & Elo, S. (2020). The trustworthiness of content analysis. In *The application of content analysis in nursing science research* (pp. 41–48). Springer.

Lee, Y.-C., Lin, Y.-C., Huang, C.-L., & Fredrickson, B. L. (2013). The construct and measurement of peace of mind. *Journal of Happiness Studies, 14*(2), 571–590. https://doi.org/10.1007/s10902-012-9343-5

Li, C. (2006). The Confucian ideal of harmony. *Philosophy East and West, 56*(4), 583–603.

Li, C. (2008). The philosophy of harmony in classical Confucianism. *Philosophy Compass, 3*(3), 423–435. https://doi.org/10.1111/j.1747-9991.2008.00141.x

Lincoln, Y. S., & Guba, E. G. (1985). *Naturalistic inquiry*. Sage.

Malterud, K. (2001). Qualitative research: Standards, challenges, and guidelines. *The Lancet, 358*, 483–488.

Metz, T. (2017). Values in China as compared to Africa: Two conceptions of harmony. *Philosophy East and West, 67*(2), 441–465. https://doi.org/10.1353/pew.2017.0034

Mkhize, N. (2008). Ubuntu and harmony. In R. Nicolson (Ed.), *Persons in community: African ethics in a global culture* (pp. 35–44). University of KwaZulu-Natal Press.
Mkhize, N. (2020). African/Afrikan-centered psychology. *South African Journal of Psychology, 51*, 1–8. https://doi.org/10.1177/0081246320972002
Mogilner, C., Kamvar, S. D., & Aaker, J. (2011). The shifting meaning of happiness. *Social Psychological and Personality Science, 2*(4), 395–402. https://doi.org/10.1177/1948550610393987
Nima, A. A., Cloninger, K. M., Lucchese, F., Sikström, S., & Garcia, D. (2020). Validation of a general subjective well-being factor using classical test theory. *PeerJ, 8*(e9193), 1–29. https://doi.org/10.7717/peerj.9193
Nima, A. A., Cloninger, K. M., Persson, B. N., Sikström, S., & Garcia, D. (2020). Validation of subjective well-being measures using item response theory. *Frontiers in Psychology, 10*(3036), 1–33. https://doi.org/10.3389/fpsyg.2019.03036
Nobles, W. W. (2013). Fundamental task and challenge of Black psychology. *Journal of Black Psychology, 39*(3), 292–299. https://doi.org/10.1177/0095798413478072
Nobles, W. W. (2015). From black psychology to Sakhu Djaer: Implications for the further development of a Pan African Black psychology. *Journal of Black Psychology, 41*(5), 399–414. https://doi.org/10.1177/0095798415598038
Nowell, L. S., Norris, J. M., White, D. E., & Moules, N. J. (2017). Thematic analysis: Striving to meet the trustworthiness criteria. *International Journal of Qualitative Methods, 16*(1), 1–13. https://doi.org/10.1177/1609406917733847
Nwoye, A. (2006). Remapping the fabric of the African self: A synoptic theory. *Dialectical Anthropology, 30*(1–2), 119–146. https://doi.org/10.1007/s10624-005-5058-x
Nwoye, A. (2013). African psychotherapy. In A. Runehov & L. Oviedo (Eds.), *Encyclopedia of sciences and religions* (pp. 32–41). Springer. https://doi.org/10.1007/978-1-4020-8265-8_1509
Nwoye, A. (2015). What is African psychology the psychology of? *Theory & Psychology, 25*(1), 96–116. https://doi.org/10.1177/0959354314565116
Oishi, S., Graham, J., Kesebir, S., & Galinha, I. C. (2013). Concepts of happiness across time and cultures. *Personality and Social Psychology Bulletin, 39*(5), 559–577. https://doi.org/10.1177/0146167213480042
Osei-Tutu, A., Dzokoto, V. A., Affram, A. A., Adams, G., Norberg, J., & Doosje, B. (2020). Cultural models of well-being implicit in four Ghanaian languages. *Frontiers in Psychology, 11*(1798), 1–10. https://doi.org/10.3389/fpsyg.2020.01798
Patton, M. Q. (1999). Enhancing the quality and credibility of qualitative analysis. *Health Services Research, 34*(5), 1189–1208.
Pflug, J. (2009). Folk theories of happiness: A cross-cultural comparison of conceptions of happiness in Germany and South Africa. *Social Indicators Research, 92*(3), 551–563.
Portocarrero, F. F., Gonzalez, K., & Ekema-Agbaw, M. (2020). A meta-analytic review of the relationship between dispositional gratitude and well-being. *Personality and Individual Differences, 164*(110101), 1–14. https://doi.org/10.1016/j.paid.2020.110101
Ryff, C. D. (2014). Psychological well-being revisited: Advances in the science and practice of eudaimonia. *Psychotherapy and Psychosomatics, 83*(1), 10–28. https://doi.org/10.1159/000353263
Ryff, C. D., & Singer, B. (1998). The contours of positive human health. *Psychological Inquiry, 9*(1), 1–28. https://doi.org/10.1207/s15327965pli0901_1
Ryff, C. D., & Singer, B. (2000). Interpersonal flourishing: A positive health agenda for the new millennium. *Personality and Social Psychology Review, 4*(1), 30–44. https://doi.org/10.4324/9780203764923-3
Sandelowski, M. (2000). Whatever happened to qualitative description? *Research in Nursing & Health, 23*(4), 334–340.
Sandelowski, M. (2010). What's in a name? Qualitative description revisited. *Research in Nursing & Health, 33*(1), 77–84. https://doi.org/10.1002/nur.20362

Seligman, M. (2011). *Flourish: A new understanding of life's greatest goals - and what it takes to reach them*. Free Press.
Sheldon, K. M. (2014). Becoming oneself: The central role of self-concordant goal selection. *Personality and Social Psychology Review, 18*(4), 349–365. https://doi.org/10.1177/1088868314538549
Sheldon, K. M., Elliot, A. J., Ryan, R. M., Chirkov, V., Kim, Y., Wu, C., ... Sun, Z. (2004). Self-concordance and subjective well-being in four cultures. *Journal of Cross-Cultural Psychology, 35*(2), 209–223. https://doi.org/10.1177/0022022103262245
Singelis, T. M. (1994). The measurement of independent and interdependent self-construals. *Personality and Social Psychology Bulletin, 20*(5), 580–591. https://doi.org/10.1177/0146167294205014
Slife, B. D., & Richardson, F. C. (2008). Problematic ontological underpinnings of positive psychology: A strong relational alternative. *Theory & Psychology, 18*(5), 699–723. https://doi.org/10.1177/0959354308093403
Tugade, M. M., Shiota, M. N., & Kirby, L. D. (2014). *Handbook of positive emotions*. Guilford Publications.
Tutu, D. (1999). *No future without forgiveness*. Random House.
Uchida, Y., & Kitayama, S. (2009). Happiness and unhappiness in east and west: Themes and variations. *Emotion, 9*(4), 441–456. https://doi.org/10.1037/a0015634
Uchida, Y., & Ogihara, Y. (2012). Personal or interpersonal construal of happiness: A cultural psychological perspective. *International Journal of Wellbeing, 2*(4), 354–369. https://doi.org/10.5502/ijw.v2.i4
Wilson Fadiji, A., Meiring, L., & Wissing, M. P. (2019). Understanding well-being in the Ghanaian context: Linkages between lay conceptions of well-being and measures of hedonic and eudaimonic well-being. *Applied Research in Quality of Life*. https://doi.org/10.1007/s11482-019-09777-2
Wissing, M. P. (2008/2012). *The prevalence of levels of psychosocial health: Dynamics and relationships with biomarkers of (ill) health in South African social contexts (FORT3)*.
Wissing, M. P. (2016). *The dance of sun and shadow in multicultural well-being: Cultures of positivity in South Africa [Invited keynote]*. Paper presented at the Italian Positive Psychology Conference, Cesena, Italy.
Wissing, M. P., Schutte, L., & Wilson Fadiji, A. (2019). Cultures of positivity: Interconnectedness as a way of being. In I. Eloff (Ed.), *Handbook of quality of life in African societies* (pp. 3–22). Springer. https://doi.org/10.1007/978-3-030-15367-0_1
Wissing, M. P., Wilson Fadiji, A., Schutte, L., Chigeza, S., Schutte, W. D., & Temane, Q. M. (2020). Motivations for relationships as sources of meaning: Ghanaian and South African experiences. *Frontiers in Psychology, 11*(2019). https://doi.org/10.3389/fpsyg.2020.02019

Chapter 15
Concordance of Goals and Meaning with Reference to the Interpersonal Relationships Domain: Associations with Sociodemographic Variables and Well-Being in a Multicultural South African Group

Christelle Liversage, Marié P. Wissing, and Lusilda Schutte

Abstract The self-concordance model proposes that the concordance of goals and meaning may be associated with higher levels of well-being. But is this the case for specific life domains such as the interpersonal relationships domain? Are the patterns of goals and meaning alignment the same for different sociodemographic sub-groups? As no studies could be sourced on this topic, this study explores these dynamics. Open-ended questions on important goals and meaningful things, a sociodemographic questionnaire, and selected well-being questionnaires were administered to a multicultural South African sample ($N = 585$) in a convergent parallel mixed methods research design. The content of the qualitative data were coded and converted to quantitative data. Associations between alignment patterns and selected sociodemographic variables were explored via contingency tables and Pearson's chi-square test. A MANOVA was performed followed by a series of one-way ANOVAs to explore associations between alignment patterns and well-being variables. Alignment patterns were found to be associated with age, gender, level of education, and work status, and the MHC-SF (total score) index of well-being. Despite the statistically significant association of alignment patterns with the MHC-SF, the self-concordance model was not supported in this study with reference to the interpersonal relationships domain, as the both-goal-and-meaning pattern did not reveal a higher level of well-being compared to other patterns as predicted by the self-concordance model.

C. Liversage (✉) · M. P. Wissing · L. Schutte
Africa Unit for Transdisciplinary Health Research, Faculty of Health Sciences, North-West University, Potchefstroom, South Africa
e-mail: Christelle.Liversage@nwu.ac.za

L. Schutte et al. (eds.), *Embracing Well-Being in Diverse African Contexts: Research Perspectives*, Cross-Cultural Advancements in Positive Psychology 16,
https://doi.org/10.1007/978-3-030-85924-4_15

Keywords Concordance · Goals · Meaning · Interpersonal relationships · Well-being

15.1 Introduction

The self-concordance model (SCM; Sheldon & Elliot, 1999) plays a prominent role in studies on psychosocial well-being and health. According to this SCM the alignment (concordance) of goals and meaning may be associated with higher levels of well-being in general, but it is not known whether this is the case in all the diverse domains of life, or whether sociodemographic factors play a role in the association of alignment patterns and well-being. In this study, we untangle these dynamics in the case where people indicated their most important goals and things that are meaningful to them, referring to wider connections in the interpersonal relationships domain of life. Our focus is not on interpersonal relationships as such, but on goals and meaningful things, and whether they are in accord or diverge in reference to the interpersonal relationships domain as defined in this study. We explore if the manner in which they are aligned or diverging is associated with sociodemographic variables and/or well-being. In the following section, we will briefly introduce the main constructs used in this study and how they may hang together according to existing research, whereafter the method of this study and findings with discussion will be presented.

15.1.1 Concordance

The self-concordance model, formulated by Sheldon and Elliot (1999), is an extension of the self-determination theory (Deci & Ryan, 2000) that defines self-concordance as the extent or degree to which goals are aligned with intrinsic values or what is meaningful to a person. It refers to the ownership that people have (or do not have) over their goals which are self-chosen (Sheldon & Houser-Marko, 2001). Self-concordant goal pursuit and the realization thereof lead to sustained effort with resulting satisfaction, which in turn lead to meaning and well-being (Deci et al., 2017; Feldman et al., 2018). As goals and meaning are integral to the SCM, this theory will be used as a theoretical foundation for this study.

In this study, the words "concordance" and "alignment" are used interchangeably, and concordance will be operationalized as determined by Wissing et al. (2017). These authors demarcated patterns of alignment/concordance of goals and meaning by considering whether specific life domains were mentioned in participants' responses to questions on what their most important goals are and why these goals are important to them, and what the most meaningful things are to them and why these are meaningful (see Method section for detail). In terms of the interpersonal relationships domain of life, which is relevant to the current study, the alignment patterns distinguished by Wissing et al. (2017) are thus: (a) no-goal-no-meaning, where interpersonal relationships did not appear in the participant's responses to the questions on goals or meaningful things; (b) both-goal-and-meaning, where interpersonal relationships appeared in the participant's responses to the questions on goals and the questions on meaningful things; (c) goal-no-meaning, where interpersonal relationships appeared in the participant's responses to the goals questions, but not the questions on meaningful things; and (d) meaning-no-goal, where interpersonal relationships appeared in the participant's responses to the questions on meaningful things, but not the questions on goals. The expectation in line with the SCM is that the goal and meaning pattern as operationalized here (both-goal-and-meaning), will be associated with higher levels of well-being than the other patterns.

15.1.2 Goals

The quality of human life is greatly defined by the choice of goals or actions to reach a desirable end result (Sheldon et al., 2019). In everyday functioning, people take control of their own lives through the setting of goals, and if these goals are aligned with what is valuable to them, working towards and realizing such goals are associated with well-being (Hennecke & Brandstätter, 2017; Steca et al., 2016). Hence, goal-related theories of well-being have been formulated by various scholars (Bandura, 1988; Baumeister, 2016; Brunstein, 1993; Dweck, 1986; Emmons, 1989, 2003; Little, 1983; Little et al., 2017).

Orehek et al. (2018) posit that goal pursuit and relationships are closely connected. Goals which relate to interpersonal relationships can influence the quality of relationships and well-being (Lee et al., 2019). The way in which these positive relational goals are maintained, in turn, influences the experience of meaning (Thomas et al., 2018).

Theorists agree that goal pursuit is not just about 'what' is being pursued, but also 'why' it is being pursued (Converse et al., 2019). An important concept within the self-determination theory of Deci and Ryan (2000) explicates the reasons why goals are being pursued. According to the self-determination theory, behavior is based on autonomous motivation, controlled motivation, or amotivation. These different forms of motivation are also predictors of well-being outcomes (Deci & Ryan, 2008). Self-concordance refers to the degree to which autonomy (internal motivation) is experienced when pursuing a goal (Werner et al., 2016). Research has found that pursuing self-concordant goals, i.e., goals that are aligned with intrinsic values, is associated with better goal progress and, ultimately, attainment (Milyavskaya et al., 2015; Sheldon & Elliot, 1999).

15.1.3 Meaning

The pursuit of meaning in life was viewed by Frankl (1963) as an innate desire to live according to values in a meaningful manner. He believed that meaning was found in creativity, interpersonal relations, and the endurance of suffering. Since this early approach, scholars in various contexts have argued that meaning is at the heart of well-being (Batthyany & Russo-Netzer, 2014; Ryff, 2014; Steger, 2018; Wong, 2017). For example, Steger (2011, Catch Basin of Consciousness, [PowerPoint slide 1]) refers to meaning as "the catch basin of consciousness". In his model of meaning, he delineates between the "presence of" and "search for" meaning. The presence of meaning is explicated as "the extent to which people comprehend, make sense of, or see significance in their lives, accompanied by the degree to which they perceive themselves to have a purpose, mission, or over-arching aim in life" (Steger et al., 2009, p. 43). The search for meaning entails the degree to which individuals are striving to understand their purpose and meaning in life (Steger et al., 2008). Antonovsky (1993) theorized meaning as a component of sense of coherence.

In many perspectives on meaning in life, goals and meaning are regarded as interconnected (Ward & King, 2017). For example, Battista and Almond (1973) conceptualized meaning as the understanding of life in general, the striving towards important goals, as well as the experience of fulfilment in goal achievement. Wong (2012) proposed the meaning mindset model which views people as "meaning-seeking" and "meaning-making" individuals, living a balanced life through meaning acquired from the achievement of goals and quality relationships. George and Park (2016) explicated meaning in life as "the extent to which one's life is experienced as making sense, as being directed and motivated by valued goals, and as mattering in the world" (p. 206). Thus, the way in which positive goals are maintained influences the experience of meaning (Thomas et al., 2018).

Connectivity and relationships remain central to meaning-making and experiences of life as meaningful (Martino et al., 2017; Van Tongeren et al., 2016; Wissing, 2014). In the same vein, interconnectedness is integral to human functioning and a key determinant of quality of life and pathways to meaning (Wissing, Schutte, & Wilson, 2019). Although conceptualizations of meaning differ in ways, all include relatedness and connectedness with people as a basic source of meaning (Delle Fave & Soosai-Nathan, 2014). The relationality-meaning model (Wissing & Delle Fave, 2013) postulates that connectedness and relationships are fundamental to meaning in life, vertical and horizontal relationships are interlinked, and context has a cardinal influence on meaning-making, relationships, and well-being.

15.1.4 Sociodemographic Variables

In a study conducted in 27 European countries, the findings suggest that sociodemographic factors can influence well-being and life satisfaction (Geldenhuys

& Henn, 2017; Rajani et al., 2019). Sociodemographic variables are regarded as valuable indicators in the interpretation, variances, and experiences of well-being (Akhtar & Kroener-Herwig, 2019; Delle Fave et al., 2016; Diener & Ryan, 2009; Khumalo et al., 2012). The present study will consider age, gender, standard of living, level of education, marital status, and work status as sociodemographic variables. Their associations with patterns of concordance of goals and meaning with reference to the interpersonal relationships domain will be explored in a multicultural South African sample.

15.1.5 Well-Being

Two broad perspectives on well-being are often distinguished, namely the hedonic and the eudaimonic perspective. The hedonic perspective defines well-being as experiencing happiness and feeling good, while the eudaimonic perspective views well-being as functioning well (Ryan & Deci, 2001; Waterman, 1993). For the purposes of this study, both hedonic and eudaimonic well-being were considered when the associations between alignment patterns and well-being were explored.

In various theoretical perspectives of well-being, especially in eudaimonic well-being approaches, goals, meaning, and relationships/connectedness feature. For example, Ryff and Singer (1998) highlighted the following core facets of Ryff's (1989) six-component well-being model, namely: leading a life of purpose/meaning (which includes a sense of directedness, intentions, and goals), quality connections to others, followed by positive self-regard, autonomy, and environmental mastery. Fowers et al. (2016) validated a eudaimonic relationship scale in which some of the essential elements of relational well-being are portrayed as goal sharing and meaning.

In spite of the theorized interrelation of goals and meaning in eudaimonic well-being, they have generally been researched as separate constructs/phenomena (Wilson et al., 2018) without much attention to the implications of their concordance. In addition, the importance of relationships/connectedness for well-being has been neglected in scientific literature, while the impact of social support in negative life events or the influence of dysfunctional relations has been studied extensively (Schotanus-Dijkstra et al., 2017).

15.1.6 Interpersonal Relationships

Positive interpersonal relationships are regarded as intrinsic components of psychological well-being and satisfaction with life (Diener & Seligman, 2009). According to Prilleltensky (2005), the well-being of humans is reliant on the quality of their relationships and the context in which they live. In this regard, well-being is defined as "a positive state of affairs in which the personal, relational and collective needs and aspirations of individuals and communities are fulfilled" (Prilleltensky, 2005, p. 54). This echoes the views of more researchers that some of the most cardinal motives and values of humans are to experience belongingness, connection, and meaningful relations (Baumeister & Leary, 1995; Deci & Ryan, 2014). Well-known scholar Christopher Peterson, when asked for a definition of positive psychology, focused on the value of relationships in his well-known phrase, "Other people matter. Period." (Peterson et al., 2008, p. 1).

Interpersonal relationships are defined in many different ways in the literature. For example, in some instances, a distinction is made between close and wider relationships and in other instances, not. In this study, the demarcation of relationships described in the Eudaimonic and Hedonic Happiness Investigation (EHHI) project (cf. Delle Fave et al., 2011) was used in which a distinction is made between life domains of close family relationships, wider interpersonal relationships, social/community relationships, and spiritual/religious relationships. The current study focused on the wider interpersonal relationships domain.

Interpersonal relationships in this study refers specifically to wider interpersonal relationships such as with friends, colleagues, and others (excluding close relationships such as with a partner or family, or more distant relationships with society/community, and a divinity/spiritual relationship). This clear delineation is different from what is mostly found in existing literature referring to relationships. Apart from specific references to family relationships, couple relationships, or romantic relationships, the type of relationship which is referred to in many studies is often not specified or is all-inclusive, indicating interconnectedness in general.

15.1.7 The Present Study

Goals and meaning have generally been researched as separate phenomena and no studies on their concordance or alignment could be sourced with reference to the interpersonal relationships domain. Thus far, concordance has only been explored in general, not in diverse domains of life, and in particular, not with reference to wider interpersonal relationships, as is the focus of the present study. In this study, the interpersonal relationships domain is conceptualized as delineated in the Eudaimonic and Hedonic Happiness Investigation (EHHI; Delle Fave et al., 2011) and captured in the developed coding system. Details are provided in the Method section. The domain of interpersonal relationships, which is the focus of the present study, excludes close relationships such as with family or distant relationships such as with society or spiritual relatedness. In view of the above, the aim of the present study was to explore the concordance of goals and meaning with reference to the wider interpersonal relationships domain, and to determine whether different patterns of alignment were associated with sociodemographic variables and hedonic and eudaimonic indicators of well-being.

15.2 Method

15.2.1 Design and Participants

This study utilized data that were collected cross-sectionally in survey format, with concurrent collection of quantitative and qualitative data as described by Delle Fave et al. (2011). To address the research question of the current study, a convergent parallel mixed methods research design was used (Creswell & Plano Clark, 2011; Plano Clark, 2017).

The inclusion criteria for the participants ($N = 585$) stipulated that they should be older than 18 years of age, with a level of education of at least Grade 12 to ensure good comprehension and reading, reflection, and writing skills. The demographic profile of the participants in this study comprised: $n = 222$ males and $n = 362$ females; $n = 51$ participants from 18 to 25 years of age, $n = 213$ from 26 to 40 years, $n = 304$ from 41 to 60 years, $n = 16$ above 60 years of age, and $n = 1$ with age not indicated. The marital status of the participants included single ($n = 145$), married ($n = 367$), divorced or separated ($n = 34$), widowed ($n = 11$), cohabitating ($n = 19$), and not indicated ($n = 9$). The level of education of participants included secondary ($n = 220$), tertiary ($n = 176$), post-graduate ($n = 185$), and not indicated ($n = 4$). The standard of living or income level was below average ($n = 32$), average ($n = 385$), above average ($n = 147$), and not indicated ($n = 1$), as subjectively indicated by participants. Work status constituted unemployed ($n = 58$), employed ($n = 258$), retired ($n = 4$), family and housekeeping ($n = 7$), and not indicated ($n = 257$).

15.2.2 Data Gathering

Quantitative data were gathered with well-known measures of hedonic and eudaimonic well-being as typically used in similar studies, and with a sociodemographic questionnaire. Qualitative data were obtained from answers to semi-structured questions. Details are as follows:

15.2.2.1 Socio-Demographic Questionnaire

Data were collected on, among others, age, gender, marital status, level of education, standard of living, and work status.

15.2.2.2 Satisfaction with Life Scale (SWLS)

The level of life satisfaction experienced by people is quantified in this scale (Diener et al., 1985). The SWLS, comprising 5 items, is not focused towards specific life domains, but depicts the person's global and holistic experience of satisfaction with life. Diener et al. (1985) found that the SWLS displayed high internal consistency reliability with a Cronbach's alpha value of .87, as well as test-retest reliability based on a correlation coefficient of $r = .82$. Validity was also supported in different South African samples (Schutte et al., 2019; Wissing et al., 2010). The Schutte et al. (2019) study applied Rasch analysis to investigate the scale's psychometric properties. In Wissing et al. (2010), the Cronbach's alpha value was 0.67. See Results section for information on the validity and reliability of scales in the present study.

15.2.2.3 Positive and Negative Affect Schedule (PANAS)

Watson et al. (1988) designed the PANAS as a scale with 20 items, of which 10 items assess positive affect (PA) and 10 items assess negative affect (NA) under different circumstances. The subscale scores of the PANAS-PA and PANAS-NA can be used in subsequent analyses. In the original study by Watson et al. (1988), the PANAS was administered to a nonclinical student sample, a nonclinical adult sample, and an inpatient sample, with consistent outcomes of Cronbach's alpha values above .85 for both the PANAS-PA and the PANAS-NA for all samples. As far as could be established, a comprehensive validation study of the PANAS has not yet been conducted using South African data.

15.2.2.4 Meaning in Life Questionnaire (MLQ)

In a 10-item questionnaire consisting of two 5-item subscales, the MLQ assesses the presence of and search for meaning in life (Steger et al., 2006). The validity of this measure was supported by Steger et al. (2006) in three studies. Cronbach's alpha values indicated support for internal consistency reliability with values of .82 and higher in the original scale development study (Steger et al., 2006). In South Africa, support was found for the reliability and validity of the MLQ in studies by Schutte et al. (2016) and Temane et al. (2014).

15.2.2.5 Mental Health Continuum-Short Form (MHC-SF)

The 14-item MHC-SF (Keyes, 2006, 2009; Keyes et al., 2008) measures positive mental health by means of three items that measure emotional well-being (EWB), six items that measure psychological well-being (PWB), and five items that measure social well-being (SWB). In this scale, the EWB subscale is associated with hedonic well-being, while the PWB and SWB subscales are associated with eudaimonic well-being. The initial validation of the 14-item MHC-SF was conducted in a Setswana-speaking South African sample where support was established for the validity and reliability of the instrument with a Cronbach's alpha value of .72 (Keyes et al., 2008). Schutte and Wissing (2017) found that a bifactor exploratory structural equation modeling model displayed best fit where participants completed the English, Afrikaans, and Setswana versions of the scale, with the global scale displaying sufficient reliability (omega coefficients between .86 and .90), but the subscales attaining marginal to low reliability (omega coefficients between .36 and .63).

15.2.2.6 Semi-Structured Open-Ended Questions on Goals and Meaning

In the Eudaimonic-Hedonic Happiness Investigation (EHHI), Delle Fave et al. (2011) formulated semi-structured open-ended questions which were included in this study. Two semi-structured open-ended questions were asked on goals and meaning, namely: (a) "Please list the three most important future goals for you", followed by "For each of them, please specify why it is important"; and (b) "Please list the three things that you consider most meaningful in your present life", followed by "For each of them, please specify why it is meaningful (try to be as specific as possible)".

15.2.3 *Procedure and Ethical Considerations*

Written informed consent was obtained from participants and participation was voluntary. Anonymized data were used. Participants were recruited in South Africa in the FORT3 project (FORT3 = The prevalence of levels of psychosocial health: dynamics and relationships with biomarkers of (ill)health in South African social contexts; Wissing, 2008/2012) that also included the EHHI data gathering instrument described by Delle Fave et al. (2011). All ethical principles as specified by the Health Research Ethics Committee of the North-West University were adhered to, and ethical approval was granted for the FORT3 project (NWU 00002-07-A2) as well as this study (NWU-00030-19-A1).

15.2.4 *Data Analysis*

15.2.4.1 Qualitative Data Analysis

The coding system developed in the EHHI international project was used to code and convert answers to the questions on goals and meaning to quantitative data (cf. Delle Fave et al., 2011). In the development of the coding system, open and inductive coding were used with codes extracted from the text and not led by theory. In the end, the coding system consisted of a large number of basic codes which are closely related to the verbatim responses of participants. The basic codes are grouped into different categories and then into life domains (including interpersonal relationships) at the highest level. For the current study, all participants' responses received a basic code as determined by the coding system and quantified for further analysis. The codes captured in the interpersonal relationships domain of life are of particular relevance to the present study.

15.2.4.2 Quantitative Data Analysis

After the qualitative data were coded and quantified, the quantified data were further processed per person in Microsoft Office Excel to determine the pattern of concordance between goals and meaning with reference to the interpersonal relationships domain, and how the distinguished substantive patterns of concordance were associated with sociodemographic variables and indicators of well-being, which formed part of the gathered quantitative data. Specifically, following Wissing et al. (2017), an alignment pattern was determined for the responses of each participant. Four alignment patterns were distinguished, namely (a) "no-goal-no-meaning", where the interpersonal relationships domain was not reflected in the important goals or the reasons therefore, nor in the meaningful things or motivations therefore per person; (b) "both-goal-and-meaning", where the interpersonal relationships domain was reflected both in the important goals or the reasons therefore, and in the meaningful things or motivations therefore per person; (c) "goal-no-meaning", where the interpersonal relationships domain was reflected in the important goals or the reason therefore, but not in the meaningful things or motivations therefore per person; and (d) "meaning-no-goal", where the interpersonal relationships domain was not reflected in the important goals or the reasons therefore, but was indicated in the meaningful things or motivations therefore per person.

The variable containing the alignment patterns for the participants was integrated per person with the quantitative data from the sociodemographic questionnaire and the Likert-type well-being questionnaires to yield the dataset for the present study. The following quantitative analyses were done using IBM SPSS Statistics Version 26, unless specified differently.

15.2.4.2.1 Determining the Validity and Reliability of the Scores for the Likert-Type Well-Being Questionnaires

The psychometric properties of the SWLS, PANAS, MLQ, and MHC-SF were evaluated to determine whether the use of scale scores in subsequent analyses was supported. Specifically, the factorial validity and the internal consistency of these measures were explored.

In terms of factorial validity, confirmatory factor analysis (CFA) was utilized to determine the factor structure of the SWLS, PANAS, MLQ, and MHC-SF. Furthermore, bifactor exploratory structural equation modeling (bifactor ESEM) was applied to the MHC-SF. The subscales of the PANAS and MLQ are not expected to be positively correlated; therefore, the bifactor ESEM model is not appropriate for these scales. For the SWLS, which is one-dimensional, this model is also irrelevant. The MHC-SF was thus the only scale where the bifactor ESEM model was applicable. Mplus 8.3 was used for these analyses (Muthén & Muthén, 1998–2019). We applied the robust maximum likelihood (MLR) estimator and full information likelihood estimation was applied in cases of missing data. For the CFA models, the cross-loadings were set to zero. For the bifactor ESEM model, orthogonal rotation was implemented and cross-loadings were estimated to be close to, but not precisely zero (Asparouhov & Muthén, 2009). The χ^2-statistic, comparative fit index (CFI), Tucker-Lewis index (TLI), root mean square error of approximation (RMSEA), and the standardised root mean square residual (SRMR) are reported. Although we report the χ^2-statistic, the CFI, TLI, RMSEA, and SRMR were utilized to interpret model fit as the value of the χ^2-statistic is dependent on sample size. CFI and TLI values higher than .90 or .95 are regarded as indicative of adequate model fit (Byrne, 2012; Hu & Bentler, 1999). A reasonable model fit is indicated by RMSEA and SRMR scores below 1.00 or .08, with good model fit indicated by values less than .05 (MacCallum et al., 1996). In terms of internal consistency reliability, omega coefficients were calculated according to the formula utilized by Sánchez-Oliva et al. (2017). Based on conventional standards, estimates of reliability above .70 are considered sufficient (Nunnally, 1978).

15.2.4.2.2 Frequencies of Alignment Patterns Referring to the Interpersonal Relationships Domain

The frequencies of the alignment patterns pertaining to the interpersonal relationships domain of life were calculated.

15.2.4.2.3 Associations Between Alignment Patterns and Sociodemographic Variables

Next, the associations between the alignment patterns and selected sociodemographic variables (age, gender, marital status, level of education, standard of living, and work status) were explored via contingency tables and Pearson's chi-square test.[1] The chi-square test relies on the assumptions that the observations are independent, and that, for sufficient power, the expected cell counts in the contingency tables should be larger than 1 with less than 20% of the expected cell counts being smaller than 5 (Field, 2018). In order to establish statistically significant associations with goal-meaning alignment patterns, the following indices were considered: p-value of the chi-square test of less than .05, and Cramer's V effect

[1] We considered also applying a multivariate adjusted approach (GLM analysis), but deemed this unnecessary due to the insignificant results obtained from the univariate analyses.

size, interpreted as per the guidelines of David and Sutton (2004), namely 0–0.19 very low association; 0.20–0.39 low association; 0.40–0.69 modest association; 0.70–0.89 high association; and 0.90–1 very high association.

15.2.4.2.4 Associations Between Alignment Patterns and Well-Being

To explore the associations between alignment patterns and well-being variables, a MANOVA was performed as a first step with alignment patterns as the independent variable and the total scores of the indicators of positive mental health (i.e., the SWLS, PANAS-PA, MLQ-P, and the MHC-SF) as outcome variables. The MLQ-S and PANAS-NA scores were not included in the MANOVA since they are not indicators of positive mental health. MANOVA relies on the assumptions that residuals are statistically independent and have multivariate normality, and that covariance matrices are homogenous.

The MANOVA was followed up by six one-way ANOVAs[2] where the total scores on the SWLS, PANAS-PA, PANAS-NA, MHC-SF, MLQ-P, and MLQ-S, respectively, were compared for the four alignment patterns. ANOVA relies on the assumption that residuals are statistically independent and have univariate normality, and on the assumption of homogeneity of variances. The practical significance of the ANOVAs was ascertained by ω^2 effect sizes, with interpretation guidelines suggesting that .01 signifies a small effect, 0.06 a medium effect, and 0.14 a large effect (Field, 2018). ANOVAs that yielded statistically significant results were followed up by Tukey's post hoc tests to compare alignment patterns pairwise on well-being outcomes. For these tests, Cohen's d-value was calculated as the effect size, where $d = .2$ indicates a small effect, $d = .5$ indicates a medium effect, and $d = .8$ indicates a large effect (Cohen, 1988).

15.3 Results

Results are presented in the following order: exploration of the validity and reliability of the Likert-type well-being questionnaires, frequencies of alignment patterns referring (or not referring) to the interpersonal relationships domain, associations between alignment patterns and sociodemographic variables, and, finally, associations between alignment patterns and well-being.

[2] Since not all assumptions of MANOVA and ANOVA were met, we also conducted a series of six non-parametric Kruskal-Wallis tests where scores on the SWLS, PANAS-PA, PANAS-NA, MHC-SF, MLQ-P, and MLQ-S, respectively, were compared for the four alignment pattern groups. The results corresponded with the results of the parametric tests.

Table 15.1 Fit Indices for the CFA Models

Model	χ^2	*df*	*p*	CFI	TLI	RMSEA	90% CI	SRMR
SWLS (1-factor CFA)	31.172	5	<.001	.963	.926	0.095	(0.065; 0.128)	0.035
PANAS (2-factor CFA)	469.176	169	<.001	.903	.891	0.055	(0.049; 0.061)	0.053
MLQ (2-factor CFA)	206.337	34	<.001	.918	.892	0.093	(0.081; 0.106)	0.075
MHC-SF (3-factor CFA)	252.744	74	<.001	.928	.911	0.067	(0.058; 0.076)	0.055
MHC-SF (3-factor bifactor ESEM)	71.952	41	<.001	.987	.972	0.037	(0.022; 0.051)	0.017

Note. SWLS = Satisfaction with Life Scale; PANAS = Positive and Negative Affect Schedule; MLQ = Meaning in Life Questionnaire; MHC-SF = Mental Health Continuum-Short Form; CFA = confirmatory factor analysis; Bifactor ESEM = bifactor exploratory structural equation modeling; χ^2 = Chi-square; *df* = degrees of freedom; *p* = probability value; CFI = Comparative fit index; TLI = Tucker-Lewis index; RMSEA = Root mean square error of approximation; 90% CI = 90% confidence interval of the RMSEA; SRMR = Standardized root mean square residual

15.3.1 Determining the Validity and Reliability of the Scores for the Likert-Type Well-Being Questionnaires

In Table 15.1, the fit indices of the SWLS, PANAS, MLQ, and MHC-SF are presented. In general, the fit indices indicated marginal to acceptable fit with CFI values larger .90 and RMSEA values smaller than 1. For the MHC-SF, the bifactor ESEM model yielded improved fit compared to the CFA model.

In the present study, the omega coefficient was .88 for the SWLS; .84 for the PANAS-PA; .88 for the PANAS-NA; .84 for the MLQ-P; and .89 for the MLQ-S. For the MHC-SF, the CFA model omega coefficient values were .85 for EWB, .85 for SWB, and .84 for PWB. The bifactor ESEM omega coefficient values were .91 for the general mental well-being factor, .75 for EWB, .75 for SWB, and .66 for PWB. As the psychometric properties of all scales were found to be adequate, the scales were deemed appropriate for use in the current study.

15.3.2 Frequencies of Alignment Patterns Referring to the Interpersonal Relationships Domain

From the total number of participants, 50.8% did not refer to interpersonal relationships in their most important goals or meaningful things, thus yielding an operationalization pattern of no-goal-no-meaning. The frequency of the substantive patterns was 6.7% for the both-goal-and-meaning pattern; 5.8% for goal-no-meaning pattern; and 30.6% for meaning-no-goal pattern. Missing responses equated to 6.2%, indicating that participants did not respond to the open-ended questions on goals and/or the questions on meaning. Thus 43.1% of participants referred to wider interpersonal relationships in their most important goals and/or meaningful things.

15.3.3 Associations Between Alignment Patterns and Sociodemographic Variables

In terms of the assumptions of the chi-square test, the observations in this study were independent. All expected cell counts exceeded 1 and less than 20% of the cells had an expected count of less than 5 for age, gender, level of education, and standard of living, indicating that the assumptions of the chi-square test held for these variables. For marital status and work status, more than 20% of the cells had expected cell counts of less than 5, with some being less than 1, suggesting that the tests did not have sufficient power and results should be interpreted with caution. Frequencies from the contingency tables are graphically depicted in Fig. 15.1, together with the p-values of Pearson's chi-square test and Cramer's V-values.

As shown in Fig. 15.1, statistically significant associations were found for age, gender, level of education, and work status. All of these associations were of very small practical significance as shown by Cramer's V. Standard of living and marital status were not significantly associated with alignment patterns.

In terms of age, the emerging adult group (18–25 years of age) had a higher percentage of participants who mentioned interpersonal relationships in their responses to the questions on meaning but not on the goal questions, and a lower percentage who did not mention interpersonal relationships at all, compared to the midlife adult groups (26–40 years and 41–60 years). The oldest group (older than 60 years) had a higher proportion of participants who mentioned interpersonal relationships as goal-no-meaning than any of the other groups.

For gender, the females had a higher percentage of participants who mentioned interpersonal relationships in their responses to the meaning questions but not the goals questions, and a lower percentage who did not mention interpersonal relationships at all, compared to males. In terms of level of education, the higher the level of education, the more likely participants were to mention interpersonal relationships in their responses to the meaning questions but not the goals questions, and the less likely they were not to mention interpersonal relationships at all.

For work status, a higher percentage of participants who indicated that they were employed indicated interpersonal relationships in their responses to the meaning questions but not the goals questions, compared to the unemployed group. The employed group were also less likely not to mention interpersonal relationships at all compared to the unemployed group. (Different patterns were observed for the retired and family and housekeeping groups, but these groups' sample sizes were very small and therefore we do not interpret these findings).

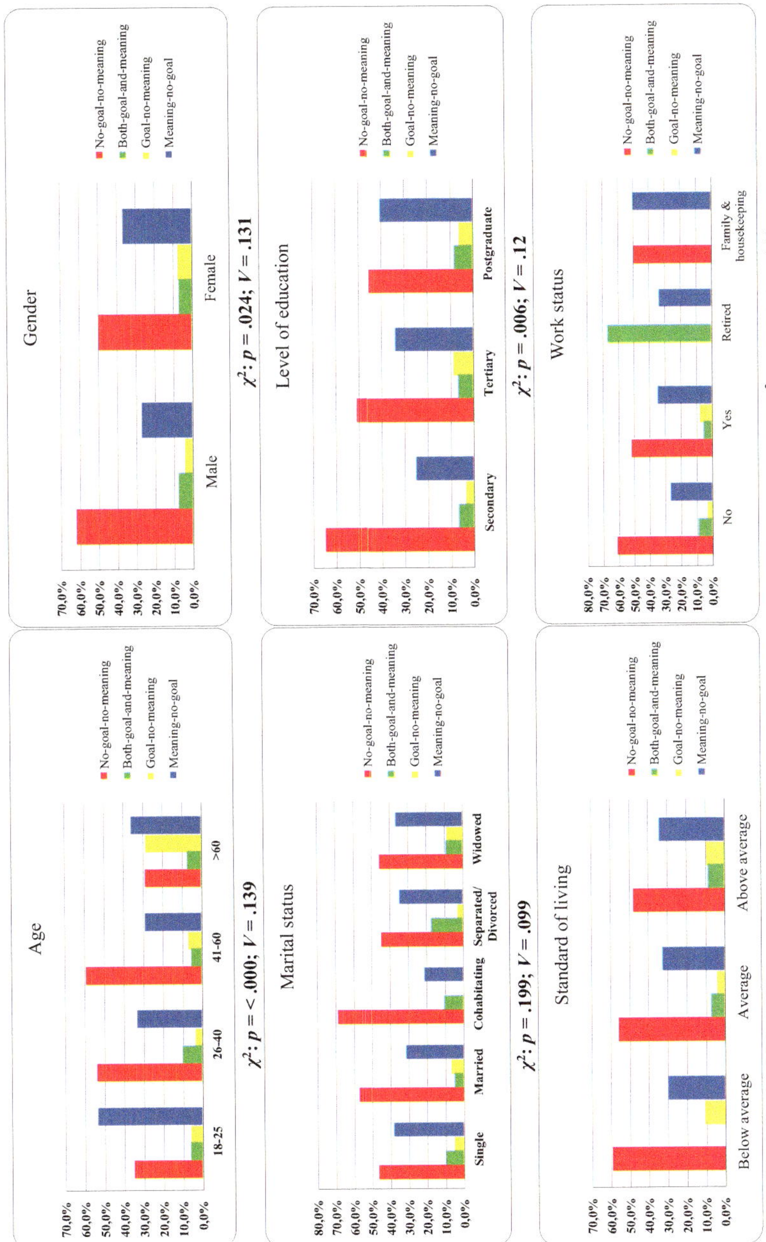

Fig. 15.1 Alignment patterns of goals and meaning in association with sociodemographic variables

Table 15.2 ANOVAs to evaluate associations between alignment patterns of goals and meaning with well-being indices

Measure	F	df_1, df_2	p	ω^2
SWLS	.100	3.544	.960	− .005
PANAS-PA	1.011	3.545	.387	.000
PANAS-NA	1.818	3.545	.143	.004
MLQ-P	.723	3.544	.539	− .002
MLQ-S	1.416	3.544	.237	.002
MHC-SF	4.588	3.502	.004	.021

Note. SWLS = Satisfaction with Life Scale; PANAS-PA = Positive and Negative Affect Schedule Positive-Affect; PANAS-NA = Positive and Negative Affect Schedule-Negative Affect; MLQ-P = Meaning in Life Questionnaire-Presence; MLQ-S = Meaning in Life Questionnaire-Search; MHC-SF = Mental Health Continuum-Short Form

15.3.4 Associations Between Alignment Patterns and Well-Being

In terms of the assumptions of the MANOVA and ANOVA, the residuals were independent. Univariate analyses (e.g., the Shapiro-Wilk test for univariate normality, probability-probability [P-P] plots, histograms, and Levene's test for homogeneity of variances) showed that the assumptions of univariate normality and homogeneity of variances did not hold in all instances. This implies that the assumptions also did not hold on a multivariate level. In view of the violation of assumptions, nonparametric Kruskal-Wallis tests were performed. In all cases, the results corresponded with the results from the parametric tests and therefore only the results from the parametric tests are presented.

For the MANOVA, using Wilk's lambda statistic,[3] the four alignment pattern groups differed significantly on well-being, with $\Lambda = 0.955$, $F = 1.924$, and $p = .028$. Results for the separate univariate ANOVAs are displayed in Table 15.2.

Table 15.2 indicates that alignment patterns differed statistically significantly only for the MHC-SF total scale score, but this association was of small practical significance. The differences between the alignment patterns for the MHC-SF total score were further explored using Tukey's post hoc test and the results are graphically depicted in Fig. 15.2.

The only statistically significant difference was found in the group who did not mention interpersonal relationships at all in their goals or meaning and scored significantly higher on well-being as measured by the MHC-SF than the group who mentioned interpersonal relationships as a meaning-no-goal ($p = .004$). This difference was not practically significant ($d = .32$). In terms of practical significance, d-values were larger when the meaning-no-goal group was compared to the group who mentioned interpersonal relationships as both-goal-and-meaning ($d = .38$) and

[3]MANOVA using Pillay's trace statistic, Hotelling's trace statistic, and Roy's largest root statistic also pointed to a statistically significant difference between the alignment pattern groups.

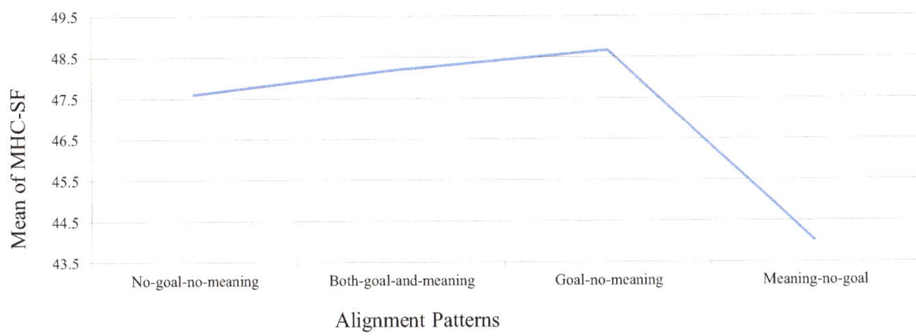

Fig. 15.2 Plot of the mean total scores of the Mental Health Continuum-Short Form for the different alignment patterns. *Note.* MHC-SF = Mental Health Continuum-Short Form

the group who mentioned interpersonal relationships as a goal-no-meaning ($d = .42$), but these were still indicative of small to medium effects.

15.4 Discussion

The aim of this study was to explore the alignment/concordance of goals and meaning of a multicultural South African sample with reference to the wider interpersonal relationships domain of life and if/how different patterns of concordance were associated with sociodemographic variables and indices of hedonic and/or eudaimonic well-being. The results showed that just over 40% of the participants mentioned wider interpersonal relationships as one of their three most important goals and/or things that are meaningful to them as reflected in the frequencies of alignment patterns. Alignment patterns were associated with the sociodemographic factors of age, gender, level of education, work status, and the MHC-SF (total score) index of well-being. Despite the statistically significant association of alignment patterns with (only) the MHC-SF, the SCM was not directly supported with reference to the interpersonal relationship domain of life. The both-goal-and-meaning pattern did not reflect a significantly higher score on the MHC-SF in comparison to the other patterns. A discussion of the results will follow.

15.4.1 Frequencies of Alignment Patterns Referring to the Interpersonal Relationships Domain

It is noteworthy that half of the participants did not mention wider interpersonal relationships as one of their three most important goals or meaningful things in life and also not in the motivations for the goals or meaning sources. An explanation may be that while wider interpersonal relationships may be important to people, other domains of life may just be more important. For example, Delle Fave et al. (2011) found in an international sample that the most important domain mentioned when participants described what happiness means to them was family, with interpersonal relationships in the second place. Delle Fave, Wissing, et al. (2013) reported, in order of priority, that family, work, and interpersonal relationships were the most prominent life domains as sources of meaning in life in an international sample, and that the most prominent goals were (in order of frequency) family, work, health, standard of living, personal life (psychological definitions), leisure, and interpersonal relationships (being only in the seventh place). Liversage (2019) conducted a study similar to the current study, but focusing specifically on the family domain of life. In her study, she found that many more participants mentioned family in their meaningful things than in their goals. Interpersonal relationships, in the sense of wider peripheral relationships as portrayed in this study, are not prioritised as a goal or meaning in the same way as family relationships, as also shown by the studies mentioned above.

The alignment pattern of meaning-no-goal had a much higher frequency (30.6%) than the pattern of goal-no-meaning (5.8%). It thus seems that people do not typically mention wider interpersonal relationships when defining or motivating their most important goals, despite such relationships being sources of meaning to many. Why would this be the case? It may be that such wider interpersonal relationships are often taken for granted with limited intentional effort made to cultivate and maintain them. Alternatively, it can be that people appreciate such wider relationships (providing meaning in life), but that they just have limited energy or too many obligations in daily life and at work which are the focus of their attention, time, and goals. A question that can be asked is whether these findings will correspond for participants who are flourishing (high levels of well-being) versus those who are languishing (low levels of well-being). It is interesting to note that the meaning-no-goal alignment pattern had the highest frequency (after the "empty" no-goal-no-meaning pattern). This implies that interpersonal relationships are very important to people, which is in line with what Christopher Peterson indicated with his statement that "Other people matter. Period." (Peterson et al., 2008, p. 1); relationships thus remain a wellspring of meaning (Stavrova & Luhmann, 2016), well-being, and happiness (Anderson & Fowers, 2020).

15.4.2 Associations Between Alignment Patterns and Sociodemographic Variables

The age group 18–25, who showed the highest frequency for the meaning-no-goal pattern compared to other age groups, are in a developmental stage of life where networks of friends and peer groups are very important, as proposed by Zhaoyang et al. (2018). Young adults can be expected to value friendships as a source of meaning in their lives being at the age where they are also searching for life partners.

Interpersonal relationships also featured more prominently in the group older than 60 years of age than in the two middle age groups. In this phase of life, which is often accompanied by retirement and children who have left home, it seems that the value of wider relationships such as friends is cherished more, perhaps in view of the changes in relationships with children and life partners.

A higher proportion of males did not mention interpersonal relationships as a goal or as something meaningful (no-goal-no-meaning pattern) compared to females. Moreover, the meaning-no-goal alignment pattern was more prevalent for females than for males. This is in line with the general notion that females have more awareness towards relationships than males, as also shown in other studies. For example, in a study by Delle Fave et al. (2016) on what happiness entailed to people, women were more likely to refer to family and interpersonal relations, whereas men were more prone to mention standard of living. Women also tend to have larger social networks than men, according to Fuhrer and Stansfeld (2002).

The higher the level of education, the more likely participants were to indicate interpersonal relationships in their responses to the meaning questions but not to the goals questions, and the lower the level of education, the more participants did not mention interpersonal relations in their indications of important goals or meaning at all. This finding is line with the results of Albert and David (2018) who found that participants with higher educational levels tended to have more friends and relationships, which could explain why interpersonal relationships featured more often in these participants' sources of meaning and the reasons therefore.

Employed participants portrayed, in comparison to unemployed participants, a lower proportion of responses in the no-goal-no-meaning pattern and a higher proportion in the meaning-no-goal pattern. Being employed may offer the opportunity to experience meaning in interpersonal relationships with colleagues even though these relationships are not necessarily prioritized in people's general life goals. Another interpretation may be that unemployment is an uncertain and stressful time in which job-searching may become the main concern and focus (Stam et al., 2016) and interpersonal relationships are put on the back burner. In a period of unemployment, lower levels of well-being may also be experienced (Gander et al., 2019) where energy is firstly committed to finding employment and not so much invested in wider relationships. The present findings dovetail with those of other studies indicating the association between employment and mental health and well-being. Employment is regarded as a material and psychological foundation for individuals to plan and build their lives freely (Bonanomi & Rosina, 2020). Employment, according to Jahoda (1981), provides social contacts and purpose. Taking this into consideration, interpersonal relationships may be more meaningful to employed participants as employment already provides an opportunity for interpersonal contact and such relationships can then also contribute to the experience of meaning.

15.4.3 Associations Between Alignment Patterns and Well-Being

Contrary to expectations from the SCM, no significant associations were found between alignment patterns and well-being variables in the case of the SWLS, the PANAS, and the MLQ. In the case of the MHC-SF total score, a statistically significant association with alignment patterns was found (of small practical significance), but the both-goal-and-meaning pattern did not show higher levels of well-being than the other alignment patterns as would be predicted by the SCM. These findings thus indicate that the SCM is not supported in the present study with focus on references to the wider interpersonal relationship domain of life.

The following possible explanations and interpretations for the present findings can be considered. It may be that alignment between goals and meaning is associated with well-being when considered in terms of life in general as was mostly explored and supported in studies with the SCM, but not in the case of specific life domains such as the wider interpersonal relationships domain of life as referred to in the present study. The same lack of association between alignment patterns and well-being was found in the family domain of life by Liversage (2019).

Another possible explanation for the lack of support for the SCM in the present study may be related to differences in the method of conceptualization and operationalization of concordance between goals and meaning. In previous studies (Gordeeva et al., 2019; Sheldon & Elliot, 1999; Sheldon et al., 2019; Zhang et al., 2018), participants were requested to formulate goals and then to rate the reason for pursuing the goal. Goal self-concordance was established in terms of four types of motivation, namely, external, introjected, identified, and intrinsic. The combined goal self-concordance score was calculated by firstly reversing the external and introjected motivation scores and then averaging all scores (Bahrami & Cranney, 2018). In other studies, a self-concordance score was determined by the sum of the identified and intrinsic ratings after which the external and introjected ratings were subtracted (Zhang et al., 2018). Participants thus subjectively rate themselves on whether goals and intrinsic values/meanings are aligned. In the present study, participants mentioned their most important goals and reasons therefore, and the most important meaningful (valued) things and reasons therefore. Through the analysis of this information, researchers "objectively" established whether goals and meanings and the reasons for these were aligned as shown by references to the interpersonal life domain offered independently in goals and meaningful things (or reasons for these). In other words, the participants did not judge for themselves whether there was concordance between important goals and valued meanings with specific reference to wider interpersonal relationships. The conceptualization and operationalization of concordance between goals and meaning as shown in reference to the interpersonal domain of life might thus have been stricter than the original method used by Sheldon and colleagues. Differences in methods of concordance conceptualization and operationalization may thus possibly explain the differences in findings between our study and those by Sheldon and colleagues (Sheldon & Elliot, 1999; Sheldon et al., 2019) as far as support for the SCM is concerned.

It is also possible that the association between patterns of alignment and well-being may differ in various life domains (and differ from what the SCM suggested). In the present study it was established that although the highest frequency of participants was found in the meaning-no-goal pattern of alignment (apart from the "empty" no-goal-no-meaning pattern), this group of participants showed the lowest well-being scores on the MHC-SF as can be seen in Fig. 15.2. This is difficult to explain. Does it mean that other people are important for one to be okay (people as means to own ends), reflecting an individualistic orientation? The pattern of goal-no-meaning was associated with the highest well-being scores on the MHC-SF. Could this result refer to people who set goals for relationships and are givers without expecting anything in return? Is it possible that this group of participants reflect a relatively more interdependent or collectivistic orientation? But why higher levels of well-being? In a study by Wissing, Schutte, Liversage, et al. (2019), the flourishing participants had more altruistic intentions to assist others and contribute to the lives of others. But why will a group in the goal-no-meaning pattern, as defined in the present study, contain more flourishers? Other studies such as that of Fowers et al. (2016), which suggests that both shared goals and meaningful experiences are part of flourishing relationships, indicate that more knowledge is to be gathered before the present findings can be understood. We contend that the present finding of an association between patterns of alignment and well-being as measured with the MHC-SF should not be over-interpreted as differences between associations of alignment patterns and well-being are of small practical significance, all scores are in the region of moderate mental health, and because other indices of mental health did not show similar findings.

15.5 Limitations and Recommendations

A limitation in this study could be that the conceptualization and operationalization of concordance between goals and meaning as shown in reference to the interpersonal domain of life might have been stricter than the original method used by Sheldon and colleagues, leading to a different result. Since participants were only required to list their top general three goals and reasons therefore, and the three most meaningful things in their lives with motivations, this approach could have disguised the importance of interpersonal relationships. As the association between patterns of alignment and well-being may differ in various life domains, similar studies in various other life domains are recommended which may lead to a deeper understanding of goals and meaning as important facets of eudaimonic well-being through the comparison of results. It can also be further explored whether participants higher in intrapersonal harmony differ from those with lower levels of experienced internal harmony with regard to the manifestation of possible associations between alignment of goals and meaning as manifested in general or in specific life domains.

Similarly, it can be explored if flourishing versus languishing people differ in association of alignment patterns and well-being manifestations (the pursuit of personal valued goals is linked to flourishing—cf. Little et al., 2017). This may further contribute to the appraisal of the self-concordance model and alternative understandings of the association between patterns of alignment on the one hand and well-being manifestations on the other hand.

15.6 Conclusion

More than 40% of the participants referred to wider interpersonal relationships when mentioning their three most important goals and/or things that are meaningful to them, or the reasons for their goals or for what is meaningful to them. Many more participants experienced wider relationships as meaningful, compared to participants who intentionally formulated goals that referred to wider relationships. However, participants who included wider interpersonal aspects in their most important goals, showed a (non-significant) tendency to a higher level of psychological well-being than those only mentioning it as meaningful. This renders the question whether facilitation of goals for, and alignment of goals and meaningful things in, wider interpersonal relationships will boost well-being levels?

Despite the statistically significant association of alignment patterns with the MHC-SF, the SCM was not supported in this study as the goal-and-meaning pattern of concordance was not associated with the highest well-being scores in comparison to other substantive patterns. This study contributed to the evaluation of the SCM and opening up of further questions to be explored with regard to the dynamics of goals and meaning with reference to the interpersonal relationships domain of life.

Acknowledgements This chapter is based on an earlier draft in the PhD of the first author. The work is based on research partially supported by the National Research Foundation (NRF) of South Africa (grant nrs. 91557, 106050, and 121948). It is acknowledged that opinions, findings, conclusions, and recommendations expressed are those of the authors and that the NRF accepts no liability in this regard. The North-West University is acknowledged for bursaries awarded to the first author. Appreciation to Suria Ellis for professional advice regarding the statistical analyses and Amanda Cromhout for valued assistance in the determination of validity and reliability indices.

Declaration of Interest The authors of this article have no conflict of interest to declare.

References

Akhtar, M., & Kroener-Herwig, B. (2019). Coping styles and socio-demographic variables as predictors of psychological well-being among international students belonging to different cultures. *Current Psychology, 38*(3), 618–626. https://doi.org/10.1007/s12144-017-9635-3

Albert, F., & David, B. (2018). Interpersonal relationships in Hungary – An overview. *Metszetec, 7*(2), 72–93.

Anderson, A. R., & Fowers, B. J. (2020). An exploratory study of friendship characteristics and their relations with hedonic and eudaimonic well-being. *Journal of Social and Personal Relationships, 37*(1), 260–280. https://doi.org/10.1177/0265407519861152

Antonovsky, A. (1993). The structure and properties of the sense of coherence scale. *Social Science & Medicine, 36*(6), 725–733. https://doi.org/10.1016/0277-9536(93)90033

Asparouhov, T., & Muthén, B. O. (2009). Exploratory structural equation modeling. *Structural Equation Modeling: A Multidisciplinary Journal, 16*(3), 397–438. https://doi.org/10.1080/10705510903008204

Bahrami, Z., & Cranney, J. (2018). Integrated conative model of well-being: From motives to well-being. *Journal of Happiness Studies: An Interdisciplinary Forum on Subjective Well-Being, 19*(4), 961–981. https://doi.org/10.1007/s10902-017-9845-2

Bandura, A. (1988). Self-regulation of motivation and action through goal systems. In *Cognitive perspectives on emotion and motivation* (pp. 37–61). Springer.

Batthyany, A., & Russo-Netzer, P. (2014). Psychologies of meaning. In A. Batthyany & P. Russo-Netzer (Eds.), *Meaning in positive and existential psychology* (pp. 3–22). Springer. https://doi.org/10.1007/978-1-4939-0308-5_1

Battista, J., & Almond, R. (1973). The development of meaning in life. *Psychiatry, 36*(4), 409–427. https://doi.org/10.1080/00332747.1973.11023774

Baumeister, R. F. (2016). Toward a general theory of motivation: Problems, challenges, opportunities, and the big picture. *Motivation and Emotion, 40*(1), 1–10. https://doi.org/10.1007/s11031-015-9521-y

Baumeister, R. M., & Leary, M. R. (1995). The need to belong: Desire for interpersonal attachments as a fundamental human motivation. *Psychological Bulletin, 117*, 497–529. https://doi.org/10.1037/0033-2909.117.3.497

Bonanomi, A., & Rosina, A. (2020). Employment status and well-being: A longitudinal study on young Italian people. *Social Indicators Research*, 1–18.

Brunstein, J. C. (1993). Personal goals and subjective well-being: A longitudinal study. *Personality and Social Psychology, 65*(5), 1061–1070. https://doi.org/10.1037/0022-3514.65.5.1061

Byrne, B. M. (2012). *Structural equation modeling with Mplus: Basic concepts, applications, and programming*. Routledge.

Cohen, J. (1988). *Statistical power analysis for the behavioral sciences* (2nd ed.). Erlbaum.

Converse, B. A., Juarez, L., & Hennecke, M. (2019). Self-control and the reasons behind our goals. *Journal of Personality and Social Psychology, 116*(5), 860–883. https://doi.org/10.1037/pspp0000188

Creswell, J. W., & Plano Clark, V. L. (2011). *Designing and conducting mixed methods research* (2nd ed.). SAGE.

David, M., & Sutton, C. D. (2004). *Social research: The basics*. Sage. Retrieved from https://trove.nla.gov.au/version/46502328

Deci, E. L., Olafsen, A. H., & Ryan, R. M. (2017). Self-determination theory in work organizations: The state of a science. *Annual Review of Organizational Psychology and Organizational Behavior, 4*, 19–43. https://doi.org/10.1146/annurev-orgpsych-032516-113108

Deci, E., & Ryan, R. (2000). The "what" and "why" of goal pursuits: Human needs and the self-determination of behavior. *Psychological Inquiry, 11*(4), 227–268. https://doi.org/10.1207/S15327965PLI1104_01

Deci, E. L., & Ryan, R. M. (2008). Self-determination theory: A macrotheory of human motivation, development, and health. *Canadian Psychology/Psychologie Canadienne, 49*(3), 182–185. https://doi.org/10.1037/a0012801

Deci, E. L., & Ryan, R. M. (2014). Autonomy and need satisfaction in close relationships: Relationships motivation theory. In N. Weinstein (Ed.), *Human motivation and interpersonal relationships: Theory, research, and applications* (pp. 53–73). Springer. https://doi.org/10.1007/978-94-017-8542-6_3

Delle Fave, A., Brdar, I., Freire, T., Vella-Brodrick, D., & Wissing, M. P. (2011). The eudaimonic and hedonic components of happiness: Qualitative and quantitative findings. *Social Indicators Research, 100*(2), 185–207. https://doi.org/10.1007/s11205-010-9632-5

Delle Fave, A., Brdar, I., Wissing, M. P., Araujo, U., Castro Solano, A., Freire, T., Hernández-Pozo, M. D. R., Jose, P., Martos, T., Nafstad, H. E., Nakamura, J., Singh, K., & Soosai-Nathan, L. (2016). Lay definitions of happiness across nations: The primacy of inner harmony and relational connectedness. *Frontiers in Psychology, 7*, 30. https://doi.org/10.3389/fpsyg.2016.00030

Delle Fave, A., & Soosai-Nathan, L. (2014). Meaning as inter-connectedness: Theoretical perspectives and empirical evidence. *Journal of Psychology in Africa, 24*(1), 33–43. https://doi.org/10.1080/17439760.2013.830761

Delle Fave, A., Wissing, M., Brdar, I., Vella-Brodrick, D., & Freire, T. (2013). Cross-cultural perceptions of meaning and goals in adulthood: Their roots and relations with happiness. In A. S. Waterman (Ed.), *The best within us: Positive psychology perspectives on eudaimonia* (pp. 227–247). American Psychological Association. https://doi.org/10.1037/14092-012

Diener, E. D., Emmons, R. A., Larsen, R. J., & Griffin, S. (1985). The satisfaction with life scale. *Journal of Personality Assessment, 49*(1), 71–75. https://doi.org/10.1207/s15327752jpa4901_13

Diener, E., & Ryan, K. (2009). Subjective well-being: A general overview. *South Africa Journal of Psychology, 39*(4), 391–406. https://doi.org/10.1177/008124630903900402

Diener, E., & Seligman, M. P. (2009). Beyond money: Toward an economy of well-being. In E. Diener (Ed.), *The science of well-being: The collected works of Ed Diener* (pp. 201–265). Springer.

Dweck, C. S. (1986). Motivational processes affecting learning. *American Psychologist, 41*, 1040–1048. https://doi.org/10.1037/0003-066X.41.10

Emmons, R. (1989). The personal striving approach to personality. In L. A. Pervin (Ed.), *Goal concepts in personality and social psychology* (pp. 87–126). Erlsbaum. https://doi.org/10.1177/0146167291176007

Emmons, R. A. (2003). Personal goals, life meaning, and virtue: Wellsprings of a positive life. In C. L. M. Keyes & J. Haidt (Eds.), *Flourishing: Positive psychology and the life well-lived* (pp. 105–128). American Psychological Association. https://doi.org/10.1037/10594-005

Feldman, D. B., Balaraman, M., & Anderson, C. (2018). Hope and meaning-in-life: Points of contact between hope theory and existentialism. In M. W. Gallagher & S. J. Lopez (Eds.), *Oxford library of psychology: The Oxford handbook of hope* (pp. 353–362). Oxford University Press.

Field, A. (2018). *Discovering statistics using IBM SPSS statistics* (5th ed.). Sage.

Fowers, B. J., Laurenceau, J. P., Penfield, R. D., Cohen, L. M., Lang, S. F., Owenz, M. B., & Pasipanodya, E. (2016). Enhancing relationship quality measurement: The development of the relationship flourishing scale. *Journal of Family Psychology, 30*(8), 997–1007.

Frankl, V. E. (1963). *Man's search for meaning: An introduction to logotheraphy*. Washington Square Press.

Fuhrer, R., & Stansfeld, S. A. (2002). How gender affects patterns of social relations and their impact on health: A comparison of one or multiple sources of support from "close persons.". *Social Science & Medicine, 54*(5), 811–825. https://doi.org/10.1016/S0277-9536(01)00111-3

Gander, F., Hofmann, J., & Ruch, W. (2019). From unemployment to employment and back: Professional trajectories and well-being. *Applied Research in Quality of Life*. https://doi.org/10.1007/s11482-019-09797-y

Geldenhuys, M., & Henn, C. M. (2017). The relationship between demographic variables and well-being of women in South African workplaces. *SA Journal of Human Resource Management, 15*(1), 1–15.

George, L. S., & Park, C. L. (2016). Meaning in life as comprehension, purpose, and mattering: Toward integration and new research questions. *Review of General Psychology, 20*(3), 205–220. https://doi.org/10.1037/gpr0000077

Gordeeva, T., Sheldon, K., & Sychev, O. (2019). Pursuing self-concordant goals breeds optimism and thus well-being. In *XVI European Congress of Psychology* (pp. 148–148). Melbourne, Australia.

Hennecke, M., & Brandstätter, V. (2017). Means, ends, and happiness: The role of goals for subjective well-being. In M. D. Robinson & M. Eid (Eds.), *The happy mind: Cognitive contributions to well-being* (pp. 235–251). Springer. https://doi.org/10.1007/978-3-319-58763-9_13

Hu, L., & Bentler, P. M. (1999). Cutoff criteria for fit indexes in covariance structure analysis: Conventional criteria versus new alternatives. *Structural Equation Modeling, 6*(1), 1–55. https://doi.org/10.1080/10705519909540118

Jahoda, M. (1981). Work, employment, and unemployment: Values, theories, and approaches in social research. *American Psychologist, 36*(2), 184–191. https://doi.org/10.1037/0003-066X.36.2.184

Keyes, C. L. M. (2006). The subjective well-being of America's youth: Toward a comprehensive assessment. *Adolescent and Family Health, 4*(1), 3–11. https://doi.org/10.1037/0002-9432.76.3.395

Keyes, C. L. M. (2009). The Black–White paradox in health: Flourishing in the face of social inequality and discrimination. *Journal of Personality, 77*(6), 1677–1706. https://doi.org/10.1111/j.1467-6494.2009.00597

Keyes, C. L. M., Wissing, M., Potgieter, J. P., Temane, M., Kruger, A., & van Rooy, S. (2008). Evaluation of the mental health continuum-short form (MHC-SF) in Setswana-speaking South Africans. *Clinical Psychology & Psychotherapy, 15*(3), 181–192. https://doi.org/10.1002/cpp.572

Khumalo, I. P., Temane, Q. M., & Wissing, M. P. (2012). Socio-demographic variables, general psychological well-being and the Mental Health Continuum in an African context. *Social Indicators Research, 105*(3), 419–442. https://doi.org/10.1007/s11205-010-9777-2

Lee, H., Lou, N. M., Johnson, M. D., & Park, S. W. (2019). A socioecological perspective to understanding mental and physical health: The mediating role of relationship mindsets and goals. *Journal of Social and Personal Relationships, 36*(10), 3117–3138. https://doi.org/10.1177/0265407518814371

Little, B. R. (1983). Personal projects: A rationale and method for investigation. *Environment and Behavior, 15*(3), 273–309. https://doi.org/10.1177/0013916583153002

Little, B. R., Salmela-Aro, K., & Phillips, S. D. (2017). *Personal project pursuit: Goals, action, and human flourishing*. Taylor & Francis. https://doi.org/10.4324/9781315089928

Liversage, M. T. (2019). *Concordance of goals and meaning in the family domain: Associations with socio-demographic variables and well-being* (Master's dissertation, North-West University, Potchefstroom, South-Africa).

MacCallum, R. C., Browne, M. W., & Sugawara, H. M. (1996). Power analysis and determination of sample size for covariance structure modeling. *Psychological Methods, 1*(2), 130. https://doi.org/10.1037/1082-989X.1.2.130

Martino, J., Pegg, J., & Frates, E. P. (2017). The connection prescription: Using the power of social interactions and the deep desire for connectedness to empower health and wellness. *American Journal of Lifestyle Medicine, 11*(6), 466–475. https://doi.org/10.1177/1559827615608788

Milyavskaya, M., Inzlicht, M., Hope, N., & Koestner, R. (2015). Saying "no" to temptation: Want-to motivation improves self-regulation by reducing temptation rather than by increasing self-control. *Journal of Personality and Social Psychology*. https://doi.org/10.1037/pspp0000045

Muthén, L. K., & Muthén, B. O. (1998–2019). *Mplus User's guide. (Version 8.3) [Computer software]*. Muthén & Muthén.

Nunnally, J. C. (1978). *Psychometric theory* (2nd ed.). McGraw-Hill.

Orehek, E., Forest, A. L., & Barbaro, N. (2018). A people-as-means approach to interpersonal relationships. *Perspectives on Psychological Science, 13*(3), 373–389. https://doi.org/10.1177/1745691617744522

Peterson, C., Park, N., & Sweeney, P. J. (2008). Group well-being: Morale from a positive psychology perspective. *Applied Psychology, 57*, 19–36. https://doi.org/10.1111/j.1464-0597.2008.00352.x

Plano Clark, V. L. (2017). Mixed methods research. *The Journal of Positive Psychology, 12*(3), 305–306. https://doi.org/10.1080/17439760.2016.1262619

Prilleltensky, I. (2005). Promoting well-being: Time for a paradigm shift in health and human services. *Scandinavian Journal of Public Health, 33*(66), 53–60. https://doi.org/10.1080/14034950510033381

Rajani, N. B., Skianis, V., & Filippidis, F. T. (2019). Association of environmental and sociodemographic factors with life satisfaction in 27 European countries. *BMC Public Health, 19*(1), 534. https://doi.org/10.1186/s12889-019-6886

Ryan, R. M., & Deci, E. L. (2001). On happiness and human potentials: A review of research on hedonic and eudaimonic well-being. *Annual Review of Psychology, 52*(1), 141–166. https://doi.org/10.1146/annurev.psych.52.1.141

Ryff, C. D. (1989). Happiness is everything, or is it? Explorations on the meaning of psychological well-being. *Journal of Personality and Social Psychology, 57*(6), 1069–1081. https://doi.org/10.1037/0022-3514.57.6.1069

Ryff, C. D. (2014). Psychological well-being revisited: Advances in the science and practice of eudaimonia. *Psychotherapy and Psychosomatics, 83*(1), 10–28. https://doi.org/10.1159/000353263

Ryff, C. D., & Singer, B. (1998). The contours of positive human health. *Psychological Inquiry, 9*(1), 1–28. https://doi.org/10.1207/s15327965pli0901_1

Sánchez-Oliva, D., Morin, A. J. S., Teixeira, P. J., Carracxa, E. V., Palmeira, A. L., & Silva, M. N. (2017). A bifactor exploratory structural equation modeling representation of the structure of the basic psychological needs at work scale. *Journal of Vocational Behavior, 98*, 173–187. https://doi.org/10.1016/j.jvb.2016.12.001

Schotanus-Dijkstra, M., Drossaert, C. H., Pieterse, M. E., Boon, B., Walburg, J. A., & Bohlmeijer, E. T. (2017). An early intervention to promote well-being and flourishing and reduce anxiety and depression: A randomized controlled trial. *Internet Interventions, 9*, 15–24. https://doi.org/10.1016/j.invent.2017.04.002

Schutte, L., Negri, L., Delle Fave, A., & Wissing, M. P. (2019). Rasch analysis of the satisfaction with life scale across countries: Findings from South Africa and Italy. *Current Psychology*, 1–10. https://doi.org/10.1007/s12144-019-00424-5

Schutte, L., & Wissing, M. P. (2017). Clarifying the factor structure of the mental health continuum short form in three languages: A bifactor exploratory structural equation modeling approach. *Society and Mental Health, 7*(3), 142–158. https://doi.org/10.1177/2156869317707793

Schutte, L., Wissing, M. P., Ellis, S. M., Jose, P. E., & Vella-Brodrick, D. A. (2016). Rasch analysis of the meaning in life questionnaire among adults from South Africa, Australia, and New Zealand. *Health and Quality of Life Outcomes, 14*(12), 1–18. https://doi.org/10.1186/s12955-016-0414

Sheldon, K. M., & Elliot, A. J. (1999). Goal striving, need satisfaction, and longitudinal well-being: The self-concordance model. *Journal of Personality and Social Psychology, 76*(3), 482–497. Retrieved from http://psycnet.apa.org/buy/1999-10261-009

Sheldon, K. M., & Houser-Marko, L. (2001). Self-concordance, goal attainment, and the pursuit of happiness: Can there be an upward spiral? *Journal of Personality and Social Psychology, 80*(1), 152–165. https://doi.org/10.1037/0022-3514.80.1.152

Sheldon, K. M., Prentice, M., & Osin, E. (2019). Rightly crossing the Rubicon: Evaluating goal self-concordance prior to selection helps people choose more intrinsic goals. *Journal of Research in Personality, 79*, 119–129. https://doi.org/10.1016/j.jrp.2019.03.001

Stam, K., Sieben, I., Verbakel, E., & de Graaf, P. M. (2016). Employment status and subjective well-being: The role of the social norm to work. *Work, Employment and Society, 30*(2), 309–333.

Stavrova, O., & Luhmann, M. (2016). Social connectedness as a source and consequence of meaning in life. *The Journal of Positive Psychology, 11*(5), 470–479. https://doi.org/10.1080/17439760.2015.1117127

Steca, P., Monzani, D., Greco, A., D'Addario, M., Cappelletti, E., & Pancani, L. (2016). The effects of short-term personal goals on subjective well-being. *Journal of Happiness Studies, 17*(4), 1435–1450. https://doi.org/10.1007/s10902-015-9651-7

Steger, M. F. (2011). *Meaning in life: Catch basin of consciousness*. In Invited lecture at the North-West University, Potchefstroom, South Africa.

Steger, M. F. (2018). Meaning and well-being. In E. Diener, S. Oishi, & L. Tay (Eds.), *Handbook of well-being*. DEF Publishers. Retrieved from https://www.nobascholar.com/chapters/50/download.pdf

Steger, M. F., Frazier, P., Oishi, S., & Kaler, M. (2006). The meaning in life questionnaire: Assessing the presence of and search for meaning in life. *Journal of Counseling Psychology, 53*(1), 80–93. https://doi.org/10.1037/0022-0167.53.1.80

Steger, M. F., Kashdan, T. B., Sullivan, B. A., & Lorentz, D. (2008). Understanding the search for meaning in life: Personality, cognitive style, and the dynamic between seeking and experiencing meaning. *Journal of Personality, 76*(2), 199–228. https://doi.org/10.1111/j.1467-6494.2007.00484

Steger, M. F., Oishi, S., & Kashdan, T. B. (2009). Meaning in life across the life span: Levels and correlates of meaning in life from emerging adulthood to older adulthood. *Journal of Positive Psychology, 4*(1), 43–52. https://doi.org/10.1080/17439760802303127

Temane, L., Khumalo, I. P., & Wissing, M. P. (2014). Validation of the meaning in life questionnaire in a South African context. *Journal of Psychology in Africa, 24*(1), 81–95. https://doi.org/10.1080/14330237.2014.904088

Thomas, N. K., Sugiyama, K., Rochford, K. C., Stephens, J. P., & Kanov, J. (2018). Experiential organizing: Pursuing relational and bureaucratic goals through symbolically and experientially oriented work. *Academy of Management Review, 43*(4), 749–771. https://doi.org/10.5465/amr.2016.0348

Van Tongeren, D. R., Green, J. D., Davis, D. E., Hook, J. N., & Hulsey, T. L. (2016). Prosociality enhances meaning in life. *The Journal of Positive Psychology, 11*(3), 225–236. https://doi.org/10.1111/ajsp.12212236

Ward, S. J., & King, L. A. (2017). Work and the good life: How work contributes to meaning in life. *Research in Organizational Behavior, 37*(24), 59–82. https://doi.org/10.1016/j.riob.2017.10.001

Waterman, A. S. (1993). Two conceptions of happiness: Contrasts of personal expressiveness (eudaimonia) and hedonic enjoyment. *Journal of Personality and Social Psychology, 64*(4), 678–691. https://doi.org/10.1037/0022-3514.64.4.678

Watson, D., Clark, L. A., & Tellegen, A. (1988). Development and validation of brief measures of positive and negative affect: The PANAS scales. *Journal of Personality and Social Psychology, 54*(6), 1063–1070. https://doi.org/10.1037/0022-3514.54.6.1063

Werner, K. M., Milyavskaya, M., Foxen-Craft, E., & Koestner, R. (2016). Some goals just feel easier: Self-concordance leads to goal progress through subjective ease, not effort. *Personality and Individual Differences, 96*, 237–242. https://doi.org/10.1016/j.paid.2016.03.002

Wilson, A., Wissing, M. P., Ndima, L., & Somhlaba, N. Z. (2018). Representations of hope, goals, and meaning from Lay person's perspectives in two African contexts. *Journal of Humanistic Psychology*. https://doi.org/10.1177/0022167818785070

Wissing, M. P. (2008/2012). *The prevalence of levels of psychosocial health: Dynamics and relationships with biomarkers of (ill) health in South African social contexts (FORT3)*. Research project with ethical approval registered at the North-West University, Potchefstroom, South Africa.

Wissing, M. P. (2014). Meaning and relational well-being: A reflection on the state of the art and a way forward. *Journal of Psychology in Africa, 24*(1), 115–121.

Wissing, M. P., Carlquist, E., Martos, T., & Schutte, L. (2017, September). Do goals walk the talk of meaning in well-being? In I. Brdar (Croatia) & M. P. Wissing (SA), Discussant Des (Ed.). *International Society for Quality of Life Conference. Symposium Presentation: In their own voices: Lay people's perceptions and dimensions of well-being facets across world regions.* Innsbruck, Austria.

Wissing, M. P., & Delle Fave, A. (2013, May). Meaning and relational well-being: Towards a model. In *Paper presented at the Second Conference on Positive Psychology (CPPC) in Brno*, Czech Republic.

Wissing, M. P., Schutte, L., Liversage, C., Entwisle, B., Gericke, M., & Keyes, C. (2019). Important goals, meanings, and relationships in flourishing and languishing states: Towards patterns of well-being. *Applied Research in Quality of Life, 2019*, 1–37. https://doi.org/10.1007/s11482-019-09771-8

Wissing, M. P., Schutte, L., & Wilson, F. A. (2019). Cultures of positivity: Interconnectedness as a way of being. In I. Eloff (Ed.), *Handbook of quality of life in African societies*. International Handbooks of Quality-of-Life. Springer. https://doi.org/10.1007/978-3-030-15367-0_1

Wissing, M. P., Thekiso, S. M., Stapelberg, R., Van Quickelberge, L., Choabi, P., Moroeng, C., Nienaber, A., Temane, M., & Vorster, H. H. (2010). Validation of three Setswana measures for psychological wellbeing. *South African Journal of Industrial Psychology, 36*(2), 1–8. https://doi.org/10.4102/sajip.v36i2.860

Wong, P. T. P. (2012).The meaning mindset: Measurement and implications. *International Journal of Existential Positive Psychology, 4*(1), 3. Retrieved from http://journal.existentialpsychology.org/index.php/ExPsy/article/view/181

Wong, P. T. P. (2017). A decade of meaning: Past, present, and future. *Journal of Constructivist Psychology, 30*(1), 82–89. https://doi.org/10.1080/10720537.2015.1119085

Zhang, H., Chen, K., & Schlegel, R. (2018). How do people judge meaning in goal-directed behaviors: The interplay between self-concordance and performance. *Personality and Social Psychology Bulletin, 44*(11), 1582–1600. https://doi.org/10.1177/0146167218771330

Zhaoyang, R., Sliwinski, M. J., Martire, L. M., & Smyth, J. M. (2018). Age differences in adults' daily social interactions: An ecological momentary assessment study. *Psychology and Aging, 33*(4), 607–618. https://doi.org/10.1037/pag0000242

Part IV
Well-Being Promotion in Africa

Chapter 16
Positive Psychological Interventions in African Contexts: A Scoping Review

Tharina Guse

Abstract Research on positive psychology interventions (PPIs) are expanding, also in non-Western contexts. This study examined literature on PPIs in African countries through a scoping review. Databases were searched for studies implemented between 2006 and 2019. The bibliographic search used a broad and inclusive definition of PPIs and yielded 23 studies for analysis. The results indicated that the majority of studies were implemented in group settings among adults in South Africa, using quantitative research designs. However, research elsewhere on the continent is starting to emerge. There is a need for more research among youth, older persons and clinical populations. Future studies should also focus on cultural adaptation of existing PPIs, and take cultural practices and traditions into account.

Keywords Positive interventions · Positive activities · African · South Africa · Scoping review

16.1 Introduction

A major aim of positive psychology is to enhance individual, group and community well-being. Accordingly, research on interventions to increase well-being, or positive psychological interventions (PPIs), has expanded rapidly in the past decade. Some meta-analyses indicated that PPIs are effective in increasing well-being and decreasing depression (Bolier et al., 2013; Sin & Lyubomirsky, 2009; Weiss et al., 2016) but most published studies were implemented in Western countries. A recent review on the origins of studies on PPIs indicated that 78% originated in Western, industrialised countries and only two originated from Africa, both from South Africa (Hendriks et al., 2019). However, this review only included randomized controlled trials (RCTs) which are less likely to be implemented in lower income countries due

T. Guse (✉)
Department of Psychology, University of Pretoria, Pretoria, South Africa
e-mail: tharina.guse@up.ac.za

L. Schutte et al. (eds.), *Embracing Well-Being in Diverse African Contexts: Research Perspectives*, Cross-Cultural Advancements in Positive Psychology 16,
https://doi.org/10.1007/978-3-030-85924-4_16

to financial and logistical constraints (Hendriks et al., 2019; Struck et al., 2014). The question arises: What interventions with the aim to enhance well-being have been implemented in African countries? This chapter examines what is known about the nature and implementation of PPIs in Africa. First, we consider what PPIs are, followed by a brief discussion of evidence regarding the effectiveness of PPIs. We then situate PPIs in the African context through a scoping review.

16.1.1 Positive Psychological Interventions

Despite the large number of studies reporting on the effect of PPIs, there is still a lack of consensus on what constitutes a PPI. In the broadest sense PPIs are activities which aim to enhance people's well-being and psychological resources. Originally, Seligman and Csikszentmihalyi (2000) broadly referred to activities which are specifically designed to build positive emotions, behaviours and psychological capacities that will ultimately lead to flourishing individuals and communities. Later Sin and Lyubomirsky (2009) defined positive psychology interventions as intentional activities designed to increase the frequency of positive emotions, behaviours, and cognitions. The authors argued that interventions aimed at decreasing pathology or deficits are not PPIs, as PPIs are more focused on building strengths than decreasing distress.

Bolier et al. (2013, p. 3) narrowed this definition by specifying that PPI's only entail interventions that "have been explicitly developed with the theoretical tradition of positive psychology". This elicited criticism from other scholars for being too narrow and excluding interventions which may not explicitly self-identify as PPIs, for example mindfulness meditation and physical exercise interventions (Schueller & Parks, 2014; Schueller et al., 2014). Parks and Biswas-Diener (2013) added a further criterion for interventions to qualify as PPIs, positing that there should be empirical evidence for increasing positive feelings, behaviours, and/or cognitions. Other terms used include positive activity interventions (Layous & Lyubomirsky, 2014; Shin & Lyubomirsky, 2017), positive interventions (Parks & Biswas-Diener, 2013) and positive psychological interventions (Schueller et al., 2014; Van Zyl et al., 2019).

While it is clear that PPIs aim to enhance well-being, Schueller and colleagues (Schueller & Parks, 2014; Schueller et al., 2014) suggested that, in addition to this goal, PPIs follow specific pathways or strategies, conceptually embedded in positive psychology theories. These are: (1) savouring experiences and sensations, which entails intensifying pleasurable experiences in the moment; (2) cultivating or expressing gratitude; (3) engaging in acts of kindness; (4) promoting positive relationship processes; and (5) pursuing and enhancing hope and meaning. Schueller et al. (2014) further argued in favour of the term "positive psychological interventions" to underscore the importance of including interventions that are theoretically or conceptually aligned with the aims of positive psychology, even if positive psychology is not explicitly mentioned in the study.

Recently, Ng and Lim (2019) proposed that definitions of PPIs should be expanded to include multiple avenues to reach well-being, including activities that are not necessarily regarded as inherently positive, but which could facilitate optimal functioning, such as building resilience. Moreover, PPIs should not be limited to intentional individual activities to increase well-being, but also include new activities more suited to collectivistic contexts, such as interventions focusing on families and communities.

In this study, we followed Schueller et al.'s (2014) definition, using the term "positive psychological interventions". We also included suggestions by Hendriks et al. (2018) as well as Ng and Lim (2019). Accordingly, we conceptualized PPIs broadly and more inclusively as interventions that aim to enhance well-being through multiple avenues, including increasing positive emotions, behaviours and cognitions, and that also utilize pathways or strategies that are conceptually based on processes that support well-being. Thus, as proposed by Ng and Lim (2019), we considered PPIs to be interventions broadly focused on enhancing psychological functioning and facilitating optimal functioning.

16.1.2 Outcomes of Implementing Positive Psychological Interventions

Numerous studies have investigated the effect of PPIs on both hedonic and eudaimonic well-being. Interventions have been evaluated in single-component studies (SPPIs) as well as multi-component studies (MPPIs). SPPIs consist of one or more activities that aim to enhance only one component of well-being (Hendriks et al., 2020), most often hedonic well-being. For example, gratitude interventions (e.g., Cunha et al., 2019; Lai & O'Carroll, 2017), the best possible selves intervention (see Loveday et al., 2018 for a review) and savouring interventions (e.g. Quoidbach et al., 2010; Smith & Hanni, 2019).

MPPIs contain several activities, often integrated in a programme which aim to promote components of both hedonic and eudaimonic well-being (Hendriks et al., 2020). These include, for example, interventions to enhance job satisfaction and well-being of physicians (Dyrbye et al., 2016), strength-based interventions to enhance well-being and alleviate depression (Gander et al., 2013) and an online intervention to promote multidimensional well-being (Myers et al., 2017). According to a recent meta-analysis, MPPIs have a small effect on subjective well-being and depression, as well as a small to moderate effect on psychological well-being (Hendriks et al., 2020).

Overall, PPIs seem to have a positive effect on well-being, but the effects may be smaller than previously suggested (White et al., 2019). Reported effect sizes of PPIs were larger in non-Western countries, compared to Western countries, which may be due to lower quality of the studies but could also be due to a good cultural fit of certain PPIs with participants in collective cultures (Hendriks et al., 2018). It is evident that more research is needed on PPIs beyond the Western context.

16.1.3 Positive Psychological Interventions in African Contexts

After its initial development in Western contexts, positive psychology has gradually expanded to other countries and regions. However, a recent review reported that 70% of positive psychology research still originates from Western countries (Kim et al., 2018). There are some indications of increasing research emanating from the Middle East and North African region (MENA) with most studies being reported from Israel, Turkey, and Iran, but African studies are still limited (Rao et al., 2015). Eloff et al. (2008) found that positive psychology was not clearly studied or practiced in six African countries surveyed. Rather, it was implicitly practiced and linked to indigenous knowledge systems. Similarly, most research on PPIs have been implemented in Western countries and were informed by Western understandings of well-being (Hendriks et al., 2019; Ng & Lim, 2019). However, this may be because previous international reviews may have been too narrow, focusing on limited definitions of PPIs and ignoring methodologies other than RCTs. Interventions to enhance well-being may have been implemented in African contexts albeit in different formats and using different research designs.

It is increasingly being accepted that PPIs may not work equally well across cultures. In particular, PPIs focused on Westernized, individualistic values such as self-enhancement, may be less effective in societies that emphasize collectivistic values and social well-being (Ng & Lim, 2019), such as African societies. Understanding the nature and breadth of PPIs in African countries is therefore important and can shed light on the outcomes and culture-activity fit of these PPIs (see Layous, 2018). Effective and relevant implementation of PPIs may make mental health care more accessible and decrease stigma associated with seeking such care (Hendriks et al., 2019), thus further exploration on PPIs in African contexts is warranted.

16.1.4 Present Study

Since previous reviews on PPIs in non-Western countries only considered RCTs, and no information exist on the extent of the implementation of PPIs in the broader sense in the African context, we implemented a scoping review (Arksey & O'Malley, 2005) to establish what is known about implementing PPIs in African countries. In particular, we report on the origin of the PPIs, the nature of the intervention, the research design, population targeted, as well as important outcomes of the interventions.

16.2 Method

Scoping reviews are appropriate to obtain an overall picture of a research field and to identify knowledge gaps. It is also useful to examine emerging evidence (Munn et al., 2018). Unlike systematic reviews, scoping reviews examine broader topics and can include different research designs (Arksey & O'Malley, 2005). In this study, our main research question was: *What is known from the existing literature about the implementation of PPIs in Africa?* The aim was to explore and describe existing research on PPIs in the African context. We did not assess research quality due to the exploratory nature of the study, as indicated in scoping review methodology.

Between May and September 2019, a bibliographic search for published journal articles was conducted on the EbscoHost, Sage-Pub, Scopus, Proquest, PsyNet, and Google Scholar databases. Additionally, a search for unpublished dissertations or theses was conducted within the institutional repositories of the North-West University (NWU), the University of Johannesburg, and the University of Pretoria. The search was restricted to the mentioned institutions as those institutions constituted the majority of references in the scoping search within the Google Scholar database. We also searched the reference lists of relevant publications. We limited our search to studies published from January 2006 to September 2019, published in English, based on practical and time constraints. We also considered the fact that international literature on positive psychology interventions started to appear from the 2000's onwards (e.g., Rashid, 2009; Seligman et al., 2006; Sin & Lyubomirsky, 2009).

Studies were considered eligible if the primary focus was on an intervention aimed at enhancing well-being or building positive psychological resources and not on symptom reduction, and if the intervention was implemented in an African country. Studies were excluded if the research reported on case studies for the development of an intervention or proposed interventions without reporting on actual implementation.

The key terms used were: "Positive Psychology" OR Wellbeing OR Well-being OR "Psychological Well-being" OR Happiness OR Resilience) AND (interventions OR Strategies OR Best Practices) AND Africa. Two independent evaluators reviewed and selected the studies. By the end of the reviewing process, 23 studies were identified for analysis, as reflected in Fig. 16.1.

We then set out to chart the data, a descriptive-analytical approach proposed by Arksey and O'Malley (2005) which involves applying a common analytical framework to all the studies obtained. We reported the information in several columns including author/s, year, title, nature of publication, country of origin, methodology, target population, nature of intervention, aims of intervention and important outcomes.

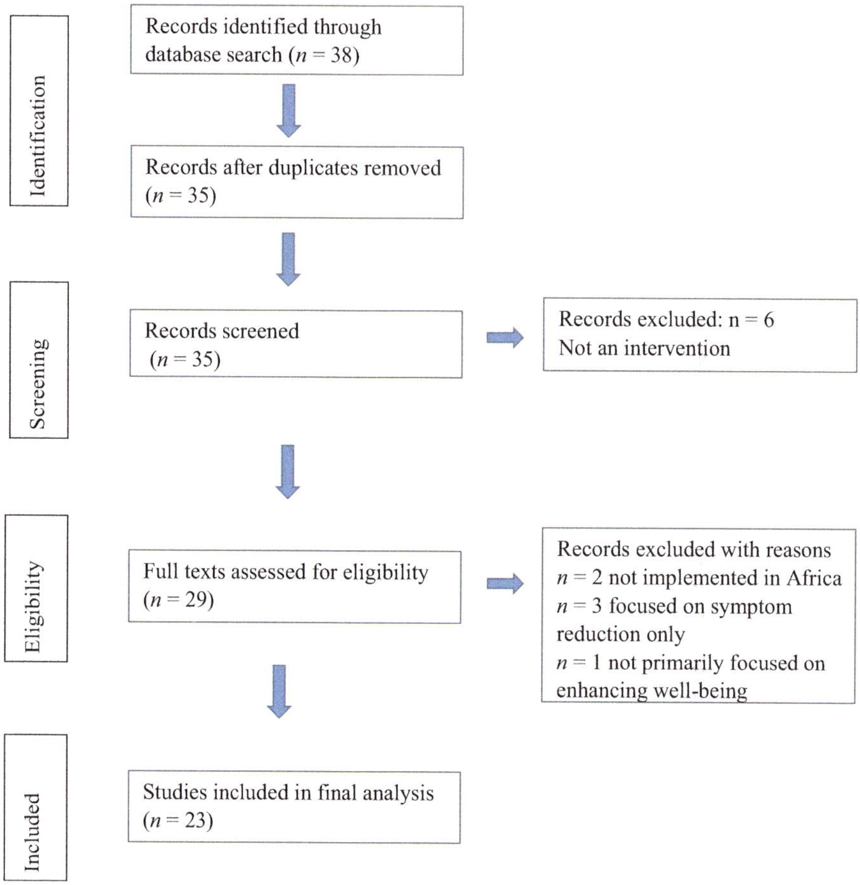

Fig. 16.1 Search strategy and results

16.3 Results

As reflected in Fig. 16.1, 38 studies were identified through the database search, and 23 were finally included in the analysis. The included studies are contained in Table 16.1. The findings will be presented along three dimensions. First, the type of research output, country of origin of participants, research design and participants. Second, the nature and aims of the intervention and specific positive activities implemented. Finally, we presented the important outcomes of the studies.

Table 16.1 Description of included studies

#	Author, year	Type	Implemented in/author origin	Design	Sample	Nature of intervention	Aims	Positive activities implemented	Outcomes
1	Guse et al., 2006	Journal article	SA	Quantitative	Females ($n = 23$)	Individual delivery of a structured six-session programme implementing hypnosis with a focus on mobilizing psychological strengths.	To evaluate the effect of a prenatal hypnotherapeutic programme on the postnatal psychological well-being of first-time mothers.		Improved in psychological well-being at 2 weeks postpartum, conceptualized as increased maternal self-confidence, sense of coherence and decreased negative affect. At 10 weeks postpartum fewer symptoms of depression.
2.	Pretorius et al., 2008	Journal article	SA	Quantitative	White young adults ($n = 8$)	A hope enhancement programme based on Snyder's Hope theory, consisting of six two-hour sessions conducted over 5 days.	To enhance dimensions of hope and evaluate its effect on well-being.		Increased hope, sense of coherence and life satisfaction.
3.	Edwards & Edwards, 2009	Journal article	SA	Quantitative	Zulu-speaking south African adults living with	A counselling program which provided person centred, group counselling interventions for inpatients infected with	To enhance dimensions of well-being in accordance with		Significant improvements in perceptions of autonomy, personal growth,

(continued)

Table 16.1 (continued)

#	Author, year	Type	Implemented in/author origin	Design	Sample	Nature of intervention	Aims	Positive activities implemented	Outcomes
					HIV/AIDS in a rural setting ($n = 30$)	HIV/AIDS. The programme was underpinned by empowerment theory.	Ryff's (1989) well-being scales		environmental mastery, positive relations with others and self-acceptance.
4.	Bonthuys et al., 2011	Journal article	SA	Mixed methods	Adults living in rural towns in the Taung community. Majority Setswana-speaking. ($n = 47$)	Implementation of the Lifeplan® programme,a combination of human development and training in life skills, in order to improve wellbeing in terms of health, nutrition and choice, thus holistic promotion of health.	To explore the effect of the Lifeplan® programme on psychological wellbeing.		Increase in general psychological and emotional wellbeing
5.	Fourie & Guse, 2011	Journal article	SA	Qualitative	One woman who experienced childhood sexual abuse.	An integrated, individual hypnotherapeutic approach applied with a specific focus on "symptoms" of health, strengths, and well-being.	To reduce symptoms associated with childhood sexual abuse and increase psychological well-being.		Self-reported decrease in symptoms of distress, increased life satisfaction and positive affect.
6	Grobler, 2012	Dissertation	SA	Mixed methods	Adults ($n = 5$)	Participants watched five movies identified as positive psychology movies.	To examine whether existing character strengths and well-being can be augmented or		Increased psychological well-being and emotional well-being; slight decrease in

							developed by viewing films that specifically portray the strengths.		social well-being. Increase in several strengths, but a decrease in others.
7	Van Zyl & Rothmann, 2012	Journal article	SA	Quantitative	University students, majority female and black. ($n = 109$)	A programme presented in three phases: (a) initial orientation, (b) a three day personal and group development programme and (b) six sessions of individual coaching.	To encourage participants to become aware of their signature strengths and apply it in their own lives in order to increase their experience of happiness.	Strengths-based activities; Gratitude activities; Savouring, Best possible self Forgiveness activity	Increase in overall happiness, in particular higher levels of overall life satisfaction, meaning, engagement, positive affect balance, authenticity, person-environment fit, autonomy, competence and relatedness.
8	Wood et al., 2012	Journal article	SA	Qualitative	Young children orphaned by HIV/Aids ($n = 32$)	Read-me-to-resilience (Rm2R) intervention, consisting of telling 22 culturally sensitive stories to children.	Explored whether and how culturally sensitive stories can encourage resilience.		Increased self-esteem as well as more positive relations with others. Bolstered indicators of resilience and resilience processes.

(continued)

Table 16.1 (continued)

#	Author, year	Type	Implemented in/author origin	Design	Sample	Nature of intervention	Aims	Positive activities implemented	Outcomes
9	Kruger, 2013	Dissertation	SA	Mixed method	Adolescents (n = 112) White (41%) Black (37%) Indian (17%) Coloured (4.5%)	Four-week gratitude intervention.	To increase gratitude, hedonic and eudaimonic well-being.	Gratitude activities	Quantitatively no increases in gratitude or well-being; qualitative indications of increased gratitude and improved interpersonal relationships.
10	Van Schalkwyk & Wissing, 2013	Chapter	SA	Mixed method	Adolescents (n = 64) White (66%) Coloured (31%) Black (3%)	Structured programme consisting of 10 sessions of 50 minutes each, based on Keyes' (2005) model of well-being as well as Peterson and Seligman's (2004) conceptualization of character strengths.	To promote psychosocial well-being and flourishing	Strengths based activities	Increased well-being and flourishing and fewer symptoms of distress.
11	Eloff et al., 2014	Journal article	SA	RCT	HIV-positive women (n = 161) and their children (n = 151)	Structured programme of 24 weekly sessions focused on parent-child communication and parenting.	To promote children's resilience.		Significant improvements in children's externalizing behaviours, communication, and daily living skills as indicators of resilience.

12	Davies, 2015	Dissertation	SA	Quantitative	Early adolescents (n = 44)	Four week multicomponent PPI delivered in group setting	To enhance hedonic and eudaimonic well-being	Gratitude exercise Acts of kindness Savouring Identifying and using strengths Best possible self	No increase in facets of well-being but decreased anxiety and depression
13	Chidrawi et al., 2015	Journal article	SA	Quantitative	People living with HIV (n = 18) People close to those living with HIV (n = 60) Majority Setswana-speaking	Comprehensive HIV stigma reduction and wellness enhancement community intervention implemented as workshops in three phases.	To evaluate well-being of both groups over over time	Identifying strengths	Well-being were more sustained in people living close to people with HIV over time following the intervention.
14	Van der Smit, 2015	Thesis	SA	Quantitative	Adolescents (n = 40)	A self-help online anger management programme implementing positive psychology activities.	To facilitate coping with anger and enhance well-being	Written gratitude exercise	Increased positive emotions, better coping skills, decreased anger.
15	Miano, 2016	Dissertation	SA	Mixed methods	Female university students at a university counselling Centre (n = 10)	A six-week group programme based on enhancing Well-being based on the PERMA model	To increase life satisfaction and decrease depression	Three good things Identifying and using strengths in a new way Acts of kindness	Increased life satisfaction and decreased depression

(continued)

Table 16.1 (continued)

#	Author, year	Type	Implemented in/author origin	Design	Sample	Nature of intervention	Aims	Positive activities implemented	Outcomes
16	Cherrington & De Lange, 2016	Journal article	SA	Qualitative	Primary school children in a rural village in QwaQwa ($n = 12$)	Visual participatory research-as-intervention to facilitate co-construction of hope.	To strengthen hope		Strengthened personal hope, enhanced relational hope, and mobilised collective hope.
17	Hatzipapas et al., 2017	Journal article	SA	Mixed method	Community care workers ($n = 10$)	Laughter therapy intervention	To examine if laughter therapy had an effect on well-being, in particular protecting against stress		Increase in positive emotions and positive coping as well as improved interpersonal relationships; deceased stress, anxiety and depression
18	Theron et al., 2017	Journal article	SA	Mixed method	African orphans and vulnerable children ($n = 345$)	A bibliotherapy intervention based on African stories	To explore if specifically chosen African stories could facilitate resilience		Increased awareness of personal and community-based protective resources.
19	Berger et al., 2018	Journal article	Tanzania	Quantitative	Primary school children ($n = 183$)	A 16-session school-based intervention including stress-reduction strategies (body-oriented and narrative therapy techniques)	To evaluate the efficacy of the programme to increase resilience and		Improved overall functioning, promoted pro-social orientation and better

						as well as pro-social strategies (based on social-emotional learning and contemplative practices); culturally adapted.	prosocial behaviour.		school adjustment.
20	Dow et al., 2018	Journal article	Tanzania	Quantitative	Adolescents living with HIV ($n = 58$)	A comprehensive mental health intervention, Sauti ya Vijana (the voice of youth); ten group sessions and two individual sessions developed around resilience domains.	To improve treatment adherence, reduce mental health symptoms, and increase youth resilience		Increased resilience as evident in new coping skills, improved interpersonal relationships, reduced stigma, and improved confidence to live positively according to personal values.
21	Marsay et al., 2018	Journal article	SA	Mixed method	Black adolescent juvenile sexual offenders ($n = 10$)	Six group sessions based on theory of fundamental hope (Scioli & Biller, 2009).	To facilitate hope and assist with making decisions about the future		Increase in three components of hope
22	Baranov et al., 2020 (first published online, 2019)	Journal article	Kenya	Quantitative	Adults residing in an informal settlement ($n = 120$)	Daily exercises to promote gratitude, self-affirmation, and prime aspirations over a period of 16 days	To increase psychological well-being and facilitate economic decision-making	Gratitude lists	Increased gratitude but no effect on self-reported happiness, life satisfaction, affect, depression or decision-making

(continued)

Table 16.1 (continued)

#	Author, year	Type	Implemented in/author origin	Design	Sample	Nature of intervention	Aims	Positive activities implemented	Outcomes
23	Teodorczuk et al., 2019	Journal article	SA	Quantitative	Adolescents living in a child and youth care Centre ($n = 29$)	A multicomponent PPI presented over 6 weeks	To increase hope and well-being.	Gratitude lists Acts of kindness Identifying and using strengths Best possible self Savouring	No effect on well-being or hope

16.3.1 Type of Research Output, Country of Origin, Participants and Research Design

The vast majority of studies ($n = 17$) were journal articles, followed by masters' dissertations. One book chapter and one thesis were identified. Most of the studies reported on interventions implemented in South Africa ($n = 20$) while two were implemented in Tanzania and one in Kenya. These latter three studies were all published since 2018 but the lead authors were affiliated with non-African universities. In terms of research design, the majority of studies ($n = 12$) implemented a quantitative approach, followed by mixed methods ($n = 8$), and qualitative studies ($n = 3$). Most interventions comprised of relatively small samples.

The participants in the studies varied substantially. From a developmental perspective, most interventions were implemented among adults ($n = 11$), followed by adolescents ($n = 7$), and children ($n = 5$). One study included children and their mothers (Eloff et al., 2014). Among the studies with adults, three comprised university students.

None of the studies were conducted in clinical settings or with clinical populations, but one study recruited participants from a student counselling centre (Miano, 2016) and one in an individual therapeutic context (Fourie & Guse, 2011). Several interventions ($n = 10$) were implemented among participants who may be more vulnerable to develop psychological distress or mental illness. These included people living with HIV/Aids ($n = 4$), orphaned children ($n = 2$), adolescents living in a youth care centre (Teodorczuk et al., 2019), juvenile sexual offenders (Marsay et al., 2018), and community care workers (Hatzipapas et al., 2017).

Only some studies reported racial or ethnic information of the participants. After reading the description of the research settings, we ascertained that 14 studies included mostly or only Black African participants.

16.3.2 Nature and Aims of the Interventions

The majority of the interventions ($n = 18$) were implemented in group settings while three studies conducted interventions with individuals. Of the remaining two studies one was implemented online (Van der Smit, 2015) and one was not clear on whether delivery occurred in group or individual format (Grobler, 2012). Most were structured programmes ($n = 20$) including one or more activities, while two were therapeutic interventions (Fourie & Guse, 2011; Hatzipapas et al., 2017) and one consisted of a visual-participatory activity (Cherrington & de Lange, 2016).

The content of the interventions varied substantially. Several ($n = 9$) included classic positive psychology activities such as gratitude activities, strength-based interventions, engaging in acts of kindness and the best possible self-intervention. Three focused on activities to enhance hope (Cherrington & de Lange, 2016; Marsay et al., 2018; Pretorius et al., 2008) while another two interventions comprised of reading stories to children (Theron et al., 2017; Wood et al., 2012). Four studies were implemented in a therapeutic context. Of these, two studies implemented hypnotherapy with a focus on clients' strengths without engaging in specific positive psychology activities (Guse et al., 2006; Fourie & Guse, 2011). A group counselling intervention was based on empowerment theory as well as Ryff's (1989) conceptualization of well-being and followed a person-centred approach (Edwards & Edwards, 2009) while another intervention implemented laughter therapy (Hatzipapas et al., 2017).

The remaining programmes focused on activities as diverse as life skills development (Bonthuys et al., 2011), parent-child-communication (Eloff et al., 2014), contemplative practice and stress-reduction strategies (Berger et al., 2018) and watching positive psychology movies (Grobler, 2012). One comprehensive intervention included activities to identify and reduce stress, foster strong familial and social relationships, and cultivate a safe and healthy environment (Dow et al., 2018).

As outlined in the criteria, all the interventions aimed to enhance one or more facets of well-being or optimal functioning, broadly defined. Most of the studies explicitly mentioned well-being as outcome ($n = 14$). Among these, five studies referred to psychological well-being specifically and two studies focused on enhancing both hedonic and eudaimonic well-being (Davies, 2015; Kruger, 2013). Five studies aimed to strengthen resilience, of which one added reducing distress and increasing medical treatment adherence (Dow et al., 2018) and another increasing prosocial behaviour (Berger et al., 2018). Two studies aimed to increase hope, without mentioning well-being (Cherrington & de Lange, 2016; Marsay et al., 2018) and one intended to increase happiness (Van Zyl & Rothmann, 2012). One study aimed to enhance life satisfaction and decrease depression (Miano, 2016).

16.3.3 Outcomes of Interventions

The majority of the studies ($n = 19$) reported increases in facets of well-being or associated constructs such as increased sense of coherence, hope, life satisfaction, positive affect, resilience, gratitude, and improved interpersonal relationships. Some studies also reported a decrease in symptoms of distress, including depression, anxiety, anger, and externalizing behaviour. Four studies failed to find increases in well-being, but only two were published in peer-reviewed journals (Baranov et al., 2020; Teodorczuk et al., 2019). In sum, most of the PPIs reported in this review did enhance well-being.

16.4 Discussion

This scoping review aimed to explore and describe existing research on implementing PPIs in African countries. The results indicated that studies are still limited, even when the search was broadened through using more flexible criteria (see Ng & Lim, 2019; Schueller et al., 2014). Most studies followed quantitative designs, among adult participants, in group settings, and were implemented in South Africa. While Hendriks et al. (2019) pointed out the lack of research on PPIs in non-Western countries in general, our study further points to limited implementation of PPIs on the rest of the African continent beyond South Africa. This may be because until now, positive psychology as a field was not explicitly studied in most African countries (Eloff et al., 2008; Kim et al., 2018; Rao et al., 2015). Another possible reason could be that psychotherapeutic interventions in general are not widely included in mental health treatments in low and middle-income countries, such as those on the African continent (Rathod et al., 2017). Yet, studies in Tanzania and Kenia are starting to emerge.

Although several interventions were implemented among participants who may be more vulnerable to develop psychological distress, no studies were done among clinical populations. This finding supports previous research reporting that PPIs in clinical contexts were mostly conducted in Western countries (Chakhssi et al., 2018). Most interventions were delivered in group settings, but the content varied substantially. Just under a third of the studies implemented the more well-known PPIs, such as increasing gratitude or strength-based interventions, while the remaining interventions varied from reading stories to children (Theron et al., 2017; Wood et al., 2012) to psychotherapeutic strategies (Edwards & Edwards, 2009; Fourie & Guse, 2011; Guse et al., 2006). It is evident that activities to promote well-being in African contexts cover a broad range, unlike earlier narrower descriptions (e.g., Bolier et al., 2013).

The majority of studies explicitly aimed to increase well-being, with some focusing on either hedonic or eudaimonic well-being, or both. Therefore, there is some evidence of emerging research on SPPIs and MPPIs (Hendriks et al., 2020). In terms of outcomes, almost all studies reported increases in well-being, broadly defined, while some also found decreased psychological distress. Only two peer-reviewed studies failed to find positive outcomes, which may be due to publication bias (Franco et al., 2014; Hendriks et al., 2018).

Taking all into consideration, this scoping study suggests that implementation and evaluation of PPIs, broadly viewed, are starting to emerge. However, several research gaps need to be addressed in future studies. First, it is unclear to which extent PPIs were adapted to suit cultural contexts. Although several well-known positive activities were included in more than half of the studies identified in this review, there was limited information regarding the language used in the interventions or considerations given to cultural traditions and practices. It was thus difficult to establish culture-activity fit (Layous, 2018). Future studies could pay more attention to these elements when implementing and reporting on interventions. In addition, research is needed on how and when PPIs could be adapted to be implemented by community health workers. Through a process of task shifting (Rathod et al., 2017), where specific tasks are moved from highly qualified health professionals to health workers who received shorter training, PPIs could be useful in mental health promotion on a broader scale. This is especially important in in resource-constrained contexts, such as those in many African countries.

Second, there seems to be a lack of studies exploring the effect of PPIs on adolescents and children and most studies were implemented among adults. While this trend is also seen in international research (Gillham et al., 2019), young people constitute more than 50% of the population on the African continent (United Nations Economic Commission for Africa, 2016). It is crucial to develop and evaluate well-being interventions among African youth as positive mental health in adolescence seem to predict adult well-being (O'Connor et al., 2017). In addition, the current review also found an absence of research on interventions to enhance the well-being of older persons. Implementing PPIs among older adults could facilitate positive aging and contribute to associated individual and societal benefits (Bartholomaeus et al., 2019; Friedman et al., 2019). In terms of demographics, there were also no studies on PPIs among people diagnosed with psychological disorders. PPIs could be useful in supplementing existing treatment approaches to psychological disorders (Johnson & Wood, 2017; Ruini, 2017). International research pointed to promising results when implemented among people diagnosed with specific disorders such as mood disorders (Chaves et al., 2017), anxiety disorders (Ruini & Fava, 2009) and psychotic disorders (Sims et al., 2015). Since culture influences the prevalence and symptomatology of psychological disorders (Kirmayer & Ryder, 2016) it is evident that more research on implementing PPIs among clinical populations in the African context is needed.

Third, as research on PPIs in African contexts move forward, it is important to take note of existing criticism on the value of PPIs (e.g., Wong & Roy, 2017), and to pay careful attention to planning, structuring and reporting on interventions. Van Zyl et al. (2019) offered extensive guidelines for best practice in implementing PPIs, and we recommend considering these guidelines in future research. Robust and replicable studies are needed to advance knowledge on the effect of PPIs in individuals and groups on the African continent.

16.5 Conclusion

This scoping review found that African research on PPIs are limited but emerging. There is a need for more studies on the cultural adaptation of PPIs as well as for research among youth and older populations. We acknowledge that this review may have omitted relevant research not published in English, or that may have used other terms than those included in our search. However, through pointing out several research gaps, this study may contribute to further exploration of well-being interventions in the African context.

Acknowledgement I would like to acknowledge Lebogang Ramalepe and Maham Hassan for their assistance with the literature search for this review.

References[1]

Arksey, H., & O'Malley, L. (2005). Scoping studies: Towards a methodological framework. *International Journal of Social Research Methodology, 8*(1), 19–32. https://doi.org/10.1080/1364557032000119616

*Baranov, V., Haushofer, J., & Jang, C. (2020). Can positive psychology improve psychological wellbeing and economic decision-making? Experimental evidence from Kenya. *Economic Development and Cultural Change, 68,* 1345–1376. https://doi.org/10.1086/702860

Bartholomaeus, J. D., Van Agteren, J. E., Iasiello, M. P., Jarden, A., & Kelly, D. (2019). Positive aging: The impact of a community wellbeing and resilience program. *Clinical Gerontologist, 42*(4), 377–386. https://doi.org/10.1080/07317115.2018.1561582

*Berger, R., Benatov, J., Cuadros, R., VanNattan, J., & Gelkopf, M. (2018). Enhancing resiliency and promoting prosocial behavior among Tanzanian primary-school students: A school-based intervention. *Transcultural Psychiatry, 55*(6), 821–845. https://doi.org/10.1177/1363461518793749

Bolier, L., Haverman, M., Westerhof, G. J., Riper, H., Smit, F., & Bohlmeijer, E. (2013). Positive psychology interventions: A meta-analysis of randomized controlled studies. *BMC Public Health, 13*(1), 119.

*Bonthuys, A., Botha, K. F., Nienaber, A. W., Freeks, F. E., & Kruger, A. (2011). The effect of the Lifeplan® programme on the psychological wellbeing of a rural community in South Africa. *Journal of Psychology in Africa,* 21(3), 421–428. https://doi.org/10.1080/14330237.2011.10820476

Chakhssi, F., Kraiss, J. T., Sommers-Spijkerman, M., & Bohlmeijer, E. T. (2018). The effect of positive psychology interventions on Well-being and distress in clinical samples with psychiatric or somatic disorders: A systematic review and meta-analysis. *BMC Psychiatry, 18*(1), 211. https://doi.org/10.1186/s12888-018-1739-2

Chaves, C., Lopez-Gomez, I., Hervas, G., & Vazquez, C. (2017). A comparative study on the efficacy of a positive psychology intervention and a cognitive behavioral therapy for clinical depression. *Cognitive Therapy and Research, 41*(3), 417–433. https://doi.org/10.1007/s10608-016-9778-9

*Cherrington, A. M., & De Lange, N. (2016). 'I want to be a hope champion!'–Research as hope intervention with rural South African children. Journal of Psychology in Africa, 26(4), 373-378. doi:https://doi.org/10.1080/14330237.2016.1208954

*Chidrawi, H. C., Greeff, M., Temane, Q. M., & Ellis, S. (2015). Changeover-time in psychosocial wellbeing of people living with HIV and people living close to them after an HIV stigma reduction and wellness enhancement community intervention. *African Journal of AIDS Research, 14*(1), 1–12. https://doi.org/10.2989/16085906.2014.961940

Cunha, L. F., Pellanda, L. C., & Reppold, C. T. (2019). Positive psychology and gratitude interventions: A randomized clinical trial. *Frontiers in Psychology, 10,* 1–9. https://doi.org/10.3389/fpsyg.2019.00584

*Davies, J. C. (2015). *The effect of a positive psychology intervention on psychosocial wellbeing among a group of early adolescents* (Unpublished master's dissertation). University of Johannesburg.

*Dow, D. E., Mmbaga, B. T., Turner, E. L., Gallis, J. A., Tabb, Z. J., Cunningham, C. K., & O'Donnell, K. E. (2018). Building resilience: A mental health intervention for Tanzanian youth living with HIV. *AIDS Care, 30*(Suppl 4), 12–20. https://doi.org/10.1080/09540121.2018.1527008

Dyrbye, L. N., West, C. P., Richards, M. L., Ross, H. J., Satele, D., & Shanafelt, T. D. (2016). A randomized, controlled study of an online intervention to promote job satisfaction and well-

[1]References preceded by an asterisk were included in the scoping review.

being among physicians. *Burnout Research, 3*(3), 69–75. https://doi.org/10.1016/j.burn.2016.06.002

*Edwards, S. D., & Edwards, D. J. (2009). Counselling for psychological well-being in persons living with HIV/AIDS. *Journal of Psychology in Africa, 19*(4), 561–563. https://doi.org/10.1080/14330237.2009.10820329

Eloff, I., Achoui, M., Chireshe, R., Mutepfa, M., & Ofovwe, C. (2008). Views from Africa on positive psychology. *Journal of Psychology in Africa, 18*(1), 189–194. https://doi.org/10.1080/14330237.2008.10820185

*Eloff, I., Finestone, M., Makin, J. D., Boeving-Allen, A., Visser, M., Ebersöhn, L., Sikkema, F. R., Briggs-Gowan, M. J., & Forsyth, B. W. (2014). A randomized clinical trial of an intervention to promote resilience in young children of HIV-positive mothers in South Africa. *AIDS, 28*(03), S347–S357. https://doi.org/10.1097/QAD.0000000000000335

*Fourie, G., & Guse, T. (2011). An integrated hypnotherapeutic model for the treatment of childhood sexual trauma: A case study. *American Journal of Clinical Hypnosis, 53*(3), 193–205.

Franco, A., Malhotra, N., & Simonovits, G. (2014). Publication bias in the social sciences: Unlocking the file drawer. *Science, 345*(6203), 1502–1505. https://doi.org/10.1126/science.1255484

Friedman, E. M., Ruini, C., Foy, C. R., Jaros, L., Love, G., & Ryff, C. D. (2019). Lighten UP! A community-based group intervention to promote eudaimonic well-being in older adults: A multi-site replication with 6 month follow-up. *Clinical Gerontologist, 42*(4), 387–397. https://doi.org/10.1080/07317115.2019.1574944

Gander, F., Proyer, R. T., Ruch, W., & Wyss, T. (2013). Strength-based positive interventions: Further evidence for their potential in enhancing well-being and alleviating depression. *Journal of Happiness Studies, 14*(4), 1241–1259. https://doi.org/10.1007/s10902-012-9380-0

Gillham, J., Leventhal, K. S., Rashid, T., Anjum, A., & Leventhal, S. (2019). Positive psychology programs for youth in diverse communities. In L. E. Van Zyl & S. Rothmann (Eds.), *Evidence-based positive psychological interventions in multi-cultural contexts* (pp. 197–225). Springer.

*Grobler, L. (2012). *An exploration of the use of positive psychology movies to enhance wellbeing* (Unpublished master's dissertation). North West University.

*Guse, T., Wissing, M., & Hartman, W. (2006). The effect of a prenatal hypnotherapeutic programme on postnatal maternal psychological well-being. *Journal of Reproductive and Infant Psychology, 24*(2), 163–177. https://doi.org/10.1080/02646830600644070

*Hatzipapas, I., Visser, M. J., & Janse van Rensburg, E. (2017). Laughter therapy as an intervention to promote psychological well-being of volunteer community care workers working with HIV-affected families. *SAHARA-J: Journal of Social Aspects of HIV/AIDS, 14*(1), 202–212. https://doi.org/10.1080/17290376.2017.1402696

Hendriks, T., Schotanus-Dijkstra, M., Hassankhan, A., De Jong, J., & Bohlmeijer, E. (2020). The efficacy of multi-component positive psychology interventions: A systematic review and meta-analysis of randomized controlled trials. *Journal of Happiness Studies, 21*(1), 357–390. https://doi.org/10.1007/s10902-019-00082-1

Hendriks, T., Schotanus-Dijkstra, M., Hassankhan, A., Graafsma, T., Bohlmeijer, E., & De Jong, J. (2018). The efficacy of positive psychology interventions from non-Western countries: A systematic review and meta-analysis. *International Journal of Wellbeing, 8*(1), 71–98. https://doi.org/10.5502/ijw.v8i1.71

Hendriks, T., Warren, M. A., Schotanus-Dijkstra, M., Hassankhan, A., Graafsma, T., Bohlmeijer, E., & De Jong, J. (2019). How WEIRD are positive psychology interventions? A bibliometric analysis of randomized controlled trials on the science of well-being. *The Journal of Positive Psychology, 14*(4), 489–501. https://doi.org/10.1080/17439760.2018.1484941

Johnson, J., & Wood, A. M. (2017). Integrating positive and clinical psychology: Viewing human functioning as continua from positive to negative can benefit clinical assessment, interventions and understandings of resilience. *Cognitive Therapy and Research, 41*(3), 335–349. https://doi.org/10.1007/s10608-015-9728-y

Keyes, C. L. M. (2005). Mental illness and/or mental health? Investigating axioms of the complete state model of health. *Journal of Consulting and Clinical Psychology, 73*, 539–548.

Kim, H., Doiron, K., Warren, M. A., & Donaldson, S. I. (2018). The international landscape of positive psychology research: A systematic review. *International Journal of Wellbeing, 8*(1), 50–70. https://doi.org/10.5502/ijw.v8i1.651

Kirmayer, L. J., & Ryder, A. G. (2016). Culture and psychopathology. *Current Opinion in Psychology, 8*, 143–148. https://doi.org/10.1016/j.copsyc.2015.10.020

*Kruger, T. (2013). *The effect of gratitude interventions on the psychological wellbeing of a group of adolescents in Gauteng* (Unpublished master's dissertation). University of Johannesburg.

Lai, S. T., & O'Carroll, R. E. (2017). 'The three good things' – The effects of gratitude practice on wellbeing: A randomised controlled trial. *Health Psychology Update, 26*, 10–18.

Layous, K. (2018). Malleability and intentional activities. In E. Diener, S. Oishi, & L. Tay (Eds.), *Handbook of well-being*. DEF Publishers.

Layous, K., & Lyubomirsky, S. (2014). The how, why, what, when, and who of happiness: Mechanisms underlying the success of positive interventions. In J. Gruber & J. Moscowitz (Eds.), *Positive emotion: Integrating the light sides and dark sides* (pp. 473–495). Oxford University Press.

Loveday, P. M., Lovell, G. P., & Jones, C. M. (2018). The best possible selves intervention: A review of the literature to evaluate efficacy and guide future research. *Journal of Happiness Studies, 19*(2), 607–628. https://doi.org/10.1007/s10902-016-9824-z

*Marsay, G., Scioli, A., & Omar, S. (2018). A hope-infused future orientation intervention: A pilot study with juvenile offenders in South Africa. *British Journal of Guidance & Counselling, 46*(6), 709–721. https://doi.org/10.1080/03069885.2018.1480011.

*Miano, P. W. (2016). *Positive psychology interventions in a student counselling centre: An exploratory study* (Unpublished master's dissertation). Nelson Mandela Metropolitan University.

Munn, Z., Peters, M. D., Stern, C., Tufanaru, C., McArthur, A., & Aromataris, E. (2018). Systematic review or scoping review? Guidance for authors when choosing between a systematic or scoping review approach. *BMC Medical Research Methodology, 18*(1), 143. https://doi.org/10.1186/s12874-018-0611-x

Myers, N. D., Prilleltensky, I., Prilleltensky, O., McMahon, A., Dietz, S., & Rubenstein, C. L. (2017). Efficacy of the fun for wellness online intervention to promote multidimensional well-being: A randomized controlled trial. *Prevention Science, 18*(8), 984–994. https://doi.org/10.1007/s11121-017-0779-z

Ng, W., & Lim, W. S. (2019). Developing positive psychological interventions: Maximizing efficacy for use in Eastern cultures. In L. E. Van Zyl & S. Rothmann (Eds.), *Positive psychological intervention design and protocols for multi-cultural contexts* (pp. 277–295). Springer.

O'Connor, M., Sanson, A. V., Toumbourou, J. W., Norrish, J., & Olsson, C. A. (2017). Does positive mental health in adolescence longitudinally predict healthy transitions in young adulthood? *Journal of Happiness Studies, 18*(1), 177–198. https://doi.org/10.1007/s10902-016-9723-3

Parks, A. C., & Biswas-Diener, R. (2013). Positive interventions: Past, present, and future. In T. Kashdan & J. Ciarrochi (Eds.), *Mindfulness, acceptance, and positive psychology: The seven foundations of well-being* (pp. 140–165). Context Press.

Peterson, C., & Seligman, M. E. P. (2004). *Character strengths and virtues: A handbook and classification*. American Psychological Association.

*Pretorius, C., Venter, C., Temane, M., & Wissing, M. (2008). The design and evaluation of a hope enhancement programme for adults. *Journal of Psychology in Africa, 18*(2), 301–308. https://doi.org/10.1080/14330237.2008.10820202

Quoidbach, J., Berry, E. V., Hansenne, M., & Mikolajczak, M. (2010). Positive emotion regulation and well-being: Comparing the impact of eight savoring and dampening strategies. *Personality and Individual Differences, 49*(5), 368–373. https://doi.org/10.1016/j.paid.2010.03.048

Rao, M. A., Donaldson, S. I., & Doiron, K. M. (2015). Positive psychology research in the Middle East and North Africa. *Middle East Journal of Positive Psychology, 1*(1), 60–76.

Rashid, T. (2009). Positive interventions in clinical practice. *Journal of Clinical Psychology, 65*(5), 461–466. https://doi.org/10.1002/jclp.20588

Rathod, S., Pinninti, N., Irfan, M., Gorczynski, P., Rathod, P., Gega, L., & Naeem, F. (2017). Mental health service provision in low-and middle-income countries. *Health Services Insights*. https://doi.org/10.1177/1178632917694350

Ruini, C. (2017). *Positive psychology in the clinical domains: Research and practice*. Springer.

Ruini, C., & Fava, G. A. (2009). Well-being therapy for generalized anxiety disorder. *Journal of Clinical Psychology, 65*(5), 510–519. https://doi.org/10.1002/jclp.20592

Ryff, C. D. (1989). Happiness is everything, or is it? Explorations on the meaning of psychological well-being. *Journal of Personality and Social Psychology, 57*(6), 1069–1081. https://doi.org/10.1037/0022-3514.57.6.1069

Schueller, S. M., Kashdan, T. B., & Parks, A. C. (2014). Synthesizing positive psychological interventions: Suggestions for conducting and interpreting meta-analyses. *International Journal of Wellbeing, 4*(1), 91–98. https://doi.org/10.5502/ijw.v4i1.5

Schueller, S. M., & Parks, A. C. (2014). The science of self-help: Translating positive psychology research into increased individual happiness. *European Psychologist, 19*(2), 145–155. https://doi.org/10.1027/1016-9040/a000181

Scioli, A., & Biller, H. B. (2009). *Hope in the age of anxiety*. Oxford University Press.

Seligman, M. E., & Csikszentmihalyi, M. (2000). Positive psychology: An introduction. *American Psychologist, 55*(1), 5–14. https://doi.org/10.1037//0003-066X.55.1.5

Seligman, M. E., Rashid, T., & Parks, A. C. (2006). Positive psychotherapy. *American Psychologist, 61*(8), 774–778.

Shin, L. J., & Lyubomirsky, S. (2017). Increasing well-being in independent and interdependent cultures. In M. A. Warren & S. I. Donaldson (Eds.), *Scientific advances in positive psychology* (pp. 11–36). Praeger.

Sims, A., Barker, C., Price, C., & Fornells-Ambrojo, M. (2015). Psychological impact of identifying character strengths in people with psychosis. *Psychosis, 7*(2), 179–182. https://doi.org/10.1080/17522439.2014.925485

Sin, N. L., & Lyubomirsky, S. (2009). Enhancing well-being and alleviating depressive symptoms with positive psychology interventions: A practice-friendly meta-analysis. *Journal of Clinical Psychology, 65*(5), 467–487. https://doi.org/10.1002/jclp.20593

Smith, J. L., & Hanni, A. A. (2019). Effects of a savoring intervention on resilience and well-being of older adults. *Journal of Applied Gerontology, 38*(1), 137–152. https://doi.org/10.1177/0733464817693375

Struck, R., Baumgarten, G., & Wittmann, M. (2014). Cost-efficiency of knowledge creation: Randomized controlled trials vs. observational studies. *Current Opinion in Anesthesiology, 27*(2), 190–194. https://doi.org/10.1097/ACO.0000000000000060

*Teodorczuk, K., Guse, T., & Du Plessis, G. A. (2019). The effect of positive psychology interventions on hope and well-being of adolescents living in a child and youth care centre. *British Journal of Guidance & Counselling, 47*(2), 234–245. https://doi.org/10.1080/03069885.2018.1504880

*Theron, L., Cockcroft, K., & Wood, L. (2017). The resilience-enabling value of African folktales: The read-me-to-resilience intervention. *School Psychology International, 38*(5), 491–506. https://doi.org/10.1177/0143034317719941

United Nations Economic Commission for Africa. (2016). *The demographic profile of African countries*. UNECA.

*Van der Smit, E. (2015). *A computer-based self-help programme facilitating anger management using positive activity interventions* (Unpublished doctoral thesis). North West University.

*Van Schalkwyk, I., & Wissing, M. P. (2013). Evaluation of a programme to enhance flourishing in adolescents. In M.P. Wissing (Ed.), *Wellbeing research in South Africa* (pp. 581–605). Springer.

Van Zyl, L. E., Efendic, E., Rothmann, S., & Shankland, R. (2019). Best-practice guidelines for positive psychological intervention research design. In L. E. Van Zyl & S. Rothmann (Eds.), *Positive psychological intervention design and protocols for multi-cultural contexts* (pp. 1–32). Springer.

*Van Zyl, L. E., & Rothmann, S. (2012). Beyond smiling: The evaluation of a positive psychological intervention aimed at student happiness. *Journal of Psychology in Africa, 22*(3), 369–384. https://doi.org/10.1080/14330237.2012.10820541.

Weiss, L. A., Westerhof, G. J., & Bohlmeijer, E. T. (2016). Can we increase psychological well-being? The effects of interventions on psychological well-being: A meta-analysis of randomized controlled trials. *PLoS One, 11*(6), e0158092.

White, C. A., Uttl, B., & Holder, M. D. (2019). Meta-analyses of positive psychology interventions: The effects are much smaller than previously reported. *PLoS One, 14*(5), e0216588. https://doi.org/10.1371/journal.pone.0216588

Wong, P. T. P., & Roy, S. (2017). Critique of positive psychology and positive interventions. In N. J. L. Brown, T. Lomas, & F. J. Eiroa-Orosa (Eds.), *The Routledge international handbook of critical positive psychology* (pp. 142–160). Routledge.

*Wood, L., Theron, L., & Mayaba, N. (2012). 'Read me to resilience': Exploring the use of cultural stories to boost the positive adjustment of children orphaned by AIDS. *African Journal of AIDS Research, 11*(3), 225–239. https://doi.org/10.2989/16085906.2012.734982.

Chapter 17
Community-Based Interventions to Improve Well-Being of Youth in a High-Risk Community in South Africa: Researcher's Experiences and Implementation Outcomes

Izanette van Schalkwyk

Abstract While the contribution of research conducted within positive psychology is acknowledged, this sub-discipline of psychology is criticised for its "limited utility" in the South African context. The researcher's continuous involvement and knowledge from practice and practical field experiences obtained from more than 10 years of connecting with community members living in a high-risk context opened doors for meaningful and engaged research. This chapter describes experiences and implementation outcomes based on positive psychology in a high-risk community in the South African context. Drawing on various well-being research studies conducted within the selected high-risk community, research findings are described to illustrate the outcomes of the implementation of a sustainable well-being programme, its progress over time, and lessons learned in the process. The well-being of children, families, and schools in a Western Cape high-risk community is seriously challenged as they are continuously exposed to a "hostile environment". While the negative effects of poverty and many social ills are confirmed by research, the need for contextually appropriate positive psychology interventions to mitigate the psychological consequences of economic deprivation is clear. Engaging with vulnerable groups is important to enable the generation of well-being interventions at the community level in the South African context.

Keywords Positive psychology intervention · Implementation · Well-being programme · High-risk community · South Africa

I. van Schalkwyk (✉)
Africa Unit for Transdisciplinary Health Research (AUTHeR), Faculty of Health Sciences, North-West University, South Africa
e-mail: 20977026@nwu.ac.za

L. Schutte et al. (eds.), *Embracing Well-Being in Diverse African Contexts: Research Perspectives*, Cross-Cultural Advancements in Positive Psychology 16,
https://doi.org/10.1007/978-3-030-85924-4_17

17.1 A Well-Being Programme

Positive psychological interventions (PPIs) offer strategies and practices in the protection and promotion of mental health (Baños et al., 2017). Van Zyl et al. (2019) refer to the need for best practices in PPI research design in order to promote the applied nature of positive psychology (PP). While the contribution of research conducted within PP is acknowledged (Mahali et al., 2018), this sub-discipline of psychology is criticised for its "limited utility" in the South African context (Kagee, 2014, p. 357). Prilleltensky (2012) connotes the ignoring of context as a shortcoming of PP, and he opines that it offers a set of tools to promote flow, meaning, and thriving for people who are enjoying favourable circumstances. Recently, Van Zyl et al. (2019) also referred to such criticism and underlying methodological concerns for quantitative research as the lack of replicability and poor effectiveness of PPIs due to specific problems, such as evaluating the effectiveness of programmes. Apart from criticism regarding PPIs and issues related to the scientific process, such statements imply that PP might be of little use in the Global South where millions of people suffer from material deprivations or serious injustice. Therefore, when we consider the application of PPIs or well-being programmes in the South African context, contextual factors must be taken into account, since the inequality within this society is extreme (Ebersöhn, 2015; Ebersöhn et al., 2018; Statistics South Africa, 2018b/2019; The World Bank, 2018).

Involvement in a voluntary capacity to facilitate various community projects aimed at encouraging resilient youth (learners in schools), positive school communities, and competent families offered this researcher valuable opportunities for the building of trust, insightful encounters, and many learnt lessons. During more than 10 years of personal encounters with community members, she obtained practical experience of and insight into the resources and risks of a particular high-risk community in the Western Cape of South Africa.

A well-being programme refers to specific scientific tools and functional strategies that focus on the enhancement of well-being and increased levels of prosocial behaviour (Keyes, 2002; Norrish & Vella-Brodrick, 2009). In alignment with the aim of PP to promote facets of well-being/mental health (van Schalkwyk & Wissing, 2013), the use of the term 'well-being programme' indicates those intentional efforts to optimise positive human health within this particular context. Setbacks in life are rather commonplace for millions of children (Masten, 2015; Theron et al., 2011; Ungar, 2015; UNICEF, 2016), especially when they are dealing with multiple adversities in their context of development (Ebersöhn et al., 2018). It is commendable that in our current socio-political framework, the legal status of South African children is given the highest priority (Savahl et al., 2015). Also, the South African government has ratified the Sustainable Development Goals (SDGs) 2030, adding to the existing efforts in this country towards promoting such development goals (Jamieson et al., 2017). Clearly, scientific efforts to enhance the well-being of South African youth warrant prime attention.

Since all intervention takes place in a specific context (Lachman et al., 2016), this researcher offers information to illustrate the impact of lack in terms of objective indicators of well-being for persons and families living in an urban disadvantaged community called Delft. The influence of lack in terms of these objective indicators of well-being is central to positive functioning, with the objective indicators referring to aspects such as monetary income, employment, shelter, safety, and health (Prilleltensky, 2012). In South Africa, the incidence of low socioeconomic position (SEP), as indicated by these objective indicators of well-being, is evident; for example, (a) The World bank report (2018) stated that absolute poverty is increasing in South Africa to the extent that between 2011 and 2015, poverty rates increased and the level of poverty became deeper and society became more unequal; (b) South Africa is one of three countries where unemployment rates have increased over the past 20 years to the extent that the unemployment rate of youth aged 15–24 years (the most vulnerable in the South African labour market) was 55.2% in the first quarter of 2019 (StatsSA, 2019) and the unemployment rate of adults was 29% in the second quarter of 2019 (StatsSA, 2019); (c) 63% of SA children are growing up in households with mostly one female adult (van Schalkwyk, 2020); (d) the seriousness of gangsterism and its offering of an economic alternative by, for example, selling drugs are increasing (Jones, 2019); (e) with approximately 20% of people living with HIV (PLWH) in the world, the largest number of PLWH in the world reside in South Africa (7.1 million; UNAIDS, 2017); and (f) in challenging contexts like Delft in the Western Cape of South Africa, problematic alcohol and other drug (AOD) use is prevalent and associated with poor HIV treatment and secondary HIV prevention outcomes (Magidson et al., 2019). In the following section, specific information is given about Delft which is a disadvantaged community where the negative impacts of the abovementioned factors are commonplace.

17.2 Delft, a Disadvantaged Community

Formerly disadvantaged communities were called townships (Theron, 2007). In South Africa, townships have their origin in the apartheid era, and this term is commonly used to describe mostly poorly resourced urban areas that were reserved for black, coloured, or Indian people (Theron & Theron, 2010). Townships are still home to mostly non-white poorer citizens (Geldenhuys & van Schalkwyk, 2019). Delft was established under the apartheid regime as part of residential racial segregation known as the Group Areas Act (Seekings, 2011). Aside from the physical segregation or "apartheid" of groups of people, the apartheid regime also aimed to accomplish a clear racial hierarchy (Seekings, 2011). Unfortunately, these townships did not disappear after 1994 and the legacy of inequality persists in such communities (Pohl, 2018). Also, post-apartheid townships consist mainly of government housing and informal settlements, which have increased significantly (Mahajan, 2014). In townships and informal settlements, the incidence of serious challenges includes poverty, unemployment, crime, and high rates of communicable diseases such as HIV (Mathews & Benvenuti, 2014; van Lennep, 2019). The compounding effects of these conditions place many communities at risk, and exert a crucial challenge for the well-being of families and, moreover, the well-being of children.

17.2.1 Delft, a High-Risk Community

Delft is classified as one of 20 identified high-risk South African communities (Delft census, 2011). While the lack of adequate infrastructure is frequently mentioned in the description of a high-risk community, serious challenges associated with unemployment and limited employment opportunities are critical issues in these communities (Felner & de Vries, 2013). In the Delft-area, specific risks include high levels of crime, gangsterism and gangster-related violence, dysfunctional families (van Schalkwyk, 2019), domestic violence, abusive drinking (May et al., 2013), murder, rape, school dropouts, and poverty (Crime Stats SA, 2018). Recently, Delft has been categorised as one of the ten most dangerous areas in South Africa (Crime Stats SA, 2018), and it was selected to be one of the ten communities in the Cape Flats for intervention by the South African Defence Force to counteract gangster violence and killing (Son Digitaal, 2019). While this information could aid to depict this community, it is important to emphasise the risks endemic to living in this high-risk context.

17.2.2 Implications of Living in a High-Risk Community

Young people, families, and schools in Delft are subject to multiple risks that include "... poor health, under- or malnourishment, an absence or erratic supply of electricity, education backlogs, disrupted schooling, an unsupportive home environment, limited social status, language barriers, violence, technological delays (e.g., limited electrical infrastructure and limited or no access to computers and the internet), substance abuse, and a dim view of the future" (van Schalkwyk, 2020, p. 62). For many families, the sudden and often untimely death of a child is not uncommon (Malherbe, 2019; Son Digitaal, 2019). In the formal 2019 South African Police Service (SAPS) annual report, it was stated that most of these murders were gangster-related (South African Police Service annual report, 2018/2019). The majority of the risks and social ills in Delft are associated with poverty, which limits access to food and shelter and is associated with poorer scholastic functioning and psychological vulnerability or low levels of well-being (Grimova & van Schalkwyk, 2016; Hamman & Kruger, 2017; Naidoo & van Schalkwyk, 2021).

Besides poverty, Delft is associated with mostly overcrowded residences and family members having little personal space (van Schalkwyk, 2019). The practical implications of such conditions are, for example, high noise levels which makes studying difficult for youth in school (Naidoo & van Schalkwyk, 2021). Despite some promising relief offered by formal education institutes, the history of violence seriously obstructs schooling in South Africa in fulfilling its mandate (Chipkin & Meny-Gibert, 2013; Heywood, 2020). In Delft, most children at primary and secondary schools have experienced some form of violence while being at school, most commonly threats of violence, robbery, and attacks. These experiences of the learners are substantiated by Delft school principals who point out that many youngsters have become socialised to cope with challenges in aggressive or violent ways (Mr Jansen, school principal in Delft, personal conversation, June, 2019; Jones, 2019).

The use of aggression also refers to women, including young women, who are involved in female gangs (social worker in Delft, personal conversation, May, 2019). When adolescent girls are dealing daily with poverty, fractured families, and mothers having problems with substance abuse or addiction, "...they get drawn in by the gangs that saturate their communities" (Pohl, 2018, p. 28). The troubling effect of gangsterism—common to most communities across the world—is linked to poverty and marginalisation (van Schalkwyk, 2020). Pinnock (2016) indicated the severely limited options of community members for making a living, especially youth, who often consider gangs as their only workable option for survival. In communities like Delft where the disintegration of community structures is evident, gangs form and recruit local youths (Roloff, 2014). Pinnock (2016) states that adolescents' need to establish a sense of belonging and identity in dysfunctional ways, such as gangsterism, is a result of society's failure to provide opportunities for youth to do so in a constructive manner.

As a result of the risks endemic to township living, such as in Delft, youth are in crisis (Jamieson et al., 2017), families are in crisis (Department of Social Development, 2013), schools are in crisis (Bylieveldt et al., in press), and communities are in crisis (Isaacs & Roman, 2018; Lazarus et al., 2014). Contextually, this provides a bleak picture for resilient youth functioning in challenging settings such as Delft, due to the ongoing crisis of structures that should serve as protective factors (Geldenhuys & van Schalkwyk, 2020).

However, while it is well-documented that many South African youth face cumulative risk, we need to heed Seligman's (2002) caution that pathologising does not move us closer to the prevention of serious disorders and dysfunction. Therefore, we argue that intentional efforts in the format of a well-being programme are crucial to encourage resilience, empowerment, and positive functioning in the face of these multiple risks (Savahl et al., 2015). South African studies show that if the well-being of youth, such as those dwelling in townships, is intentionally protected and promoted, they can be equipped with skills enabling them towards higher levels of psychological, social, and relational well-being (Van Schalkwyk & Wissing, 2013; Geldenhuys & van Schalkwyk, 2019). The fundamentals of PP imply that the dynamics of human strengths are most likely to enhance higher levels of wellness while safeguarding against mental illness (Seligman, 2011).

Drawing on various well-being research studies conducted within Delft, research findings are described to illustrate the outcomes of the implementation of a sustainable well-being programme, its progress over time, and lessons learned in the process.

17.3 Method

17.3.1 Positive Psychology, the Theoretical Framework

The broad conceptual framework of PP allows for the development of interventions focusing on human strengths and individuals' potential, and Seligman and Csikszentmihalyi (2000) clarified that PP is about the study of the conditions and processes that contribute to the flourishing or optimal functioning of people, groups, and institutions. The main areas of study can be grouped into four categories: (a) positive emotions (e.g., happiness, gratitude, and flow) and their effects on psychological and physical functioning; (b) positive individual traits (e.g., values and talents) and their protective role in different physical and psychological disorders; (c) positive interpersonal relationships (e.g., friendship, romantic relations, and marriage); and (d) positive institutions (e.g., family, school, and business/workplace; Baños et al., 2017). PPIs represent those intentional activities that aim to cultivate positive feelings, cognition, and behaviours (Sin & Lyubomirsky, 2009; van Zyl et al., 2019). The use of specific activities (e.g., counting your blessings, practising kindness, expressing gratitude, and using personal strengths) which have demonstrated empirically to increase positive emotions, satisfaction with life, or other positive states is integral to PPIs. In this sense, these planned interventions contribute to the promotion of well-being and health through activities focusing on positive emotions and behaviours (Lyubomirsky, 2008).

17.3.2 Evidence-Based Programme

An evidence-based well-being programme was designed and evaluated in the South African context (van Schalkwyk, 2009; van Schalkwyk & Wissing, 2013). The focal point of the well-being programme was to encourage higher levels of well-being and, in time, sustainable well-being in adolescents by means of the deliberate development of selected psychological strengths (Park & Peterson, 2009; Peterson, 2006). The well-being strategy consisted of ten sessions and was based on Keyes's (2005, 2006, 2007) model of complete well-being, with special emphasis on the psychological dimension: Session 1: Grand strategy and functional strategies; session 2: Dimensions of well-being: psychological/personal, social and emotional; session 3: Psychological strengths and the role of values; session 4: Self-acceptance (psychological dimension) and gratitude (strength); session 5: Autonomy (psychological well-being) and self-regulation (strength); session 6: Positive relations with others (psychological well-being) and kindness (strength); session 7: Environmental mastery (psychological well-being) and wisdom (strength); session 8: purpose-in-life (psychological dimension) and persistence (strength); session 9: Personal growth (psychological well-being) and enthusiasm (strength); and session 10: Recapitulation of well-being components and psychological strengths (van Schalkwyk & Wissing, 2013, p. 585).

The content of the well-being programme as a plan of action was built on existing knowledge (Baltes & Freund, 2003; Deci & Ryan, 2002; Fredrickson, 2009; Keyes, 2005, 2006, 2007, 2009; Linley et al., 2006; Lyubomirsky, Sheldon, & Schkade, 2005; Peterson, 2006; Smith, 2006; Yates & Masten, 2004). Strengths were selected from six categories of character strengths and virtues (see Peterson & Seligman in van Schalkwyk & Wissing, 2013, p. 585), namely gratitude, self-regulation, kindness, perspective, persistence, and enthusiasm. These strengths were considered to be of primary importance for the promotion of sustainable well-being in youth. The programme was based on the principle that the building of personal resources entails the mastering of specified skills, which should be implemented on a daily basis. Habit formation was central to this process to acquire high well-being over time.

Since 2009, this programme has been adapted and implemented in most Delft school communities to enhance learners'/students' resilient living, and has been extended progressively to encourage competent families, better performing schools, and, ultimately, a stronger and safer community. The implementation of the well-being programme also generated various research studies conducted within Delft using the theoretical framework of PP. These research studies (discussed below) used quantitative, qualitative, and mixed methods approaches to investigate personal, relational, and collective well-being, and their findings informed adaptations to the well-being programme towards more relevant implementation and sustainability.

17.3.3 Research Studies Conducted in Delft

Research conducted in Delft investigated core components related to adolescents' positive functioning and those structures/institutions central to their well-being, namely adolescents' personal and relational well-being (Geldenhuys & van Schalkwyk, 2019; Geldenhuys & van Schalkwyk, 2020); adolescents' experiences of fatherlessness (Louw, 2014); the involvement of early adolescents' primary caregivers in their school community (Cronjé-Malan & van Schalkwyk, 2015); educators' experiences of their relationships with adolescents involved in drug use in the Delft community (Walton et al., 2016); exploring the resilience of female educators who are in leadership positions (Bylieveldt et al., in press); adolescent learners' perceptions and experiences of respect in educator-learner relationships (Grimova & van Schalkwyk, 2016); grade 9 learners and the role of career maturity for academic success (Naidoo et al., 2019); research about families, exploring the challenges and strengths of mothers with substance-problems to strengthen these female-headed households (van Schalkwyk, 2019), and married couples' perceptions of relational strengths (Nortjé et al., submitted). In summary, research looked at adolescents' levels of personal well-being; learners dealing with substances (complications for personal well-being and health); relational well-being and relations within the school community regarding the role of parents/legal guardians or caregivers; the role of educators and educators' well-being with particular reference to their resilient coping; and the challenges and strengths of families in Delft.

17.3.4 Facets and Outcomes of the Well-Being Programme

Since PP is about those factors that encourage well-being and the active development of personal, relational, and collective strengths or resources (see Seligman, 1998), the proposed facets and outcomes of the well-being programme entail particular aspects relating to this context, namely (a) mastering the language of well-being and strengths (including skills) in contrast to a vernacular focused on ill-being, lack, and deficiency—this focus entails the capacity-building processes founded upon character strengths and virtues conceived as moral competencies to guide this progression; (b) the continuous growth of the well-being programme with the aim of ensuring sustainability and overcoming constant challenges; (c) the key role of relational competencies; (d) long-term progress and positive outcomes in terms of learners'/students' school and life success; (e) strengthening the family unit; and (f) building a strong community (inside out). This growth-focused process in the presentation of the well-being programme to the Delft community in the long term is in contrast to a framework associated mainly with ill-being and deficiency.

17.3.4.1 Mastering of the Language of Well-Being and Strengths

The primary outcome of the implementation of the well-being programme in Delft can be rendered as mastering the language of well-being and strengths in a context of ill-being and lack. Particular practices of psychological strengths offer the key to establish a fortogenic approach in this community. This point of departure provides a foundation to all projects of the well-being programme and represents the motivation for all research conducted up to date in Delft within the framework of PP as "the scientific study of optimal human functioning that aims to discover and promote the factors that allow individuals and communities to thrive" (Seligman & Csikszentmihalyi, 2000, p. 13).

Despite wide acknowledgement that individuals should be informed on the best available evidence about living well, translating research into practice is challenging (Curtis et al., 2016). Therefore, the implementation of the evidence-based well-being programme in Delft requires some continued adjusting by taking into account practical concerns or structural barriers (see Sect. 17.3.5). While the programmatic content is valid, we converted or translated the identified objectives (identified character strengths) into specific targets (well-being practices). This process was guided by an interactive participatory approach to allow the input of community members. The following character strengths were considered to be positive principles for a life well lived: respect, honesty, helpfulness, excellence, empowerment, and self-discipline (Park & Peterson, 2009; Peterson, 2006; Peterson & Seligman, 2004; Smith, 2006). These were used in a first and fundamental project called the "Positive Principle Project" (Wissing et al., 2020).

The well-being practices are implemented via particular projects, called clubs, to encourage a healthy sense of belonging and mattering (Lambert et al., 2013). Keys for success are integral to these clubs, such as the deliberate use of positive emotions, social support, timing and variety, plus commitment and repetition (cf. Lyubomirsky, 2008). The effective application of these keys is the determining factor to guide adolescents' decision making and behaviour. The intentional use of character strengths and virtues (see positive principles), conceived as moral competencies, is central to guide this process to attain prosocial behaviour (Haidt, 2006; Lent, 2004). This point of departure is based on the systematic development of psychological strengths by means of specific activities to acquire the skills as associated with selected strengths (Fredrickson, 2009; Lyubomirsky, 2008; Lyubomirsky & Layous, 2013; Seligman, 2011). For example, learners/students obtain information in a concrete way about strengths, such as self-regulation, and this strength is developed by the mastering of specific skills, taking into account the role of extra-psychological factors, such as contextual vulnerabilities and children's poor concentration caused by being hungry (objective indicators of well-being). In brief: The use of a well-being-focused language entails an strong and honest awareness of factors related to flourishing as factors promoting well-being (Keyes, 2005).

17.3.4.2 Emergence of Projects

The main content of the well-being programme, that is, building psychological, emotional, and social capacity through the intentional use of selected character strengths, resulted in various other projects (on demand of the community). The following projects have emerged in Delft since 2010: the Positive Principle Project to direct positive functioning and prosocial behaviour (Park & Peterson, 2009; Peterson, 2006; Peterson & Seligman, 2004; Smith, 2006); Princess Club to encourage pregnant adolescents towards healthy behaviour and the avoidance of substance use (Smith, 2006); Music and Choir Club to support learners towards the actualisation of life potential (Peterson & Seligman, 2004; Seligman, 2011); Prayer Club to encourage learners' spiritual well-being and purpose in life (Keyes, 2005, 2007); Reading Club (primary schools) and Success Club (secondary schools) to enhance learners' academic performance (Keyes, 2007); Mothers Clubs to strengthen families (Department of Social Development, 2013), mothers' personal functioning (Peterson & Seligman, 2004), and mothers' parenting skills (Wessels et al., 2016); Maths Club to encourage learners' academic success, particularly in terms of improved mathematical success (Park & Peterson, 2009; Smith, 2006); Stars Club for female adolescents towards positive womanhood; Kings Club for male adolescents toward positive man- and fatherhood; and Rugby Club to develop male and female adolescents' physical health and rugby skills (Keyes, 2005, 2007; Smith, 2006). The growth of the projects of the well-being programme in Delft can be illustrated, for example, by describing how the Kings Club developed. Most South African children do not live with both parents (Statistics South Africa, 2018a) and in Delft, children mostly grow up with their mothers and/or grandmothers (van Schalkwyk, 2019). This means that many children in this community experience either a father being "absent", or fatherlessness; that is, not knowing the biological father at all. Louw (2014) conducted research about adolescents' experiences of fatherlessness and indicated that adolescents living in Delft often have negative experiences related to the absence of fathers: *"First of all we made our own statistics we put it in 85% fathers in Delft are irresponsible, careless, selfish, useless, cowards"* (Louw, 2014, p. 21). Louw (2014) also indicates adolescents' positive outlook on some fathers in the Delft community as father figures: *"A father figure here around in Delft is and in my community are not only fathers to their children but as well into the community"* (p. 22). These findings imply the need for father figures to step up and lead the way for the development of strong and healthy adolescents. Louw's (2014) research sparked the need for a project called Kings Club where male adolescents are part of a well-being project aimed at promoting healthy manhood and fatherhood. The Kings Club is an example of a project where artwork is used to encourage these skills, offering project-partakers a creative space and inviting other disciplines towards the building of capacity (Daykin et al., 2006). In similar ways, projects for female adolescents were created, such as the Stars Club for female adolescents aimed at promoting healthy womanhood.

17.3.4.3 Key Role of Relational Competencies

Research conducted in Delft investigated core components related to adolescents' relational well-being, seen by Gergen (2009) as an innately free gift to all humans as relational beings. Geldenhuys and van Schalkwyk (2019) found that adolescents' relational well-being in this community is seriously challenged, and although adolescents view belonging as important, this outlook does not automatically equal relational skills. While positive relationships are central to well-being and healthy functioning, a specific focus on healthy interaction is vital for well-being projects in this risk-laden community with its numerous incidences of violence. Research conducted by Grimova and van Schalkwyk (2016) explored the learners' perceptions and experiences of respect in educator-learner relationships, and found that learners principally value respect within this context. About educator-learner relationships, Xhosa learners expressed the experience of respect in the following way: "Respect is for example, when you are talking or sharing your opinions in the class then the teacher doesn't disturb you, he or she listens to you when you are talking" (Participant #10/3, male learner, Xhosa); and "Respectful behaviour is when teachers do listen to me when I talk, they don't shut me down" (Participant #15/3, male learner, Xhosa). Adolescent learners referred to the dynamics of respect and good manners in daily interacting in their real-life settings (Grimova & Van Schalkwyk, 2016).

These studies demonstrate the importance of relational competencies in all persons who are partaking in well-being projects, and the mastering of skills related to the language of positive respect versus negative respect and fear. Also, project-members are sensitised to their cultural practices under which such behaviour is seen as respectful encounters, since this can be greatly influenced by the social environment (Rosa & Tudge, 2013; Wissing & Temane, 2008).

Walton et al. (2016) looked at educators' relationships with adolescent learners who are dealing with substance use/abuse in Delft. Increasing substance abuse rates—especially among the youth—is a significant problem "...with a fifth of school learners having tried a drug by the time they finish primary school" (Walton et al., 2016, p. 1). In other words, thousands of learners in Delft have been initiated to drug use by the age of 12 years. Educators' relationships with learners are critical for the possible progression of drug use to drug abuse and addiction, because learners' behaviour related to continued drug use may come to the attention of educators who then need to deal with these challenges. Besides, there is a high incidence of Foetal Alcohol Syndrome (FAS) and Foetal Alcohol Spectrum Disorder (FASD) in the Western Cape province of South Africa (Olivier et al., 2013; van Schalkwyk & Marais, 2017). Also, the incidence of teenage pregnancy and risky sexual behaviour is common in Delft (Odimegwu et al., 2018). In view of these challenges, research conducted by Walton et al. (2016) highlighted the need for well-being projects that can buffer the risk and encourage much-needed support networks for adolescents in this high-risk community.

In contrast to this negative or even dysfunctional relational functioning, healthy interaction within the school and family context are viewed as priceless opportunities for enhancing daily well-being. In view of this, all well-being project facilitators (called project leaders) deliberately highlight positive relatedness and its complexities, as well as the long- and short-term effects of impaired relationships. Therefore, all well-being projects in this programme include guidelines on how to counteract risks for personal and relational well-being, such as poor self-regulation and substance use, risky sexual activities and teenage pregnancies, and/or poor school performance and dropping out (Seligman, 2011; van Schalkwyk & Marais, 2017). Practices of positive relating and prosocial interacting are central to all well-being projects.

17.3.4.4 Progress of the Well-Being Programme Over Time: Resilient Coping and School Success

Originally, the well-being programme and some projects were only presented at one secondary school in Delft. Due to the positive impact of this programme, this led to the expansion of projects to most of the 23 schools in this community by 2019. Another remarkable effect of the successful implementation of the well-being programme is that numerous teachers and parents/legal guardians/caregivers became involved. All the well-being clubs of the many school communities involve teachers who act as coordinators/key persons between the project leaders/facilitators and the learners/project-partakers. In this sense, the well-being programme joins the schools and educators to achieve positive outcomes (Naidoo & van Schalkwyk, 2021). For example, the Success Clubs, active in most schools in this community, function to encourage and equip learners towards improved school success.

It is well known that poor academic achievement among disadvantaged groups is a grave concern in South Africa (Romero et al., 2018). Louw et al. (2011) report that many learners in the Cape Flats are struggling with the motivation to complete their school education in an environment with a drop-out ratio of more than 50% and with extremely high levels of youth unemployment. The focus of the Success Club was to improve academic performance by targeting the known barriers to education in this environment, such as learners' lack of motivation and poor study skills, and by overcoming external barriers related to poverty traps (Burger et al., 2014) in a resilient way. For example, Success Club learners are trained to use keys for success, namely positive emotions and strengths, such as honesty, love of learning, and hope (Lyubomirsky, 2008; Lyubomirsky, King, & Diener, 2005) in various practical ways to activate positive spirals. The effective use of these learning aids is critical to infuse the individual's decision-making and other behaviours as strength-congruent activities. Also, students from the Delft community studying at institutions of higher education in the Western Cape act as facilitators of this well-being project, and they are examples of young people living towards fulfilling their dreams (Naidoo & van Schalkwyk, 2021). Since Delft is well known for its poorly performing schools, learners' resilient coping and teachers' strengths to overcome continuous difficulties are of the utmost importance in building youth well-being in these risk-saturated communities.

Bylieveldt (2019) explored the resilience of female educators/teachers who are in leadership positions in Delft schools. Teachers from Delft schools face enormous challenges because their learners come mostly from families who face enduring poverty and these schools are typically categorised as poorly resourced learning communities. For example, gangsters do not exempt the 25 schools in Delft and their learners of their violent activities, and these dangers add to the vulnerabilities of the community's learning environments. Due to these circumstances and based on the recommendations from this research, a well-being project is being generated to focus on school well-being. This project aims at promoting the well-being of entire school communities by focusing on the drivers of healthy behaviours in school settings. This project links well with efforts or initiatives of the well-being programme to enable parents—that is, mostly mothers of the school communities—towards the building of well-being. This need was motivated by the statement: "*The learners are mastering these principles of positive living, but their parents do not know the language*" of Mr. Manchest, vice-principal at Hindle High (2012).

17.3.4.5 Strengthening the Family Unit

Although schools are viewed as valuable resources in Delft, parent involvement in the learning environment of their children remains weak (Louw et al., 2011). Research conducted by Cronjé-Malan and van Schalkwyk (2015) in Delft shows the detrimental impact when early adolescents' parents/legal guardians are mostly uninvolved in their children's school communities. Interestingly, the demographic information of this study revealed that most participants' caregivers were not their biological parents, but rather the grandparents, an aunt, or an older sibling. This research indicates that learners view their parents/legal guardians' involvement as a basic need and as primary for their school success. For example, a learner participant stated: *"Nou bly hy (pa) anderkant, as ek na hom toe gaan dan jaag hy my weg van sy huis af, hy stuur nie vir my geld nie, ek is nie so much oor hom nie."/"Now my dad he lives on the other side, when I go to him he chases me away from his house, he does not send me money, I am not so fond of him."* Findings also showed that parents' perceptions about school involvement are often negative, as illustrated, for example, by the fact that learners often do not complete their school assignments. A learner participant explained: "Omdat ek gee nie al my werk ingee nie. . .is soos my juffrou miskien vir ons werk gegee het en dan vergeet ek. . . dan vergeet ek om dit te doen."/"Because I do not give in my (home)work, for example, my teacher maybe gave us homework and then I forget. . .then I forget to do this."

Findings of the abovementioned study offered a strong motivation to initiate well-being projects to bring school learners and parents/legal guardians/caregivers together. For example, a celebration of womanhood (celebrated in the month of August in South Africa) is done in a festive manner by means of "mother and daughter events". This is a yearly event where various schools partake, for example, learners are invited to write a special letter/poem of gratitude for her/his mother/legal guardian/caregiver; these letters are given to adult caregivers during the festive event on a Saturday. While teachers of the many Delft schools are also invited as guests to these events, it offers a friendly space for learners and their parents/caregivers and educators to meet. This project also allows women of all races and socio-economic levels to enjoy strengths associated with personal beauty, relational connecting, and collective wisdom.

Since youth are part of families, and many families in Delft can be described as female-headed households (single-parent families), van Schalkwyk (2019) conducted research to explore how female-headed households (FHHs) in the Delft community can be strengthened when mothers are dealing with substance problems. This research shows that these households are seriously challenged. Van Schalkwyk (2019) stated that ". . .the circular effects of familial breakdown were obvious as the children of these mothers are more likely to engage in risky behaviour and contribute to societal breakdown" (p. 20). The immense impact of poverty on family life (Holborn & Eddy, 2011) was confirmed (van Schalkwyk, 2019). This is important evidence since families present a unique context for the promotion of children's psychological development (Ryan et al., 2016) as well as parents' well-being through the dynamics of daily interactions and relational exchanges.

For this reason, the need for the generation of well-being projects to encourage mothers' personal health and parenting competencies was clear. PPIs in family contexts have shown that bolstering family strengths as opposed to ameliorating risks was beneficial for child and parental well-being (Newland, 2015). Various well-being projects/clubs exist for mothers in Delft, to comply with mothers' needs (van Schalkwyk & Naidoo, 2021). For example, a club called Angel Mothers promotes the spiritual well-being of Delft mothers which supports them to act as guardians of their families; a club called Power Mothers focuses on the strengthening of mothers' personal and parenting competencies; and a club called Delft Daisies is for mothers with children of 2–5 years old, where both mothers and their children partake to enhance the children's positive development.

17.3.4.6 Building a Resilient Community

Community well-being entails the contribution of knowledge partners, namely professional persons' skills and expertise, as well as the active participation of community members and their collective wisdom (Lazarus et al., 2014). Therefore bottom-up and top-down approaches are used (National Drug Master Plan, 2019–2024) to nurture personal well-being and competent families. One of these recommendations is to use religious practices such as prayer. For this reason, it is part of the strategic partnering inherent to the well-being programme's effective implementation to work with various faith communities within and outside of Delft. A team of project leaders organises these opportunities for communal prayer towards the strengthening of Delft families and protection against identified destructive elements in the community. Standing together in such a way offers a stance of unity towards a positive collective. It is not uncommon for South African communities to display a high ranking of spirituality and religious practices in relation to happiness and meaningfulness (Delle Fave et al., 2010).

In summary, the findings of well-being research conducted within Delft show the effective implementation of the well-being programme and its progress over time towards significant outcomes. This method allows for a bottom-up (input from the community-members) and a top-down approach (scientific method and research) towards sustainability and numerous lessons learned. These experiential lessons are important to guide effective implementation.

17.3.5 Lessons Learned

All community engagement can be described as the blending of science and art. While disciplines such as psychology, political science, social work, and cultural anthropology represent the scientific contribution, the art is composed of skills and sensitivity together with understanding to apply and adapt the science in suitable ways for the particular community of interest (National Institutes of Health, 2011). This viewpoint is helpful seeing that the scientific stance provides the systematic background for the well-being programme in the Delft community and the skilful application as well as innovative adaption which are important for efficient implementation. The growth and sustainability of the various projects in the Delft community since 2010 can indeed be summarised as the blend of science and art with the needed bravery and inventive twists on the basic theme. Character strengths and virtues (cf. Peterson & Seligman, 2004) offer powerful guidelines towards the perseverance needed to keep on trying in spite of many creative changes to the original plan(s), to be committed to connect versus the discontentment of numerous disappointments, and not to be side-tracked by plentiful risks, such as drop-out or death of learners, robberies, suicide of mothers, or problems with taxi transport. Over and above these matters, the quality of relationships and trustworthiness, in spite of the complexities of these mentioned difficulties, are essential. According to the researcher's experience, trustworthiness cannot be attained without paying close attention to practicalities.

17.3.5.1 Practicalities

The effective implementation of a PPI in Delft embraces the intentional use of valuable human and communal resources for positive functioning. Practical aspects of the programme involve a standard of procedure when introducing the projects to school communities; for example, the director of projects will organise a formal meeting with a school's principal and will offer information about the aim and outcomes of the project(s), the specific modus operandi with regard to the day and time of the planned project, the project leader acting as a facilitator, the number of learners per project, and the requirement for the principal to appoint an educator to act as the co-ordinator for the particular project. Due to the building of trust over time, these meetings also serve to strengthen relationships and celebrate positive outcomes. Once these meetings are conducted, the project leader/facilitator of the proposed club will contact the co-ordinator (appointed educator) of the school to arrange the practicalities of the project. For instance, the project leader (retired mathematics educator) of the proposed Maths Club at the school will contact the appointed educator at the local school to organise the following: (a) to select 15–20 top performers at mathematics from the grade 11 learners (three learners per each of the seven class groups in grade 11); (b) to give letters to these selected learners to inform their parents about their participation in the Maths Club and all the needed information about the day and time of the weekly Maths Club meeting; the parents' written permission will be obtained; and (c) to make arrangements about a classroom and snacks for the learners. The content of the weekly Maths Club is determined by the project leader in co-ordination with the head of department of the selected grade at the school, and a weekly feedback report is sent in electronic format to the director of projects of the well-being programme in Delft.

In this community, it is of the utmost importance to always take into account matters related to structural, personal, and programmatic barriers as well as facilitators to success. For example, Wessels et al. (2016) found that although most parents in a South African disadvantaged community were eager to receive parenting programmes, more than just "interest in attending" is required (p. 3). Since most learners in Delft are not familiar with extra-mural activities, it is crucial that, apart from the need for well-being programmes, the contexts where the interventions are delivered are considered (Baños et al., 2017). For example, PPIs presented at schools can be more effective if adolescents view the activity as an additional school task (Burckhardt et al., 2015). However, it is our experience that for some learners, the school building is associated with effort and these learners will not be likely to attend due to a negative association with "school" and hard work. Therefore, it is critical to make precautions on a practical level to prevent dropout. Nonetheless, most learners view school buildings as "a safe space" to meet in Delft, since, currently, all schools are assisted by law enforcement (that is, two or three police officers are present at all school buildings to ensure safety and prevent, for example, gangster activities on the school grounds). Furthermore, learners have the assurance that all well-being projects are presented with the needed permission from community leaders (school principals) for the implementation of the projects. Also, we tap into the notion that schools provide important environments for life success by embracing positive academic outcomes.

17.3.5.1.1 Barriers

Structural Barriers In the Delft community, low socio-economic status is the most significant structural barrier for learners and parents/mothers taking part in projects. The most common matters related to this barrier are transport and safety (public transport/taxis), food (hunger implies poor concentration), family support, and the lack of items such as stationery. For example, when learners take part in Maths Club for improved academic success in mathematics, money for transport, e.g., taxi fare, snacks, and items such as books, pens, etc. must be provided by the project organisers.

Personal Barriers Poor health is a barrier to participation in projects. For example, when a learner taking part in the music club and choir performances suffers from a cold/flu, he/she usually does not have access to medicine and the cold could become a serious infection with long-lasting symptoms. As another example, when youngsters face psychological stressors associated with fractured families and poor physical health due to hunger, their attendance and participation in well-being projects are influenced negatively.

Lack of motivation to commit to a project in the long term is another personal barrier with sad consequences. While project-partakers enjoy elements of fun and external motivation such as rewards (food parcels), lack of interest (locus of control) is a serious barrier to prolonged engagement. For example, although learner partakers would voice the need for projects, many are known not to commit the time and effort required for positive outcomes.

Programmatic Barriers All projects are presented in groups, and certain challenges associated with group dynamics must be taken into account. For example, project-leaders must be sensitive to male adolescents partaking in the Kings Club who are uncomfortable to share personal information with the group. Also, frequent attenders might feel disheartened when others drop out of the project as this could affect the trust developed in the group over multiple meetings. Likewise, since projects are presented as extra-mural activities, learners' safety must always be protected; for example, sometimes a learner taking part in the reading club does not attend school because his/her family was threatened and/or attacked by gangsters in the past week.

17.3.5.1.2 Facilitators

Structural Facilitators Learners are encouraged to attend well-being programme sessions at their school buildings either immediately after school on a weekday (reading clubs, success clubs, music clubs, Kings Club), or on a Saturday morning (for example, Maths Club). Mothers prefer to meet in the morning at a school building for safety reasons. When projects are delivered in the morning, this fits in with mothers dropping off and fetching children from school. Also, living close to the project venue is a facilitator as parents can walk to the school building.

Personal Facilitators Family support appears to be an important facilitator of attendance. High attenders frequently mention how their families and their school support their attendance. For example, learners who are partaking in music club activities, such as choir performances and/or shows, appreciate the encouragement of their parents/legal guardians and educators/teachers. However, this support needs to be continuously encouraged by project leaders.

What also seemingly sets high attenders apart from the low attenders is a greater sense of commitment and readiness to engage. This factor is of crucial importance; therefore, intentional efforts to encourage participants' long-term participation to achieve meaningful outcomes require continuous support for intrinsic motivation. When reflecting on why they first became involved in projects, learner or mother participants often refer to the programme's aims and how this could address their needs. For example, mothers attending a well-being project to enhance their personal and parenting skills would talk about changes they can see in themselves and their children, which they attribute to the programme. When project members experience this benefit, high attenders often mention how they reschedule other commitments if necessary.

Programmatic Facilitators The fundamental aspects of well-being and the nurturing thereof is a vital programmatic facilitator. Apart from the powerful content of the well-being programme used within the various well-being clubs, the application of this perspective is vital. This means that even when project members are dealing with traumatic events, such as the sudden death of a friend being shot by gangsters, or the suicide of a mother, the dynamics of positive interacting offers a safe space which is very meaningful to participants (Myers, 2018, SAAMS conference).

Openness to paying attention to recommendations offered by community members is indispensable for a well-being programme in this high-risk community, and to adjust project plans; for example: (a) to accommodate adolescents' traumatic and adverse experiences, such as a step-father's murder, or a mother's drunkenness on the streets the previous night, or the family being robbed, or domestic violence; (b) to identify coping mechanisms of the past (e.g., parenting and substance use) and to discuss alternative coping mechanisms (versus drugs); (c) to identify poor physical and mental health behaviour (e.g., using risky sex to obtain money for food); (d) to actively resist re-traumatisation through continuous conversations about these incidences of terror; (e) using many activities and visuals (also video—especially relevant for the South African context); (f) obtaining regular feedback from the project members as experts of their lived experiences; (g) to use many visual symbols for projects to reinforce, for example, the positive principles acting as a code of conduct for all projects of the well-being programme.

It is important to add some information about the human facilitators—also called project leaders—for the successful implementation of a well-being programme. They are vital for the growth and sustainability of the well-being programme in Delft. Project leaders fulfil various roles; for example, facilitators of success club projects at various schools in the Delft community are students at universities and are also positive role-models for Delft learners; project leaders of reading clubs are mothers of the school community who are trained once a term/quarter to act as facilitators. These mothers' involvement in their school communities is highly valued, and their continuous feedback informs better performance and the overcoming of challenges. Other projects, such as music club, maths club, Kings club, and Delft Daisies club (mothers and early child development training) require that facilitators have the needed expertise to act as project leaders. These facilitators act as volunteers of a specific non-profit organisation. Apart from expertise, it is crucial that all project leaders act as positive role models to demonstrate to project members (e.g., learners or mothers) real-life prosocial behaviour guided by positive principles.

In summary, the effective implementation of the well-being programme and its various projects in Delft requires much more than the offering of outstanding information or research. Beyond the structure of the various projects and project leaders' expertise, the programme is action-based (Isaacs & Roman, 2018). In this section, some barriers and facilitators were presented towards the effective implementation of the well-being programme (Holtzkamp, 2012). Effective implementation requires addressing many barriers in the context of a high-risk community, and enhancing enabling factors towards facilitation.

17.4 Conclusion

Research findings indicate that the well-being of children, families, and schools in a Western Cape high-risk community is seriously challenged. While the sad reality of the negative effects of poverty and many social ills is not overlooked, the distinct need for intentional efforts by means of the well-being programme is emphasised. Within the theoretical framework of PP, and including ecological and multi-disciplinary approaches, the effective implementation of a well-being framework in this high-risk context embraces a process where the community and committed persons join efforts. Continued research is essential to this process of effective implementation.

Ultimately, longitudinal research and other rigorous methodologies are recommended to examine the long-term impact of PPIs, such as the well-being programme and its various projects in Delft. We need research to look at the time factor, since in this population, every step of the process towards the enhancement of psychosocial wellness is vital towards changes in habitual thought, feeling, and behaviour. Also, intentional building of strong communities in a South African context where families are dealing with numerous needs is vital, especially since the South African government has ratified the Sustainable Developmental Goals (SDGs) 2030 (Hall & Sambu, 2017). Research could uncover the strengthening structures of competent families in contrast to spirals of destruction perpetuating poverty traps in high-risk communities.

In conclusion, effective implementation of this well-being programme is a process directed by well-being. The people of Delft themselves are the living examples of the positive outcomes, growth, and sustainability of the well-being programme. This was expressed in a local newspaper as follows: "These projects in the Delft community are influencing true change in the lives not only of young people but an entire community by successfully creating a sustainable system from the school to the household" (The DelftSTAR news, August 2019, p. 8).

References

Baltes, P. B., & Freund, A. M. (2003). Human strengths as the orchestration of wisdom and selective optimization with compensation. In L. G. Aspinwall & U. Staudinger (Eds.), *A psychology of human strengths: Fundamental questions and future directions for a positive psychology* (pp. 23–47). American Psychological Association Press.

Baños, R. M., Etchemendy, E., Mira, A., Riva, G., Gaggioli, A., & Botella, C. (2017). Online positive interventions to promote well-being and resilience in the adolescent population: A narrative review. *Frontiers in Psychiatry, 8*(10), 1–9. https://doi.org/10.3389/fpsyt.2017.00010

Burckhardt, R., Manicavasagar, V., Batterham, P. J., Miller, L. M., & Talbot, E. A. (2015). Web-based adolescent positive psychology program in schools: Randomized controlled trial. *Journal of Medical Internet Research, 17*(7). https://doi.org/10.2196/jmir.4329

Burger, R., van der Berg, S., Gustafsson, M., Adams, C., Coetzee, M., Moses, E., et al. (2014). *Poverty traps and social exclusion among children in South Africa: A report to the South African Human Rights Commission* (pp. 1–198). SAHRC.

Bylieveldt, L. (2019). *Resilience in a high-risk community: Experiences of female educators in leadership positions* (Unpublished master's dissertation). North-West University, Potchefstroom.

Bylieveldt, L., van Schalkwyk, I., & de Jager, L. (in press). Resilience in a high-risk community: Experiences of female educators in leadership positions. *Journal of Africa Education.*

Chipkin, I., & Meny-Gibert, S. (2013). *Understanding the social justice sector in South Africa. A Report to the RAITH Foundation and Atlantic Philanthropies.*

Crime Stats SA. (2018). *Crime Stats.* Delft census. Retrieved from http://www.crimestatssa.com/topten.php

Cronjé-Malan, L., & van Schalkwyk, L. (2015). Vroeë adolessente se persepsies van hulle primêre versorgers se betrokkenheid by die skoolgemeenskap in 'n hoë-risiko gemeenskap. *Koers: Bulletin for Christian Scholarship, 80*(2), 1–10.

Curtis, K., Fry, M., Shaban, R. Z., & Considine, J. (2016). Translating research findings to clinical nursing practice. *Journal of Clinical Nursing, 26*(5–6), 862–872. https://doi.org/10.1111/jocn.13586

Daykin, N., Evans, D., Orme, J., Salmon, D., McEachran, M., & Brain, S. (2006). The effects of participation in performing arts for health on young people. *Environmental Sciences.* Retrieved from http://www.ahsw.org.uk/userfiles/Research/Young_People_Review_copy.pdf

Deci, E. L., & Ryan, R. M. (2002). The 'what' and 'why' of goal pursuits: Human needs and the self-determination of behaviour. *Psychological Inquiry, 11*(4), 227–268.

Delft census. (2011). Retrieved from http://www.capetown.gov.za/Local%20and%20communities/Education-and-research-materials/Data-statistics-and-research/Cape-Town-census

DelftSTAR News. (2019, August). *Delft Star of the Month: Dr Izanette van Schalkwyk.* Retrieved from https://www.hitimemedia.co.za/newspaper

Delle Fave, A., Brdar, I., Freire, T., Vella-Brodrick, D., & Wissing, M. P. (2010). The eudaimonic and hedonic components of happiness: Qualitative and quantitative findings. *Social Indicators Research, 100*(2), 185–207. https://doi.org/10.1007/s11205-010-9632-5

Department of Social Development Republic of South Africa. (2013). *White paper on families in South Africa.* Government Printers.

Ebersöhn, L. (2015). Making sense of place in school-based intervention research. *Contemporary Educational Psychology, 40*, 121–130. https://doi.org/10.1016/j.cedpsych.2014.10.004

Ebersöhn, L., Loots, T., Mampane, R., Omidire, F., Malan-Van Rooyen, M., Sefotho, M., & Nthontho, M. (2018). An indigenous psychology perspective on psychosocial support in Southern Africa as collective, networking, and pragmatic support. *Journal of Community & Applied Social Psychology, 28*(5), 1–16. https://doi.org/10.1002/casp.2371

Felner, R. D., & de Vries, M. L. (2013). Poverty in childhood and adolescence: A transactional–ecological approach to understanding and enhancing resilience in contexts of disadvantage and developmental risk. In S. Goldstein & R. B. Brooks (Eds.), *Handbook of resilience in children* (2nd ed., pp. 105–126). Springer.

Fredrickson, B. L. (2009). *Positivity.* Random House.

Geldenhuys, O., & van Schalkwyk, I. (2019). Investigating the relational well-being of a group of adolescents in a South African high-risk community. *Psychology and Behavioral Science International Journal, 12*(2), 20–23. https://doi.org/10.19080/PBSIJ.2019.12.555835

Geldenhuys, O., & van Schalkwyk, I. (2020). *Verhoudingwelstand van adolessente in 'n Suid-Afrikaanse hoë-risiko gemeenskap.* LitNet Akademies (Geesteswetenskappe). Retrieved February 4, 2020 from https://www.litnet.co.za/relational-well-being-of-adolescents-in-a-south-african-high-risk-community/

Gergen, K. J. (2009). *Relational being: Beyond self and community.* Oxford University Press.

Grimova, L., & van Schalkwyk, I. (2016). Learners' perceptions and experiences of respect in educator-learner relationships. *Journal of Psychology in Africa, 26*(4), 343–350.

Haidt, J. (2006). Elevation and the positive psychology of morality. In C. L. M. Keyes & J. Haidt (Eds.), *Flourishing: Positive psychology and the life well-lived* (pp. 275–289). American Psychological Association Press.

Hall, K., & Sambu, W. (2017). *Demography of South Africa's children*. In South African Child Guage, pp. 100–104. Retrieved from http://www.ci.uct.ac.za/sites/default/files/image_tool/images/367/Child_Gauge/South_African_Child_Gauge_2017/Child_Gauge_2017_lowres.pdf

Hamman, C., & Kruger, L. M. (2017). Gossip girls: The power of girls' gossip in a low-income south African community. *Critical Arts, 31*(1), 1–17. https://doi.org/10.1080/02560046.2017.1300822

Heywood, M. (2020). The transformative power of civil society in South Africa: An activist's perspective on innovative forms of organizing and rights-based practices. *Globalizations, 17*(2), 294–316. https://doi.org/10.1080/14747731.2019.1652466

Holborn, L., & Eddy, G. (2011). *First steps to healing the South African family. A research paper by the South African Institute of Race Relations*. Retrieved from https://irr.org.za/reports/occasional-reports/files/first-steps-to-healing-the-south-african-family-final-report-mar-2011.pdf

Holtzkamp, J. (2012). *The development and assessment of a family resilience enhancement programme* (Unpublished doctoral thesis). University of Stellenbosch.

Isaacs, S. A., & Roman, N. V. (2018). The development of a family resilience-strengthening programme for families in a South African rural community. *Journal of Community Psychology*, 1–20. https://doi.org/10.1002/jcop.21962

Jamieson, L., Berry, L., & Lake, L. (2017). *South African child gauge*. Children's Institute, University of Cape Town.

Jones, C. (2019, March 23). *Die monopolie van geweld* (p. 11). Die Burger.

Kagee, A. (2014). South African psychology after 20 years of democracy: Criticality, social development, and relevance. *South Africa Journal of Psychology, 44*(3), 350–363. https://doi.org/10.1177/0081246314534147

Keyes, C. L. M. (2002). The mental health continuum: From languishing to flourishing in life. *Journal of Health and Social Behavior, 43*, 207–222.

Keyes, C. L. M. (2005). Mental illness and/or mental health? Investigating axioms of the complete state model of health. *Journal of Consulting and Clinical Psychology, 73*(3), 539–548. https://doi.org/10.1037/0022-006X.73.3.539

Keyes, C. L. M. (2006). Subjective well-being in mental health and human development research worldwide: An introduction. *Social Indicators Research, 77*, 1–10. https://doi.org/10.1007/s11205-005-5550-3

Keyes, C. L. M. (2007). Promoting and protecting mental health as flourishing: A complementary strategy for improving national mental health. *American Psychologist, 62*(2), 95–108.

Keyes, C. L. M. (2009). The nature and importance of positive mental health in America's adolescents. In R. Gilman, E. S. Huebner, & M. J. Furlong (Eds.), *Handbook of positive psychology in schools* (pp. 9–24). Routledge.

Lachman, J. M., Sherr, L. T., Cluver, L., Ward, C. L., Hutchings, J., & Gardner, F. (2016). Integrating evidence and context to develop a parenting program for low-income families in South Africa. *Journal of Child and Family Studies, 25*(7), 2337–2352. https://doi.org/10.1007/s10826-016-0389-6

Lambert, N. M., Stillman, T. F., Hicks, J. A., Kamble, S., Baumeister, R. F., & Fincham, F. D. (2013). To belong is to matter: Sense of belonging enhances meaning in life. *Personality & Social Psychology Bulletin, 39*(11), 1418–1427. https://doi.org/10.1177/0146167213499186

Lazarus, S., Naidoo, A. V., May, B., Williams, L., Demas, G., & Filander, F. J. (2014). Lessons learnt from a community-based participatory research project in a South African rural context. *South Africa Journal of Psychology, 44*(2), 149–161. https://doi.org/10.1177/0081246314528156

Lent, R. W. (2004). Toward a unifying theoretical and practical perspective on well-being and psychosocial adjustment. *Journal of Counselling Psychology, 51*(4), 482–509.

Linley, P. A., Joseph, S., Harrington, S., & Wood, A. M. (2006). Positive psychology: Past, present, and (possible) future. *The Journal of Positive Psychology, 1*(1), 3–16. https://doi.org/10.1080/17439760500372796

Louw, J. (2014). *Adolescents' experience of absent fathers in a high-risk community* (Unpublished master's dissertation). University of South Africa.

Louw, W., Bayat, A., & Eigelaar-Meets, I. (2011). *A report on underperforming secondary schools in die Western Cape*. Institute of Social Development, University of the Western Cape.

Lyubomirsky, S. (2008). *The how of happiness: A scientific approach to getting the life you want*. Penguin Press.

Lyubomirsky, S., King, L., & Diener, E. (2005). The benefits of frequent positive affect: Does happiness lead to success? *Psychological Bulletin, 131*(6), 803.

Lyubomirsky, S., & Layous, K. (2013). How do simple positive activities increase well-being? *Current Directions in Psychological Science, 22*(1), 57–62.

Lyubomirsky, S., Sheldon, K., & Schkade, D. (2005). Pursuing happiness: The architecture of sustainable change. *Review of General Psychology, 9*, 111–131. https://doi.org/10.1037/1089-2680.9.2.111

Magidson, J. F., Joska, J. A., Regenauer, K. S., Satinsky, E., Andersen, L. S., Seitz-brown, C. J., Borba, C. P., Safren, S. A., & Myers, B. (2019). "Someone who is in this thing that I am suffering from": The role of peers and other facilitators for task sharing substance use treatment in South African HIV care. *International Journal of Drug Policy, 70*, 61–69. https://doi.org/10.1016/j.drugpo.2018.11.004

Mahajan, S. (2014). *Economics of South African townships: Special focus on Diepsloot*. World Bank.

Mahali, A., Lynch, I., Fadiji, A. W., Tolla, T., Khumalo, S., & Naicker, S. (2018). Networks of well-being in the global south: A critical review of current scholarship. *Journal of Developing Societies, 34*(4), 373–400. https://doi.org/10.1177/0169796X18786137

Malherbe, N. (2019, June 27). *Die Burger, 2 300 Moorde in 29 weke ruk Wes-Kaap*, p. 1.

Masten, A. S. (2015). *Ordinary magic: Resilience in development*. The Guilford Press.

Mathews, S., & Benvenuti, P. (2014). Violence against children in South Africa: Developing a prevention agenda. In S. Mathews, L. Jamieson, L. Lake, & S. Smith (Eds.), *South African child gauge* (pp. 81–92). Children's Institute, University of Cape Town.

May, P. A., Blankenship, J., Marais, A. S., Gossage, J. P., Kalberg, W. O., Barnard, R., . . . Seedat, S. (2013). Approaching the prevalence of full spectrum of fetal alcohol spectrum disorders in a South African population-based study. *Alcoholism: Clinical & Experimental Research, 37*(5), 818–830. https://doi.org/10.1111/acer.12033

Myers, B. (2018, August). *Addressing trauma, substance use and sexual risk among young South African women*. In Paper presented at South African Addiction Medicine Society (SAAMS), Cape Town, South Africa.

Naidoo, A. V., Visser, M., de Wet, M., Rabie, S., van Schalkwyk, I., Boonzaier, M., de Bruin, G., Shirley, L., & Venter, C. (2019). A group-based career guidance intervention for South African high-school learners from low-income communities. In J. G. Maree (Ed.), *Handbook of innovative career counselling* (pp. 665–685). Springer.

Naidoo, L., & van Schalkwyk, I. (2021). Pathways to academic success of disadvantaged undergraduate university students from a high-risk community in the Western Cape. *South African Journal of Higher Education, 35*(4), 180–204. https://dx.doi.org/10.20853/35-4-4175

National Drug Master Plan. (2019-2024). Government Press.

National Institutes of Health - Clinical and Translation Science Awards Consortium, Community Engagement Key Function Committee Task Force on the Principles of Community Engagement. (2011). *Principles of community engagement*. NIH Publication No. 11-7782.

Newland, L. A. (2015). Family well-being, parenting, and child well-being: Pathways to healthy adjustment. *Clinical Psychologist, 19*(1), 3–14.

Norrish, J. M., & Vella-Brodrick, D. A. (2009). Positive psychology and adolescents: Where are we now? Where to from here? *Australian Psychologist, 44*(4), 270–278. https://doi.org/10.1080/00050060902914103

Nortjé, V., van Schalkwyk, I., & de Jager, L. (submitted). Married couples' perceptions of relational strengths in the context of a South African high-risk community. *Journal for Family Relations: Interdisciplinary Journal of Applied Family Science*.

Odimegwu, C. O., Amoo, E. O., & de Wet, N. (2018). Teenage pregnancy in South Africa: Where are the young men involved? *South African Journal of Child Health, 12*(2), 44–50. https://doi.org/10.7196/SAJCH.2018.v12i2.1523

Olivier, L., Urban, M., Chersich, M., Temmerman, M., & Viljoen, D. (2013). Burden of fetal alcohol syndrome in a rural west coast area of South Africa. *South African Medical Journal, 103*(6), 402–405. https://doi.org/10.7196/SAMJ.6249

Park, N., & Peterson, C. (2009). Strengths of character in schools. In R. Gilman, E. S. Heubner, & M. J. Furlong (Eds.), *Handbook of positive psychology in schools* (pp. 65–76). Routledge.

Peterson, C. (2006). The values in action (VIA) classifications of strengths. In M. Csikszentmihalyi & I. S. Csikszentmihalyi (Eds.), *A life worth living: Contributions to positive psychology* (pp. 29–48). Oxford University Press.

Peterson, C., & Seligman, M. E. P. (2004). *Character strengths and virtues: A handbook and classification*. Oxford University Press.

Pinnock, D. (2016). *Gang town*. Tafelberg.

Pohl, S. M. (2018). *Exploring the experiences of programme graduates of a pilot preventative intervention for adolescent girls at risk to gang activity* (Master's dissertation). Stellenbosch University.

Prilleltensky, I. (2012). Wellness as fairness. *American Journal of Community Psychology, 49*(1–2), 1–21. https://doi.org/10.1007/s10464-011-9448-8

Roloff, N. S. (2014). *Gang typologies of the Western Cape (Research report)*. Retrieved from http://www.safetylab.co.za/gang-inquiry/

Romero, R. H., Hall, J., Cluver, L., & Meinck, F. (2018). Can supportive parenting protect against school delay amongst violence-exposed adolescents in South Africa? *Child Abuse & Neglect, 78*, 31–45. https://doi.org/10.1016/j.chiabu.2017.09.025

Rosa, E. M., & Tudge, J. (2013). Urie Bronfenbrenner's theory of human developments: Its evolution from ecology to biotechnology. *Journal of Family Theory and Review, 5*(4), 243–258.

Ryan, R. M., Deci, E. L., & Vansteenkiste, M. (2016). Autonomy and autonomy disturbances in self-development and psychopathology: Research on motivation, attachment, and clinical process. *Development and Psychopathology*, 1–54.

Savahl, S., Adams, S., Isaacs, S., September, R., Hendricks, G., & Noordien, A. (2015). Subjective well-being amongst a sample of South African children: A descriptive study. *Journal of Child Indicators Research, 8*(1), 211–226. https://doi.org/10.1007/s12187-014-9289-8

Seekings, J. (2011). Race, class and inequality in the south African city. In G. Bridge & S. Watson (Eds.), *The new Blackwell companion to the City* (pp. 532–546). Wiley-Blackwell.

Seligman, M. E. P. (1998). President's column: Building human strength: Psychology's forgotten mission. *APA Monitor, 29*(1), 1.

Seligman, M. E. P. (2002). *Authentic happiness*. Free Press.

Seligman, M. E. P. (2011). *Flourish: A visionary new understanding of happiness and well-being*. Free Press.

Seligman, M. E. P., & Csikszentmihalyi, M. (2000). Positive psychology. *American Psychologist, 55*, 5–14.

Sin, N. L., & Lyubomirsky, S. (2009). Enhancing well-being and alleviating depressive symptoms with positive psychology interventions: A practice-friendly meta-analysis. *Journal of Clinical Psychology, 65*(5), 467–487. https://doi.org/10.1002/Jclp.20593

Smith, E. J. (2006). The strength-based counselling model. *The Counselling Psychologist, 34*(1), 13–79. https://doi.org/10.1177/0011000005277018

Son Digitaal. (2019, July 11). *Army word in Kaap losgelaat*. Retrieved from https://www.son.co.za/Nuus/Kaapsenuus/army-in-kaap-losgelaat-20190711

South African Police Service Annual Report. (2018/2019). Retrieved March 31, 2020 from https://www.saps.gov.za/about/stratframework/annualreports.php

Statistics South Africa. (2018a). *Four facts about our provincial economies*. Retrieved from http://www.statssa.gov.za/?p=12056

Statistics South Africa. (2018b/2019). *Statistics South Africa to release Gross domestic product (GDP) Q3*. Retrieved from http://www.statssa.gov.za/?m=2018

Statistics South Africa. (2019). *Statistics South Africa to release the Quarterly Labour Force Survey (QLFS), Second Quarter*. Retrieved from http://www.statssa.gov.za/?p=12358

The World Bank. (2018). *Overcoming poverty and inequality in South Africa: An assessment of drivers, constraints and opportunities*. The World Bank.

Theron, L. C. (2007). Uphenyo ngokwazi kwentsha yasemalokishini ukumelana nesimo esinzima: A South African study of resilience among township youth. *Child and Adolescent Psychiatric Clinics of North America, 16*(2), 357–375. https://doi.org/10.1016/j.chc.2006.12.005

Theron, L., Cameron, A. C., Didkowsky, N. L. C., Liebenberg, L., & Ungar, M. (2011). A "day in the lives" of four resilient youths: Cultural roots of resilience. *Youth & Society, 43*(3), 799–818. https://doi.org/10.1177/0044118X11402853

Theron, L. C., & Theron, A. M. C. (2010). A critical review of studies of South African youth resilience, 1990-2008. *South African Journal of Science, 106*(7–8), 1–8. https://doi.org/10.4102/sajs.v107i7/8.252

Ungar, M. (2015). *Working with children and youth with complex needs: 20 skills to build resilience*. Routledge.

United Nations Children's Fund (UNICEF). (2016). *The state of the world's children*. UNICEF.

United Nations Programme on HIV/AIDS (UNAIDS). (2017). *UNAIDS data 2017*. Retrieved from Joint United Nations Programme on HIV/AIDS (UNAIDS) http://www.unaids.org/sites/default/files/media_asset/20170720_Data_book_2017_en.pdf

Van Lennep, T. (2019, January 29). Cape Town gangs: Political dimensions. *Politicsweb*. Retrieved from https://www.politicsweb.co.za/opinion/cape-town-gangs-political-dimensions

Van Schalkwyk, I. (2009). *Flourishing in a group of South African adolescents* (unpublished doctoral thesis). North-West University.

Van Schalkwyk, I. (2019). Strengthening female-headed households: Exploring the challenges and strengths of mothers with substance-problems living in a high-risk community. *Journal of Family Studies, 2019*, 1–23. https://doi.org/10.1080/13229400.2019.1584122

Van Schalkwyk, I. (2020). *A wellness programme for mothers living in a high-risk community in the Western Cape to promote their personal and parental competencies (Unpublished doctoral thesis)*. Stellenbosch University.

Van Schalkwyk, I., & Marais, S. (2017). Educators' relational experiences with learners identified with fetal alcohol spectrum disorder. *South African Journal of Education, 37*(3), 1–9. https://doi.org/10.15700/saje.v37n3a1278

Van Schalkwyk, I., & Naidoo, A. V. (2021, July). Evaluating the impact of a wellness programme for mothers living in the context of a South African high-risk community. Paper presented at the 7th International Positive Psychology Association (IPPA) virtual world congress.

Van Schalkwyk, I., & Wissing, M. P. (2013). Evaluation of a programme to enhance flourishing in adolescents. In M. P. Wissing (Ed.), *Well-being research in South Africa* (pp. 581–606). Springer.

Van Zyl, L. E., Efendic, E., Rothman, S. R., & Shankland, R. (2019). Best-practice guidelines for positive psychological intervention research design. In L. E. van Zyl & S. Rothmann Sr. (Eds.), *Positive psychological intervention design and protocols for multi-cultural contexts* (pp. 1–32). Springer. https://doi.org/10.1007/978-3-030-20020-6_1

Walton, K. L., Avenant, J., & van Schalkwyk, I. (2016). Educators' experiences of their relationships with adolescents involved in drug use. *South African Journal of Education*. https://doi.org/10.15700/saje.v36n3a1188

Wessels, I., Lester, S., & Ward, C. L. (2016). *Engagement in parenting programmes: Exploring facilitators of and barriers to participation*. Institute for Security Studies, Policy Brief 82 (March 2018), University of Cape Town.

Wissing, M. P., Nel, L., Guse, T., Liversage, C., Wilson-Fadiji, A., Appiah, R., & Monyeko, A. (2020). Towards well-being in diverse contexts. In M. P. Wissing, J. Potgieter, T. Guse, T. Khumalo, & L. Nel (Eds.), *Towards flourishing: Embracing well-being in diverse contexts* (2nd ed., pp. 375–432). Van Schaik.

Wissing, M. P., & Temane, Q. M. (2008). The structure of psychological well-being in cultural context: Towards a hierarchical model of psychological health. *Journal of Psychology in Africa, 18*(1), 45–56.

Yates, T. M., & Masten, A. S. (2004). Fostering the future: Resilience theory and the practice of positive psychology. In P. A. Linley & S. Joseph (Eds.), *Positive psychology in practice* (pp. 521–539). Wiley.

9783030859237